Decision Making in Transfusion Medicine

AABB PRESS

Decision Making in Transfusion Medicine

Eleftherios C. Vamvakas, MD, PhD, MPH
Department of Pathology and Laboratory Medicine
Cedars-Sinai Medical Center
Los Angeles, California

AABB Press
Bethesda, Maryland
December 2011

AABB
8101 Glenbrook Road
Bethesda, Maryland 20814-2749

ISBN NO. 978-1-56395-828-1
Printed in the United States

Library of Congress Cataloging-in-Publication Data

Vamvakas, Eleftherios C.
Decision making in transfusion medicine / Eleftherios C. Vamvakas.
p. ; cm.
Includes bibliographical references and index.
ISBN 978-1-56395-828-1
I. AABB Press. II. Title.
[DNLM: 1. Blood Transfusion. 2. Blood Banks--organization & administration. 3. Decision Making. 4. Evidence-Based Medicine. 5. Risk Assessment. WB 356]

615.3'9--dc23

2011051112

Table of Contents

Preface xi

About the Author xiii

1. Can Policy Decisions in Transfusion Medicine Be Evidence Based? 1

A Case in Point: WBC Reduction 1
Evidence-Based Medicine 5
Best Research Evidence 5
Application of the Precautionary Principle in Transfusion Medicine 11
The Debate over TRIM and Universal WBC Reduction 12
Competing Risks and Decision Making in Transfusion Medicine 24
References 25

2. Causes of Mortality Related to Allogeneic Blood Transfusion 31

Passive Surveillance Studies of ABT-Related Mortality 34
Transfusion-Associated Sepsis 39
TRALI 45
HTRs 57
Poorly Understood Causes of Death Attributed to ABT by RCTs 61
The Impact of the Next Fatal TTI 64
Conclusions 74
References 77

3. Assessment of the Risk of Emerging Transfusion-Transmitted Infections 87

Emerging TTIs 88
Prevalence of Subclinical vCJD in the United Kingdom 90
Transfusion-Transmitted Cases of Clinical vCJD 95
Prion-Reduction Filters 100
Has Ordinary WBC Reduction Prevented Transfusion Transmission of vCJD? 103
Are Further Measures Needed to Prevent Transfusion Transmission of vCJD? 104
Summary 107
References 107

4. Strategies to Further Reduce Allogeneic-Blood-Transfusion-Related Mortality 113

Reduction in the Risk of TTIs Through PR of Platelet and Plasma Components 116

Reduction in Ill-Defined ABT-Associated Adverse Effects Through WBC Reduction of RBCs Transfused in Cardiac Surgery 124
Reduction in the Risk of TTIs Through Replacement of Pooled Blood Components by Apheresis (Single-Donor) Components 125
Prevention of HTRs 129
Prevention of TRALI Through Reduction in the Number of Immunologic Exposures to Blood Donors 130
Decrease in the Risk of all ABT Complications by Reducing the Number of Donor Exposures Through Avoidance of Unnecessary Transfusions 134
Conclusions 151
References 151

5. Applications of Meta-Analysis in Transfusion Medicine 161

The Unit of Observation in Meta-Analysis 165
Assessment of the Eligibility of Original Reports for Inclusion in a Meta-Analysis 174
Assessment of the Quality of RCTs Included in a Meta-Analysis 176
Rationale for Quantitative Research Synthesis 179
Assessment of the Combinability of the Reports Included in the Meta-Analysis 181
The Medical Interpretation of Overviews 185
Bias in Meta-Analytic Research 192
Conclusions 193
References 195

6. Have Policy Makers Been Selectively Precautionary in Indefinitely Deferring Men Who Have Had Sex with Men (MSM) from Donating Blood? 201

Currently Tolerated ABT Risk in the United States That Exceeds the ALARA Risk 203
Scope of the Comparison 204
TTIs for Which Blood Donors Are Tested 207
HHV-8 Transmission by ABT 216
Emerging Agents 218
Discussion 218
References 227

7. Equipoise and the Continued Transfusion of "Old" Blood 235

Equipoise as a Prerequisite for Undertaking RCTs 237
Preliminary Results from RCTs 241
Observational Studies 243
RCTs Currently Under Way in the United States and Canada 253
Discussion 258
References 259

8. Paradigm Shifts in Transfusion Medicine 265

Patient Blood Management in RBC Transfusion 270
Multicomponent Apheresis 280
Patient Blood Management in Platelet Transfusion 288

Pathogen Reduction of Platelet Components . . . 293
Conclusions . . . 296
References . . . 299

Index . . . 307

Electronic Supplement

The CD-ROM included with this textbook contains three chapters from *Evidence-Based Practice of Transfusion Medicine* by Eleftherios C. Vamvakas, MD, PhD (AABB Press, 2001).

1. Basic Concepts

Introduction to Statistical Terms
Measures of Disease Frequency
Measures of Association
References
Additional Reading

2. Statistical Associations and Cause-and-Effect Relationships

Association between Treatment (or Exposure) and Outcome
Valid Statistical Associations vs Causal Relationships
Refuting the Role of Chance
Refuting the Role of Bias
Refuting the Role of Confounding Factors
Conclusions
References
Additional Reading

3. Diagnostic Accuracy and Clinical Value of Laboratory Tests Used to Screen the Allogeneic Blood Supply for Infectious Disease Markers

Sensitivity
Specificity
Diagnostic Accuracy vs Clinical Value of a Laboratory Test
Predictive Value
Laboratory Tests Reported on a Continuous Scale
Parallel Testing
Serial Testing
Meta-Analyses of Studies of the Diagnostic Accuracy of Laboratory Tests
Summary
References
Suggested Reading

Preface

THIS BOOK CONTINUES A DIScussion that began with the author's previous AABB Press book *Evidence-Based Practice of Transfusion Medicine.* After reviewing, in Chapter 1, whether decisions concerning transfusion-safety interventions can be truly evidence-based, the book examines the most hotly contested policy directions in transfusion medicine today. Such directions include those that 1) may be competing with one another for any additional funds that the US health-care system could make available in the future toward optimally meeting the transfusion needs of all patients, 2) may involve transfers of funds from blood centers to hospitals or vice versa, and 3) may require very major changes in the way that transfusion medicine is practiced.

This book examines the policy directions that are currently (late 2011) being considered in blood safety and often amount to such radical changes in transfusion medicine as to be called "paradigm shifts." These changes include:

- Moving from allogeneic blood transfusion (ABT) to patient blood management and also from transfusion of *stored* Red Blood Cells (RBCs) to transfusion of *fresh* RBCs, the patient's own freshly shed blood, or even fresh whole blood (Chapters 4 and 7).
- Administering ABT only when empirical evidence indicates that actual (as opposed to postulated) benefit can be expected from the transfusion for a particular patient (Chapter 4).
- Transitioning from the whole-blood collections of the 20th century to the multi-component apheresis collections of the 21st century—whereby RBCs along with platelets and/or plasma could be collected from the same donor at the same time, with all the various components harvested from the same multicomponent apheresis collection reserved for transfusion to the same transfusion recipient (Chapter 4).
- Implementing pathogen reduction for plasma, platelets, and (eventually) RBCs—that is, inactivating microorganisms in blood components with only a modest (and deemed acceptable) decrease in the function of blood cells and plasma proteins (Chapter 5).

To appreciate, and perhaps rank, the expected benefits from these currently debated policy alternatives, Chapters 2 and 3 review the causes of ABT-related mortality. Chapter 5 describes the research method (meta-analysis) developed for disciplined research synthesis and used throughout this book, and Chapter 7 explores the concept of equipoise, which is a prerequisite for undertaking randomized controlled trials.

Chapter 6 examines a policy alternative postulated to increase the infectious risks of ABT, however minimally. This regulatory intervention would call for reducing the donor deferral for men who have had sex with men (MSM) from an indefinite deferral to a 12-month deferral. The intent of that chapter is to illustrate the magnitude of an increase in ABT risk not deemed to be "tolerable" by policy-makers, so as to compare this postulated increase in risk (from reducing the MSM deferral) to the reduction in risk expected from the other examined policy directions. Chapter 8 presents a synthesis of the different "paradigm shifts" developing in transfusion medicine today. In so doing, it categorizes the various proposals for enhancing transfusion safety as being most compatible with a "patient-centric" vs "component-centric" approach to meeting patient transfusion needs. It also attempts to define what represents a "paradigm shift" in transfusion medicine.

Four recurring principles have been enunciated by the US Food and Drug Administration (FDA): 1) zero risk is a goal—not a mandate; 2) acceptance of risk is a political decision; 3) acceptance of cost is also a political decision; and 4) decision-making must be transparent. This book is intended to serve the fourth principle and it appraises the evidence vis-à-vis the reduction in the risk of ABT that can be obtained from the various policy alternatives currently being considered in the United States. Although the book concludes that policy decisions in transfusion medicine are based on a wider range of inputs than solely the best research evidence, the orientation of the book is always *evidence-based.* For readers who wish to undertake a direct assessment of the quality of the original studies referenced in this book, three additional chapters are provided in the electronic supplement. The latter chapters present the technical information on how to perform independent assessments of the quality of published studies, and they are reproduced from the author's previous AABB Press book *Evidence-Based Practice of Transfusion Medicine.*

The book may well be controversial, reflecting as it does on questions that amount to major changes in transfusion medicine and on issues that represent long-standing controversies operating at the intersection of medicine, society, and public health (such as blood donation by MSM). Parts of the book may make some transfusion-medicine colleagues uncomfortable, with different parts of the book causing discomfort in different sectors. In pursuing all arguments based on the quality of the available empirical research, the book may even offend some readers—a possibility for which the author apologizes in advance. Nonetheless, the book is intended to be thought-provoking and supportive of open and unfettered debate. The author presents what would be in the transfusion recipient's best interest given our current capabilities, in the author's own opinion and based on a synthesis of the available research evidence undertaken personally by him—not what might be cost-effective, operationally welcomed, or equally acceptable by all stakeholders. Thus, the conclusions reached here do not represent any official AABB position, but rather the author's own opinions. They should not be regarded as AABB recommendations, but as proposals to be subjected to further scrutiny and debate.

The author is grateful to the members of the AABB Press Editorial Board for initially approving the concept for such a controversial book, for reviewing the individual chapters, and for offering him valuable feedback for revisions. The author also declares upfront that he has no conflict of interest of any kind, and that—other than his *previous* employment by Canadian Blood Services, membership on the Blood Systems Research Institute Scientific Advisory Board, and membership on various AABB committees—he also has no involvement with any organization that has (or could be perceived as having) a financial stake in the outcome of any of the policy directions examined in this book.

The author is indebted to the philanthropists of the Lenore S. and Bernard A. Greenberg Fund who—by endowing the Rita and Taft Schreiber Chair in Transfusion Medicine at the Cedars-Sinai Medical Center—permitted him to both have the protected time for writing this book and maintain his independent voice (free of any real or perceived conflict of interest) throughout the appraisal and exposition of the evidence. I am also deeply thankful to Laurie Munk, Nina Hutchinson, Jennifer Boyer, and Carolinda Hales for working tirelessly to ensure publication very promptly after the appraisal of the evidence and the description of the status of the policy debates reviewed here.

Eleftherios C. Vamvakas, MD, PhD

About the Author

Eleftherios C. Vamvakas is Professor and Vice-Chair for Clinical Pathology, Department of Pathology and Laboratory Medicine, Cedars-Sinai Medical Center, in Los Angeles where he has also served as the Rita and Taft Schreiber Chair in Transfusion Medicine. He received his MD from the University of Athens, Greece; an MPH in epidemiology from Harvard University; and an MPA in health services management and an MPhil and PhD in health policy analysis from New York University. He completed a residency in anatomic and clinical pathology at the New York University Medical Center and a fellowship in transfusion medicine at the Mayo Clinic.

Before joining Cedars-Sinai Medical Center, Dr. Vamvakas was Executive Vice-President, Medical, Scientific and Research Affairs at Canadian Blood Services and Adjunct Professor of Pathology at the University of Ottawa. Previously, he had practiced transfusion medicine at the Massachusetts General Hospital and the New York University Medical Center, with dual appointments as Assistant Professor of Pathology at Harvard Medical School and Associate Professor of Pathology at the New York University School of Medicine. He was also Chief of the Pathology and Laboratory Service of the New York VA Medical Center.

Since 1990, Dr. Vamvakas has studied the purported deleterious immunomodulatory effects of transfusion, the epidemiology of blood transfusion, and the survival of transfusion recipients. With more than 150 publications, his first-authored work on these themes includes 30 original reports, 54 peer-reviewed review articles and book chapters, co-editorship of *Immunomodulatory Effects of Blood Transfusion*, and authorship of *Evidence-Based Practice of Transfusion Medicine*. The purpose of Dr. Vamvakas' work is integrating and evaluating the evidence on the composite risks of allogeneic blood transfusion to assist in public-policy decision-making. His work quantifies and ranks all the disparate risks of transfusion, so as to: 1) advocate the implementation of interventions for enhancing blood safety in the order of the number of transfusion-related deaths that each intervention is expected to prevent; and 2) promote decision making based on empirical evidence from systematically appraised studies, to maximize the resulting safety improvement and also to dispel myths and resolve long-standing controversies vis-à-vis measures to enhance blood safety.

In: Vamvakas EC.
Decision Making in Transfusion Medicine
Bethesda, MD: AABB Press, 2011

1

Can Policy Decisions in Transfusion Medicine Be Evidence Based?

Evidence-based medicine integrates best research evidence with clinical expertise and patient values. It de-emphasizes intuition, unsystematic clinical experience, and pathophysiologic rationale as sufficient grounds for clinical decision making.

IN TREATING AN INDIVIDUAL patient, physicians must decide what criteria to use for the administration of red cell (RBC), platelet, or plasma transfusion; what platelet dose to administer; whether to routinely obtain a measurement of the posttransfusion platelet count after a platelet transfusion; whether (or for how long) to monitor a patient for adverse reactions after the start of a transfusion; and so on. At a societal level, another set of decisions must be made that concern the safety of a country's entire blood supply. Examples of these decisions include the decision to adopt or not adopt any of the following proposed safety initiatives: pathogen reduction (PR) of plasma and platelet components; universal white-cell (WBC) reduction of all cellular blood components; continued screening for cytomegalovirus (CMV) when universal WBC reduction has already been implemented; and so on.

A Case in Point: WBC Reduction

WBCs in units of non-WBC-reduced blood components do not contribute to product efficacy, and they may be regarded as contaminants that potentially reduce transfusion safety. Prestorage WBC reduction of cellular blood components removes donor WBCs before they undergo apoptosis or necrosis and before they release breakdown products at 4 C or cytokines at room temperature. It appears that, aside from specific device (filter) failures, no clinically significant adverse effects are associated with leukocyte reduction.[1] A transfused cellular blood component [eg, a pool of whole-blood-derived (WBD) platelets, an apheresis platelet concentrate, or an RBC concentrate] is considered to be WBC-reduced if it contains $<5 \times 10^6$ residual donor WBCs *and* retains $\geq$85% of the therapeutic blood element (platelets or red cells) intended for transfusion.

Both basic and clinical studies have documented the efficacy of WBC reduction in reducing the risk of three complications of allogeneic blood transfusion (ABT). These are 1) the occurrence of febrile nonhemolytic transfusion reactions (FNHTRs); 2) refractoriness to random-donor platelet transfusions secondary to HLA alloimmunization; and 3) transmission of CMV.[2] These benefits from WBC reduction can be secured through selective WBC reduction of the cellular blood components destined for transfusion to specific categories of patients: 1) patients with a history of FNHTRs; 2) patients at risk of platelet refractoriness because of the receipt of multiple platelet transfusions; and 3) patients at risk of CMV disease.

In the absence of considerations of cost, universal WBC reduction of all transfused cellular blood components could extend to all patients these three proven benefits of WBC reduction.[1,3] Although patients who have not suffered FNHTRs, are not receiving long-term platelet transfusions, and are not at risk of developing CMV disease may derive no immediate benefit from prestorage WBC reduction, it is possible that these patients may receive some tangible benefit in the future. However, before the possibility of introducing PR of platelet components started to be debated, WBC reduction represented the greatest incremental increase in the cost of manufacturing blood components in the history of blood banking.[4]

In 1999, the United Kingdom, Ireland, and Portugal implemented universal WBC reduction of all transfused cellular blood components, on the basis of the hypothesis—supported by experimental evidence of the effect of B-cell depletion in an animal model[5]—that this intervention would prevent transmission by transfusion of the agent of variant Creutzfeldt-Jakob disease (vCJD). France and Canada also implemented universal WBC reduction in 1998 and 1999, respectively, to enhance overall transfusion safety, and universal WBC reduction has since been listed among the precautionary measures implemented in France to prevent transmission of vCJD by transfusion. Some countries neighboring France successively adopted the policy, at least in part owing to the risk of transfusion transmission of vCJD. All European countries in which cases of vCJD have been reported (ie, Spain, The Netherlands, and Italy), as well as neighboring countries in which no vCJD cases have yet arisen (eg, Germany), are currently employing universal WBC reduction.

At the beginning of the 21st century, as these developments unfolded in Europe, there was a considerable period of public debate in the United States and elsewhere about the appropriateness of introducing universal WBC reduction. In North America, the debate focused mainly, but not exclusively, on an examination of the efficacy of WBC reduction in preventing the purported adverse immunomodulatory effects of ABT. The reason for this focus is that prevention of the purported deleterious effects of ABT-related immunomodulation [generally called the transfusion-related immunomodulatory (TRIM) effect][6,7] would apply to all patients and would thus justify universal WBC reduction. In the end, Canada implemented universal WBC reduction but the United States did not, and the proportion of WBC-reduced components transfused by US hospitals today reflects availability more than clinical preference. More specifically, US hospitals use WBC-reduced components either universally or selectively, depending primarily on a hospital's location and the practice of the local blood provider (which may manufacture only WBC-reduced or both WBC-reduced and non-WBC-reduced cellular blood components).

ABT results in numerous immunologic alterations that may represent mere laboratory curiosities or may reflect some clinically relevant aberration in the recipient's immune function—the so-called "immunomodulatory" effect of ABT.[8] The acronym TRIM was initially introduced to designate the constellation of ABT-associated laboratory alterations as well as clinical effects [eg, enhanced survival of renal allografts, increased rate of recurrence of resected malignancies, increased incidence of postoperative bacterial infections, and activation of endogenous CMV and human immunodeficiency virus (HIV) infection] that could be attributed to ABT by immunologic mechanisms. More recently, the term has been used more broadly, to encompass additional effects that could be related to ABT by means of both immunomodulatory and proinflammatory (as opposed to only immunomodulatory) mechanisms. Proinflammatory effects (and other poorly understood ABT effects) have been invoked, for example, to explain the association between ABT and increased short-term (up to 3 months) posttransfusion mortality.

Figures 1-1 and 1-2 show the evidence available to policymakers today as to whether it is

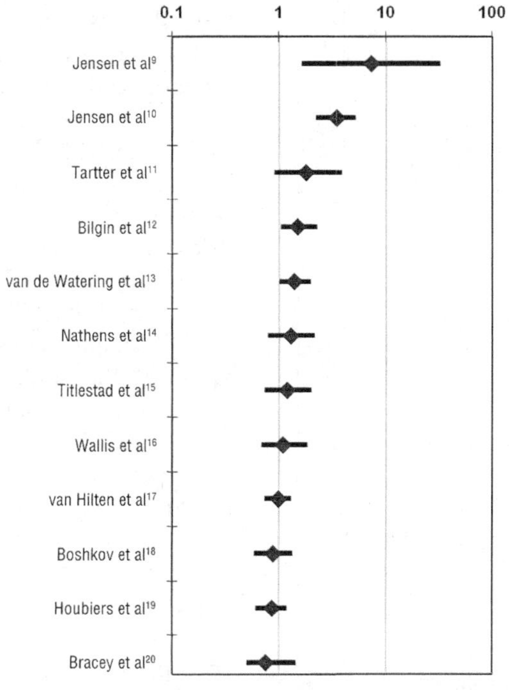

Figure 1-1. Randomized controlled trials (RCTs) investigating the association of white blood cell (WBC)-containing allogeneic blood transfusion (ABT) with bacterial infection, ranked according to the magnitude of the ABT effect that they reported (from largest to smallest).[9-20] For each RCT, the filled diamond shows the odds ratio (OR) of bacterial infection in patients who were randomly assigned preoperatively to receive non-WBC-reduced or WBC-reduced allogeneic RBCs or whole blood in the event that they needed perioperative ABT. Each OR is surrounded by its 95% CI. If the 95% CI of the OR includes the null value of 1, the transfusion-related immunomodulatory (TRIM) effect is not statistically significant ($p>0.05$). A deleterious effect of ABT is indicated by an OR >1, provided that the associated 95% CI does not include the null value of 1. Jensen et al[9] and Tartter et al[11] had not reported the data needed for an intention-to-treat analysis, presenting instead an observational comparison between recipients of non-WBC-reduced (or WBC-reduced) allogeneic RBCs[11] or whole blood[9] and patients who did not need perioperative transfusion. For the intention-to-treat analysis shown in the figure, patients not needing transfusion who developed postoperative infection were allocated to the two randomization arms. Boshkov et al[18] followed up after randomization (and recorded the outcome for) the transfused patients only; therefore, the comparison depicted in the figure represents a comparison of recipients of non-WBC-reduced and recipients of WBC-reduced RBCs. With the exception of a cardiac-surgery RCT,[12] only studies completed before 1999 had reported a significant TRIM effect in intention-to-treat[9,10] or as-treated[11] analyses.[3]

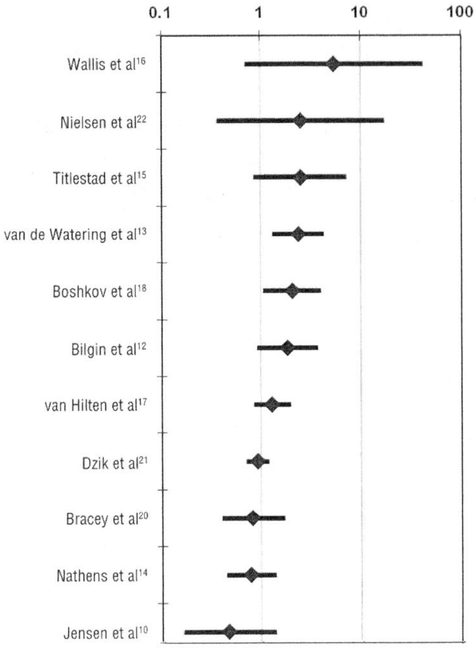

Figure 1-2. Randomized controlled trials (RCTs) investigating the association of white blood cell (WBC)-containing ABT with short-term (up to 3 months after transfusion), *all-cause* mortality, ranked according to the magnitude of the allogeneic blood transfusion (ABT) effect that they reported (from largest to smallest).[10,12-18,20-22] With the exception of Boshkov et al[18] (who compared patients transfused with non-WBC-reduced or WBC-reduced RBCs), all odds ratios (ORs) depicted in the figure are based on intention-to-treat analyses. Of the seven RCTs[12-14,17,18,21,22] that reported specifically on mortality, two cardiac surgery studies[13,18] reported a significant ($p<0.05$) adverse ABT effect.[3]

appropriate to introduce universal WBC reduction for the prevention of the purported deleterious TRIM effects. Randomized controlled trials (RCTs) that examined the association of perioperative non-WBC-reduced (vs WBC-reduced) ABT with postoperative bacterial infection have produced highly contradictory findings (Fig 1-1). Estimates of the TRIM effect have varied from a 7.3-fold increase in the risk of postoperative infection in association with the receipt of non-WBC-reduced (vs WBC-reduced) ABT[9] to no TRIM effect.[13-20] With the sole exception of the cardiac surgery RCT of Bilgin et al,[12] all RCTs conducted in the 21st century[14-20] have consistently produced negative findings. Figure 1-2 presents the findings of RCTs reporting on the association between non-WBC-reduced (vs WBC-reduced) ABT and all-cause, short-term (up to 3 months after transfusion) mortality. With the exception of the RCT of Bilgin et al and two other cardiac surgery RCTs,[13,18] all studies produced negative findings. Given this evidence (Figs 1-1 and 1-2) from all reported clinical experiments,[9-22] the question arises: Should US policymakers opt to introduce universal WBC reduction to abrogate the purported deleterious TRIM effects, thereby potentially reducing the risks of both posttransfusion bacterial infection and mortality?

This chapter considers two perspectives for assessing the soundness of the available evidence and for making policy decisions in transfusion medicine: the evidence-based approach and the precautionary principle. It also debates whether policy decisions in transfusion medicine can truly be evidence-based. The discretion of policymakers in making decisions in transfusion medicine is often limited by regulatory mandates, societal expectations, fear of future litigation, public perceptions of ABT as being an inherently unsafe intervention, public expectations about transfusion safety, and proposals for applying the precautionary principle in transfusion medicine. Such constraints reduce the applicability of evidence-based medicine (EBM) as a means for optimizing policy decisions in transfusion medicine. To examine the relevance of the evidence-based approach (compared with the precautionary principle) in the making of policy decisions, this chapter uses as an example the debate about the introduction of universal WBC reduction to prevent TRIM. This debate, which took place in the United States early in this century, was selected for this purpose because it is—at this point—mostly of historical, rather than current, relevance and because fewer regulatory, societal, and medico-legal pressures likely exist vis-à-vis the prevention of the poorly understood and purported TRIM effects compared with the pressures that affect policy decisions in the context of ABT-transmitted infectious diseases. In addition, the chapter defines EBM and presents a hierarchy of the strength of evidence.

Evidence-Based Medicine

EBM is a term coined in the early 1990s by a clinical epidemiologist at McMaster University (Hamilton, ON, Canada).[23] The term originally described a concept in which physicians were "aware of the evidence on which one's practice is based, the soundness of the evidence, and the strength of the inference the evidence permits."[24] As happens in most areas of medicine, the concept has evolved. Initially, EBM focused on the best research evidence that was relevant to the clinical problem being addressed. More recently, the traditional determinants of clinical practice have been incorporated into the model, along with the recognition that patient preferences and values, along with societal issues facing health-care systems, also are important components.[25]

Thus, EBM integrates best research evidence with clinical expertise and patient values. It deemphasizes intuition, unsystematic clinical experience, and pathophysiologic rationale as sufficient grounds for clinical decision making and requires the application of formal rules of evidence in the evaluation of the clinical literature. To solve specific patient problems, physicians practicing EBM need to select the best of the relevant studies, identify their strengths and weaknesses, and extract the clinical message. Alternatively, physicians need to rely on rigorous systematic reviews and meta-analyses that—as discussed in Chapter 5—perform those functions. Whether physicians make independent assessments of the available evidence or rely on systematic reviews, the EBM approach dictates that the management of each patient should be based on the best available evidence.[26]

The concept of EBM can be applied to both the individual and societal levels. Clinicians engage in a decision-making process that balances the benefits and risks for an individual patient, taking into account the preferences and values of that particular patient. To balance benefits and risks, clinicians must critically appraise the quality of reports of clinical research (or evaluate the quality of systematic reviews of the reports of clinical research if they rely on such reviews to assess the evidence and extract the clinical message). They also must determine the relevance of published findings to the clinical problem and setting of their own patient. In contrast, policymakers have to consider the roles that society and health-care organizations play in providing, and in limiting, resources for health care. In this context, issues of cost-effectiveness and local resources enter the decision-making process, and the application of EBM at the policy level requires that policymakers have the capacity to critically appraise reports of cost-effectiveness analyses. Such analyses incorporate "average" patient values, and these averages may not reflect the values or preferences of an individual patient.[27] Despite these additional considerations that enter the policy-making process, the concept of EBM would dictate that—much like clinical decisions—policy decisions should also be made on the basis of the best available research evidence.

Best Research Evidence

Several rankings of the strength of evidence generated by different types of clinical research designs have been presented. In addressing a particular policy problem (about which the reported evidence in the literature is inconsistent or contradictory), policymakers can base their decision making on the types of clinical reports that have been presented (Tables 1-1 through 1-4), along with an assessment of the strengths and weaknesses of each study.

Hierarchy of Strength of Evidence

Green and Byar[28] presented a hierarchy of evidence ranging from anecdotal case reports to confirmed RCTs (Table 1-1). They thought of that list as an eight-level pyramid. As one pro-

Table 1-1. Green and Byar's Hierarchy of Strength of Evidence about Efficacy of Therapeutic Interventions[28] (from weakest to strongest)

1. Anecdotal case reports
2. Case series without controls
3. Series with literature controls
4. Analyses using computer databases
5. Case-control observational studies
6. Series with historical controls
7. Single randomized controlled trial
8. Confirmed randomized controlled trial

ceeds down the list, there is a broader and broader base on which to establish one's conclusions. All of the studies listed in Table 1-1 have played a role in the development of medical science. All of them are useful, and they all have a role in EBM. However, the issue is which type of report one should believe the most.

When the undertaking of large, double-blind RCTs (ie, of definitive clinical experiments) is deemed unlikely, meta-analyses of individual patient data (ie, of the data recorded previously on the subjects enrolled in published, small RCTs) may allow investigators to address issues of possible biases and residual confounding factors in the earlier studies and may permit them to make a judgment of a cause-and-effect relationship between a treatment and an improved clinical outcome.[29] Thus, Sackett[30] proposed that the evidence generated from meta-analyses of individual patient data could be regarded as being equivalent in strength to evidence generated from a large RCT (Table 1-2). Table 1-3 presents a variation of the same hierarchy as that shown in Table 1-2, making the point that the importance attached to the available evidence should vary according to the magnitude of the demonstrated treatment effect. A treatment effect can be real, but it may be too small to be clinically relevant.[31]

Table 1-4 presents a more recent hierarchy of strength of evidence, prepared by the same team of investigators that pioneered the concept of EBM.[24] The "N of 1" RCT is at the top of this hierarchy, followed by systematic reviews of RCTs, a single RCT, systematic reviews of observational studies, and a single observational study. The "N of 1" RCT is a randomized crossover design used in just one person. The patient undergoes pairs of treatment periods, of which one period is the experimental treatment while the other is either a placebo or an alternative treatment, and the treatment periods are randomly allocated within each pair. The "N of 1" RCT provides the strongest level of evidence about the existence of a cause-and-effect relationship between a treatment and an improved outcome, but it permits no generalization of the findings of the study to any patient population other than the individual enrolled in the study.

RCTs

RCTs are controlled clinical experiments in which patients are randomly allocated by the investigators to receive (or not receive) a treatment under study. If randomization is used, all participants are equally likely to be allocated to either the treatment or the control arm of the RCT. RCTs should be distinguished from observational studies, in which investigators passively observe patients who happen to receive (or not receive) a treatment under study.

Confounding refers to the situation in which an unrecognized variable is associated with both the outcome of interest and its putative cause, which produces a spurious association (or conceals a true relationship) between the treatment and the outcome when the data are analyzed and reported. Because the allocation of patients to the treatment and control arms of an RCT is random, the play of chance should distribute all confounding factors equally between these two arms. Thus, the treatment and control arms of an RCT should be equivalent with respect to the levels of all confounding factors, except for the receipt of the treatment under study.

Table 1-2. Sackett's Levels of Scientific Evidence about the Efficacy of Therapeutic Interventions*

Level	Type of Study
Level 1	1a) Randomized controlled trials (RCTs) that are sufficiently large to be either • positive, with a small risk of being falsely positive. • negative, with a small risk of being falsely negative. 1b) Meta-analyses of individual patient data (ie, analyses of raw, unprocessed data on individual patients enrolled in previously conducted RCTs).
Level 2	2a) RCTs that are not sufficiently large to confidently detect (or rule out) a treatment effect. 2b) Meta-analyses of the literature (ie, systematic reviews integrating the processed findings of previously published RCTs).
Level 3	Cohort observational studies comparing treated patients with concurrent, nonrandomized controls.
Level 4	Cohort observational studies comparing treated patients with historical controls.
Level 5	5a) Case series describing the experience of treated patients and using no controls. 5b) Expert opinion.

*Modified from Sackett.[30]

Table 1-3. Cook's Levels of Scientific Evidence about the Efficacy of Therapeutic Interventions*

Level	Type of Study
Level 1	Randomized controlled trails (RCTs) or meta-analyses of RCTs in which the lower 95% confidence interval (CI) of the treatment effect exceeds the minimal clinically important benefit.
Level 2	RCTs or meta-analyses of RCTs in which the lower 95% CI for the treatment effect overlaps the minimal clinically important benefit.
Level 3	Observational studies with concurrent controls.
Level 4	Observational studies with historical controls.
Level 5	Case series without controls.

*Modified from Cook et al.[31]

Table 1-4. Guyatt's Hierarchy of Strength of Evidence Concerning Efficacy of Therapeutic Interventions*

Hierarchy
1. "N of 1" randomized controlled trial†
2. Systematic reviews of randomized controlled trials†
3. Single randomized controlled trial†
4. Systematic reviews of observational studies†
5. Single observational study†
6. Physiologic studies‡
7. Unsystematic clinical observations

*Modified from Guyatt.[24]
†Measuring a "patient-important" clinical outcome (eg, mortality, recovery, cancer recurrence, and/or postoperative infection).
‡Measuring a physiologic endpoint (eg, blood pressure, cardiac output, exercise capacity, and/or bone density), rather than a clinical outcome.

Bias is any systematic error in the design of a study (or execution of the study protocol) that may result in a systematic deviation from the truth when the data are analyzed and reported. (A deviation is "systematic" when it is not random—that is, when it always occurs in the same direction.) Selection bias refers to systematic differences between patients who receive the treatment under study and those who do not. Observation bias refers to systematic differences in the investigators' diagnoses of subsequent disease activity among patients who receive the treatment under study and those who do not. Randomization removes the effect of selection bias, because neither the investigator nor the participant knows what the treatment allocation will be before the patient's decision to enter the study. (Thus, sicker patients cannot be systematically channeled to one arm or the other.) When an RCT is double-blind, the effect of observation bias is removed as well, because preconceived notions about benefit from the treatment cannot color the reporting of symptoms by the patient or the assessment of disease activity by the investigator.

Thus, a randomized, double-blind study yields the strongest evidence that an observed association is one of cause-and-effect. This is because other (alternative) explanations for the observed association—such as bias and baseline differences between the treatment and control arms—can be excluded by a large, double-blind RCT. These alternative explanations can never be entirely ruled out by any observational research design (see Chapter 2 in the electronic supplement).

Meta-Analyses and Systematic Reviews of RCTs

Meta-analysis, or statistical overview, is the structured and systematic integration of information from different studies of a given problem.[32] It refers to a disciplined synthesis of previous research findings in which the results of multiple reports on the efficacy of an intervention are compared, contrasted, and re-analyzed. When the results are discrepant, the purpose of an overview is to investigate reasons for disagreements among studies. When the results are concordant, the goal of meta-analysis is to derive, through the application of a number of quantitative techniques, a measure of the effect of the intervention across the combined investigations. This measure is referred to as the "average" or "summary" effect of the treatment under study. The component parts of a meta-analysis and the medical interpretation of the findings of such overviews are considered in Chapter 5.

Meta-analysis is the epidemiology of study results. Clinical studies use the individual patient as the unit of observation. In contrast, the unit of observation in meta-analysis is the effect of an intervention or exposure, as calculated from each individual original report. From each study included in the analysis, the meta-analysts extract one estimate of the effect of the intervention—usually in the form of an odds ratio (OR). The "summary" effect of the intervention calculated by the meta-analysis across the combined studies is referred to as the summary OR. Thus, a meta-analysis of the literature (MAL) integrates the processed findings of previously published RCTs, by extracting information on the estimate of effect of each study from the published report of that study.

A meta-analysis of individual patient data (IPD) analyzes raw, unprocessed data on individual patients enrolled in previously published RCTs. The data on such individual patients are received directly from the primary investigators, and the availability of these data permits meta-analysts to redress shortcomings in the analyses of the original reports. Thus, the conclusion of an IPD meta-analysis often differs from that of an MAL. Stewart and Parmar conducted both an MAL and an IPD meta-analysis, using the data on patients enrolled in RCTs of cisplatin-based therapy for ovarian cancer.[29] Unlike the MAL, the IPD meta-analysis produced a result that was not statistically significant. In addition, the treatment effect calculated from the IPD meta-analysis was one-third that obtained from the MAL.[29]

Systematic reviews differ from meta-analyses, but they often do include results of meta-analyses.[33] A systematic review presents a tabulation of the characteristics of the studies included in the review, along with information relevant to an assessment of the methodologic quality of each study. It also includes a tabulation of the results of the studies, with presentation of the findings of meta-analyses only if statistical integration is both possible and appropriate.

Are RCTs Necessary for Establishing Cause-and-Effect Relationships?

Because of the known risks of ABT (Chapter 2), trialists cannot possibly randomly allocate patients to receive ABT if such transfusion is not expected to benefit a patient to an extent that exceeds the known risks of ABT. Neither can they withdraw ABT when evidence-based criteria indicating a need for ABT are met. Thus, some clinical experimental designs necessary for the study of purported TRIM effects nonspecifically mediated by ABT (rather than attributed to a specific blood constituent such as the WBCs) are not feasible. EBM does not rely exclusively on RCTs and meta-analyses of RCTs, however. When RCTs and systematic reviews of RCTs (Tables 1-1 to 1-4) are not feasible because an intervention (such as ABT) is already used in clinical practice and/or has established risks, clinicians and policymakers have to fall back on "weaker" evidence and base their conclusions on observational studies or even uncontrolled clinical observations. The same rule applies, at least provisionally, when RCTs are feasible but not yet available. Even when findings from RCTs have been presented, EBM requires that all available evidence be considered in a disciplined and hierarchical manner. Such assessments of the available evidence are accomplished by systematic reviews and meta-analyses and by consensus conferences that compile and evaluate all available literature (as opposed to canvassing "expert opinion").

If chance, bias, and confounding factors are reasonably refuted as alternative explanations for the findings of a study, a valid statistical association (see Chapter 2 in the electronic supplement) can be reported from either an observational study or an RCT. A judgment of a cause-and-effect relationship is then based on the totality of all available evidence—that from both observational studies and RCTs in the case of therapeutic interventions or that from observational studies alone in the case of deleterious exposures. Hypotheses investigated in clinical medicine are usually amenable to experimentation, and EBM requires that any postulated benefit from a proposed new treatment (such as WBC-reduced ABT) compared with standard therapy (non-WBC-reduced ABT) must be shown by RCTs before the new treatment is adopted for routine use. Different considerations apply to risk-factor epidemiology in which an inference of cause from passive observation (such as the establishment of a causal link between cigarette smoking and lung cancer from observational studies) is frequent. Because it is impossible to administer a deleterious exposure to humans, only results from observational studies are available when effects of deleterious exposures are considered.[34,35] Criteria for inferring cause from passive observation have been developed for use in such situations, which often arise in risk-factor epidemiology.[36]

The relative strengths and weaknesses of observational studies and RCTs have been discussed in the medical literature for a long time.[37-39] In the absence of randomization, selection bias in the allocation of subjects to treatment and control arms is unavoidable, and any adjustment for differences in the levels of confounding factors occurring in patients who did or did not receive a new therapy is incomplete. Observational studies use statistical techniques to adjust for such baseline differences, and they control only for the effects of known and measurable confounders. The effects of unknown and/or poorly quantified confounding factors cannot be controlled statistically, and these variables always compromise, to some extent, the findings of observational studies.

Need for transfusion reflects severity of illness—a factor that cannot be adequately quantified and controlled by statistical techniques. Either a need for transfusion (ie, more severe illness) or the receipt of transfusion can then be responsible for the various adverse outcomes seen in association with ABT in observational studies. In fact, observational studies have associated ABT with all of the following: increased risk of morbidity and mortality, postoperative infection, acute respiratory distress syndrome (ARDS), multi-organ failure, and prolongation of both intensive-care unit (ICU) and hospital stay.[40] Such a nonspecific association of ABT with virtually any adverse outcome(s) studied probably indicates that ABT is an excellent surrogate factor for illness severity.[41] Alternatively, it can be argued—as was recently done by Isbister et al[40]—that these common adverse outcomes have a multifactorial etiology, with ABT being one of multiple factors contributing to the occurrence of each adverse outcome.

Neither interpretation of the origin of the nonspecific association between ABT and all studied adverse outcomes can be proven (or disproven) by observational studies, because illness severity and the need for ABT are highly correlated, which makes it impossible to use statistical methods to adjust for the effect of illness severity on any apparent association between ABT and such adverse outcomes (see Chapter 2 in the electronic supplement). To definitively determine which of the two interpretations[40,41] of the origin of the nonspecific association of ABT with all studied adverse outcomes is correct, one would have to randomly assign patients to receive (or not receive) ABT—a study design that is not feasible, for the reasons already mentioned.

When it is possible to conduct both observational studies (that incorporate the effects of selection bias and confounding factors) and RCTs (that can be devoid of the effects of selection bias and confounding factors), it is possible to compare the results of observational studies with the results of RCTs. By removing the influence of selection bias and confounding factors, randomization reduces the magnitude of calculated treatment effects.[42,43] For example, Chalmers et al[44] calculated a 20% reduction in mortality due to acute myocardial infarction in patients receiving anticoagulant therapy in the context of RCTs, as compared with a 50% benefit due to this treatment reported from observational studies. The excess benefit attributed to anticoagulant therapy by the latter investigations reflects the effects of bias and confounding factors. In other words, nonrandomized studies could have detected a 20% to 30% benefit from anticoagulant therapy even if the treatment had no effect.

That observation has important implications for the need for RCTs, especially in situations such as the multifactorial etiology of the common adverse outcomes of ABT, which have been extensively studied in observational studies and have been nonspecifically attributed to the purported, and ill-defined, "TRIM" effects of ABT.[45] If observational studies are invariably compromised by the effects of bias and uncontrolled confounding factors, which can register as a 20% to 30% treatment effect, intervention effects as small as or smaller than a 20% to 30% change in disease outcome cannot be established reliably from observational studies because—when a nonrandomized investigation detects a 20% to 30% treatment effect—it is impossible to be certain that the measured effect is truly due to the intervention, rather than to the effects of bias and uncontrolled confounding factors. Therefore, if the objective of a study were to establish a 20% to 30% change in disease outcome (as would presumably be the case for each of the multiple factors—including ABT—contributing to the occurrence of a multifactorial adverse outcome), a randomized controlled design would be necessary.

After numerous observational studies comparing transfused and untransfused patients were conducted in the 1980s and 1990s, 14 RCTs compared the risks of postoperative infection and/or mortality between patients allocated to receive non-WBC-reduced or WBC-reduced RBCs.[9-22] Similarly, as discussed in Chapter 7, RCTs of patients allocated to receive "old" or "fresh" RBCs are currently under way in both the United States and Canada.

Application of the Precautionary Principle in Transfusion Medicine

The precautionary principle states that when a purported risk represents a threat of "serious or irreversible damage," complete evidence of risk does not have to exist to justify the institution of measures to protect individuals and society from that risk. The precautionary principle was initially applied to environmental issues, such as ocean dumping of pollutants, that are characterized by a sparseness of the scientific data that are useful for making policy decisions. Use of the principle was then expanded to include environmental health risks for which extensive toxicologic and/or epidemiologic data were available, notwithstanding gaps and inconsistencies in the presented evidence.[46] Use of the principle in the environmental sector has varied, however, from a requirement for absolute proof of safety before new technologies are adopted[47] to an allowance for making policy decisions in the absence of any scientific evidence at all.[48] Because the precautionary principle has been enshrined in European Union law, a communication by the European Commission[49] can be referred to for guidance in the appropriate use of the principle. That communication stresses the need for "reliable scientific data and logical reasoning" when the precautionary principle is applied. Before the use of the principle is "triggered," the communication requires identification of a potentially hazardous effect, with "all effort" being made to "evaluate the available scientific information." Such analysis must include an assessment of the uncertainties in the scientific data, and it must also consider the wide range of actions that might be taken under the principle, *including no action at all.* Finally, the communication says that the principle must be applied in a politically "transparent" manner—a statement that acknowledges that decisions to act (or not act) once the precautionary principle has been triggered are essentially political.[46]

Once the precautionary principle has been triggered, the standards of proof that are needed for taking regulatory action differ from those needed in other contexts in which regulatory decisions are based on evidence. Although some standard of proof is still needed after the precautionary principle has been triggered, this standard need not be as high as what scientists would require in their own discourses. In the United States, where few (if any) laws cite the precautionary principle, courts have upheld the government's ability to base regulatory decisions on substantial evidence that is "less than a preponderance, but more than a scintilla."[50] This ruling should not preempt the need for basing decisions on a careful analysis of the available scientific data—which clearly has not occurred in some applications of the precautionary principle.[46] The debate continues over 1) the appropriateness of applying the precautionary principle at all; 2) the question of whether the use of the principle as a policy tool is a threat to science; and 3) the conditions under which the precautionary principle could (or should) be appropriately triggered.[51-53]

Policymakers in the environmental sector have often introduced a purely precautionary measure to eliminate a perceived risk.[54] In doing so, they have chosen to accept a trade-off between the economic costs of introducing a precautionary measure and the potential environmental or health benefits that the proposed measure might provide. Such a conceptual framework assumes that a proposed intervention is free of risk. When the precautionary principle is applied to transfusion medicine, policymakers generally encounter a trade-off between the health benefit of introducing a precautionary measure and the health risk of introducing that same measure.[55] For example, in implementing geographic donor deferral policies for vCJD, policymakers must weigh the potential health benefit of protecting the blood supply from an infectious risk against the potential health impact of a reduction in the blood supply. Because this process involves such "competing risks," it can be viewed as more of a risk-management approach than a purely precautionary approach. Risk management is the attempt to anticipate, and to prevent or mitigate, harms that may be avoidable.

Even if we were to accept such a weak interpretation of the precautionary principle as being suitable for transfusion medicine, policy decisions based on the resulting risk-management approach could differ from the ones that would be made based on an evidence-based approach. The evidence-based approach defers introduction of a measure for protecting the safety of the blood supply until definitive clinical or epidemiologic evidence of risk and/or benefit becomes available. (For example, if the rationale for introducing universal WBC reduction were to prevent adverse TRIM effects, the evidence-based approach would defer introduction of universal WBC reduction until the evidence became definitive that the TRIM effects are real and can be ameliorated by WBC reduction.) In contrast, the risk management approach favors the introduction of a precautionary measure that is designed to balance risk prevented by the implementation of the measure and risk created by the introduction of the measure.[55] Thus, the risk management approach would favor introduction of universal WBC reduction if the risk(s) of WBC reduction did not exceed the uncertain (or unproven) risk(s) of TRIM. Even if the latter remained unproven, evidence of safety of WBC reduction alone could be used to justify a policy of universal WBC reduction.

The Debate over TRIM and Universal WBC Reduction

Figure 1-3 summarizes the postulated immunomodulatory (TRIM) effects of ABT, the postulated mediators, and the proposed interventions for abrogating the adverse effects.[56-58] TRIM effects mediated by WBCs may also be mediated by immunologically competent allogeneic mononuclear cells[59-61] and/or WBC-derived soluble mediators that progressively accumulated in the supernatant fluid of RBC units during storage.[62-65] Transfusion of WBC-reduced RBCs filtered before storage should prevent all WBC-mediated TRIM effects.[59-65] In contrast, transfusion of WBC-reduced RBCs filtered after storage should prevent TRIM effects mediated by immunologically competent allogeneic mononuclear cells,[59-61] but not TRIM effects mediated by WBC-derived soluble mediators that are progressively released from deteriorating WBCs during storage.

Twelve RCTs[9-20] comparing subjects randomly assigned to receive non-WBC-reduced or WBC-reduced allogeneic RBCs or whole blood and reporting on the development of bacterial infection were published between 1992 and 2005 (Fig 1-1 and Table 1-5). Eleven RCTs[10,12-18,20-22] reported on short-term (up to 3 months after transfusion) mortality from all causes (Fig 1-2 and Table 1-5). The RCTs showed significant medical heterogeneity (Table 1-5) in the RBC component given to the treatment or the control arm and in the clinical setting in which the transfusions were conducted. Heterogeneity also existed in the proportion of the patients who were randomly assigned before the procedure who needed to receive perioperative transfusion and the proportion of the subjects who developed bacterial infection or died during the hospitalization or up to 3 months after transfusion.

All but four RCTs, including all RCTs published after 1998, transfused to patients in the WBC-reduced arm allogeneic RBCs filtered *before* storage (Table 1-5). Thus, for patients in the WBC-reduced arm, these RCTs abrogated both any ABT effects mediated by immunologically competent allogeneic mononuclear cells[59-61]

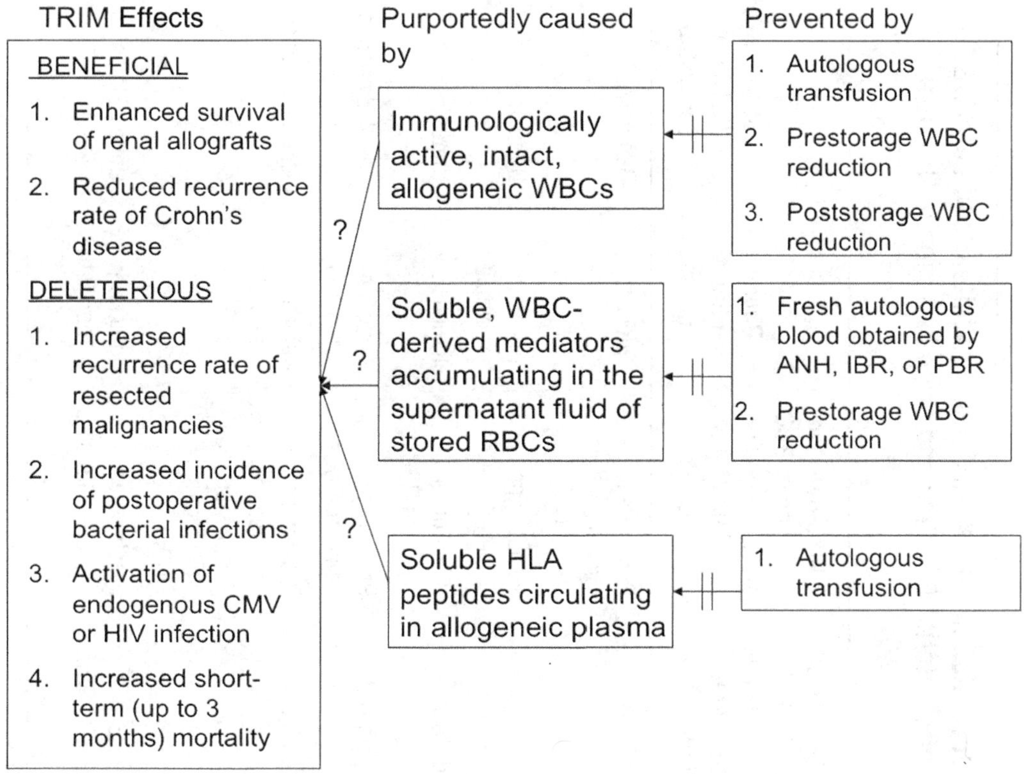

Figure 1-3. The purported deleterious transfusion-related immunomodulatory (TRIM) effects are mediated by an unknown constituent(s) of allogeneic blood that may (or may not) include one (or more) of the mediators shown. Stored autologous blood obtained by preoperative autologous blood donation is replete with white blood cell (WBC)-derived soluble mediators, because both autologous and allogeneic WBCs deteriorate equally during storage, releasing such mediators. Fresh autologous blood, transfused within hours of collection and processing, is free of WBC-derived soluble mediators and can be produced by acute normovolemic hemodilution (ANH), intraoperative blood recovery (IBR), or postoperative blood recovery (PBR). WBC-reduction filters do not retain WBC-derived soluble mediators, which accounts for the difference between prestorage and poststorage WBC reduction in abrogating the TRIM effects mediated by such mediators. Initially published by Vamvakas in Am J Clin Pathol 2006;126(Suppl 1):S71-S75.[57]
CMV = cytomegalovirus; HIV = human immunodeficiency virus; RBC = Red Blood Cells.

and any ABT effects mediated by WBC-derived soluble mediators that progressively accumulate in the supernatant fluid of RBC units during storage.[62-65] In contrast, three RCTs published between 1992 and 1998,[9-11] as well as one of three randomization arms employed in the RCT of van de Watering et al,[13] transfused to patients in the WBC-reduced arm allogeneic RBCs or whole blood filtered after storage. For patients in the WBC-reduced arm, these RCTs[9-11,13] prevented effects mediated by immunologically competent allogeneic mononuclear cells,[59-61] but not effects mediated by WBC-derived soluble mediators that accumulate during storage.[62-65]

Five RCTs[12,13,16,18,20] were conducted in the setting of cardiac surgery and five[9-11,15,19] in that of gastrointestinal surgery. The ABT effect may be enhanced in the setting of cardiac surgery, because WBC-derived soluble mediators and/or allogeneic mononuclear cells may act as a sec-

Table 1-5. Design of Randomized Controlled Trials (RCTs) Investigating the Association of White Blood Cell (WBC)-Containing Allogeneic Red Blood Cell (RBC) Transfusion with Bacterial Infection and/or up to 3-Month All-Cause Mortality

Study	Clinical Setting	Sample Size (n)	Non-WBC-Reduced Allogeneic RBC Component Given to Treatment Arm Patients	WBC-Reduced Allogeneic RBC Component Given to Control Arm Patients	Reported Clinical Outcomes	Country in which RCT Was Conducted
Jensen et al[9]	Colorectal surgery	197	Unmodified whole blood	Poststorage-filtered whole blood	Infection	Denmark
Jensen et al[10]	Colorectal surgery	586	Buffy-coat-reduced allogeneic RBCs	Poststorage-filtered RBCs	Infection mortality	Denmark
Tartter et al[11]	Gastrointestinal surgery	221	Unmodified RBCs	Poststorage-filtered RBCs	Infection	United States
Bilgin et al[12]	Cardiac surgery	474	Buffy-coat-reduced RBCs	Prestorage-filtered RBCs	Infection mortality	The Netherlands
van de Watering et al[13]	Cardiac surgery	914	Buffy-coat-reduced RBCs	Prestorage-filtered (n = 305) or poststorage-filtered (n = 303) RBCs	Infection mortality	The Netherlands
Nathens et al[14]	Trauma patients	324*	Unmodified RBCs stored for <25 days	Prestorage-filtered RBCs	Infection mortality	United States

Titlestad et al[15]	Colorectal surgery	279	Buffy-coat-reduced RBCs	Prestorage-filtered RBCs	Infection mortality	Denmark
Wallis et al[16]	Cardiac surgery	597	Buffy-coat-reduced (n = 204) or plasma-reduced† (n = 198) RBCs	Prestorage-filtered RBCs	Infection mortality	United Kingdom
van Hilten et al[17]	Acute (n = 79) or elective (n = 413) aortic aneurysm repair; resection of gastrointestinal malignancy	1052	Buffy-coat-reduced RBCs	Prestorage-filtered RBCs	Infection mortality	The Netherlands
Boshkov et al[18]	Cardiac surgery	562‡	Unmodified RBCs	Prestorage-filtered RBCs	Infection mortality	United States
Houbiers et al[19]	Colorectal cancer resection	697	Buffy-coat-reduced RBCs	Prestorage-filtered RBCs	Infection	The Netherlands
Bracey et al[20]	Cardiac surgery	443	Unmodified RBCs	Prestorage-filtered RBCs	Infection mortality	United States
Dzik et al[21]	All hospitalized patients	2780	Unmodified RBCs	Prestorage-filtered RBCs	Mortality	United States
Nielsen et al[22]	Burn trauma patients	24	Buffy-coat-reduced RBCs	Prestorage-filtered RBCs	Mortality	Denmark

*All randomly assigned patients (n = 324) were used in the analysis of mortality; patients who did not refuse consent (n = 268) were used in the analysis of infection.
†In terms of its WBC content, this component is equivalent to non-buffy-coat-reduced (ie, unmodified) RBCs.
‡Transfused patients only (rather than all randomly assigned patients).

ond inflammatory insult, compounding the diffuse inflammatory response to the extracorporeal circuit and predisposing patients to postoperative complications.[66] Alternatively, the ABT effect may be enhanced in the "unclean" setting of gastrointestinal surgery. Either way, it is possible for a deleterious ABT effect to become manifest only in the presence of co-factors, such as the special conditions that exist in cardiac or gastrointestinal surgery.

In addition, there was great variation among the RCTs in the amount of blood transfused and the frequency of a diagnosis of postoperative infection. As little as 26.7% of randomly assigned patients needed perioperative transfusion in some gastrointestinal surgery studies[15]; in contrast, up to 94.7% of randomly assigned subjects needed perioperative transfusion in some cardiac surgery studies.[13] In gastrointestinal surgery, the frequency of postoperative infection ranged from 8.1%[9] to 33.4%.[19] The differences in the proportion of transfused patients reflected patient-related selection factors (severity of underlying illness) as well as setting- and surgeon-related selection factors (subjective application of liberal or conservative transfusion criteria during an operation–when objective laboratory indicators of the need for transfusion are unavailable). The differences in the frequency of postoperative infection reflected differences in the patients' severity of illness and the employed diagnostic criteria for infection, differences in the types of infections evaluated in each study, and perhaps also differences in the effects of observation and/or selection bias [because not all RCTs were double-blind and, in most cases, the details of the randomization procedure(s) were not reported].

Thus, it is most unlikely that all RCTs studied an increase in the risk of postoperative infection or all-cause mortality mediated by a deleterious ABT effect that was biologically the same in all the cases. Instead, these RCTs[9-22] most likely studied effects of a non-WBC-reduced ABT that differed in magnitude and/or nature. Such effects could have been mediated by either allogeneic mononuclear cells[59-61] or WBC-derived soluble mediators accumulating during storage[62-65] or both. In addition, such effects could have been compounded (or not) by other co-factors, such as a diffuse inflammatory response to the extracorporeal circuit used in cardiac surgery.[66] Accordingly, a meta-analysis integrating the results of all available RCTs would not establish a homogeneous effect attributed to a specific biologic mediator or mechanism. In other words, the medical heterogeneity of the available RCTs made it inappropriate to combine the results of all available RCTs in a meta-analysis.[67]

This medical heterogeneity of the studies was reflected in extreme statistical heterogeneity. In Fig 1-1, the reported TRIM effect varied from a 20% reduction[20] to a 630% increase[9] in the risk of postoperative infection. In Fig 1-2, for the seven RCTs that reported specifically on mortality,[12-14,17,18,21,22] the ABT effect varied from a 20% reduction[14] to a 140% increase[13] in short-term mortality. In both cases, there was a probability of <1 per 1000 that the variation in the findings of all the available studies might have arisen by chance ($p<0.001$ for the Q test statistic).

Meta-Analyses of the RCTs of the Purported TRIM Effects

Meta-analyses of clinically homogeneous subsets of RCTs of WBC reduction and bacterial infection by a random-effects method[68] produced results diametrically opposed to the findings expected from the immunomodulation theory that attributes the effect of non-WBC-reduced ABT to WBC-derived soluble mediators[62-65]: there was a reduction in the risk of postoperative infection in association with poststorage (as opposed to prestorage) WBC reduction.[69] More specifically, across nine relatively homogeneous RCTs[12-20] that transfused allogeneic RBCs filtered before storage to patients in the WBC-reduced arm, no increase in the risk of postoperative infection was detected in association with non-WBC-reduced ABT (summary OR = 1.06; 95% CI = 0.91-1.24; $p>0.05$–Part B in Fig 1-4). If the ABT effect were mediated by WBC-derived soluble mediators, prestorage filtration should have abrogated an increased infection risk associated with non-WBC-reduced ABT,

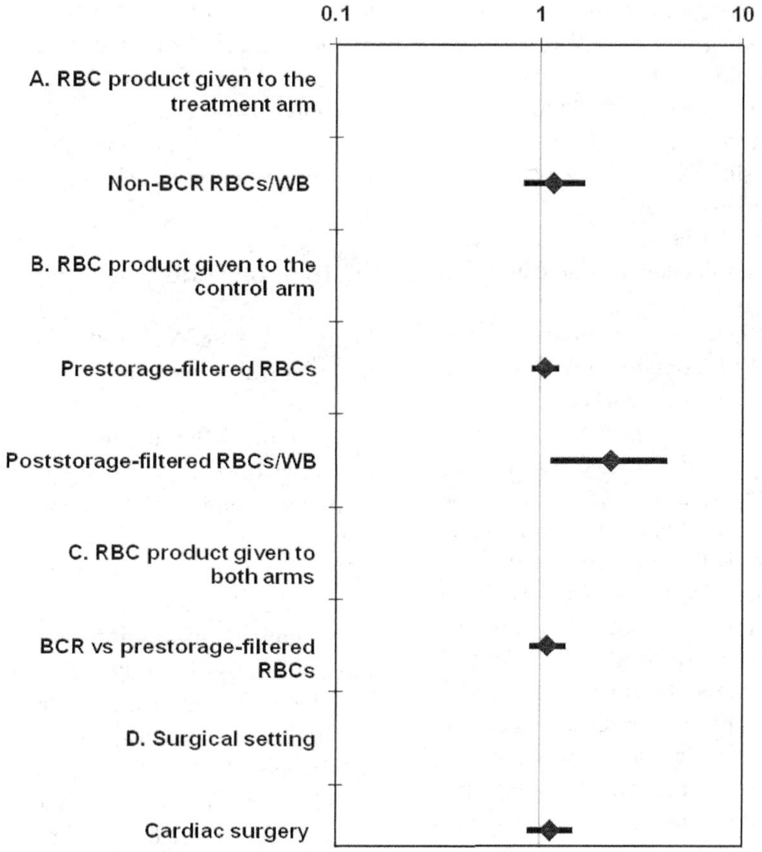

Figure 1-4. Possible sources of variation in the findings of randomized controlled trials (RCTs) investigating the association between white blood cell (WBC)-reduced (or non-WBC-reduced) allogeneic blood transfusion (ABT) and bacterial infection. Stratified meta-analyses are presented for RCTs that administered the same Red Blood Cell (RBC) component to patients in their treatment or control arm, or to both the arms, or that were conducted in the same clinical setting, provided that there was ≥5% probability that the variation in the findings of the studies from within each stratum might have arisen by chance (ie, $p>0.05$ for the Q test statistic). Only the subgroup analysis of the studies that administered *poststorage-filtered* allogeneic RBCs or whole blood to patients in the control arm produced a statistically significant ($p<0.05$) ABT effect [summary odds ratio (OR) = 2.25; 95% CI = 1.12-4.25]. Thus, the transfusion-related immunomodulatory (TRIM) effect of WBC-containing ABT appeared to be prevented by the transfusion of WBC-reduced RBCs filtered after—but not before—storage. The subgroup of four studies[9-11,13] that transfused poststorage-filtered allogeneic RBCs[10,11,13] or whole blood[9] to patients in the control arm included a total of 1616 patients and consisted of early studies published before 1999. Transfusion of poststorage-filtered allogeneic RBCs or whole blood is rarely (if ever) used any longer in the United States.[3] BCR = buffy-coat-reduced; WB = whole blood.

because it would have removed the allogeneic WBCs from the components given to patients in the WBC-reduced arm of each study before the WBCs could release any significant amounts of mediators into the supernatant fluid of the components.

In contrast, across four RCTs[9-11,13] that transfused RBCs filtered after storage to the WBC-reduced arm, there was an increase of more than twofold in the risk of infection in association with non-WBC-reduced ABT (Part B in Fig 1-4). If the ABT effect were mediated by WBC-derived soluble mediators, poststorage filtration should not have abrogated an increased infection risk associated with non-WBC-reduced ABT, because it would not have removed such mediators from the supernatant fluid of the stored RBCs given to patients in the WBC-reduced arm of the studies. Yet this was the only clinically homogeneous subset of studies in which an adverse TRIM effect of WBC-containing ABT on bacterial infection was detected (Fig 1-4).

Investigation of the sources of variation in the results of RCTs of WBC-containing ABT and all-cause mortality did generate a clinically meaningful result, however (Part D in Fig 1-5). Across the (also statistically homogeneous) cardiac surgery studies,[12,13,16,18,20] there was a 72% increase in mortality in association with non-WBC-reduced (compared with WBC-reduced) ABT. This result conforms to what would have been expected from the immunomodulation theory[66] (that there would be more of a TRIM effect in cardiac surgery, where the pro-inflammatory effect of the extracorporeal circuit acts as a co-factor, than in other settings), and it was also calculated in adherence to the rule of integrating only medically and statistically homogeneous studies.[69] This example is the only statistically valid and clinically meaningful adverse TRIM effect detected from the 14 available RCTs[9-22] (Figs 1-1, 1-2, 1-4, 1-5, and 1-6).[69]

Previous meta-analyses[70,71] of a subset of the RCTs (ie, those published through 2002) reached radically different conclusions, however, supporting the existence of a large deleterious TRIM effect, regardless of clinical setting and RBC component(s) administered to the treatment and/or control arm(s) of the studies. Accordingly, these meta-analyses[70,71] concluded that universal WBC reduction should be implemented to protect all transfusion recipients from the deleterious TRIM effect of ABT. Although the technical merits of the meta-analyses[69-71] have been extensively, and sometimes acrimoniously,[72,73] debated on methodologic grounds,[74-76] Fig 1-6 shows that the reason for the disagreements[69-71] was simply the inclusion in the meta-analysis[77] of all available RCTs,[69] rather than only a subset of the RCTs initially made available.[70,71] When all RCTs available today[9-22] are integrated, despite their significant medical and extreme statistical heterogeneity, an adverse TRIM effect on either bacterial infection or short-term mortality is not detected, no matter whether the meta-analysts integrate results from intention-to-treat[69] or as-treated[70,71] analyses.

"Before-and-After" Studies

When universal WBC reduction is implemented, the opportunity to conduct further RCTs—to rule in (or out) the existence of a deleterious TRIM effect(s) of WBC-containing ABT—is removed, and only observational studies are possible for further evaluation of the appropriateness of the policy. The observational studies from the 1980s and 1990s compared transfused and untransfused patients, thus including much-sicker patients in the transfused (compared with the untransfused) group and introducing a selection factor too difficult to control by statistical methods. In contrast, the "before-and-after" observational studies compared patients transfused before or after the implementation of universal WBC reduction in France,[78] the United Kingdom,[79] Canada,[80,81] or the United States,[82,83] thus including in both comparison groups patients sick enough to need ABT.

When all of the before-and-after studies were considered together in a meta-analysis[84] and the findings of the univariate analyses from five studies[78-82] were integrated, there was an unadjusted association of WBC reduction with a decreased risk of postoperative infection (summary OR = 0.93; 95% CI = 0.88-0.99; $p<0.05$). However, this association did not persist when findings from multivariate analyses that had been adjusted for the effects of confounding factors were integrated (summary OR = 0.94; 95% CI = 0.85-1.04; $p>0.05$). There was neither an unadjusted (Fig 1-7) nor an adjusted (Fig 1-8) association of WBC reduction with decreased short-term (up to 3 months after hospitalization) mortality (summary OR = 0.94; 95% CI = 0.71-1.23; $p>0.05$; and OR = 0.92; 95% CI = 0.80-1.05; $p>0.05$, respectively).[84]

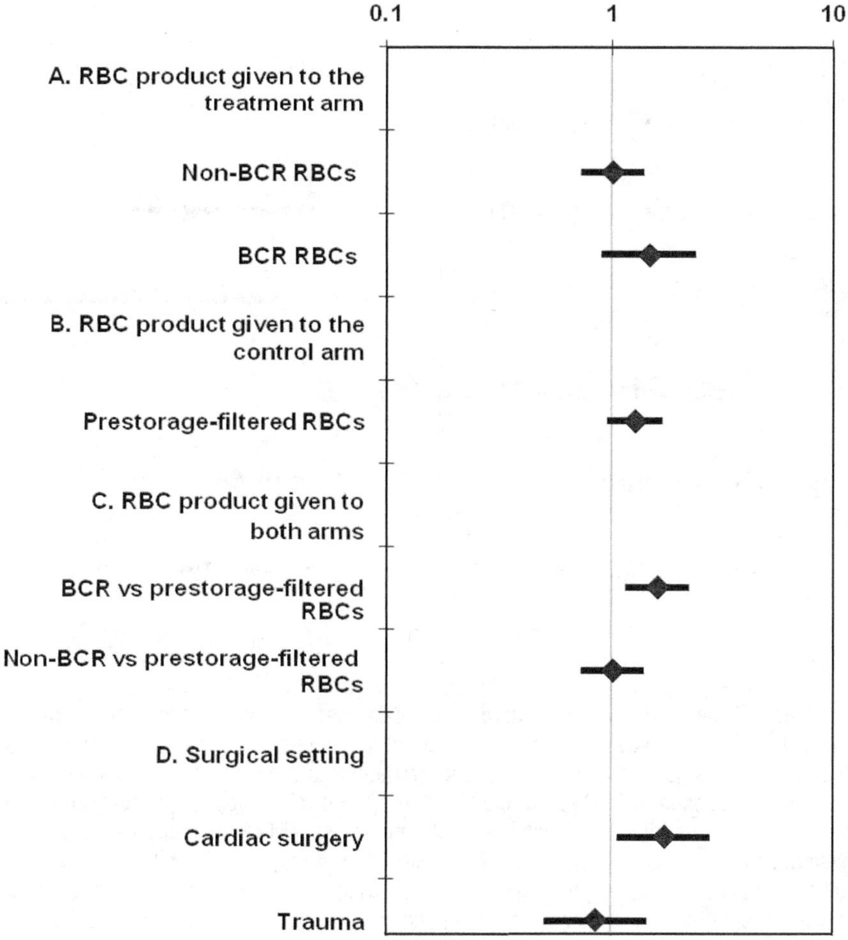

Figure 1-5. Possible sources of variation in the findings of randomized controlled trials (RCTs) investigating the association between white blood cell (WBC)-containing allogeneic blood transfusion (ABT) and short-term (up to 3 months after transfusion), *all-cause* mortality. Stratified meta-analyses are presented of studies that administered the same red blood cell (RBC) component to patients in their treatment and control arms, or both of the arms, or that were conducted in the same clinical setting, provided that there was ≥5% probability that the variation in the findings of the studies from within each stratum might have arisen by chance (ie, $p>0.05$ for the Q test statistic). The subgroup analysis of RCTs conducted in the setting of cardiac surgery[12,13,16,18,20] produced a statistically significant ($p<0.05$) ABT effect [summary odds ratio (OR) = 1.72; 95% CI = 1.05-2.81]. Across the remaining RCTs conducted at other settings, the summary OR was 0.99 (95% CI = 0.73-1.33). The subgroup analysis of RCTs comparing recipients of buffy-coat-reduced (BCR) and of prestorage-filtered RBCs (six studies[12,13,15-17,22] enrolling 2838 patients) also produced a statistically significant ($p<0.05$) ABT effect (summary OR = 1.60; 95% CI= 1.14-2.24). These studies were conducted in various clinical settings: cardiac surgery,[12,13,16] gastrointestinal surgery,[15] trauma,[22] or other.[17] Moreover, although the same RBC component (prestorage-filtered RBCs) was administered to the control arm of both subgroups of studies integrated in Part C of the figure, only across the studies that transfused BCR (as opposed to non-BCR) RBCs was a deleterious effect of WBC-containing ABT detected. Because non-BCR RBCs contain approximately three times as many allogeneic WBCs as BCR RBCs, the opposite result (ie, an ABT effect mediated by the non-BCR—as opposed to the BCR—RBCs) would have been expected. Reprinted with permission from Vamvakas.[3]

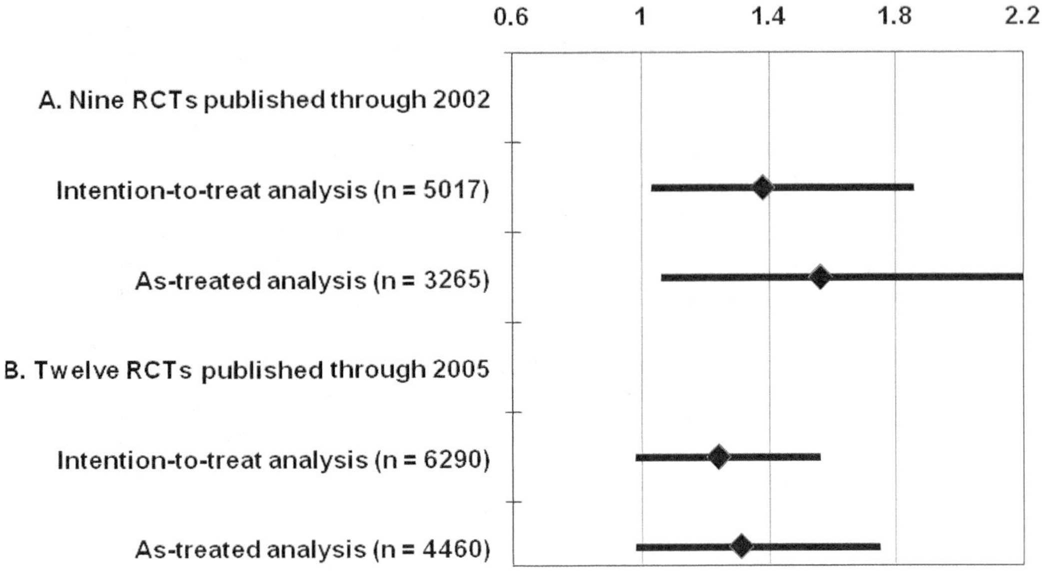

Figure 1-6. Resolution of the disagreements regarding the existence of a deleterious effect of white blood cell (WBC)-containing allogeneic blood transfusion (ABT) between the meta-analyses of randomized controlled trials (RCTs) that compared the risk of bacterial infection between subjects randomly assigned to receive non-WBC-reduced or WBC-reduced allogeneic RBCs or whole blood. If all nine RCTs reported through 2002 (see Fig 1-1) were integrated, despite their significant clinical and extreme statistical heterogeneity ($p<0.001$ for the Q test statistic), a deleterious effect of WBC-containing ABT would be detected, no matter whether the meta-analysts combined findings from the intention-to-treat (ITT) or the as-treated (AT) analyses. In contrast, if all 12 RCTs available today were integrated—again, despite their significant clinical and extreme statistical heterogeneity—a deleterious effect of WBC-containing ABT would not be detected, no matter whether the meta-analysis combined findings from the ITT or the AT analyses. Thus, the disagreements between meta-analysts[69-71] over whether to integrate[70,71] or not integrate[69] results in the presence of significant clinical (see Table 1-5) and extreme statistical (see Fig 1-1) heterogeneity and over whether to integrate ORs from RCTs based on the ITT[69] or the AT[70,71] analysis were resolved by the reporting of additional RCTs.[14,18,20] Readers should disregard the optical illusion created by the graph—that there may exist a marginally significant ($p\geq0.05$) deleterious TRIM effect across the studies—because the integrations of all nine (upper part of the figure) and all 12 (lower part) previously and currently available RCTs are invalid mathematical exercises devoid of medical meaning.[77] The results of medically and statistically homogeneous meta-analyses are shown in Fig 1-4, and those are the only valid conclusions[77] that can be reached from the 12 available RCTs.[9-20] Reprinted with permission from Vamvakas.[3]

It is especially telling that no adverse TRIM effect(s) were detected by this meta-analysis, because the overview[84] used fixed-effects methods[85] to integrate the adjusted findings from the reported multivariate analyses. Because fixed-effects methods take into account only within-studies variation (as opposed to between-studies variation; Chapter 5), they maximize the probability of detecting any treatment effect.[86]

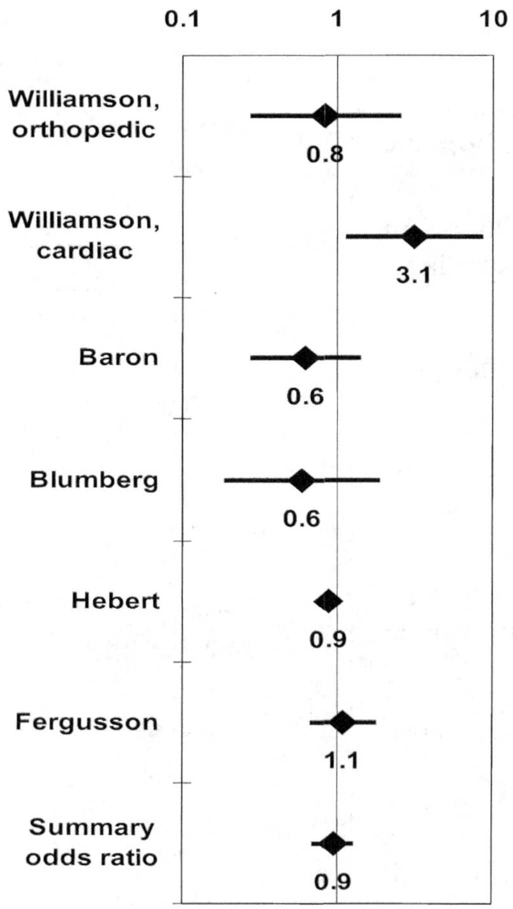

Figure 1-7. Unadjusted results of five observational, "before-and-after" studies that reported on all-cause, short-term (up to 3 months after hospitalization) mortality,[78-81,83] and unadjusted summary odds ratios (ORs) of short-term mortality calculated across these five studies. For each study, the figure shows the OR of mortality in patients transfused after (compared with before) implementation of white blood cell (WBC) reduction, before adjustment for the effects of confounding factors. Each OR is surrounded by its 95% CI. If the 95% CI of the OR does not include the null value of 1, there is a statistically significant difference in mortality between patients transfused before and those transfused after implementation of WBC-containing ABT ($p<0.05$). In that case, an OR <1 indicates a beneficial effect of WBC reduction. This differs from the data in Figs 1-1, 1-2, 1-4, 1-5, and 1-6, in which an OR >1 indicates a deleterious effect of WBC-containing ABT. Originally published by Vamvakas in Vox Sang 2004;86:111-19.[84] (At the time of that meta-analysis,[84] the results of Llewelyn et al[79] had been presented only in abstract form by Williamson et al. Those investigators studied two separate patient populations—patients undergoing either orthopedic or cardiac surgery—and reported two separate analyses. Hébert et al[80] also studied separate patient populations—of intensive care unit, cardiac, and orthopedic patients—but they reported only one unadjusted OR for all their patients combined. This "overall" unadjusted OR is depicted in this figure.)

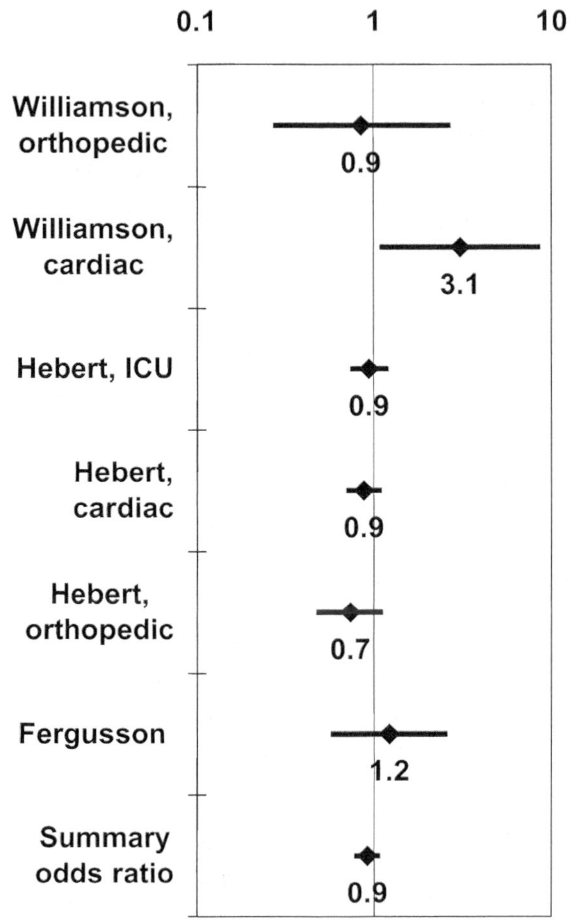

Figure 1-8. Adjusted results of three observational, "before-and-after" studies that reported on all-cause, short-term (up to 3 months after hospitalization) mortality[79-81] and adjusted summary odds ratios (ORs) of short-term mortality calculated across the three studies. For each patient group from these studies, the figure shows the adjusted OR of mortality in patients transfused after (compared with before) implementation of white blood cell (WBC) reduction, as calculated from the authors' multivariate analysis. The latter adjusted for patient co-morbidities considered and measured by the authors for their patients, albeit not for differences between the attributes of the medical care delivered before the implementation of universal WBC reduction and that delivered after the implementation of universal WBC reduction.[84] Each OR is surrounded by its 95% CI. If the 95% CI of the OR does not include the null value of 1, there is a statistically significant difference in mortality between patients transfused before and those transfused after implementation of WBC reduction ($p<0.05$). In that case, an OR <1 indicates a beneficial effect of WBC reduction. Originally published by Vamvakas in Vox Sang 2004;86:111-19.[84] (At the time of that meta-analysis,[84] the results of Llewelyn et al[79] had been presented only in abstract form by Williamson et al. Both Llewelyn et al[79] and Hebert et al[80] studied separate patient populations—orthopedic and cardiac patients[79] and intensive care unit, cardiac, and orthopedic patients,[80] respectively—and reported separate analyses for each patient population.)

Should Universal WBC Reduction Be Introduced in the United States?

Donor WBCs present in cellular blood components have been linked to a wide range of complications in transfusion recipients.[4] Nonetheless, RCTs have documented benefit from WBC reduction for only limited patient populations—namely, those at risk of FNHTRs,[87,88] refractoriness to random-donor platelet transfusions,[89-91] or CMV disease[92-95] and patients undergoing cardiac surgery.[13,18] The first three of these four indications were already established in the 1990s, while the fourth indication emerged relatively recently, through the RCTs[13,18] discussed. Targeted patient populations who must receive WBC-reduced cellular blood components because of the three established indications for WBC reduction include recipients of hematopoietic or solid-organ transplants; patients with hematologic malignancies, congenital immunodeficiencies, or acquired cellular immunodeficiencies; recipients of intrauterine transfusions and low-birth-weight neonates; and patients in whom a chronic transfusion requirement is anticipated for any reason. The results of the available RCTs, however, suggest that all patients undergoing cardiac surgery should also be included among the "targeted" patient populations.

In addition to the clinical evidence of benefit, other considerations (such as logistics, public policy, public perception, and mechanisms for funding WBC reduction) have played a role in the making of different public-policy decisions about adopting universal WBC reduction in Europe and Canada than in the United States. Nonetheless, the development of high-performance WBC reduction filters and cell separators that can adequately separate platelets from WBCs (thus obviating the need for filtration) have made WBC-reduced cellular blood components available to all transfusing facilities. The technology represents an important advance in the preparation of blood components, substantially increasing recipient safety. Perhaps the best argument for continuing the practice of universal WBC reduction in North America (in regions where it has been implemented) is the (real or perceived) difficulty in identifying, in real time, all the "targeted" patients who will benefit from WBC reduction. In contrast, the best argument for continuing the practice of universal WBC reduction in Western Europe (in the manner that it is currently employed) is that no case of vCJD has yet been documented (Chapter 3) in a recipient of a WBC-reduced cellular blood component collected from a donor who later developed vCJD.

Although a case for maintaining the status quo on both sides of the Atlantic Ocean could thus be made, the question of whether to introduce universal WBC reduction in the United States today remains unanswered. Because prestorage WBC reduction is not associated with any untoward effects, a logical argument was made in Canada and many Western European countries in the late 1990s or in the first decade of the 21st century that universal WBC reduction could be introduced—on a precautionary basis—to mitigate the purported adverse TRIM effects. The subsequent before-and-after observational studies showed that such an implementation of the policy—without proof of its efficacy to abrogate any adverse ABT effects; that is, on a precautionary basis—was not associated with any (unanticipated) harmful effects. At the same time, a beneficial effect was not shown across all of the before-and-after studies.[84] Although a beneficial effect specifically in cardiac surgery would have been expected from the results of the RCTs (Part D in Fig 1-5), the before-and-after studies were not conducted specifically in cardiac surgery.

Only one RCT[19] compared the risk of (colorectal) cancer recurrence between patients randomly assigned to receive non-WBC-reduced or WBC-reduced RBCs and found no association of non-WBC-reduced ABT with cancer recurrence. In addition, only one RCT, the Viral Activation Transfusion Study (VATS),[96] investigated the possibility of virus activation secondary to non-WBC-reduced (compared with WBC-reduced) ABT. That study transfused unmodified allogeneic RBCs stored for less than 2 weeks (and thus containing relatively undamaged allogeneic mononuclear cells) to patients in the arm exposed to allogeneic WBCs. Moreover, the two study arms were controlled for comparable duration of storage of the transfused units. There was no difference between the study arms in the HIV or CMV virus load, the length of survival, or any other outcome measure studied. Median survival was 13.0 months in recipients of WBC-reduced (prestorage-filtered) allogeneic RBCs, as compared with 20.5 months in recipients of non-WBC-reduced (buffy-coat-rich) allogeneic RBCs ($p = 0.12$).

Given the evidence available today concerning adverse TRIM effects (Figs 1-1 and 1-2), one may well ask questions. Was the application of the precautionary principle that led to the introduction of universal WBC reduction in some Western European countries and in Canada justified? Did the evidence of no harm from universal WBC reduction, provided later from the before-and-after studies, vindicate the use of the precautionary principle? Should universal WBC reduction be regarded as the standard of care? The answers to these questions remain a matter for debate, and this author can offer only his own opinion.

Competing Risks and Decision Making in Transfusion Medicine

In this author's opinion, the United States and other countries that have not introduced universal WBC reduction would do well to direct their resources and attention to reducing other, proven risks of ABT.[97] Transfusion-related acute lung injury (TRALI), mistransfusion, and bacterial contamination of platelet components (Chapter 2) are probably the "top three" proven, but not yet fully addressed, risks of ABT.[98] Because all residual risks of ABT cannot be confronted simultaneously, policymakers must carefully select which risk to confront next, so as to accrue the greatest possible societal gain in terms of improved transfusion safety.[98] The greatest competing risk when a new safety measure is implemented is the risk due to what other possible safety improvement(s) is/are left behind because public resources and attention have been directed to the measure that has been selected for implementation. In this regard, it is noted that the risks of bacterial contamination of platelets[99] and of TRALI[100] were confronted in the United States only after the debate over the appropriateness of universal WBC reduction had abated.

Because prioritization is necessary,[98] transfusion risks should be ranked objectively by means of the evidence-based approach, and the tenets of EBM should be applied with the same vigor to transfusion medicine as they already are adhered to in other fields of medicine. A cost-effectiveness threshold that differs from that used in other clinical areas applies de facto to transfusion medicine.[101] However, the approach to assessing the soundness of the evidence should be the same in transfusion medicine as it is in other clinical disciplines.

Furthermore, the assessment of the evidence should be separate from the making of policy decisions. The assessment of the soundness of the evidence does not depend on the appropriateness of applying (or not applying) the precautionary principle. Debates about the soundness of the evidence should therefore be distinguished from debates about the appropriateness of invoking the precautionary principle. The precautionary principle may have to be invoked if the purported ABT risk represents a threat of "serious or irreversible damage." Whether the precautionary principle should be applied in the absence of concrete evidence of risk may depend on public perceptions (or expectations) about transfusion safety.

The public may not perceive every ABT risk as an "HIV-like" threat for which any safety enhancement, however small or uncertain, can be deemed worth the cost.[98] Accordingly, for most purported ABT risks, policy decisions can be based on a thorough assessment of the strength of the evidence. In the context of the debate over the appropriateness of introducing universal WBC reduction, the outcomes of mortality, cancer recurrence, virus activation, or severe postoperative infection qualify as "serious or irreversible damage" and could justify application of the precautionary principle. FNHTRs, transmission of CMV, or HLA alloimmunization (in patients who are not, respectively, at increased risk of FNHTRs or at risk of CMV disease or platelet refractoriness) may not meet this criterion.

With regard to cancer recurrence, virus activation, or postoperative infection (Fig 1-1), current evidence suggests that the possibility of adverse TRIM effects is unlikely. Should the precautionary principle be invoked to prevent such serious or irreversible damage as ABT-related mortality, cancer recurrence, virus activation, or postoperative infection? Perhaps it should. (After all, nothing can be more serious than death!) However, policymakers should state explicitly that they opted to take action on a precautionary basis, instead of trying to justify their decision on the basis of the soundness of the evidence.

The essence of the precautionary principle is to take action despite uncertainty. Action founded on incomplete information, however, has some finite risk of being unnecessary or even harmful. Goldstein[102] argued that taking action in circumstances of uncertain benefits and significant costs can be socially or scientifically responsible only if it is followed up with appropriate research to examine whether the precautionary principle has dealt effectively with the threat of serious or irreversible damage that led to its application. Before-and-after studies concerning the introduction of universal WBC reduction were conducted in this spirit, and they showed that implementation of universal WBC reduction has had no effect on mortality.[84]

Universal WBC reduction introduced for the prevention of vCJD in the United Kingdom, Ireland, and Portugal likely was not subject to debate based on the merits of the evidence, and its implementation would exemplify the difficulties in relying on empirical evidence for making policy decisions in transfusion medicine. Despite such difficulties, it should be noted that most clinical decisions in transfusion medicine can be evidence-based. The ethics of conducting RCTs in clinical transfusion medicine are the same as those in any other clinical discipline.[103,104] Thus, at least in this author's opinion, there are no insurmountable regulatory, legal, ethical, or societal constraints that would prohibit the undertaking of RCTs to answer clinical transfusion medicine questions. The evidence-based approach should be applied to transfusion medicine whenever real (as opposed to perceived) regulatory, legal, ethical, or societal constraints do not prohibit its application.[41] In fact, the following is a list of clinical transfusion medicine questions currently being considered (or that have recently been considered) in RCTs, as discussed further in Chapter 4: 1) thresholds for RBC transfusion in premature, low birthweight neonates; 2) RBC transfusion thresholds in acute coronary syndromes and cardiac surgery; 3) use of a "high" (close to 1:1) plasma-to-RBCs ratio in massive transfusion for trauma; and 4) use of therapeutic (rather than prophylactic) platelet transfusions in hemato-oncology patients with hypoproliferative thrombocytopenia.

References

1. Vamvakas EC, Blajchman MA. Universal white-cell reduction: The case for and against. Transfusion 2001;41:691-712.
2. Dzik S, AuBuchon J, Jeffries L, et al. Leukocyte reduction of blood components: Public policy and new technology. Transfus Med Rev 2000; 14:34-52.
3. Vamvakas EC. Leukoreduction of blood components. In: Lozano M, Blajchman MA, Cid J, eds. Blood component preparation. Bethesda, MD: AABB Press, 2011:157-207.
4. Triulzi DJ, Dzik WH. Leukocyte-reduced blood components: Laboratory and clinical aspects. In: Simon TL, Snyder EL, Solheim BG, et al, eds. Rossi's principles of transfusion medicine. 4th ed. Bethesda, MD: AABB Press, 2009:228-46.
5. Klein MA, Friggs N, Fleschig E, et al. A crucial role for B cells in neuroinvasive scrapie. Nature 1997;390:687-90.
6. Blajchman MA. Allogeneic blood transfusions, immunomodulation and postoperative bacterial infection. Do we have the answers yet? Transfusion 1997;37:121-5.
7. Blajchman MA. Transfusion-associated immunomodulation and universal white cell reduction: Are we putting the cart before the horse? Transfusion 1999;39:665-70.
8. Vamvakas EC, Bordin JO, Blajchman MA. Immunomodulatory and proinflammatory effects of allogeneic blood transfusion. In: Simon TL, Snyder EL, Solheim BG, et al, eds.

Rossi's principles of transfusion medicine. 4th ed. Bethesda, MD: AABB Press, 2009:699-717.
9. Jensen LS, Andersen AJ, Christiansen PM, et al. Postoperative infection and natural killer cell function following blood transfusion in patients undergoing elective colorectal surgery. Br J Surg 1992;79:513-6.
10. Jensen LS, Kissmeyer-Nielsen P, Wolff B, Quist N. Randomized comparison of leukocyte-depleted versus buffy-coat-poor blood transfusion and complications after colorectal surgery. Lancet 1996;348:841-5.
11. Tartter PI, Mohandas K, Azar P, et al. Randomized trial comparing packed red cell blood transfusion with and without leukocyte depletion for gastrointestinal surgery. Am J Surg 1998;176:462-6.
12. Bilgin YM, van de Watering LMG, Eijsman L, et al. Double-blind, randomized controlled trial on the effect of leukocyte-depleted erythrocyte transfusions in cardiac valve surgery. Circulation 2004;109:2755-60.
13. van de Watering LMG, Hermans J, Houbiers JGA, et al. Beneficial effect of leukocyte depletion of transfused blood on post-operative complications in patients undergoing cardiac surgery: A randomized clinical trial. Circulation 1998;97:562-8.
14. Nathens AB, Nester TA, Rubenfeld GD, et al. The effects of leukoreduced blood transfusion on infection risk following injury: A randomized controlled trial. Shock 2006;26:342-7.
15. Titlestad IL, Ebbesen LS, Ainsworth AP, et al. Leukocyte-depletion of blood components does not significantly reduce the risk of infectious complications: Results of a double-blind, randomized study. Int J Colorectal Dis 2001;16: 147-53.
16. Wallis JP, Chapman CE, Orr KE, et al. Effect of WBC reduction of transfused RBCs on postoperative infection rates in cardiac surgery. Transfusion 2002;42:1127-34.
17. van Hilten JA, van de Watering LMG, van Bockel JH, et al. Effects of transfusion with red cells filtered to remove leukocytes: Randomized controlled trial in patients undergoing major surgery. Br Med J 2004;328:1281-4.
18. Boshkov LK, Furnary A, Morris C, et al. Prestorage leukoreduction of red cells in elective cardiac surgery: Results of a double-blind randomized controlled trial (abstract). Blood 2004;104:112a.
19. Houbiers JGA, Brand A, van de Watering LMG, et al. Randomized controlled trial comparing transfusion of leucocyte-depleted or buffy-coat-depleted blood in surgery for colorectal cancer. Lancet 1994;344:573-8.
20. Bracey AW, Radovancevick R, Nussimeier NA, et al. Leukocyte-reduced blood in open-heart surgery patients: Effects on outcome (abstract). Transfusion 2002;42(Suppl):5S.
21. Dzik WH, Anderson JK, O'Neill EM, et al. A prospective, randomized clinical trial of universal WBC reduction. Transfusion 2002;42:1114-22.
22. Nielsen HJ, Hammer J, Kraup AL, et al. Prestorage leukocyte filtration may reduce leukocyte-derived bioactive substance accumulation in patients operated for burn trauma. Burns 1999;25:162-70.
23. Guyatt GH. Evidence-based medicine. ACP J Club 1991;114:A16.
24. Guyatt G. Preface. In: Guyatt G, Rennie D, eds. Users' guides to the medical literature: A manual for evidence-based clinical practice. Chicago, IL: AMA Press, 2002:xiv.
25. Haynes RB, Devereaux PJ, Guyatt GH. Clinical expertise in the era of evidence-based medicine and patient choice. ACP J Club 2002;136:A11.
26. Evidence-Based Medicine Working Group. Evidence-based medicine: A new approach to teaching the practice of medicine. JAMA 1992; 268:2420-5.
27. Drummond MF, Richardson WS, O'Brien BJ, et al. Users' guides to the medical literature: XIII. How to use an article on economic analysis of clinical practice. A. Are the results of the study valid? JAMA 1997;277:1552-7.
28. Green SB, Byar DP. Using observational data from registries to compare treatments: The fallacy of omnimetrics. Stat Med 1984;3:361-70.
29. Stewart LA, Parmar MKB. Meta-analysis of the literature or individual patient data: Is there a difference? Lancet 1993;341:418-22.
30. Sackett DL. Rules of evidence and clinical recommendations on the use of antithrombotic agents. Chest 1989;95(Suppl 2):2S-4S.
31. Cook DJ, Guyatt GH, Laupacis A, et al. Clinical recommendations using levels of evidence for antithrombotic agents. Chest 1995;108(4 Suppl):227S-30S.
32. L'Abbé KA, Detsky AS, O'Rourke K. Meta-analysis in clinical research. Ann Intern Med 1987; 107:224-33.
33. Chalmers I. The Cochrane Collaboration: Preparing, maintaining, and disseminating systematic reviews of the effects of health care. Ann N Y Acad Sci 1993;703:156-65.

34. Doll R, Hill AB. The mortality of doctors in relation to their smoking habits: A preliminary report. Br Med J 1954;1:1451-5.
35. Doll R, Hill AB. Lung cancer and other causes of death in relation to smoking: A second report on the mortality of British doctors. Br Med J 1956;2:1071-81.
36. Howick J, Glasziou P, Aronson JK. The evolution of evidence hierarchies: What can Bradford Hill's "guidelines for causation" contribute? J Roy Soc Med 2009;102:186-94.
37. Benson K, Hartz AJ. A comparison of observational studies and randomized controlled trials. N Engl J Med 2000;342:1878-86.
38. Concato J, Shah N, Horwitz RI. Randomized controlled trials, observational studies, and the hierarchy of research designs. N Engl J Med 2000;342:1887-92.
39. Pocock SJ, Elbourne DR. Randomized trials or observational tribulations? N Engl J Med 2000; 342:1907-9.
40. Isbister JP, Shander A, Spahn DR, et al. Adverse blood transfusion outcomes: Establishing causation. Transfus Med Rev 2011;25:89-101.
41. Vamvakas EC. Establishing causation in transfusion medicine and related tribulations. Transfus Med Rev 2011;25:81-8.
42. Colditz GA, Miller JN, Mosteller F. How study design affects outcomes in comparisons of therapy: I. Medical. Stat Med 1989;8:441-54.
43. Miller JN, Colditz GA, Mosteller F. How study design affects outcomes in comparisons of therapy. II. Surgical. Stat Med 1989;8:455-66.
44. Chalmers TC, Matta RJ, Smith H, Kunzler AM. Evidence favoring the use of anticoagulants in the hospital phase of acute myocardial infarction. N Engl J Med 1977;297:1091-6.
45. Vamvakas EC, Blajchman MA, eds. Immunomodulatory effects of blood transfusion. Bethesda, MD: AABB Press, 1999:1-295.
46. Foster KR, Vecchia P, Repacholi MH. Science and the precautionary principle. Science 2000; 288:979-81.
47. United Nations General Assembly. World Charter for Nature. Resolution 37/7. New York, NY: United Nations, 1982. [Available at: http://www.un.org/documents/ga/res/37/a37r007.htm (accessed August 1, 2011).]
48. Third International Conference on the Protection of the North Sea. Ministerial Declaration of the Third International Conference on the Protection of the North Sea, The Hague, 8 March 1990: Preamble. [Available at: http://www.seas-at-risk.org/1mages/1990 Hague Declaration.pdf (accessed August 1, 2011).]
49. Commission of the European Communities. Communication from the Commission on the Precautionary Principle. Brussels: European Commission, 2000.[Available at: http://ec.europa.eu/dgs/health_consumer/library/pub/pub07_en.pdf (accessed August 1, 2011).]
50. Cellular Telephone Company v. Town of Oyster Bay, 166F.3d 490, 494 (2nd Cir. 1999).
51. Institute of Medicine Roundtable on Environmental Health Sciences, Research and Medicine. Environmental health sciences decision making: Risk management, evidence, and ethics–workshop summary. Washington, DC: National Academies Press, 2009.
52. Lo CF. Risks, scientific uncertainty and the approach of applying the precautionary principle. Med Law 2009;28:283-300.
53. Goldstein BD, Carruth RS. Implications of the precautionary principle: Is it a threat to science? Int J Occup Med Environ Health 2004;17:153-61.
54. UN Conference on Environment and Development. Rio Declaration on Environment and Development (Publ. no. E.73II.A.14).New York: United Nations, 1992. [Available at: www.unep.org/Documents.Multilingual/Default.asp?documentid=78&articleid=1163 (accessed August 1, 2011).]
55. Wilson K, Wilson M, Hébert PC, Graham I. The application of the precautionary principle to the blood system: The Canadian blood system's vCJD donor deferral policy. Transfus Med Rev 2003;17:89-94.
56. Blajchman MA, Bordin JO. Mechanisms of transfusion-associated immunosuppression. Curr Opin Hematol 1994;1:457-61.
57. Vamvakas EC. Deleterious clinical effects of transfusion-associated immunomodulation: Fact or fiction? An update through 2005. Am J Clin Pathol 2006;126(Suppl 1):S71-S75.
58. Vamvakas E, Blajchman MA. Transfusion-related immunomodulation: An update. Blood Rev 2007;21:327-48.
59. Blajchman MA, Bardossy I, Carmen R, et al. Allogeneic blood transfusion-induced enhancement of tumor growth: Two animal models showing amelioration by leukodepletion and passive transfer using spleen cells. Blood 1993;81:1880-2.
60. Mincheff MS, Meryman HT, Kapoor V, et al. Blood transfusion and immunomodulation: A possible mechanism. Vox Sang 1993;65:18-24.

61. Kao KJ. Induction of humoral immune tolerance to major histocompatibility complex antigens by transfusions of UV-B irradiated leukocytes. Blood 1996;88:4375-82.
62. Ghio M, Contini P, Mazzei C, et al. Soluble HLA class I, HLA class II, and Fas ligand in blood components: A possible key to explain the immunomodulatory effects of allogeneic blood transfusion. Blood 1999;93:1770-7.
63. Bordin JO, Bardossy L, Blajchman MA. Growth enhancement of established tumors by allogeneic blood transfusion in experimental animals and its amelioration by leukodepletion: The importance of timing of the leukodepletion. Blood 1994;84:344-8.
64. Nielsen HJ, Reimert CM, Pedersen AN, et al. Time-dependent spontaneous release of white cell- and platelet-derived bioactive substances from stored human blood. Transfusion 1996; 36:960-5.
65. Innerhofer P, Luz G, Spotl L, et al. Immunologic changes following transfusion of autologous or allogeneic buffy-coat-poor versus leukocyte-depleted blood in patients undergoing arthroplasty. I. Proliferative T-cell responses and T-helper/T-suppressor cell balance. Transfusion 1999;39:1089-96.
66. Fransen E, Maessen J, Denterner M, et al. Impact of blood transfusion on inflammatory mediator release in patients undergoing cardiac surgery. Chest 1999;116:1233-9.
67. [No author]. Diversity and heterogeneity. Oxford: the Cochrane Collaboration, 2002. [Available at http://www.cochrane-net.org/openlearning/HTML/mod13-5.htm (accessed August 1, 2011).]
68. DerSimonian R, Laird N. Meta-analysis in clinical trials. Control Clin Trials 1986;7:177-88.
69. Vamvakas EC. White-blood-cell containing allogeneic blood transfusion and postoperative infection or mortality: An updated meta-analysis. Vox Sang 2007;92:224-32.
70. Fergusson D, Khanna MP, Tinmouth A, Hébert PC. Transfusion of leukoreduced red blood cells may decrease postoperative infections: Two meta-analyses of randomized controlled trials. Can J Anaesth 2004;51:417-24.
71. Blumberg N, Zhao H, Wang H, et al. The intention-to-treat principle in clinical trials and meta-analyses of leukoreduced blood transfusions in surgical patients. Transfusion 2007;47:573-81.
72. Blumberg N. Deleterious clinical effects of transfusion immunomodulation: Proven beyond reasonable doubt. Transfusion 2005;45(Suppl): 33S-9S.
73. Vamvakas EC. Deleterious clinical effects of transfusion immunomodulation: Proven beyond reasonable doubt. Transfusion 2006;46:492-4.
74. Fergusson D, Aaron SD, Guyatt G, Hébert P. Post-randomization exclusions: The intention-to-treat principle and excluding patients from the analysis. Br Med J 2002;325:652-4.
75. Kunz R, Guyatt G. Which patients to include in the analysis? Transfusion 2006;46:881-4.
76. Vamvakas EC. Rationale for randomized controlled trials and for the intention-to-treat principle in transfusion medicine: Are they one and the same? Vox Sang 2008;95:165-73.
77. Vamvakas EC. Why have meta-analyses of the randomized controlled trials of the association between non-white-blood-cell reduced allogeneic blood transfusion and postoperative infection produced discordant results? Vox Sang 2007;93:196-207.
78. Baron JF, Gourdin M, Bertrand M, et al. The effect of universal leukodepletion of packed red blood cells on postoperative infections in high-risk patients undergoing abdominal aortic surgery. Anesth Analg 2002;94:529-37.
79. Llewelyn CA, Taylor RS, Todd AA, et al. The effect of universal leukoreduction on postoperative infections and length of stay in elective orthopedic and cardiac surgery. Transfusion 2004;44:489-500.
80. Hébert PC, Fergusson D, Blajchman MA, et al. Clinical outcomes following institution of the Canadian universal leukoreduction program for red blood cell transfusions. JAMA 2003;289: 1941-9.
81. Fergusson D, Hébert PC, Lee SK, et al. Clinical outcomes following institution of universal leukoreduction of blood transfusions for premature infants. JAMA 2003;289:1950-6.
82. Volkova N, Klapper E, Pepkowitz SH, et al. A case-control study of the impact of WBC reduction on the cost of hospital care for patients undergoing coronary artery bypass graft surgery. Transfusion 2002;42:1123-6.
83. Blumberg N, Heal JM, Cowles JW, et al. Leukocyte-reduced transfusions in cardiac surgery: Results of an implementation trial. Am J Clin Pathol 2002;118:376-81.
84. Vamvakas EC. White-blood-cell containing allogeneic blood transfusion, postoperative infection, and mortality: A meta-analysis of observational, "before-and-after" studies. Vox Sang 2004;86:111-19.

85. Yusuf S, Peto R, Lewis J, et al. Beta blockade during and after myocardial infarction: An overview of the randomized trials. Prog Cardiovasc Dis 1985;27:335-71.
86. Cooper H, Hedges LV, eds. The handbook of research synthesis. New York: Russell Sage Foundation, 1994.
87. Heddle NM, Klama L, Meyer R, et al. A randomized control trial comparing plasma removal with white cell reduction to prevent reactions to platelets. Transfusion 1999;39: 231-8.
88. Heddle NM, Klama L, Singer J, et al. The role of the plasma from platelet concentrates in transfusion reactions. N Engl J Med 1994;331:625-8.
89. TRAP Study Group. Leukocyte reduction and ultraviolet B irradiation of platelets to prevent alloimmunization and refractoriness to platelet transfusions. N Engl J Med 1997;337:1861-9.
90. Heddle NM. The efficacy of leukodepletion to improve platelet transfusion response: A critical appraisal of clinical studies. Transfus Med Rev 1994;8:15-28.
91. Vamvakas EC. Meta-analysis of randomized controlled trials of the efficacy of white cell reduction in preventing HLA-alloimmunization and refractoriness to random-donor platelet transfusions. Transfus Med Rev 1998;12:258-70.
92. Bowden RA, Slichter SJ, Sayers MH, et al. A comparison of filtered leukocyte reduced and cytomegalovirus (CMV) seronegative blood products for the prevention of transfusion-associated CMV infection after marrow transplant. Blood 1995;86:3598-606.
93. Pamphilon DH, Rider JR, Barbara JAJ, Williamson LM. Prevention of transfusion-transmitted cytomegalovirus infection. Transfus Med 1999; 9:115-23.
94. Preiksaitis JK. The cytomegalovirus-"safe" blood product: Is leukoreduction equivalent to antibody screening? Transfus Med Rev 2000;14: 112-36.
95. Vamvakas E. Is white-blood-cell reduction equivalent to antibody screening in preventing transmission of cytomegalovirus by transfusion? A review of the literature and meta-analysis. Transfus Med Rev 2005;19:181-99.
96. Collier A, Kalish L, Busch M, et al. Leukocyte-reduced red-blood-cell transfusions in patients with anemia and human immunodeficiency virus infection. JAMA 2001;285:1592-601.
97. Corwin HL, AuBuchon JP. Is leukoreduction of blood components for everyone? JAMA 2003; 289:1993-5.
98. AuBuchon JP, Petz LD. Making decisions to improve transfusion safety. In: AuBuchon JP, Petz L, Fink A, eds. Policy alternatives in transfusion medicine. Bethesda, MD: AABB Press, 2001:193-226.
99. Further guidance on methods to detect bacterial contamination of platelet components. AABB Association Bulletin #03-12 (October 1, 2003). Bethesda, MD: AABB, 2003. [Available at: http://www.aabb.org/resources/Publications/bulletins/Documents/obsolete/AB03-12 OBSOLETE.pdf.]
100. Transfusion-related acute lung injury. AABB Association Bulletin #06-07 (November 3, 2006). Bethesda, MD: AABB, 2006. [Available at: http://www.aabb.org/resources/Publications/bulletins/Pages/ab06-07.aspx.]
101. AuBuchon JP, Birkmeyer JD, Busch MP. Safety of the blood supply in the United States: Opportunities and controversies. Ann Intern Med 1997;127:904-9.
102. Goldstein BD. The precautionary principle and scientific research are not antithetical. Environ Health Perspect 1999;107:A594-5.
103. Passamani E. Clinical trials: Are they ethical? N Engl J Med 1991;324:1589-91.
104. Culpepper L, Gilbert TT. Evidence and ethics. Lancet 1999;353:829-31.

In: Vamvakas EC.
Decision Making in Transfusion Medicine
Bethesda, MD: AABB Press, 2011

2

Causes of Mortality Related to Allogeneic Blood Transfusion

WELL INTO THE 1990s, THE attention of transfusion medicine professionals remained concentrated on allogeneic blood transfusion (ABT)-related morbidity and mortality secondary to transfusion-transmitted infections (TTIs). Although only 3 years had elapsed between the recognition of the threat that the human immunodeficiency virus (HIV) posed to blood safety (1982) and the implementation of donor testing (1985), approximately 12,000 cases of transfusion-acquired HIV infection were estimated to have occurred in the United States.[1] When the interval between recognition and introduction of testing was longer, the number of TTIs was correspondingly higher. Thus, from 1970 to 1990, there were 4.8 million cases of hepatitis C virus (HCV) transmission through ABT.[2] Even if only 3% of these cases resulted in fatal cirrhosis or hepatocellular carcinoma in long-term survivors,[3] and even if only 30% of transfusion recipients survived long enough to develop such complications,[4] 43,200 ABT-related deaths still could have ensued.[5]

This mortality from TTIs before the 1990s dwarfed the concomitant mortality from transfusion-related acute lung injury (TRALI), transfusion-associated sepsis (TAS), and hemolytic transfusion reactions (HTRs), thereby focusing blood-safety efforts toward the prevention of TTIs. As a result, the past two decades have witnessed an impressive reduction in the probability of transmission of HIV and HCV through ABT, by up to 4 log.[6] Although the risks of TTIs have been greatly reduced, the risk of a new, or poorly understood, infectious disease with a long incubation period that can be transmitted by ABT while the disease is accumulating in the blood-donor base before its clinical consequences become apparent, remains a “fixed and inevitable property of transfusion medicine,”[7] and novel transfusion-transmitted, or potentially transfusion-transmitted, pathogens continue to emerge.[8]

In 2005, TRALI, HTRs, and TAS ranked, respectively, as the first, second, and third most frequent cause of transfusion-related mortality in the United States.[9] Together, these three causes of death accounted for 95% (59 of 62) of all fatalities associated with ABT that were reported to the US Food and Drug Administration (FDA) and deemed to be transfusion-related.[9] The remaining deaths passively reported to the FDA and deemed to be transfusion-related in 2005 were due to transfusion-associated circulatory overload (TACO; two deaths), transfusion-associated graft-vs-host disease (TA-GVHD; one death), and one error associated with therapeutic plasma exchange (immunoadsorption—namely, use of a column for selective removal of plasma constituents in a patient for whom use of the column was contraindicated).[9]

Of the transfusion-related deaths passively reported to the FDA in 2005,[9] TRALI was implicated in 29 (47%), HTRs in 22 (36%), and TAS in eight (13%). Along with the reports of deaths passively made to the FDA,[9-14] the hemovigilance reports from France,[15] the United Kingdom,[16,17] and the Canadian province of Quebec[18] focused attention in the early 21st century on TRALI, HTRs, and TAS as the leading causes of transfusion-related deaths and led to the implementation of measures[19,20] to at least partly confront the risks of TAS[19] and TRALI.[20] With the measures introduced in the United States in 2004 and 2006 to mitigate the risk of TAS from platelet transfusion[19] and the risk of TRALI from plasma transfusion,[20] respectively, 145 (47%) of transfusion-related deaths reported to the FDA from 2005 to 2010 were due to TRALI, 75 (24%) to HTRs, and 24 (8%) to TAS (Fig 2-1). Of the deaths reported in 2010 alone, 18 (45%) were due to TRALI, seven (18%) to HTRs, and one (3%) to TAS. TACO emerged as the second greatest cause of transfusion-related deaths in 2010, causing eight (20%) deaths.[9]

The United Kingdom (UK) introduced measures to mitigate the risk of TRALI secondary to plasma transfusion in the fall of 2003 but did not implement measures to mitigate the risk of TAS secondary to platelet transfusion until the fall of 2010.[16] Figure 2-2 gives data for 2008 to contrast the causes of 46 fatalities deemed to be transfusion-related in the United States[9] and 10 deaths in which ABT was considered, by the UK Serious Hazards of Transfusion (SHOT) System, to have a causal or contributory role.[16] Only one death (secondary to a septic reaction to platelets) was deemed to have been caused by an ABT in that year in the United Kingdom.[16] In all other

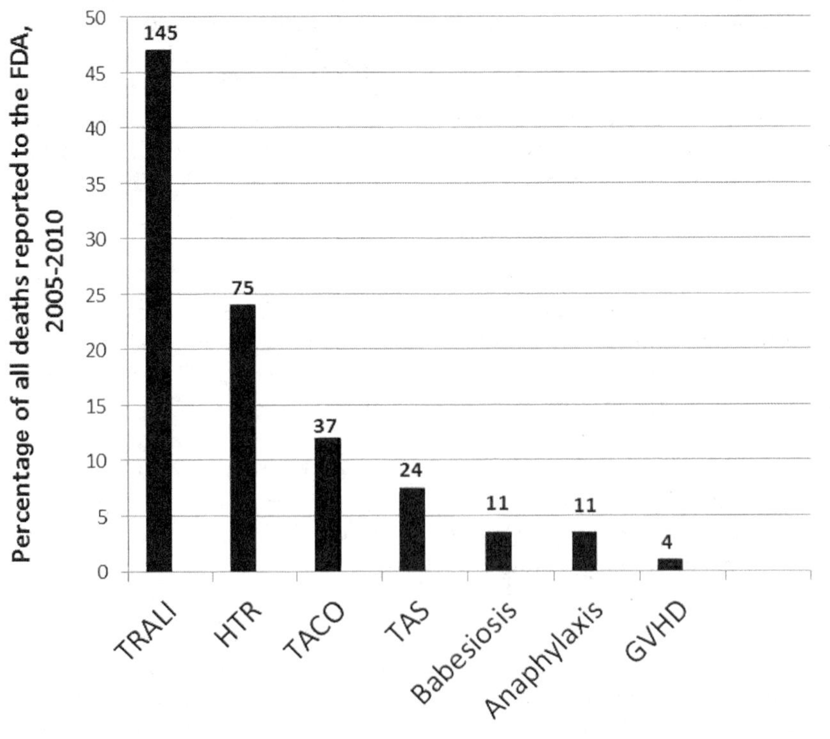

Figure 2-1. Causes of ABT-related deaths reported to the United States Food and Drug Administration (FDA) from 2005 through 2010. The actual number of deaths from each cause is shown above the corresponding column. GVHD = graft-vs-host disease; HTR = hemolytic transfusion reaction; TACO = transfusion-associated circulatory overload; TAS = transfusion-associated sepsis; TRALI = transfusion-related acute lung injury.

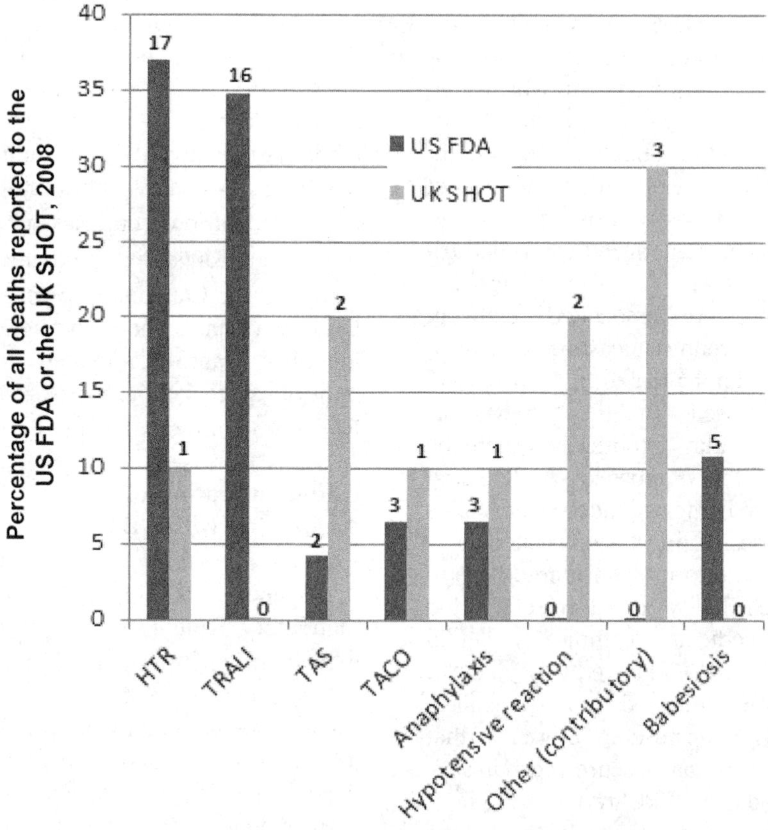

Figure 2-2. Causes of allogeneic blood transfusion (ABT)-related deaths as a proportion of all deaths reported to the United States Food and Drug Administration (US FDA) or the United Kingdom Severe Hazards of Transfusion (UK SHOT) in 2008. The actual number of deaths related to transfusion (US FDA) or in which transfusion was deemed to have a causal or contributory role (UK SHOT) is shown above each column.
HTR = hemolytic transfusion reaction; TACO = transfusion-associated circulatory overload; TAS = transfusion-associated sepsis; TRALI = transfusion-related acute lung injury. Initially published by Vamvakas and Blajchman in Transfus Med Rev 2010;24:77-124.[5]

cases, transfusion was deemed only to have contributed to a patient's death. These latter deaths included one more case of TAS, one of HTR, one of anaphylaxis, two cases of hypotensive reactions to transfusion, one of febrile nonhemolytic transfusion reaction, and two cases of inappropriate transfusion.[16] In 2008, 5 years after the introduction of measures to prevent TRALI in the United Kingdom, no death associated with ABT was due to TRALI in the United Kingdom,[16] whereas 16 TRALI deaths were recorded in the United States. At the same time, there were two deaths due to TAS in the United States (where measures to prevent TAS had been implemented 4 years previously) and two deaths due to TAS in the United Kingdom (where measures for the prevention of TAS had not yet been introduced).

Because the population of the United States is five times that of the United Kingdom, the two passive surveillance systems (the US FDA[9] and the UK SHOT[16]) seem to have recorded a similar number of ABT-related deaths per million population. Babesiosis occurs only in the United States, and the other transfusion-related deaths from specific causes represent events so rare that the differences in the frequency with which such causes of death were recorded in each country in 2008 (Fig 2-2) could probably be ascribed to chance. This chapter reviews the incidence of deaths caused by ABT as well as attributed to ABT by the results of randomized controlled trials (RCTs).[21-23] This chapter also relates the reported number of ABT-associated deaths in each country to preventive measures that have (or have not) been implemented in each respective jurisdiction, as well as to the "passive surveillance artifact" that produces systematic underreporting of the number of ABT-related deaths recorded by hemovigilance systems. The three leading causes of transfusion-related mortality in the 21st century are considered here in the order in which they were addressed by the US transfusion-medicine community: TAS (addressed in 2004), followed by TRALI (addressed in 2006), followed by HTRs (still to be addressed). The increase in mortality that RCTs have attributed, via obscure mechanisms, to non-white-blood-cell (WBC)-reduced ABT[21,22] or to ABT in general[23] is also considered, along with the threat posed to blood safety by the next fatal TTI that may appear in the future.

Passive Surveillance Studies of ABT-Related Mortality

Data on transfusion complications, including deaths from transfusion complications, come from active surveillance studies, passive surveillance ("hemovigilance") studies, RCTs, and observational studies. The latter two types of studies evaluate consecutive transfused patients at a particular setting(s) as part of a research protocol and—in theory—would be expected to produce the most reliable data. Their downside, however, is that they usually enroll a cohort of transfused patients that is much too small to allow documentation of the incidence of rare transfusion complications (or the risk of death due to ABT). Active surveillance studies are conducted at a particular hospital or at "sentinel" sites where there is heightened awareness of, and special arrangements have been made for detecting, a specific transfusion complication. Passive surveillance systems rely on passive (and often voluntary) reporting of adverse events associated with ABT, including ABT-related deaths. Such hemovigilance systems have been in place in various countries—including France,[15] the United Kingdom,[16,17] other European countries, and the Canadian province of Quebec.[18] In the United States, the reporting to the FDA of all identified transfusion-related deaths has been required since 1976. Moreover, a pilot hemovigilance program was recently introduced.[24]

Underestimation of Adverse Events Associated with ABT

Reporting to hemovigilance systems can be mandatory (as it is in France[15]) or voluntary (as it was originally in the United Kingdom[16]). Adverse events, including deaths, captured by these systems depend on whether a particular adverse event caused by a transfusion was suspected of being, investigated as possibly being, and/or deemed to be transfusion-related on the basis of the criteria employed locally for the diagnosis of each specific transfusion complication. Whether ABT is considered as the possible cause of an adverse event or death varies with the medical and nursing staff awareness of transfusion complications at each particular clinical setting, as well as with local culture, resources, and logistics vis-à-vis the extent of the investigation and the reporting of such adverse events along the designated channels of the hemovigilance system.

Thus, hemovigilance systems tend to greatly underestimate the incidence of ABT-related adverse events. When TRALI was identified by a passive surveillance system,[25] the frequency of TRALI cases (as opposed to deaths) was in the range of 1 per 16,000 units of transfused plasma, 1 per 43,000 units of transfused platelets, and 1 per 44,000 units of transfused red blood cells (RBCs). When TRALI was diagnosed as part of an active surveillance study,[26] the frequency of TRALI cases was in the range of 1 per 1000 units of transfused platelets, 1 per 4400 units of transfused RBCs, and 1 per 20,000 units of transfused plasma. However, a prospective observational study in an intensive care unit (ICU) where most transfused patients had received multiple blood components (RBCs, plasma, and/or platelets) diagnosed TRALI in 1 (8.2%) of 12 critically ill patients.[27] The hemovigilance[25] and observational[27] studies based their diagnoses of TRALI on the Canadian consensus criteria[28] promulgated by the Canadian Consensus Conference (CCC) in 2004, whereas the study employing an active surveillance system[26] had been conducted earlier—at a time when there was no standard definition of the constellation of findings that qualified as definite or possible TRALI. The two surveillance studies[25,26] encompassed all transfused patients, whereas the observational study of ICU patients[27] included only critically ill patients.

That difference is especially important, because TRALI is believed to result from an interplay of both patient- and transfusion-related factors and may thus be much more common in critically ill patients than in other transfused patients. Critically ill patients also may have a lower threshold for TRALI than does the average transfusion recipient,[29] because of sepsis, trauma, and other factors that may represent the "first hit" in the "two-hit" hypothesis of TRALI pathogenesis.[30,31] In such critically ill patients, too, many cases of acute lung injury (ALI)—occurring in the presence of one or several alternative causes of ALI—can be misdiagnosed as TRALI, because of a temporal association with ABT.

Thus, the >1000-fold difference in the reported incidence of TRALI between the hemovigilance[25] and observational[27] studies is due partly to the design employed (passive surveillance or observational) and partly to patient factors and/or to misdiagnosis of cases of ALI as TRALI in multitransfused patients (in whom respiratory distress happens to manifest itself within 6 hours of a transfusion). Notwithstanding the relevance of the patient factors, because both studies[25,27] used the same criteria[28] for diagnosing TRALI, the >1000-fold difference in the reported TRALI frequency underscores the extent to which passive surveillance data may underestimate the incidence of serious ABT complications.

When awareness of transfusion complications increases, or when resources are expended to detect transfusion complications, the reporting of transfusion complications to hemovigilance systems increases. Both of these conditions were satisfied, before the implementation of bacterial detection in platelets, at the Johns Hopkins Hospital (Baltimore, MD).[32,33] Over 12 years, Ness et al[32] had implemented a system of prospective monitoring, whereby all febrile transfusion reactions to platelets were assessed by culture. Starting from a baseline of 51.7% of the therapeutic platelet doses at their hospital provided as apheresis (single-donor) platelets, Ness et al observed that—as the proportion of therapeutic platelet doses provided as apheresis (single-donor) platelets [as opposed to whole-blood-derived (WBD) platelet pools] increased from 51.7% to 99.4%—the risk of TAS declined from 1 in 4818 to 1 in 15,098 platelet transfusions.[32] This 68% decrease in risk could be extrapolated to an 80% reduction (with an expected risk of TAS of 1 per 3000 platelet pools) had the authors started from a baseline of providing no therapeutic platelet doses as apheresis (single-donor) platelets.[32,33] A virtually identical risk (1 per 2282 platelet pools in 2000 and 1 per 4149 platelet pools in 2001) was observed during the first 2 years of the Quebec hemovigilance program, which relied on hospitals that cultured 40.4% to 51.6% of platelet pools implicated in transfusion reactions and that were staffed with transfusion officers.[18] In contrast, from 1994 to 1998, the French hemovigilance system—probably the most comprehensive passive surveillance system that entailed mandatory reporting—observed a risk of sepsis secondary to platelet transfusion (if pools of six platelet concentrates are assumed) of only 1 per 13,000 platelet pools.[15] The reported risk was far lower in the UK hemovigilance program.[16,17]

Preferential Reporting of Adverse Events Associated with ABT

Data from hemovigilance systems must therefore be interpreted in the light of this "passive surveillance artifact" that results in the underreporting of the overall adverse transfusion events, as well as the relative overreporting of specific transfusion complications (of which the medical and nursing staffs become more aware at one time or another), compared with all other transfusion complications. Influential publications in the literature, and high-profile preventive efforts initiated by national blood-safety agencies or professional societies, heighten clinicians' awareness of specific ABT complications, which generates more diagnoses of those particular ABT-related adverse events and more reporting of such events to the hemovigilance systems.

This situation is highlighted by the fact that—when the numbers of deaths due to the three leading causes of transfusion-related mortality in the United States from 2004 to 2008 and from 2001 to 2003 were compared—TRALI appeared to have displaced HTRs as the greatest of these causes. The mean annual number of deaths passively reported to the FDA and deemed to be due to TRALI doubled between the 2001-2003 (14/year) and 2004-2008 (28/year) spans.[5] In contrast, the number of deaths from HTRs was reduced by half (from 23/year to 11/year).[5] On October 19, 2001, the FDA had alerted transfusion medicine professionals in the United States to the possibility that transfused patients may be at risk of TRALI.[34] Between 1992 and 2001, the FDA had received 45 reports of transfusion-related fatalities secondary to TRALI; at that time, TRALI was thought to be the third leading cause of transfusion-related mortality in the United States. Because the FDA had not received any reports of TRALI fatalities before 1992, they ascribed the increase in the number of received reports of deaths due to TRALI to better recognition and reporting of TRALI.[34] The overall limited awareness of TRALI as a transfusion complication and as a clinical entity separate from the acute respiratory distress syndrome[35-37] (ARDS)—from which TRALI[38] is often clinically indistinguishable—is underscored by the fact that TRALI was not even identified as a specific transfusion complication by the French hemovigilance system between 1994 and 1999.[15]

Around 2004, TRALI awareness was increased by three events: the publicity associated with the UK decision in October 2003 to convert to "male-only" plasma to mitigate the risk of TRALI,[16] the publicity associated with the CCC on TRALI that was convened in April 2004 to generate a standardized definition of TRALI, and the promulgation in December 2004 of the consensus criteria for the diagnosis of TRALI.[28] Then, in March 2004, the AABB standard that blood establishments limit and detect bacterial contamination in all platelet components became effective.[19] Various process improvements were thus implemented to reduce the risk of TAS secondary to platelet transfusion.[39] The presumed increases in TRALI awareness and in the measures available to reduce TAS were temporally associated with an increase in the reporting of deaths from TRALI, as well as a reduction in the reporting of deaths from TAS (from eight/year in 2001-2003 to slightly under five/year in 2004-2008).[5]

Awareness of the risk of TAS had been increasing before 2001, culminating in a September 1999 FDA/Center of Biologics Evaluation and Research Workshop at which the data on 26 fatalities from transfusion of contaminated RBCs and 51 fatalities from transfusion of contaminated platelets between 1976 and 1998 were presented.[40] Already in 1996, as the risks of transfusion-transmitted HIV and HCV infection had declined, the AABB had alerted transfusion medicine professionals that the risk of receiving bacterially contaminated platelets might be 50- to 250-fold the combined risk of HIV, hepatitis B virus (HBV), HCV, and human T-cell lymphotropic virus (HTLV) transmission through transfusion.[41]

The reduction in the reporting of deaths from TAS to the FDA starting in 2004 is evident both for all transfused products and, specifically, for apheresis (single-donor) platelets (Fig 2-3). In March 2004, automated bacterial-culture systems were available only for platelets collected by apheresis. Hospitals releasing pooled WBD

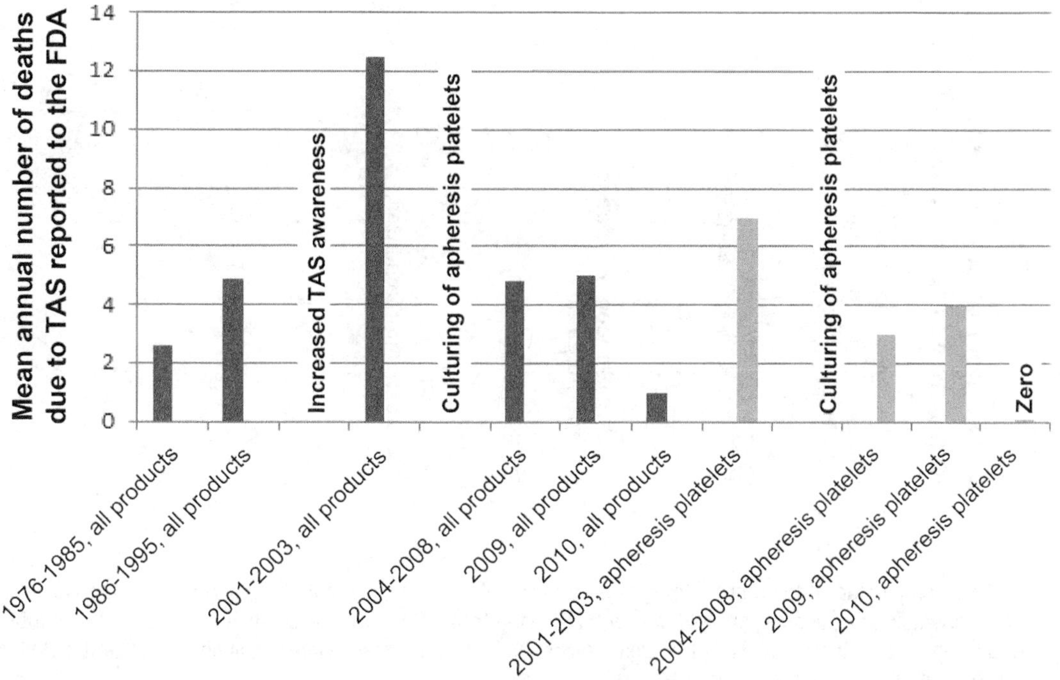

Figure 2-3. A comparison of the number of deaths from transfusion-associated sepsis (TAS) from 2001 through 2003 and from 2004 through 2010, shown separately for all transfused blood components (dark bars) and for apheresis platelets (light bars). For each period, the figure shows the mean number of deaths deemed to be due to TAS each year based on the reports of transfusion-related fatalities made to the United States Food and Drug Administration (FDA). Data are also shown for the earlier periods of 1976 through 1985 and 1986 through 1995, but the data for 1996 through 2000 have not been made available.

platelets for transfusion had to employ surrogate methods for bacteria detection[39]; the sensitivity of those methods was 4.6 times less than that of bacteria culture.[42] Accordingly, to comply with the "spirit" rather than the "letter" of the March 2004 AABB standard, US blood establishments moved voluntarily toward the provision of apheresis (rather than WBD) platelets for transfusion. Thus, in 2006, 87.5% of all therapeutic platelet doses transfused in the United States were provided as apheresis (single-donor) platelets.[43] By November 2007, virtually all plasma transfused in the United States was collected from male donors,[20] but the AABB recommendation that apheresis (single-donor) platelets be collected from male donors or from female donors without a history of pregnancy or shown not to have WBC antibodies was not implemented by November 2008 (as had originally been intended[20]). The impact of the November 2006 AABB recommendations for TRALI prevention[20] can be gleaned from the TRALI cases recorded since 2008 in association with transfusion of plasma.

Figure 2-4 shows that the conversion to male-only plasma in the United States was temporally related to a reduction in the number of TRALI deaths associated with plasma transfusion that were reported to the FDA. The variation in the number of TRALI deaths attributed to plasma reported between 2005 and 2010 could be due to chance or, alternatively, to

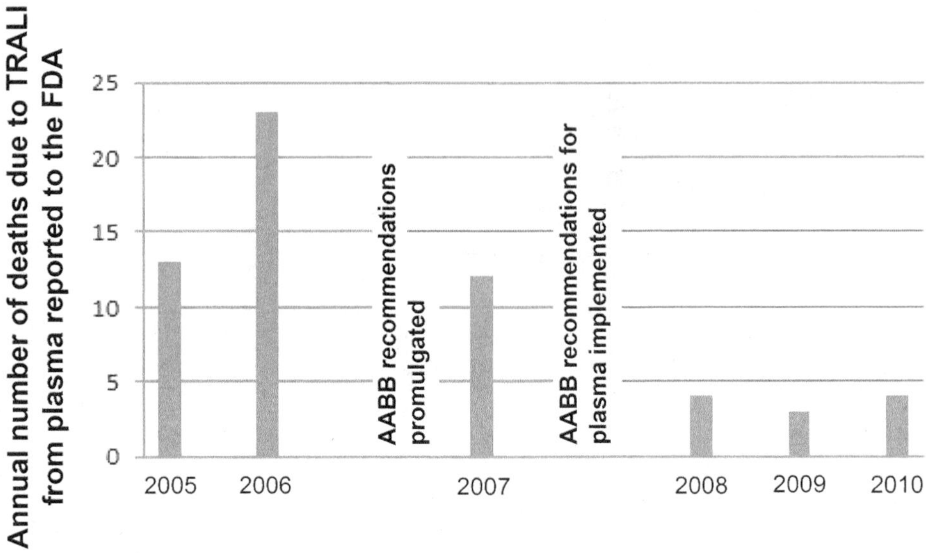

Figure 2-4. Comparison of the number of deaths from transfusion-related acute lung injury (TRALI) associated with the transfusion of plasma from 2005 through 2007 and from 2008 through 2010. For each year, the number of deaths reported to be due to TRALI is based on reports of transfusion-related fatalities made to the United States Food and Drug Administration (FDA).

increasing awareness in 2005-2006 of the risk of TRALI specifically associated with plasma transfusion, followed by a reduction in the number of TRALI deaths in 2007-2010, when female plasma was replaced by male plasma. Increasing awareness in 2005-2006 of the risk of TRALI specifically related to transfusion of plasma is likely—associated with the publicity generated from the United Kingdom, which converted to the use of male-only plasma in 2003-2004, and from the UK studies of TRALI that had considered patients who had received only plasma as the "at-risk" patient population.[44]

A reduction in the number of deaths from TRALI had already been observed in the United Kingdom, where the gradual move to male-only plasma had not been accompanied by a replacement of existing plasma inventories (or a mandating of 100% compliance with the policy that plasma for transfusion be collected solely from male donors). Awareness of the risk of TRALI in the United Kingdom may thus have preceded that in the United States by approximately 3 years, as did the policy to convert to male-only plasma. After the conversion, the annual number of deaths from TRALI reported to the SHOT system declined until, in 2008, for the first time since reporting to the SHOT system started in 1996, no death from TRALI was recorded in the United Kingdom.[16] Three nonfatal cases of TRALI were reported in 2008, all of which were due to transfusion of plasma from female donors in England (where the use of male donors for plasma is not yet universal).[16] By comparison, seven of the 12 transfusion-related deaths reported to the SHOT system in 2003 had been due to TRALI.[16]

Comparisons of the figures obtained from the different hemovigilance systems are difficult because 1) the definitions of transfusion complications vary between systems (and sometimes also between reporting facilities from the same system); 2) the denominators necessary for the estimation of the risk of a transfusion-related death are often unavailable or inconsistent between systems; and 3) the criteria used to definitely, probably, or possibly attribute a death to ABT also vary. Moreover, all hemovigilance systems are especially ineffective at capturing deaths due to TTIs. Transfusion-transmitted diseases must be reported, but such systems are designed to identify acute adverse outcomes of ABT, and they do not capture deaths from chronic infections acquired through an ABT received years before it resulted in the death of the transfusion recipient.

The recording by the SHOT system of deaths from transfusion-acquired variant Creutzfeldt-Jakob disease (vCJD) is due to the active surveillance efforts made in the United Kingdom to identify cases of transmission of vCJD through ABT. Thus, passive surveillance systems are likely to miss even some acute infections transmitted through ABT, as has been shown for TAS,[45] and as was likely the case with some West Nile virus (WNV) infections occurring in New York in the summer of 1999 (when no transfusion-transmitted cases were reported) and with some dengue fever virus (DFV) infections occurring in endemic areas over many decades. The effectiveness of the current surveillance systems thus may be low, particularly at the point of recognition of events by physicians and their subsequent reporting to transfusion services.[46] Clinicians seeing a patient with DFV infection during outbreaks are unlikely to consider ABT as a possible source of that patient's infection and to obtain the critical history of recent transfusions. As a result, the transmission of DFV through ABT had gone undetected until recently.[47,48]

Other than TAS, since 2005, the only TTI detected in the United States through the passive reporting to the FDA as causing deaths from transfusion has been babesiosis (Fig 2-1). After 7 years with no reported deaths due to transfusion-transmitted babesiosis, the FDA received reports of 11 deaths from ABT secondary to transfusion-transmitted babesiosis from 2006 through 2010.[49-51] Thus, 11 (3.6%) of 307 of transfusion-related deaths reported to the FDA from 2005 through 2010 have been due to a TTI (other than TAS; Fig 2-1).[9] When TTIs and TAS are considered together, 35 (11.4%) of 307 of transfusion-related deaths from 2005 through 2010 have been due to microbial infection.[9] When the data from the French hemovigilance system,[15] the UK SHOT system,[16,17] and the US FDA[9] are considered together, transfusion-related deaths from infectious diseases represent less than 15% of all transfusion-related mortality.[5]

Transfusion-Associated Sepsis

Bacterial contamination of blood components results most frequently from the introduction of low concentrations of skin bacteria at the time of phlebotomy, less commonly from asymptomatic donor bacteremia, and rarely during blood processing.[39] Transfusion of a bacterially contaminated blood component may result in absence of clinical symptoms (asymptomatic bacteremia), an immediate septic transfusion reaction, a delayed posttransfusion infection, or a death due to TAS. Before various process improvements started to be introduced around 2004, platelets and RBCs were responsible, respectively, for 70% and 30% of fatalities from TAS.[39] The reasons for this outcome are that platelets are stored at room temperature, which allows for bacteria proliferation, and because platelets are more often given to patients who are susceptible to bacterial infection—that is, to neutropenic subjects who also often have an impaired immune system. Accordingly, most efforts to reduce the risk of TAS have hitherto specifically targeted platelet components.[19]

The etiology of TAS has been known for years,[52] and measures to prevent TAS had been advocated[53] more than a decade before they were adopted by the AABB.[19] Before the introduction of bacteria detection for apheresis (single-donor) platelets in the United States in March 2004, TAS ranked third among the causes of transfusion-associated fatalities reported to the FDA. Since then, the number of reported TAS deaths has been reduced by more than half (Fig 2-3), and TAS no longer ranks third among the causes of transfusion-associated fatalities (Fig 2-1). Before 2004, estimates of the incidence of TAS varied widely, from approximately 1 per 3000 platelet transfusions[18,33] to 1 per 100,000.[54,55] Actual bacterial contamination rates of platelet components were substantially higher.

The data compiled by McDonald and Blajchman[39] from seven studies of apheresis (single-donor) platelets and 12 studies of pooled WBD platelets showed contamination rates of 0.09% (31/35,122) and 0.43% (376/87,922), respectively. This nearly fivefold difference was presumably due to the number of venipunctures (1 or 4-6) involved in the collection of apheresis (single-donor) or pooled WBD platelets. In five reviewed studies, the RBC contamination rate was 0.1% (60/61,136),[39] probably because the 4 C storage temperature of RBCs inhibits bacterial growth during storage. Given that skin bacteria are the major source of contamination, the difference between measured contamination rates in stored components and septic reactions in transfused patients likely can be explained by low-level contamination that does not evoke a clinical response, concomitant antibiotic therapy that blunts a clinical response, and/or failure to (correctly) attribute sepsis to the platelet transfusion in patients with neutropenia or fever.

Of the organisms that caused 16 fatalities due to contaminated platelet transfusions in the United States,[55] France,[54] and the United Kingdom,[17] 37% (six cases) were gram-positive and 63% (10) were gram-negative.[39] Of the organisms that caused all 72 episodes of TAS,[17,54,55] however, 68% were gram-positive and 32% were gram-negative. The most frequently implicated organisms were *Staphylococcus epidermidis, Escherichia coli, Staphylococcus aureus,* and *Bacillus cereus.*[39] Of the organisms that caused seven fatalities due to contaminated RBC transfusions,[17,54,55] six were gram-negative and one was gram-positive.[39] Three fatalities from contaminated RBC transfusions were also reported to the US FDA in 2005-2006, but no deaths secondary to RBC TAS have been reported since 2007.[9] At the 22 C storage temperature of platelets, a wide range of bacteria are capable of proliferation to levels of 10^6 to 10^{11} CFU/mL,[56,57] and, with growth to these levels, contaminated blood-component units can lead to significant morbidity and mortality.

In the SHOT reports,[16] of the cases in which the age of the platelet component was known, 75% of episodes of TAS occurred when the product was 4 to 5 days old. The allowed period of platelet storage was thus reduced to 3 days in Japan and 4 days in Germany. Reducing the allowable storage time to 3 days in the United States would prevent such TAS episodes but would likely result in supply problems. Moreover, 50% of the SHOT fatalities were due to platelet components 2 to 3 days old. Reducing the storage time to 3 days would not prevent fatal cases such as these. In some European centers, the introduction of bacteria detection for platelets using automated culture systems enabled the storage time to be extended to 7 days. The FDA had allowed the storage time of platelets to be extended to 7 days in 1983, but it soon returned the shelf life limit to 5 days, because of a reported increased incidence of fatal TAS episodes.[58] Recently, experimental protocols considering extension of the storage time of platelets to 7 days (after the introduction of automated bacterial-culture systems) were halted in the United States, because of an increased incidence of TAS.[59]

The same relationship between prolonged storage and increased risk of TAS has been reported for RBCs contaminated with *Yersinia enterocolitica. Yersinia* grows well at 4 C, uses the citrate of the preservative solution as a source of energy, and—owing to its lack of siderophores—requires iron for optimal growth. It can also cause asymptomatic infection in donors, while it can produce endotoxin. For all these reasons, *Yersinia* has been responsible for some 70% of fatalities secondary to TAS from RBC transfusion. Stored RBCs thus provide an ideal growth medium for this microorganism. In almost all serious reactions to RBCs containing *Y. enterocolitica,* the RBCs had been stored for >3 weeks.[60]

Interventions Introduced Around 2004 to Mitigate the Risk of Platelet TAS

By 2004, improved donor selection (intended to exclude prospective donors with bacteremia), improved donor-arm disinfection, diversion of the initial flow of donor blood (presumed to contain most skin contaminants) from the collection bag into a pouch, overnight hold of the collected whole blood, and/or WBC reduction had reduced, but not eliminated, the risk of bacterial contamination of blood components.[39] In 2004, the AABB required measures to limit and detect bacterial contamination in all platelet components. At that time, suitable automated bacterial-culture systems were available only for apheresis platelets in the United States, but they have since become available for use with pooled WBD platelets as well.

More specifically, in 2004, the BacT/Alert bacterial-culture technology (bioMerieux, Hazelwood, MO) was available for use on apheresis platelets. Later, the eBDS culture technology (Pall Corporation, Short Hills, NY) became available for use on WBD platelets. Both technologies could be used only as quality-control assays—that is, neither technology was approved by the FDA as a release test (for labeling a component as having tested negative for bacteria). Their status remains the same today. BacT/Alert relies on the generation of carbon dioxide by bacteria, and thus it can detect both aerobic and anaerobic bacteria. The eBDS technology relies on oxygen consumption by bacteria, and thus it can detect only aerobic bacteria.

Although both systems had excellent analytical sensitivity, their *clinical* sensitivity was only about 50%,[61-63] due to the exceedingly low starting concentration of bacteria in each collected platelet component. The starting number of bacteria was so low that it was possible for the small sample (<10 mL) of platelet product submitted for culture to contain no bacteria at all, even if there were enough bacteria in the rest of the unit to proliferate during storage and produce TAS in the recipient. Moreover, a sample was taken for culture at about 24 (ie, 18-36) hours, before the logarithmic phase of bacteria growth had started in the platelet component.

The impact of these two factors (the volume of product submitted for culture and the interval between collection of the unit and collection of the sample for culture) on the predicted culture results was explored in a mathematical model.[62] The model assumed that 1) 4-8 mL of product was submitted for culture, and 2) a sample was taken for culture at 24 hours. On the basis of these assumptions, the model predicted false-negative culture rates ranging between 11% and 74%. BacT/Alert had been validated as a quality-control measure to detect 1 to 10 CFU/mL. Platelet components producing false-negative results in the model of Benjamin and Wagner[62] had undetectable bacteria concentrations (ranging from <0.02 CFU/mL to 0.15 CFU/mL).

An inoculation experiment[63] produced results consistent with this predicted clinical sensitivity of about 50%.[62] Apheresis platelet components were contaminated shortly after collection with 1-10, 10-100, or 100-1000 CFU /component of seven different species of bacteria. Because the volume of these apheresis platelets was fixed at 285 mL, the initial concentration of bacteria ranged between 0.003 CFU /mL and 3 CFU / mL. At low contamination levels (1-10 CFU / component), 86% of cultures produced false-negative results 24 hours later. At intermediate contamination levels (10-100 CFU /component), 57% of cultures produced false-negative results with samples taken 24 hours after the collection of each unit.[63]

From 2004 through 2006, the American Red Cross (ARC) performed bacterial-culture testing on 1 million apheresis (single-donor) platelet donations.[64] Of these, 186 (1 in 5400) had confirmed-positive culture results, and transfusion of all but 1 of the associated 293 components was prevented. During this period, however, 20 episodes of TAS secondary to (screened) apheresis (single-donor) platelets were reported, including three fatalities (1 per 498,711 distributed components). Most TAS episodes were associated with components stored for 5 days.[64] Comparison of the risk of TAS and TAS-related death due to apheresis (single-donor) platelets before and after implementation of bacterial-culture testing of apheresis (single-donor) platelets indicated approximately 50% decreases in reported events (1 per 75,000 vs 1 per 40,000) and fatalities (1 per 500,000 vs 1 per 240,000 components).

The clinical implications of this declining trend ($p = 0.11$) were unclear. It could reflect poor sensitivity of the automated bacterial-culture testing systems,[61-63] increased recognition and reporting of TAS over time, or both. Most likely, it meant that the risk of TAS before March 2004 was greater than was generally appreciated at that time and also that a significant risk remains, despite the implementation of bacterial-culture testing systems. Septic reactions and TAS fatalities after the introduction of bacterial-culture testing have also been reported from other blood systems and with both available culture systems.[65-68] In Canada, two TAS episodes and one fatality occurred among recipients of 82,004 cultured apheresis (single-donor) platelet units.[66]

After reporting the 2004 to 2006 results for apheresis (single-donor) platelets,[64] the ARC in 2007-2008 conducted a follow-up study[69] of the impact of the optimization of the collection conditions and the doubling (from 4 mL to 8 mL) of the volume of the sample submitted for culture. The reported rate of events (1 per 87,000) did not differ significantly from that in the previous period (1 per 75,000). It is interesting that, during this latter period, culture-negative apheresis (single-donor) components were passively reported to the ARC as having caused TAS in the recipient in 1 per 87,000 platelet transfusions. Another estimate of the magnitude of the risk was reported from the Johns Hopkins Hospital, which maintains active surveillance for TAS. One per 50,000 culture-negative apheresis (single-donor) platelet components caused TAS between March 1, 2004 and August 31, 2007.[70] However, only one episode of TAS occurred in this study, which predated the process improvements implemented by the ARC[69] in 2007-2008.

Recent Studies

The studies that compared the frequency of bacterial contamination between pooled WBD and apheresis (single-donor) platelets in settings that had implemented bacterial-culture testing of both components simultaneously were subjected to a meta-analysis.[71] Across three studies conducted in the United States,[72-74] pools of five WBD platelet concentrates had a frequency of bacterial contamination 5.6 times higher than that of apheresis (single-donor) platelets [summary odds ratio (OR) = 5.58; 95% confidence interval (CI) = 2.60-11.98; $p<0.05$; Fig 2-5]. In contrast, across four studies conducted in Europe,[61,67,75,76] there was no difference in the risk of bacterial contamination between pooled WBD and apheresis (single-donor) platelets (summary OR = 0.99; 95% CI = 0.63-1.57; $p>0.05$). The two subsets of studies were highly homogeneous statistically ($p>0.90$ for the Q test statistic), despite the fact that the processes of component collection and preparation, as well as the culture conditions, sampling volumes, use of anaerobic bottles, and the criteria for determining true-positive results differed across the studies.

Whether the difference between the findings of the two analyses was due to the different methods of platelet preparation [platelet-rich-plasma (PRP) platelets in the United States and buffy-coat platelets in Europe] or to factors associated with the method of platelet preparation (eg, overnight hold of the collected whole blood in Europe) could not be determined by the meta-analysis, because the method of platelet preparation overlapped with all of the other sources of heterogeneity.[71] A theoretical justification for a lower bacterial risk associated with buffy-coat platelets has been advanced.[77] A synthesis of all seven studies[61,67,72-76] could not be undertaken, owing to significant statistical ($p<0.005$ for the Q test statistic) and medical heterogeneity.[71] The result of the meta-analysis concerning the difference in risk between pooled WBD and apheresis (single-donor) platelets in the United States was what would logically have been expected from the difference in the number of venipunctures performed.[32,33]

Figure 2-6 shows the risk of bacterial contamination of platelets (either WBD or apheresis) in studies conducted after process improvements and bacteria culture had been implemented around 2004. Despite the implementation of various process improvements in the depicted studies, initial cultures showed an average bacterial contamination rate of approximately 1 per 1500.[59,61,69,76,78] This high rate was found because, compared with the studies previ-

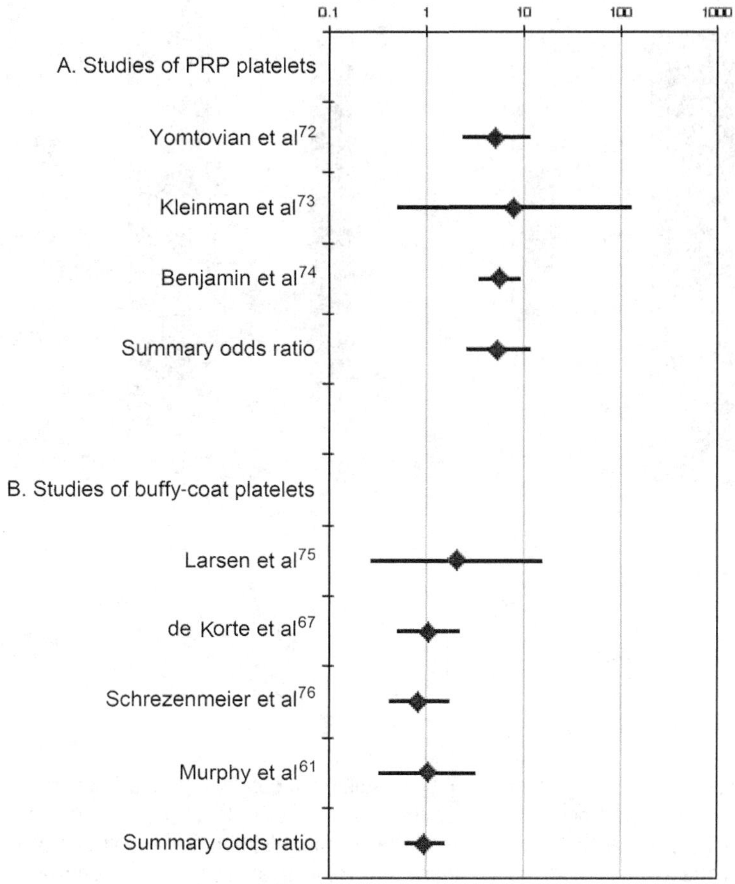

Figure 2-5. True bacterial contamination of whole-blood-derived platelets compared with apheresis (single-donor) platelets cultured simultaneously under the same conditions.[71] Whole-blood-derived platelets were manufactured by the platelet-rich plasma (PRP) method in the United States (Part A) or by the buffy-coat method in Europe (Part B). The figure shows the results of the studies available as of the end of 2008,[71] as well as the summary odds ratio (OR) of bacterial contamination in pooled whole-blood-derived [compared with apheresis (single-donor)] platelets calculated separately across studies manufacturing PRP or buffy-coat pools. An OR of >1 indicates a higher risk of true bacterial contamination in whole-blood-derived platelets than in apheresis (single-donor) platelets, provided that the difference is statistically significant (ie, provided that the corresponding 95% CI [confidence interval] does not contain the null value of 1).[71]

ously reviewed by McDonald and Blajchman,[39] these more-recent studies used larger volumes of product cultured, took a sample for culture later after collection of the unit, and used an anaerobic (in addition to aerobic) bottle, thus doubling the volume of product submitted for culture. More important, despite the fact that these components were negative for bacteria on initial culture, surveillance cultures (taken on outdated components)[59,61,78,79] showed bacterial contamination rates averaging approximately 1 per 1000. Thus, for platelet components transfused after 5 days of storage, the risk of a septic transfusion reaction could, in theory, be as high

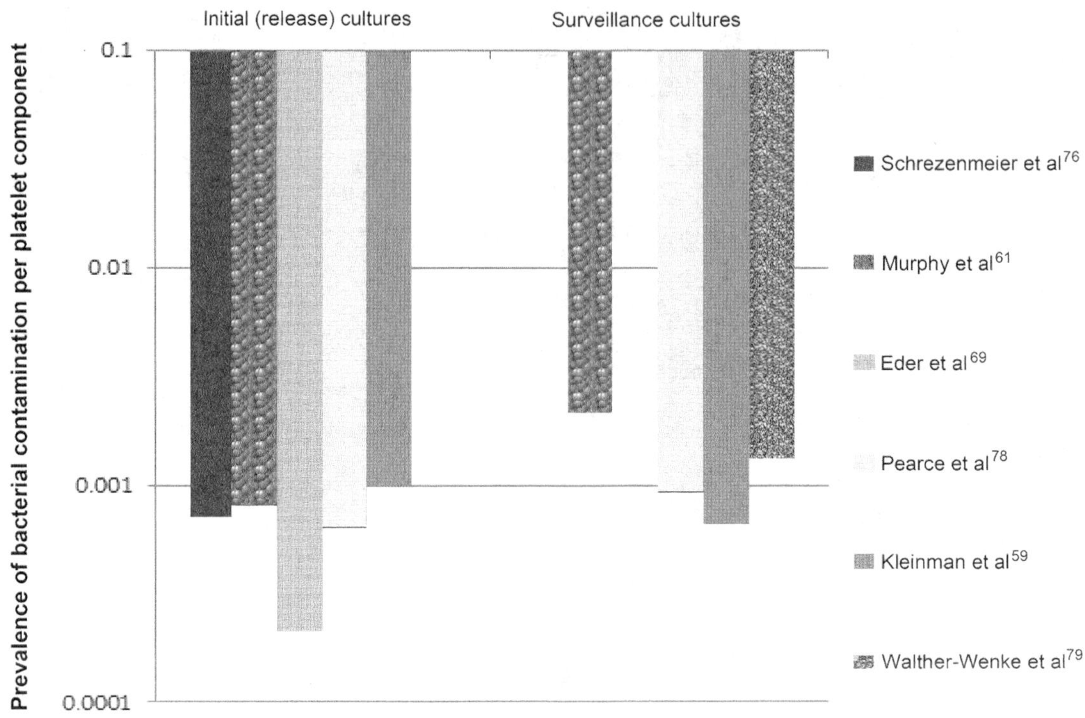

Figure 2-6. Prevalence of bacterial contamination per platelet component reported from studies conducted after the implementation of various process improvements, as well as bacterial culture, around 2004. If available, results are shown both for initial cultures (on samples taken about 24 hours after collection) and for surveillance cultures (on samples taken from outdated components) from the studies of Schrezenmeier et al,[76] Murphy et al,[61] Eder et al,[69] Pearce et al,[78] Kleinman et al,[59] and Walter-Wenke et al.[79]

as 1 per 1000 platelet transfusions if every transfusion of a contaminated unit manifested itself clinically as an immediate or delayed septic reaction in the recipient.

With the surveillance cultures positive at 1 per 1000 platelet components, a second test for bacteria detection (at time of issue) might appear to be warranted. A qualitative immunoassay for the detection of bacteria membrane constituents (PanGenera Detection, Verax, Worcester, MA) has in fact been licensed as an adjunct quality-control test for WBC-reduced apheresis platelets that have already tested negative for bacteria by a different method. The test is not licensed for platelet pools. Moreover, the test has been licensed only as an adjunct test, because it has a low analytical sensitivity for bacteria, and it can detect contamination levels of 10^3 to 10^5 CFU/mL only. In the ordinary case of bacteria contaminating a unit during phlebotomy, such levels of contamination are reached only after the logarithmic phase of bacterial growth has occurred during storage. Therefore, the immunoassay can be of clinical value only at the time of issue of a component.

The results on the performance of this (time-of-issue) second bacteria detection test on plateletpheresis units[80] parallel the figures from the surveillance cultures shown in Fig 2-6. Nine of 27,620 (1 per 3069) apheresis platelets that had tested negative for bacteria on initial culture were found to be contaminated with the second bacteria detection test at time of issue.[80] Two contaminated units that tested negative on the second bacteria detection test were also identified by bacterial culture among 10,424 units administered at participating hospitals where concurrent cultures were being performed. One further contaminated unit missed by the second test was identified through an investigation of a transfusion reaction. Thus, the second bacteria detection test identified nine of the 12 (75%) contaminated units found in this study. Furthermore, 12 of 27,620 (1 per 2302) plateletpheresis units were known to be contaminated with bacteria, while the true prevalence of bacterial contamination at time of issue was most likely higher than 1 per 2302 units (since concurrent cultures were performed on only 10,424 of the 27,620 units subjected to the second bacteria detection test). If five (rather than two) additional contaminated units testing negative on the second bacteria detection test had been uncovered through concurrent cultures performed on all 27,620 (rather than 10,424) units, the prevalence of bacterial contamination in apheresis platelets issued for transfusion in the US today would be 1 contaminated unit per 1841 transfused units (compare with the surveillance-culture figures shown in Fig 2-6).

Seven of the 9 units detected by the second bacteria detection test had high bacterial titers based on quantitative culture and/or positive Gram's stain results, making it likely that transfusion of these plateletpheresis units could have resulted in a transfusion reaction. Four of the 7 units with high bacterial titers were 3 days old and two were 4 days old. The unit that resulted in a transfusion reaction in this study (despite the use of the second bacterial test at time of issue) was contaminated with *Streptococcus oralis* (a viridans group *Streptococcus*) at the level of 2×10^7 CFU/mL. Thus, eight contaminated units among 27,620 transfused plateletpheresis units (1 per 3453) could be expected to result in a transfusion reaction.

Jacobs et al[80] commented on the difference between active and passive surveillance in detecting contaminated plateletpheresis units. Active surveillance by means of the use of a second (point-of-issue) bacteria detection test identified nine contaminated units among just 27,620 units released by blood centers as (initial) culture-negative. In comparison, the far larger ARC study[69] of 781,936 (initial) culture-negative plateletpheresis units had detected nine contaminated units through passive surveillance. Active surveillance (by means of a second bacteria detection test[80]) would appear to detect 28 contaminated units for every contaminated unit identified through passive surveillance.[69] Even if only a fraction of the contaminated units results in TAS, the results of Jacobs et al[80] suggest that there must be hundreds of cases of transfusion reactions indicative of TAS per year in the US that can be associated with several transfusion-related fatalities each year.

TRALI

Efforts to reduce the risk of TRALI (implemented in the United Kingdom since the fall of 2003 and in the United States since the fall of 2006) have specifically targeted plasma and apheresis (single-donor) platelets.[20] The reason for this focus is that, depending on how TRALI is defined,[38] WBC alloantibodies are identified in 25% to 90% of the donors implicated in TRALI cases.[81] Furthermore, such WBC-alloantibody-mediated cases represent the large majority of fatal cases according to data from the SHOT system,[16,17,82] ARC,[83] and German hemovigilance,[84] as well as the largest case series from the pre-2004 literature.[85] Such donor antibodies are believed to attack the recipient's WBCs in the microcirculation of the lungs, causing noncardiogenic pulmonary edema.[86,87] Most donors implicated in TRALI in the pre-2004 literature had been multiparous women alloimmunized to paternal WBC alloantigens during pregnancy.[88] Blood products containing a large volume of plasma from an individual donor thus could contain a large amount of a WBC antibody directed against a cognate WBC antigen of a particular transfusion recipient. As a result, if transfused into a recipient carrying the corresponding WBC alloantigen, such products could be more likely to cause TRALI than would products containing a small volume of plasma.[87] This possibility led to the recommendation that plasma and apheresis (single-donor) platelets be collected solely from male donors or from female donors without a history of pregnancy or shown not to have WBC antibodies.[20]

TRALI has emerged as the leading cause of transfusion-related mortality in the United States (Figs 2-1 and 2-2).[9] TRALI is a new ALI occurring within 6 hours after a transfusion in patients without risk factors for ALI other than transfusion.[28,38,89] Thus, the CCC definition of TRALI[28] was based on the American-European Consensus conference definition of ALI[35] and a temporal relationship to the transfusion. The definition of ALI requires that the possibility of circulatory overload (ie, left atrial hypertension) be excluded. Once circulatory overload has been excluded, however, the consensus definition of TRALI[28] allows for a diagnosis of "possible" TRALI in patients who have other risk factors for ALI that are temporally related to the transfusion.[28] These factors include sepsis, aspiration, pneumonia, toxic inhalation, lung contusion, near drowning, multiple trauma, burn injury, acute pancreatitis, cardiopulmonary bypass, and drug overdose.

TRALI has a clinical presentation mirroring ARDS[35-37] following ABT.[28,38,89] In contrast to patients with ARDS, however, patients with TRALI typically recover with resolution of their pulmonary infiltrates within 96 hours, and the case-fatality rate was only 5% to 10% in the intial reports.[86] To avoid 1) spurious associations between TRALI and transfusions of blood components collected from female donors or donors with circulating WBC antibodies, or 2) a diagnostic suspicion bias for TRALI when WBC antibody tests on female donors show WBC antibodies in the plasma of a donor(s) of a component(s) given to a patient with ALI in the presence of other risk factors for ALI, the diagnosis of TRALI is to be made solely on the basis of the clinical presentation, regardless of any subsequent laboratory tests and their results.[28]

Before the CCC criteria for diagnosing TRALI[28] were introduced, many US blood transfusion services did not perform TRALI work-ups on all donors of blood components transfused proximately to an episode of ARDS, but rather selected for a TRALI work-up the female donors of the plasma-rich [ie, plasma and apheresis (single-donor) platelet] components. They did so because the initial reports of TRALI had associated TRALI with female donors of plasma-rich components[86] and had recommended avoidance of these donors.[87] Furthermore, in the pre-2004 literature, work-ups for TRALI were usually limited to the detection of WBC alloantibodies in a donor, as opposed to including the demonstration of a positive WBC crossmatch between donor and recipient or the demonstration of a donor WBC alloantibody specifically directed to a recipient antigen. The result of such observation (ie, diagnostic suspicion) bias was a consistent association of female gender, plasma-rich components, and donor WBC alloantibodies with TRALI.[5]

This association likely was partly real, but—to a large extent—it was doubtless spurious. TRALI usually develops in patients who have received many units of various blood components (RBCs, plasma, and/or platelets).[27] For example, in the Dutch hemovigilance study,[90] patients who met the CCC criteria for TRALI had each received on average 5.3 units of blood components (Fig 2-7). If such multitransfused patients develop ARDS, some of the implicated donors are bound to be women who previously were pregnant. Because 24.4%[88] to 33%[91] of women with a history of pregnancy have HLA antibodies,[88] and 3% have neutrophil antibodies,[91] some of the implicated donors likely will be women with circulating WBC antibodies. Moreover, some of these implicated female donors with circulating WBC antibodies likely will have donated plasma-rich [ie, plasma and apheresis (single-donor) platelet] components that are administered to these multitransfused patients. If TRALI work-ups are selectively performed on the female donors of plasma-rich components, an association of female gender, plasma-rich components, and donor WBC alloantibodies with TRALI will be detected, even if no such association exists.[5] Furthermore, even when donors are not selected for TRALI work-ups on the basis of their gender or the blood component that they have donated, TRALI work-ups identifying a

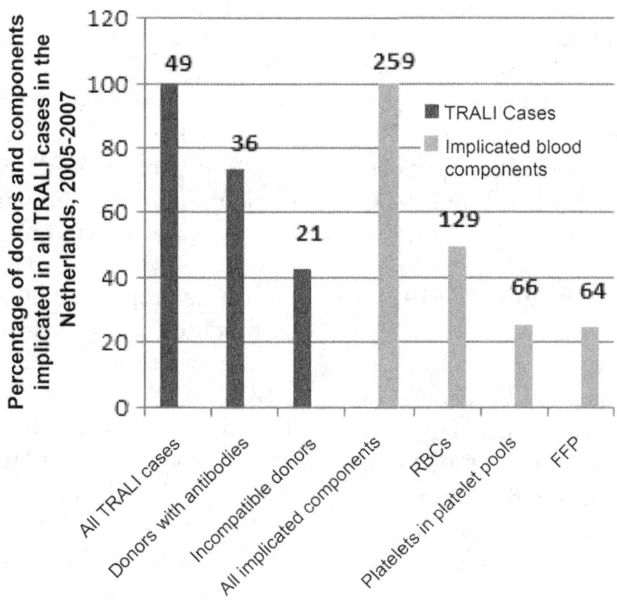

Figure 2-7. TRALI in the Netherlands before the introduction of the use of "male-only" plasma. Proportion of donors with white cell (WBC) alloantibodies and donors with WBC alloantibodies specifically directed to a recipient antigen(s) are shown by dark bars. Red cell (RBC), platelet, and fresh frozen plasma (FFP) components implicated in 49 cases meeting the Canadian consensus criteria[28] for transfusion-related acute lung injury (TRALI) or "possible" TRALI are shown by the light bars.[90] Initially published by Vamvakas in Clin Lab 2010;56:263-79.[90]

blood component with WBC alloantibodies will overestimate the association of WBC alloantibodies with TRALI, simply because transfusion recipients developing TRALI have received more than one blood component.[92]

The true incidence of TRALI is thus unknown, because a standardized definition[28,38] was not available until relatively recently. Early reports quoted an incidence of 1 per 5000 transfused blood components,[86] and subsequent reports have ranged from 1 per 432 platelet pools[26] to 1 per 557,000 RBCs.[17] TRALI has been reported with the use of all types of blood components. Most blood components implicated in published case-reports and small case-series have contained more than 50 mL of plasma, and plasma units had been the most frequently implicated component.[83,85,86] However, TRALI also occurs with WBD platelets[93-97] and with components containing as little as 10 mL of plasma.[98] It is important that not all of the pre-2004 literature indicated that plasma units or components containing large volumes of plasma are the principal culprits.[18,26]

TRALI can be due to WBC antibodies, soluble biologic response mediators accumulating during the storage of cellular blood components, or other, still unidentified agents contained in transfused blood components.[38] WBC antibodies in transfused plasma can be directed against the recipient's WBC antigens and can interact with antigens on the patient's WBCs in the microcirculation of the lungs.[86] Neutrophil-specific antibodies, especially antibody to the human neutrophil antigen-3a (HNA-3a),[99] appear to be important in European studies,[100-102] but perhaps not in US studies.[103] Nonetheless, as discussed in the next section, the presence of a WBC antibody in a donor does not predict the occurrence of TRALI in the recipient. The vast majority of

WBC antibody infusions do not cause TRALI, which makes it possible that alloantibodies—although they are present in the majority of TRALI cases—could be a surrogate for another etiologic factor. The clinical evidence that relates TRALI to WBC antibodies can indeed be explained by the spurious associations discussed above, and the link between TRALI and WBC antibodies remains circumstantial.[104]

Risk of TRALI from Transfusion of WBC Antibodies

Eight studies[105-112] of the transfusion outcomes of recipients of blood components containing HLA antibodies have been published. Four of those studies[105-108] reported on HLA-antibody-positive donors who had previously been implicated in causing TRALI in a recipient. Three of the studies[109-111] reported on donors who were positive for HLA antibodies but had not been implicated in causing TRALI. The remaining study[112] did not detect TRALI in any of 265 recipients of either HLA-antibody-positive or HLA-antibody-negative apheresis (single-donor) platelets. All eight studies[105-112] were consistent in reporting a very low risk of TRALI in recipients of blood components containing HLA antibodies. Studies of donors who were positive for HLA antibodies but had not previously been implicated in causing TRALI[109-111] reported TRALI in one of 211,[109] zero of 167,[110] and seven of 1195[111] recipients of components containing HLA antibodies. Studies of donors positive for HLA antibodies who had been previously implicated in TRALI[105-108] reported five new cases of TRALI in 171 (2.9%) recipients of components from such donors.

Possible reasons for the low risk of TRALI secondary to transfusion of blood components containing HLA alloantibodies (if indeed HLA alloantibodies have a role in the pathogenesis of TRALI) include 1) the absence from the recipient of the cognate HLA antigen to which the donor alloantibody is directed; 2) undefined characteristics of the transfused donor HLA alloantibody and corresponding cognate antigen (eg, titer of the antibody or density of the antigen on the WBC surface); and 3) the absence of an underlying risk factor predisposing the recipient to developing TRALI. Prevailing opinion on the pathogenesis of TRALI maintains that "two hits" are usually necessary for TRALI to occur. The first possible hit is a recipient condition that results in neutrophil priming, and the second is the infusion of a biologic-response modifier that activates primed neutrophils.[29,31,113] The biologic-response modifier can be an HLA antibody, a human neutrophil antibody, or several nonantibody substances, such as bioactive lipids.

The Leukocyte Antibody Prevalence Study (LAPS) II[111] reported on the occurrence of TRALI in the recipients of 1196 plasma-rich components containing HLA antibodies and the recipients of 1233 plasma-rich components not containing HLA antibodies. The study was limited to recipients of plasma-rich components [ie, apheresis (single-donor) platelets and plasma]. TRALI was diagnosed retrospectively on the basis of a review of the medical records by expert reviewers. In accordance with the CCC criteria,[28] TRALI was diagnosed based on clinical (rather than laboratory) data. Nine patients met the diagnostic criteria of TRALI; seven had received components containing HLA antibodies, and two had received components not containing HLA antibodies. Eight of the nine patients with TRALI required mechanical ventilation; in four cases, the diagnosis was made clinically at the time of the transfusion. Of the seven cases developing in recipients of components containing HLA antibodies, two had occurred in patients in whom the recipient had a cognate HLA antigen to which the donor alloantibody was directed. For the remaining five cases, the recipient's HLA type was not available.

Only one of 171 (9/1195) recipients of a plasma-rich component containing HLA antibodies developed TRALI.[111] Moreover, one of 616 (2/1233) recipients of a plasma-rich component not containing HLA antibodies developed TRALI (Fig 2-8). The difference between these groups did not attain significance ($p = 0.10$)—despite the study's large sample—but there was a trend toward a greater risk of TRALI in recipients of HLA-antibody-positive components.

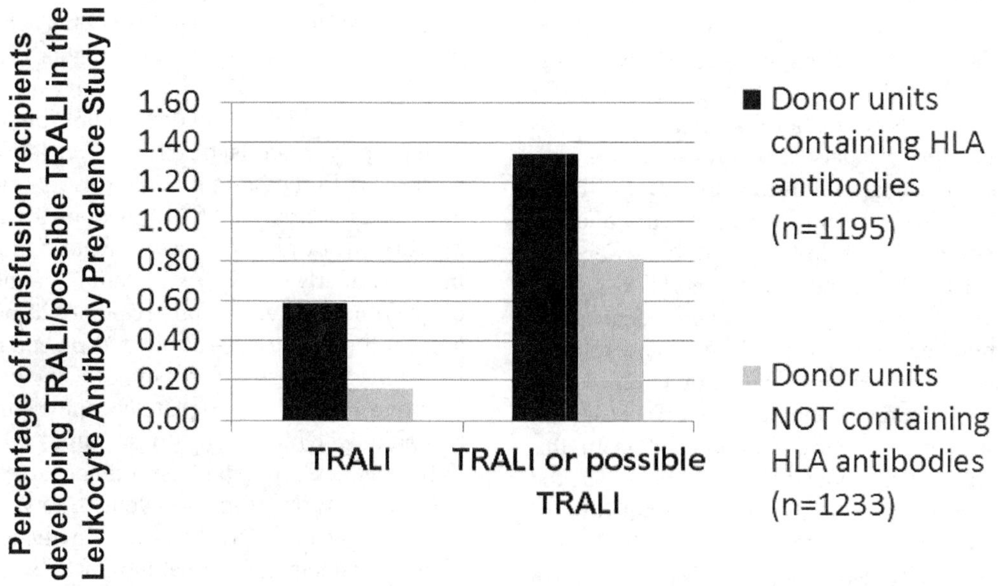

Figure 2-8. Prevalence of transfusion-related acute lung injury (TRALI) and possible TRALI in recipients of plasma-rich components (ie, plasma and apheresis platelets) containing or not containing HLA antibodies.[111] There is a trend toward a a greater risk of TRALI in association with the receipt of plasma-rich components containing HLA antibodies than with receipt of such components not containing HLA antibodies. This risk is lessened by the inclusion of the "possible" TRALI cases in the analysis (see text).

Kleinman et al acknowledged the possibility that the difference might have been due to chance, but they favored the possibility that a larger sample could have established a statistically significant difference in TRALI risk between recipients of components from HLA-antibody-positive and HLA-antibody-negative donors.[111]

Sixteen of 1196 recipients of a plasma-rich component containing HLA antibodies developed TRALI or possible TRALI, compared with 10 of 1233 recipients of a plasma-rich component not containing HLA antibodies (Fig 2-8; $p = 0.24$). When possible, TRALI was considered alone; however, no trend toward a greater risk of possible TRALI in association with receipt of HLA-antibody-positive components was evident (9/1195 compared with 8/1233; $p = 0.81$). The category of possible TRALI was included in the CCC criteria to permit consideration of a diagnosis of TRALI in the presence of an alternative risk factor for ALI.[28] The results of the LAPS II study suggest that such "possible" TRALI may be more likely due to the alternative risk factor for ALI than to a transfusion received proximately to the development of ARDS; or, alternatively, that the development of such possible TRALI does not depend on the infusion of HLA antibodies but is mediated by other mechanisms.

Risk of TRALI from Platelet Transfusion

Forty-five percent of the plasma-rich components transfused in LAPS II[111] were apheresis (single-donor) platelets, yet only one of the nine detected cases of TRALI was diagnosed in a recipient of apheresis (single-donor) platelets. Because plasma and apheresis (single-donor) platelets contain equivalent amounts of plasma from a single donor, it had been expected on theoretical grounds that they would be associated with a similar risk of TRALI; thus, avoidance of female donors with a history of pregnancy was recommended for collections of both plasma and apheresis (single-donor) platelets.[20] The LAPS-II[111] study results showed that the receipt of plasma was associated with a risk of TRALI 7.1 times higher than that of apheresis (single-donor) platelets—a difference that almost attained statistical significance ($p = 0.06$). However, the difference disappeared in the analysis of possible TRALI ($p = 0.63$) or when the results for TRALI and possible TRALI were combined ($p = 0.43$). Nonetheless, because the total number of recorded TRALI cases (nine) was small, the authors opted not to draw any inference regarding the association of TRALI with specific transfused components from this marginally significant difference between the recipients of plasma and apheresis (single-donor) platelets in their study.[111]

Apheresis (single-donor) platelets have been compared with PRP WBD platelets (such as the pooled platelets manufactured in the United States) in studies diagnosing TRALI by the CCC criteria[28] and conducted in settings simultaneously transfusing both pooled WBD and apheresis (single-donor) platelets to the same patients under the same conditions.[25,27,83] These comparisons show that the risk of TRALI is the same for both types of platelet components (see Table 4-2 in Chapter 4).[71] Briefly, in the passive surveillance (hemovigilance) studies of Robillard et al[25] and Eder et al,[83] the risk of TRALI was, respectively, 1/40,452 and 1/279,805 transfused platelet pools as compared with 1/46,995 and 1/285,630 transfused apheresis (single-donor) platelets.[71] Gajic et al[27] presented a nested case-control study within an observational study of 901 consecutive ICU patients (74 cases developing TRALI and 74 controls remaining free of TRALI). Cases received 10 apheresis (single-donor) platelets and six platelet pools; controls received three apheresis (single-donor) platelets and three platelet pools. Thus, the TRALI cases received more platelet transfusions than did the controls, but the type of platelet concentrate did not differ between the cases and the controls.[71]

The equal risk of TRALI with apheresis (single-donor) platelets and with platelet pools found in these three studies[25,27,83]—the only studies to meet the eligibility criteria for inclusion in a systematic review[71]—is what would be expected. The reason is that the higher probability of exposure to 50 mL of plasma from each alloimmunized US blood donor contributing to a platelet pool manufactured by the platelet-rich plasma (PRP) method probably carries—on average—as much risk of TRALI as does the receipt of 300 mL of plasma from a single donor who may similarly have circulating antibodies directed to the transfusion recipient's WBC antigens. If there is donor-recipient WBC incompatibility in the case of apheresis (single-donor) (compared with pooled) platelets, the transfusion recipient will receive up to six times as much WBC alloantibody, making the occurrence of TRALI more likely in the event of low antigen density, low antibody titer, etc. In the case of pooled platelets, the probability of WBC incompatibility between one of the four to six donors contributing to the pool and the recipient is up to six times as high as that of incompatibility between the single donor of an apheresis (single-donor) platelet component and the recipient. In the presence of a recipient factor(s) predisposing to TRALI, even the small amount of antibody found in the 50 mL of donor plasma contained in a PRP platelet unit could precipitate TRALI. In fact, there have been published cases of TRALI attributable to plasma amounts as small as ≤20 mL as follows:

- Plasma from a female donor not screened for WBC antibodies and contributing toward a buffy-coat platelet pool suspended in male plasma in the United Kingdom.[98]
- Donor plasma remaining in RBCs manufactured in The Netherlands by the buffy-coat method and stored in additive solution.[90]

Theories of TRALI Pathogenesis

In support of the antibody hypothesis of TRALI pathogenesis, the infusion of WBC antibodies in an ex-vivo animal model precipitated TRALI in the absence of other factors precipitating TRALI.[114] Most donors implicated in TRALI have been multiparous women, and 14 (87.5%) of 16 TRALI cases in one series[85] demonstrated

WBC antigen-antibody correlation. Eder et al[83] reviewed 550 reports of suspected TRALI (including 72 fatalities) submitted to the ARC from 2003 through 2005. Thirty-eight fatalities were categorized as attributable to "probable" TRALI, and 24 (63%) of them had occurred after plasma transfusion. A WBC-antibody-positive female donor was involved in 27 (71%) of all TRALI fatalities and in 18 (75%) of 24 deaths implicating plasma transfusion. Data from the UK SHOT system[82] reported donor WBC antibodies recognizing a cognate WBC antigen in the transfusion recipient in 62 (65%) of 96 completely investigated TRALI cases. Three clinical studies[115-117] have shown an association between female plasma and impaired pulmonary function/hypoxia, albeit not TRALI.

More specifically, a crossover RCT in 105 ICU patients showed impaired pulmonary function occurring more frequently in patients receiving plasma from multiparous women than in controls.[115] Following the conversion to male-only plasma in the United Kingdom, a before-and-after observational study in multitransfused patients undergoing abdominal aortic aneurysm repair showed a lower risk of hypoxia when male-only plasma was exclusively administered.[116] A prospective observational study comparing 55 recipients of male-only plasma with 27 recipients of mixed (ie, both male and female) plasma in Japan[117] observed the development of pulmonary distress meeting the threshold required by the CCC criteria in a research setting[28]—that is, a ratio of PaO_2 to FiO_2 of <300 mmHg—in 19 subjects within 6 hours of the transfusion: five patients with possible TRALI, seven with TACO, and seven with no apparent pulmonary edema. The receipt of male-only plasma was associated with a lower ($p = 0.02$) risk of such pulmonary distress. However, two (3.6%) subjects receiving male-only plasma developed possible TRALI, compared with three (11.1%) patients receiving "mixed" plasma ($p = 0.18$).[117]

As already discussed, Gajic et al[27] presented a prospective cohort study of 901 patients sequentially admitted to the medical ICU and evaluated for TRALI according to the CCC criteria,[28] which capture both suspected TRALI cases (with no identifiable pre-existing risk factor for ALI) and possible TRALI cases (where at least one alternate risk factor for ALI is present). Seventy-four patients developed TRALI. Of these 74, 62% had another risk factor for ALI, a fact that highlights the interaction among transfusion, patient factors, and the development of TRALI. This finding underscores the risk of ARDS (diagnosed as either ALI or TRALI) in critically ill patients with preexisting risk factors for ALI who receive transfusion of even a single unit of blood.[118] Gajic et al[27] compared 74 TRALI cases with 74 controls drawn from among the patients who did not develop worsening respiratory status within 24 hours of the transfusion. As compared with controls, the cases received more units from female donors and from donors with previous pregnancies, as well as more plasma overall and plasma from female donors with more pregnancies. In contrast, the number of RBC transfusions did not differ between the cases and controls. Both WBC antibodies and bioactive lipids accumulating during storage were higher in the components received by the cases than in those received by the controls.

Thus, Gajic et al[27] concluded that, although sepsis was the risk factor most commonly associated with the 74 diagnoses of ALI in this population of critically ill patients, modifiable transfusion factors (ie, donor gender, parity, and WBC alloimmunization) were also associated with TRALI; this conclusion indicated opportunities for prevention. WBC antibodies were not associated with TRALI in the multivariate analysis that included the various patient-related risk factors for ALI, yet the most straightforward opportunity for TRALI prevention would be the exclusion of female donors from making donations of plasma.

WBC antibodies were associated with the development of TRALI in the univariate—albeit not the multivariate—analyses of the hitherto-reported prospective observational studies that have included consecutive transfused patients.[27,117] Those studies therefore suggest that male-only plasma will be advantageous for post-transfusion pulmonary function, although other patient-related factors such as sepsis and fluid balance (as opposed to the receipt of female plasma) are the primary determinants of ALI in multitransfused patients.

In fact, alternatively (or additionally) to WBC antibodies, the two-hit model proposed by Silliman et al[31] may explain the development of TRALI in transfusion recipients with various pre-existing risk factors for ALI. As already discussed (to explain the low risk of TRALI when components containing WBC antibodies are transfused), the initial hit is an insult to the vascular endothelium (due to infection, surgery, trauma, or massive transfusion) that attracts and primes neutrophils that adhere to the endothelium.[29,31,113] A second hit is then mediated by biologic response modifiers contained in transfused plasma [eg, lipid-priming molecules found in the plasma supernatant of stored (as opposed to fresh) RBCs and platelets; cytokines; CD40 ligand; and/or WBC antibodies]. These molecules activate the sequestered neutrophils to release oxidases and proteases that damage the endothelium and produce capillary leak and ALI. A rat model showed that TRALI is the result of two factors, the first being the clinical condition of the patient and the second being the antibodies that prime neutrophils and/or plasma from stored blood.[30] The findings of the completed prospective observational studies[27,117] (which underscored the role of patient-related factors) are also consistent with this two-hit (or bioactive-lipid/neutrophil-priming) hypothesis.

Vlaar et al[119] also recently reported a retrospective cohort study identifying patients meeting the CCC criteria for TRALI from among all patients admitted to the ICU for longer than 48 hours. Patients developing TRALI were matched (on the basis of age, gender, and admission diagnosis) to transfused controls who developed ALI for other reasons. The volume of platelets and plasma transfused was associated with TRALI in the univariate analysis, but the association disappeared in the multivariate analysis. The only risk factors for TRALI that occurred more frequently in the TRALI cases than in the ALI controls were sepsis and a high Acute Physiology and Chronic Health Evaluation (APACHE) II score.[119]

If the diagnostic criteria for TRALI required that all alternative risk factors for ALI be excluded before a diagnosis of TRALI could be made, virtually no cases of TRALI mediated by such a two-hit mechanism would be diagnosed as TRALI. Such an approach to the diagnosis may explain the very high prevalence of WBC antibodies (as well as the female gender of the donors of the implicated blood components) in the pre-2004 literature on TRALI. Accordingly, the CCC criteria[28] permit the diagnosis of "possible" TRALI in patients who have other risk factors for ALI, and yet the clinical setting makes the diagnosis of TRALI likely. If the consensus criteria[28] are not adhered to, many clinicians and laboratorians will be dissuaded from making a diagnosis of TRALI either in the absence of donor WBC antibodies or in the presence of alternative risk factors for ALI.

Donor WBC Antibodies and Mortality Due to TRALI

The UK SHOT,[16,17,82] ARC,[83] and German hemovigilance[84] data have consistently supported the thesis that, although non-WBC-alloantibody-mediated cases of TRALI may well exist, the WBC-alloantibody-mediated cases represent the large majority of clinically severe and/or fatal cases of TRALI. The German hemovigilance study,[84] for example, indicated that collection of plasma exclusively from male donors could be expected to prevent 87.5% of all TRALI deaths. Of 44 cases of TRALI occurring in Germany in 2006-2007 (and confirmed as TRALI by the European Hemovigilance Network criteria), 80% were antibody-mediated and 20% were non-antibody-mediated. WBC antibodies matching a recipient antigen were found in 28 (63.6%) donors. All of these donors were female; 26 had donated plasma, one had donated platelets, and one had donated red cells. There were eight (18%) fatal cases, with all of these cases being WBC-alloantibody-mediated and linked to female donors. Seven (87.5%) deaths were due to plasma transfusion and one was due to RBC transfusion. The SHOT data[82] have in fact shown such a dramatic reduction in the number of deaths from TRALI in the United

Kingdom after the implementation of the male-only plasma rule. Hemovigilance data from The Netherlands[90,120] and Canada,[25] however, indicate that the benefit from converting to male-only plasma will be significantly smaller than that predicted by data from the UK SHOT,[82] the ARC study,[83] or the German hemovigilance study.[84]

Forty-nine cases of TRALI were diagnosed in The Netherlands between January 2005 and July 2007, by both adhering strictly to the CCC criteria[28] and performing a complete TRALI work-up (which included both tests for WBC antibodies in the sera of all implicated donors and a test for WBC incompatibility between the implicated donors and the recipient).[90] Forty-four of 49 patients underwent such complete laboratory work-ups, whose purpose was not to make the diagnosis of TRALI per se, but to identify the subcategory of cases of "alloimmune" TRALI. Consistent with the results of the German hemovigilance study,[84] in 36 (73.5%) cases, at least one implicated donor had WBC antibodies. In 21 (43%) cases, as compared with 63.6% of the cases in the German study,[84] serologic incompatibility was shown between at least one donor and the recipient—that is, there was a positive crossmatch, or the donor's antibody was directed to a cognate WBC antigen of the recipient.

These cases of "alloimmune" TRALI showed more-severe morbidity than did the remaining 28 cases, although mortality was not higher in patients with WBC-alloantibody-mediated TRALI than in those with non-WBC-alloantibody-mediated TRALI. Two hundred fifty-nine components (129 RBCs, 66 platelet pools, and 64 units of FFP) had been administered to these 49 multitransfused patients (Fig 2-7). When the analysis was limited to the 21 cases of "alloimmune" TRALI—which involved 31 donors with demonstrated serologic incompatibility between donor and recipient—25 (81%) donors were female (compared to 100% of the donors in the German study[84]), and six (19%) donors were male. Of the 31 implicated components, 14 (45%) were FFP, 14 (45%) were RBCs, and three (10%) were platelets in platelet pools (Fig 2-9). In contrast, in the German study,[84] 26 of 28 donors implicated in such "alloimmune" TRALI had donated plasma.

The Netherlands converted to the administration of male-only plasma in July 2007 when the study was terminated. Had male-only plasma been used during the 30 months of the study, 12 (24.5%) of the 49 TRALI cases and two (20%) of the 10 TRALI deaths could have been prevented. Seven of the 10 patients who died of TRALI had received only RBCs, however, and one patient had received pooled platelets (Fig 2-10). Male-only donations of both plasma and platelets could thus have prevented 30% of all TRALI deaths. To prevent the majority (70%; Fig 2-10) of the TRALI deaths, however, measures to mitigate the risk of TRALI from RBC transfusion would have been required. RBCs in this study had been manufactured by the buffy-coat method and stored in additive solution, containing ≤20 mL of residual plasma. To prevent TRALI cases (and deaths) associated with RBC transfusion, blood centers would have to screen female donors of whole blood for a history of pregnancy and/or WBC antibodies. Such screening could be performed at the same time as donor testing for TTIs. Alternatively, RBCs would have to be washed before transfusion to remove any donor WBC antibodies as well as other mediators (eg, bioactive lipids) accumulating during storage.

The January 2005 to July 2007 Dutch study[90] had several advantages over other hemovigilance reports. Most important, as already stated, that study[90] included a complete work-up of all implicated donors, thereby avoiding the observation bias introduced by selectively working up only the female donors (or, worse yet, only the donors of plasma-rich components or the female donors of plasma-rich components). Furthermore, the Dutch study[90] adhered strictly to the CCC criteria in evaluating all cases of ARDS suspected by Dutch clinicians as perhaps representing TRALI. It also employed a country-wide database and consisted of a large series of 49 consecutive cases (compared with 16 cases in the largest case series of the pre-2004 literature[85] and 38 cases in the ARC study[83]). As in the German study of 44 cases,[84] donors were screened for the pres-

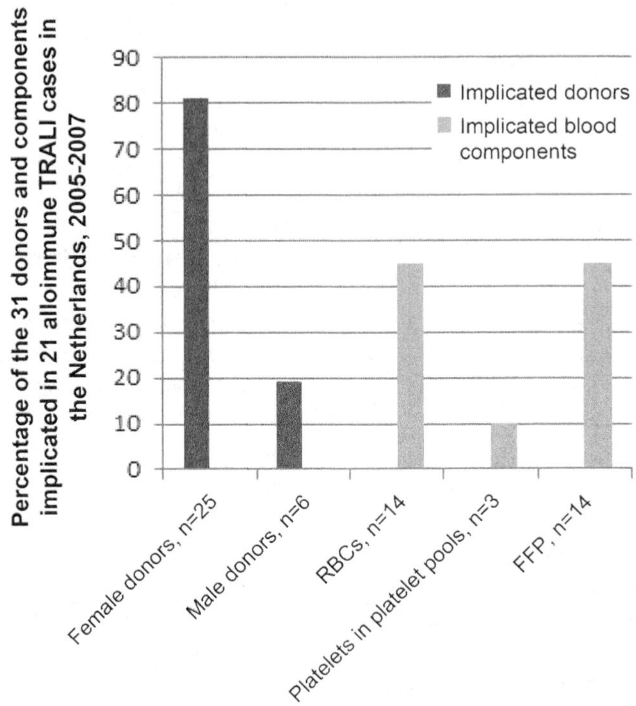

Figure 2-9. Proportion of female and male donors and of red cell (RBC), platelet, and plasma components implicated in 21 "alloimmune" cases of transfusion-related acute lung injury (TRALI) in the Netherlands before the introduction of the use of "male-only" plasma.[90] TRALI cases meeting the Canadian consensus critera[28] were designated as "alloimmune" if there was known white cell (WBC) incompatibility between donor and recipient (either a positive crossmatch or a donor WBC alloantibody directed to a recipient antigen; see text).
FFP = fresh frozen plasma.

ence of both HLA and neutrophil antibodies by using a combination of antibody-detection methods.[90]

A follow-up Dutch hemovigilance study[120] found that the introduction of male-only plasma in The Netherlands was associated with a 33% reduction in TRALI cases. A total of 110 cases of TRALI reported to the national hemovigilance office met the CCC criteria[28] from 2002 to November 2009. Of 68 cases occurring before the exclusive use of male-only plasma was introduced in July 2007, 36 had involved plasma. Thirty-one cases occurred after the implementation of male-only plasma, of which eight involved transfusion of plasma. Eleven cases occurred during the transitional period, of which four involved plasma. Although plasma was responsible for 53% of cases before the implementation of male-only plasma (compared with 26% of cases afterward), 31 cases nonetheless did occur after the implementation of this preventive measure, eight of which were attributed to plasma.[120]

Also adhering strictly to the CCC criteria,[28] the Canadian Transfusion-Transmitted Injuries Surveillance System (TTISS) reported on 105 TRALI cases that had occurred in 2004-2005.[25] Of 372 respiratory complications of ABT reported to the TTISS, 257 were deemed to represent TACO, eight transfusion-associated dyspnea, two possible TRALI, and 105 probable TRALI. Of the 105 cases of probable TRALI,

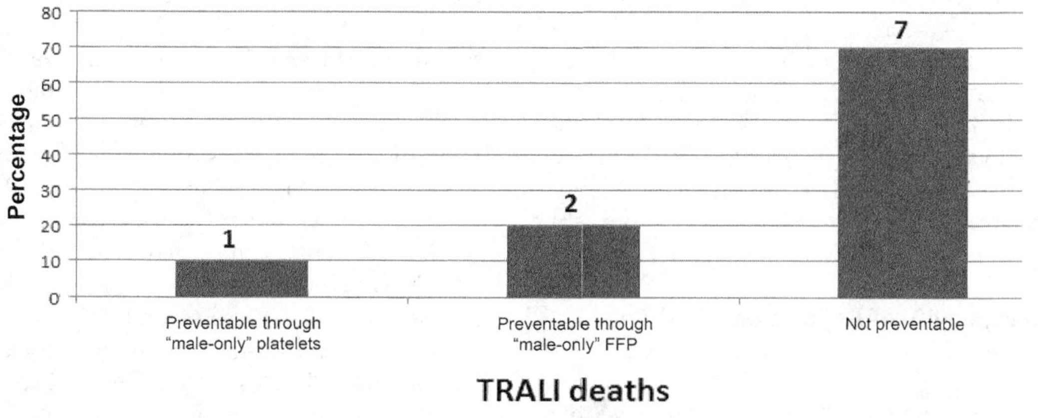

Figure 2-10. Proportion of deaths from transfusion-related acute lung injury (TRALI) occurring in The Netherlands in association with transfusion of any blood component before the introduction of "male-only" Fresh Frozen Plasma (FFP) that could have been prevented by the implementation of the use of male-only FFP and/or male-only platelets.[90] TRALI deaths attributed to red cell (RBC) transfusion would not be prevented by such measures targeting "plasma-rich" components. Blood components transfused in this Dutch study[90] included RBCs stored in additive solution and containing ≤20 mL of residual donor plasma; units of plasma containing approximately 325 mL of plasma from a single donor; and buffy-coat platelets pooled from five whole-blood donors and suspended in either platelet additive solution (with some 20 mL of residual plasma from each donor) or in approximately 200 mL of plasma from one of the five donors (whether male or female), along with some 20 mL of residual plasma from each of the other donors.

57.1% were associated with RBCs, 21.0% with plasma, 7.6% with pooled WBD platelets, and 3.8% with apheresis (single-donor) platelets. There were five deaths (case-fatality ratio of 4.8%); four deaths were attributed to transfusion of RBCs and one to transfusion of plasma.

The UK SHOT system had not been using the CCC criteria[28] for diagnosing TRALI, and thereby it included cases not occurring sufficiently near in time to a transfusion and also perhaps excluded cases in which WBC antibodies were not found (or relegated them to a "possible-TRALI" category). The UK SHOT criteria were modified in 2006[82] to limit TRALI to cases of ARDS occurring within 6 (as opposed to 24) hours of a transfusion. Some of the dramatic reduction subsequently recorded by the SHOT system in the number of TRALI cases and deaths[82] is doubtless attributable to the change in the definition of TRALI. In a similar vein, 2 years after the publication of the consensus definition,[28] 45% to 66% of US hospitals were basing their diagnoses of TRALI on a combination of clinical and serologic findings.[121] Work-ups regularly included HLA Class I and II antibodies and sometimes neutrophil antibodies as well. Which donors were screened for WBC antibodies often hinged on a donor's gender, and policies bearing on the diagnosis of TRALI were decided upon on a case-by-case basis.

Even in the recent literature, the CCC definition has not been consistently adhered to. For example, in an RCT[122] of the efficacy of WBC-reduced blood components in preventing TRALI, none of the diagnoses of TRALI assigned in either arm of the trial pertained to ALI occurring within 6 hours of a transfusion.[123] Because ALI is very common in critically ill multitransfused patients, many cases of ALI can be misdiagnosed as "TRALI" because of a temporal association with a transfusion. The demonstration of WBC incompatibility between an implicated donor and the recipient (as opposed to the mere presence of WBC antibodies in an implicated donor's serum) strengthens the evidence that a particular case of ALI (in which all consensus criteria[28] have been met and the diagnosis of TRALI has been made before the laboratory work-up) represents TRALI. However, whether TRALI is mediated by its own pathogenetic mechanisms (distinct from the generic mechanisms of ALI) remains unknown.[124]

Heterogeneity of Reports on TRALI Mortality

Studies reporting on TRALI mortality have thus been highly heterogeneous, because they used varied criteria to define TRALI and/or because they included a varied case-mix of patients with more- or less-severe ARDS. Even when the CCC criteria[28] are adhered to, a diagnosis of TRALI represents a best clinical judgment rather than a firm diagnosis buttressed by a pathognomonic diagnostic test, because the criteria[28] are broad and subjective, and they do not specify how the principal differential diagnosis of TACO is to be made from TRALI in routine clinical settings. The subjective nature of the diagnosis is highlighted when clinically and serologically "documented" cases of TRALI not meeting the consensus definition are reported.[125] Furthermore, the CCC criteria[28]—although now widely used—lack validation.[92] A study investigating the applicability of this definition of TRALI[28] to a cardiac surgery registry showed that approximately two-thirds of the patients admitted to the ICU had a PaO_2:FiO_2 ratio of <300 mmHg (ie, a ratio meeting the threshold for hypoxemia according to the CCC criteria[126]). Using those criteria to diagnose TRALI may thus be inappropriate for cardiac surgery patients.[126]

The increasing proportion of deaths secondary to TACO that were passively reported to the FDA between 2005 and 2010[9] highlights the impact of the wider adoption of the CCC criteria.[28] Deaths due to TACO likely were either missed before 2005 or were considered to represent TRALI. The CCC[28] brought attention to TRALI, and it also gradually drove home the message that, for the diagnosis of TRALI to be made, left atrial hypertension (ie, TACO) must be ruled out upfront. Both the increased attention to TRALI and the requirement that TACO be ruled out early in the process of establishing a diagnosis of TRALI likely resulted in a higher proportion of transfusion-related deaths reported to the FDA being diagnosed as TACO.[9] In 2009, TACO and HTRs were each responsible for 12 transfusion-related deaths. In 2010, TACO (with eight deaths, compared to seven deaths from HTRs) was second only to TRALI as a cause of transfusion-related mortality, and it had displaced TAS as the third highest cause of transfusion-related mortality for the period from 2005 through 2010 (Fig 2-1). As discussed in Chapter 4, TACO can be prevented only by avoiding overtransfusion and unnecessary transfusion.

Even when studies of TRALI mortality have used the CCC criteria,[25,90] they may well have included patients with more-severe[90] or less-severe[25] ARDS or TRALI. Such case-mix considerations (eg, the inclusion of a large proportion of "possible" TRALI cases that may not represent "real" TRALI) can explain the variation in mortality reported by studies using the CCC criteria[28]—for example, 4.8% in the Canadian hemovigilance study[25] compared with 20.4% in the Dutch hemovigilance study.[90] However, case-mix considerations alone cannot account for the different conclusions reached by such studies concerning the anticipated efficacy of male-only plasma in preventing deaths from TRALI. For example, the Dutch[90] and German[84] hemovigilance studies had included TRALI cases of similar severity (judging from mortality rates of 20%[90] and 18%,[84] respectively), yet they produced different results regarding the expected benefit from male-only plasma. Even though 1) consensus about the appropriateness of converting to male-only plasma has not been achieved,[127] 2) not all studies have shown a reduction in the risk of TRALI through avoidance of female donors,[128,129] and 3) many complexities are involved in the interpretation of the published data, most of the hitherto adduced evidence supports the thesis that ending the collections of plasma-rich components from women who have previously been pregnant or who have circulating WBC antibodies will enhance blood safety.[92,130]

HTRs

In HTRs, the transfused donor red cells are attacked by the recipient's "naturally occurring" antibodies to ABO antigens and/or antibodies to other red cell antigens, produced after immunization through a previous transfusion or pregnancy. Most acute HTRs occur within 24 hours of the ABT, although, in the case of an ABO-incompatible transfusion, an HTR usually begins during the transfusion. A delayed HTR (DHTR) begins after there has been an anamnestic (secondary) immune response to a donor red cell antigen to which the recipient has been alloimmunized by a previous transfusion or pregnancy. From 19.5% to 48.6% of clinically significant red cell alloantibodies to non-ABO antigens disappear over time, which predisposes a transfusion recipient to the development of DHTR.[131] It is very rare for a DHTR to cause death, although deaths have been reported.[132] The outcome of an immediate HTR depends on the potency of the (usually ABO) recipient antibody and the volume of blood transfused; infusion rate may also be a factor. Most fatalities have been associated with transfusions of ≥200 mL, and mortality approaches 44% for transfusions exceeding 1000 mL.[10,11]

Fatalities Due to HTRs

Of 44 fatalities reported to the FDA because of HTR from 1976 through 1978, 38 were due to ABO incompatibility.[10] The most common cause of HTR was failure to identify the intended recipient correctly, and most such incorrect blood component transfusions had occurred in the operating room. Of the deaths reported to the FDA from 1976 through 1985,[11] 158 were due to acute HTRs (131 to ABO incompatibility) and 26 to DHTRs (mostly due to c and Jk^a antibodies). If all of these deaths were attributed to the ABT, mortality due to HTRs would approximate 1 per 250,000 RBC units transfused during the decade of 1976 through 1985.

A 10-year (1990-1999) study in New York State documented the transfusion of incorrect blood component(s) in 1 per 19,000 transfused RBC units, ABO-incompatible transfusion in 1 per 38,000, and acute HTR (or laboratory evidence of hemolysis) in 1 per 76,000. Five deaths were reported (case:fatality ratio of 2%), resulting in a mortality due to acute HTR of 1 per 1.8 million transfused RBC units.[133] This figure is identical to that calculated from French hemovigilance data[15] (1 per 1.8 million transfused RBC units; 95% CI: 1/5 million-1/773,000) and similar to the figure of 1 per 1.4 million components issued for transfusion obtained from the SHOT system[17] (Fig 2-11).

From 2005 through 2010, there were slightly fewer than five deaths due to ABO HTRs per year (Fig 2-12)[9] or one death due to ABO HTR passively reported to the US FDA per 3 million transfused RBC units.[43] The recent decrease in deaths[9] was temporally associated with the February 2004 FDA requirement that machine-readable information be included on blood-container labels by April 2006.[134] A similar reduction in ABO-related fatalities was recently recorded by the UK SHOT system.[17] When ABO and non-ABO HTRs are considered together, however, there have been 12.5 deaths per year from 2005 through 2010 (Fig 2-12).[9] Owing to the increase in the reported number of deaths due to non-ABO HTRs, mortality due to HTRs[9] appears to have remained largely unchanged since the 1990s.[133] In the decade of 1976 through 1985,[11] there was an average of 13.1 fatal ABO HTRs and 2.7 fatal non-ABO HTRs each year. The mean annual number of fatal non-ABO HTRs increased approximately threefold between the periods 1976-1985[11] and 2005-2010 (Fig 2-12).[9]

Prevention of HTRs

Proper identification of the transfusion recipient (at the time of transfusion) and of the pretransfusion blood specimen (at the time of specimen collection) are critical for the prevention of ABO HTRs. It is human errors that cause transfusion

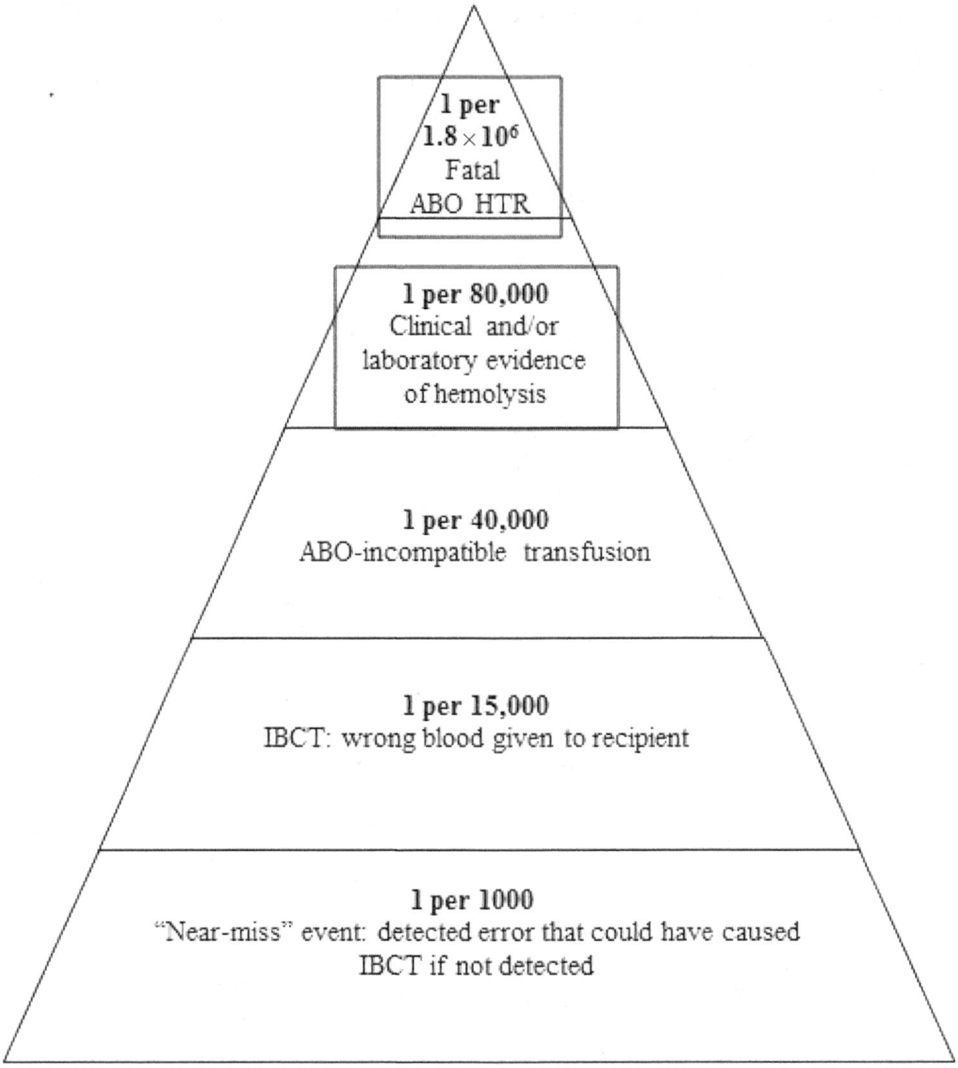

Figure 2-11. Likelihood of a serious ABO hemolytic transfusion reaction (HTR), shown in the form of a pyramid whose base represents the probability of events predisposing to incorrect blood component transfusion (IBCT), whose rising layers show the likelihood of increasingly more hazardous (as well as less likely) events sometimes leading to death from ABO HTR, and whose tip represents mortality. The figures shown within the boxes at the top pertain to the risk of actual hemolysis. The likelihoods indicated in the figure are based on data reported by surveillance systems operating in New York State, France, and the United Kingdom (see text), and they are expressed per number of Red Blood Cell (RBC) units transfused. Initially published by Vamvakas and Blajchman in Blood 2009;113:3406-17.[130]

of the wrong unit or miscollection (or mislabeling) of the pretransfusion specimen. Therefore, administrative systems have been developed to analyze errors and prevent their recurrence.[135] Moreover, because proper identification of the transfusion recipient is crucial, barrier systems intended to physically prevent the transfusion of blood without correct identification of the

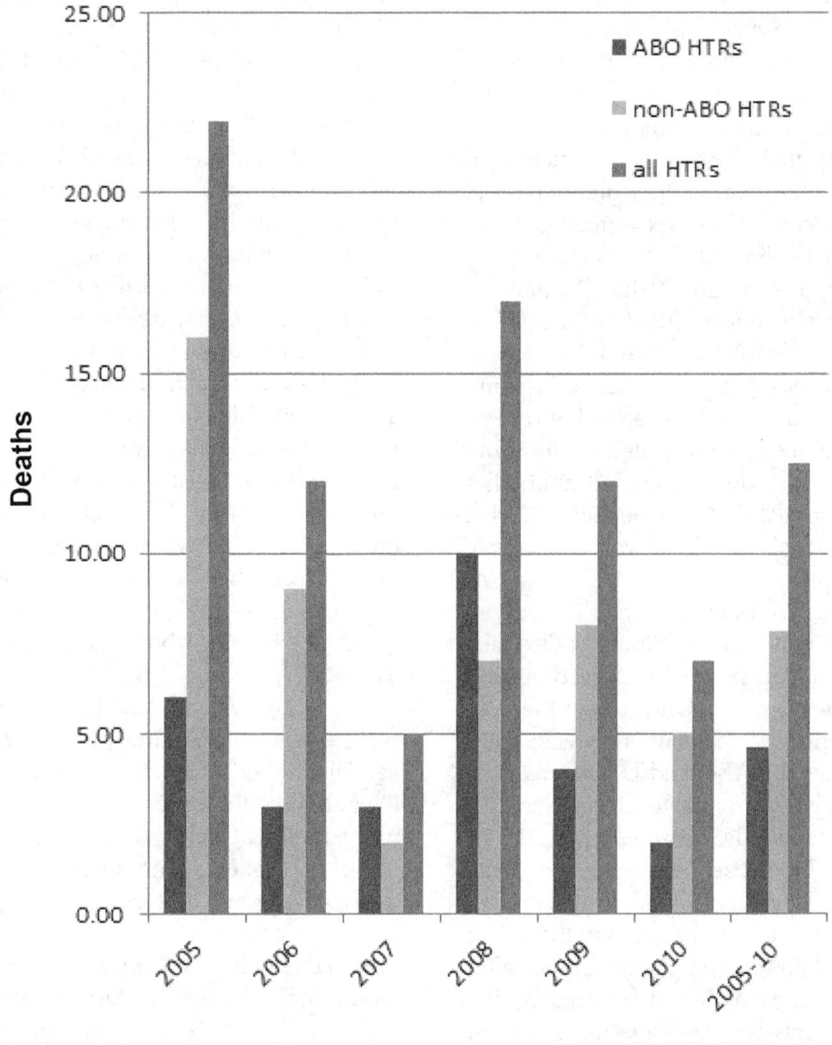

Figure 2-12. The number of deaths from ABO, non-ABO, and combined ABO and non-ABO hemolytic transfusion reactions (HTRs) passively reported to the United States Food and Drug Administration in each year from 2005 through 2010 and the mean annual number of HTRs reported over that 6-year period. Overall, from 2006 through 2010, the annual number of deaths from non-ABO HTRs exceeded the number of deaths from ABO HTRs.

patient have been devised. These systems include a plastic lock that must be unlocked by the entry of the correct identification code,[136] the use of a special wristband for identification of transfusion recipients,[137,138] the use of multiple barcodes (on patient wristbands, blood sample tubes, blood component bags, and nurses' identification badges) along with point-of-transfusion reading devices to verify identity,[139,140] and other, similar approaches.[141,142] These tools require an investment in information technology, but they can be integrated with other systems, such as medication administration. To guard against miscollection (or mislabeling) of the pretransfusion specimen, some US transfusion services require verification of the recipient's ABO group by the collection of two independent pretransfusion samples.[143]

As already stated, despite the reduction in ABO fatalities, the mean annual number of all deaths due to acute HTRs has remained virtually stable from 1976 through 1985 (15.8/year) and from 2005 through 2010 (12.5/year), because reported fatalities due to acute HTRs secondary to non-ABO antibodies have increased in recent years.[9] The increasing number of such reports to the FDA probably reflects improved awareness of the potential for non-ABO HTRs to cause death. Red cell antibodies implicated in non-ABO HTRs include Jk^b, Jk^a, Kell, Fy^a, Fy^b, E, Js^a, and I, as well as multiple antibody specificities.

Although the possibility has been considered that the formation of red cell alloantibodies may represent a random process,[144] that does not appear to be the case.[145-151] Only 1% of the nonchronically transfused patients receiving RBC units matched for the ABO and D antigens form red cell alloantibodies,[145] but the formation of a first red cell alloantibody identifies a patient as a "high responder" to subsequent red cell alloantigen challenges. Thus, once a patient has formed red cell alloantibodies, the probability that he or she will form additional red cell antibodies after further RBC transfusions is 20% to 25%.[146,147]

Remarkably, this probability is the same for hemato-oncology[147] and non-hemato-oncology[146] patients, despite the fact that hemato-oncology patients receive intensive immunosuppressive treatments. In the retrospective cohort studies of Schonewille et al[146,147] that spanned a period of approximately 20 years, hemato-oncology patients received more RBC units in more ABT episodes (seven units in three episodes) than did non-hemato-oncology patients (two units in one episode) before additional red cell alloantibodies were detected. However, hemato-oncology patients generally experience multiple transfusion events in a short period, which probably leads to an overestimation of the number of transfusions needed for additional antibody formation in these patients, as compared with obstetrical, surgical, and other medical patients.

The current standard of care requires provision of only ABO- and D-matched RBC units for patients who have not made alloantibodies to other red cell antigens. For patients who have formed alloantibodies, transfused red cells must be negative for all antigens to which a prospective recipient has detectable antibodies. Thus, when multiple antibodies are present (or are in the process of being formed), complex serologic work-ups are necessary before compatible RBC units can be issued by the blood bank. No antibody detection method is capable of identifying all clinically significant red cell alloantibodies, however. Acute HTRs still occur, either because a clinically significant red cell alloantibody is missed or because fully compatible RBC units are not available when needed. In such cases, hemolysis of the transfused red cells because of pre-existing red cell alloantibodies to non-ABO antigens can cause both morbidity and mortality.

Currently, we cannot identify patients who will respond to RBC transfusions by forming red cell alloantibodies. Once a patient has formed an alloantibody, the probability of him or her forming additional red cell antibodies is 20% to 25%.[146,147] Patients with hemoglobinopathies are especially prone to form multiple alloantibodies,[151] which generate complex serologic workups, cause delay in the provision of compatible blood, and may lead to DHTRs and sometimes also acute HTRs. To prevent such problems, the standard of care has been elevated at many US hospitals for patients with hemoglobinopathies.[152] These multitransfused patients receive units matched for the C, E, and K antigens (and sometimes also for the Jk^a and Fy^a antigens), for the purpose of preventing the formation of alloantibodies to those antigens.[152-155] Such extended antigen matching between donor and recipient is generally performed phenotypically—that is, by using the traditional serologic techniques of hemagglutination.[156,157] A driving force for performing extended antigen matching for patients with hemoglobinopathies has been the difference between donor and recipient phenotypes that is due to ethnic-pool gene diversity.[156,157]

Extended phenotypic antigen matching generally is not performed for other multitransfused patients, either because the clinical benefit from such an elevated standard of care has not been empirically documented or because the additional effort generated by the extended phenotypic matching is considered to be prohibitive. Genotyping for C, E, K, Jk,[a] Fy,[a] and other clinically significant red cell antigens is now available, however, and it can be performed on patients as well as donor units (using DNA extracted from the residual WBCs in WBC-reduced RBC units).[158-162] The feasibility of providing extended antigen matching between donor and recipient through genotyping was recently shown in a multi-center US study for several categories of patients (in addition to patients with sickle cell disease).[163] That study used RBC donor units from existing inventories, and it used a computerized inventory management system to create and maintain an inventory of genotyped units, as well as identify compatible blood for transfusion recipients at increasingly stringent levels of antigen matching.

Poorly Understood Causes of Death Attributed to ABT by RCTs

The Transfusion Requirements in Critical Care (TRICC) RCT[23] found that, compared with a restrictive RBC transfusion strategy, a liberal strategy may be associated with increased in-hospital mortality in normovolemic, critically ill patients. These investigators randomly assigned 418 ICU patients to a restrictive-strategy arm and 420 patients to a liberal-strategy arm. The former patients were transfused if the hemoglobin concentration fell to ≤7.0 g/dL and the latter if it fell to ≤10.0 g/dL. Patients allocated to the restrictive-strategy arm received on average 3.0 fewer RBC units than did those in the liberal-strategy arm (mean ± SD: 2.6 ± 4.1 and 5.6 ± 5.3 RBC units, respectively, per patient); overall, 33% compared with 0% of the patients, respectively, avoided ABT altogether ($p<0.01$).

The primary outcome of the TRICC trial, 30-day mortality, was 18.7% in the restrictive-strategy arm and 23.3% in the liberal-strategy arm ($p = 0.11$). The adjusted multiple-organ dysfunction score (MODS) differed between the arms (mean ± SD: 10.7 ± 7.5 and 11.8 ± 7.7, respectively; $p = 0.03$), as did the change in score from baseline (3.2 ± 7.0 and 4.2 ± 7.4, respectively; $p = 0.04$). In subgroup analyses, patients who were less acutely ill (APACHE II score of ≤20) and patients who were younger than 55 experienced a significant survival benefit from being allocated to the restrictive-strategy arm. Among the former, 30-day mortality was 8.7% in the liberal-strategy arm compared with 16.1% in the restrictive-strategy arm ($p = 0.03$); among the latter, it was 5.7% and 13.0%, respectively ($p = 0.02$). Mortality during the entire hospitalization was significantly lower in the restrictive-strategy arm (22.2%) than in the liberal-strategy arm (28.1%) ($p \geq 0.05$). The absolute risk difference in in-hospital mortality between the arms was 5.8% (95% CI = –0.3%-11.7%; $p \geq 0.05$). As discussed in Chapter 4, however, 12 years after the publication of the TRICC RCT,[23] the TRICC findings, which raised the possibility of a worse outcome in the liberal- than in the restrictive-strategy arm, have not been replicated by another randomized study.

In the TRICC RCT,[23] compared with the restrictive-strategy-arm, the liberal-strategy arm also experienced significantly worse outcomes in terms of the risk of myocardial infarction ($p = 0.02$) and pulmonary edema ($p<0.01$), as well as any cardiac complication ($p<0.01$); the difference in the risk of ARDS approached statistical significance ($p = 0.06$). Of 27 clinical outcomes analyzed by the authors, only four favored the liberal-strategy arm, and 23 favored the restrictive-strategy arm, with the difference being significant in the aforementioned cases. Although the greater risk of pulmonary edema in the liberal-strategy arm could be explained by the fluid overload caused by the RBC transfusion, these findings contradict what would be expected if a liberal-transfusion strategy resulted in improved oxygen delivery to the myocardium, with the enhanced oxygen consumption by the myocardium producing improved myocardial function. Because the RBCs transfused to the subjects enrolled in the TRICC RCT[23] were non-WBC-reduced, plausible reasons for any increase in in-hospital mortality, MODS, or specific adverse clinical outcomes could involve pathophysiologic mechanisms relying on either WBCs[164-169] or RBCs.

RBC-Dependent Mechanisms for Poorly Understood Adverse ABT Effects

For the particular situation of the critically ill patients with systemic inflammatory response syndrome (SIRS) and oxidative stress enrolled in the TRICC RCT,[23] Forceville et al[170] invoked the potentially deleterious effect of the iron-containing protein (hemoglobin) that is supplied by the transfused red cells. They reasoned that the red cells contain iron, which can amplify oxidative stress, and that an increase in oxygen delivery—the purpose of a RBC transfusion—in patients with SIRS may also increase the production of toxic reactive oxygen species.[171-173] Consequently, an excess production of reactive oxygen species in patients in the liberal-transfusion arm (who received 3 more RBC units, or 600 mg of extra iron, than did the patients in the restrictive-transfusion arm compared with a total body iron of 2.8 g) may have worsened the pre-existing oxidative stress.[170]

One unit of blood contains more than 100 times the quantity of iron absorbed daily from the diet (200 mg as compared with just over 1 mg), and the iron overload and toxicity from multiple RBC transfusions are well documented.[174] A patient with a transfusion-dependent anemia requiring 2 RBC units per month would receive 24 units per year, or about 100 units over 4 years, thereby accumulating 20 g of iron in her/his body. Transfused red cells have a relatively short life span compared with the approximately 120-day life span of normal red cells. Transfused red cells undergo erythrophagocytosis, with the release of iron, which eventually overloads macrophages. When this excess iron re-enters the plasma, it overwhelms the iron-carrying capacity of transferrin and is deposited in tissues as free iron. Increased iron levels become detectable 17 to 22 days after RBC transfusion. Iron overload from chronic transfusions damages the liver, heart, pancreas, thyroid, and other endocrine glands.

Forceville et al[170] therefore posited that, in a setting of SIRS, deficient antioxidant systems, and overwhelmed haptoglobin/hemopexin/transferrin systems (as could potentially have been the case in the critically ill ICU patients enrolled in the TRICC RCT[23]), the increased iron burden from the excess RBC transfusions could result in tissue injury in the acute (rather than chronic) setting (Fig 2-13). A different RBC-dependent mechanism is currently being investigated in RCTs to explain the association of (non-WBC-reduced or WBC-reduced) RBC transfusion with increased mortality. This postulated mechanism attributes the effects of RBC transfusion on mortality and major morbidity to changes that the allogeneic RBCs undergo during storage. This recent controversy about the effect of RBC storage is reviewed in Chapter 7.

WBC-Dependent Mechanisms for Poorly Understood Adverse Effects of (non-WBC-Reduced) ABT

The RCT of van de Watering et al,[21] which was designed to investigate an association between non-WBC-reduced ABT and postoperative infection, found, instead, an association between non-WBC-reduced ABT and 60-day mortality from all causes. All platelets transfused in that study[21] were WBC-reduced, but RBCs were either non-WBC-reduced or WBC-reduced, depending on the randomized study arm to which each patient had been assigned. The association between non-WBC-reduced ABT and mortality was reported as a data-derived hypothesis,[21] and the authors postulated that non-WBC-reduced ABT may predispose a patient to multiple-organ failure (MOF), which might, in turn, predispose him or her to death. Bilgin and Brand undertook another RCT that confirmed the association between ABT and short-term mortality but did not find an association between non-WBC-reduced ABT and increased MOF.[22]

Eleven RCTs comparing recipients of non-WBC-reduced and of WBC-reduced allogeneic RBCs have presented information on short-term (up to 3 months after transfusion) mortality from

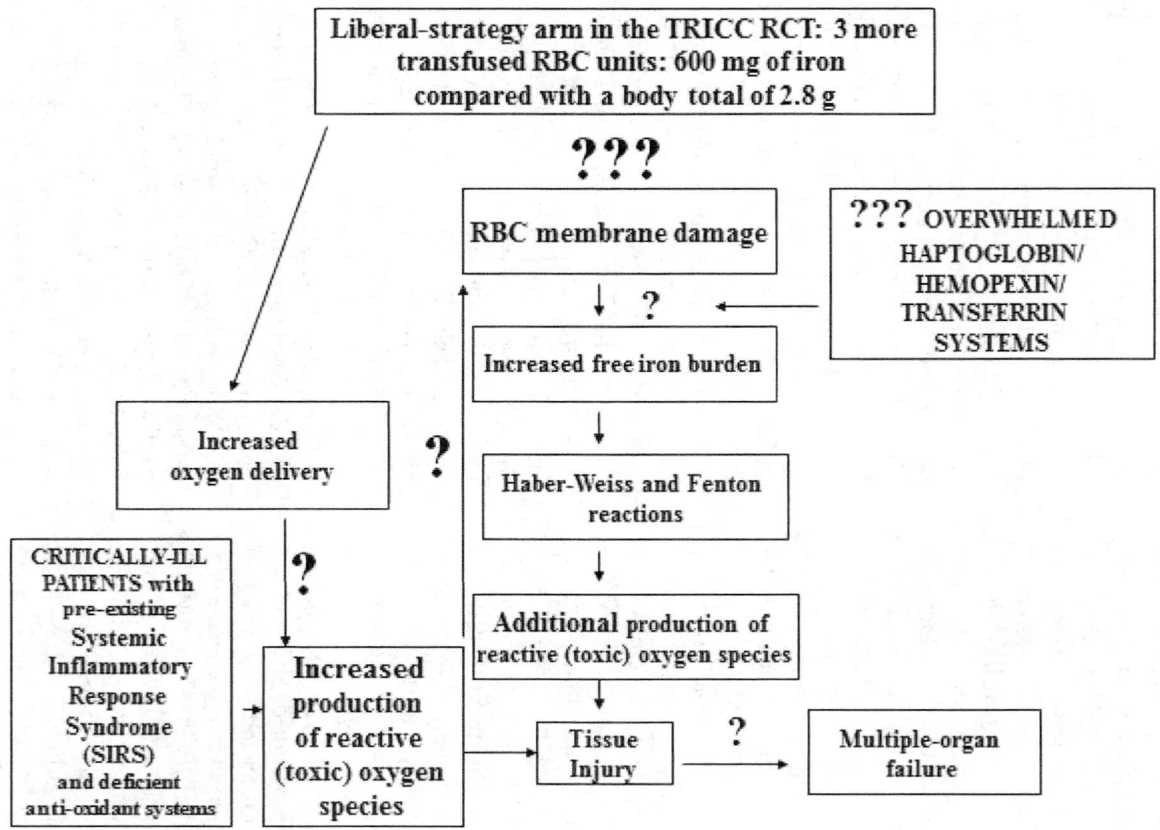

Figure 2-13. A plausible Red Blood Cell (RBC)-dependent mechanism invoked by Forceville et al[170] to explain the increase in all-cause mortality, multiple-organ dysfunction score, and specific complications reported by the Transfusion Requirements in Critical Care (TRICC)[23] randomized controlled trial (RCT) in association with any [whether non-white cell (WBC)-reduced or WBC-reduced] allogeneic blood transfusion (see text).

all causes.[21,22,175-183] Across five RCTs conducted in cardiac surgery patients[21,22,179,181,182] that transfused RBCs filtered before storage to the WBC-reduced arm, non-WBC-reduced ABT was associated with 72% greater postoperative mortality than was WBC-reduced ABT (summary OR = 1.72; 95% CI = 1.05-2.81; $p<0.05$).[184] In contrast, across six RCTs conducted in other settings,[175-178,180,183] non-WBC-reduced (compared with WBC-reduced) ABT was not associated with any increase in postoperative mortality.[184] The adverse effect seen across the open-heart surgery studies (but not in studies conducted in other settings; Fig 2-14) may be associated with factors that are prevalent among patients undergoing cardiac surgery.

During cardiac surgery, exposure to the extracorporeal circuit, hypothermia, and reperfusion injury may generate a SIRS that is counteracted by a compensatory anti-inflammatory response syndrome (CARS).[185] Any intervention by biologic response modifiers (eg, the soluble mediators contained in stored non-WBC-reduced RBCs[164-166]) during an already-existing inflammatory cascade could thus produce an imbalance in the SIRS-CARS equilibrium toward SIRS. An overwhelming SIRS causes a dormant state of cell metabolism referred to as MODS, which can ultimately lead to MOF and death (Fig 2-15).[185] However, an association between non-WBC-reduced ABT and MOF has not been reported by any RCT, and the mechanism by which non-WBC-reduced ABT (but not WBC-reduced ABT) is associated with increased mortality in cardiac surgery remains unknown.[186] In the completed RCTs,[21,22,179,181,182] non-WBC-reduced ABT was not associated with any particular cause of death, yet the aggregate mortality was higher in the non-WBC-reduced arm than in the WBC-reduced arm.[186]

Concerning soluble mediators contained in stored non-WBC-reduced RBCs (Fig 2-15), Silliman et al[164] proposed that ABT may exercise a neutrophil-priming effect mediated by bioactive lipids that accumulate during storage. Those investigators postulated that rapidly deteriorating WBCs in stored RBCs release cytotoxic enzymes that may act on fragmented red cell membranes to produce mediators responsible for neutrophil priming and endothelial cell activation. Silliman et al[164] and Zallen et al[165] showed that plasma obtained from stored RBCs primes neutrophils for superoxide production and enhanced cytotoxicity and also activates pulmonary endothelial cells in dose- and age-dependent fashions. The length of storage was important in these studies, because no evidence of neutrophil priming was obtained when plasma stored for short periods was used. Similarly, Chin-Yee et al[166] reported that plasma supernatant from stored RBCs activates neutrophils, while WBC reduction of the RBC units abrogates the effect. Studies investigating the benefits obtained from placing a WBC-reduction filter in the arterial line of the cardiopulmonary bypass circuit[167-169] suggested that non-WBC-reduced ABT may provoke cardiac and/or pulmonary failure.

If the lower mortality during the hospitalization (22.2% compared with 28.1%; $p\geq0.05$) observed in the restrictive-strategy arm compared with the liberal-strategy arm of the TRICC RCT[23] was indeed due to the receipt of an average of 3 more RBC units in the former than in the latter group of patients, ABT would appear to be causing the death of 1 of every 16.9 transfused, critically ill patients admitted to the ICU. Similarly, if the lower mortality (3.5% compared with 7.8%; $p<0.05$) observed in recipients of WBC-reduced RBCs than in recipients of non-WBC-reduced RBCs, respectively, in the RCT of van de Watering et al[21] was indeed due to the different type of RBC component administered, non-WBC-reduced ABT would appear to be causing the death of 1 of every 23.3 transfused cardiac surgery patients. Although overall mortality has been lower in the US studies[182] than that reported in the Dutch RCTs,[21,22] such potentially WBC-mediated adverse ABT effects (Fig 2-15) could account for a far larger number of ABT-related deaths than do all of the currently established complications of ABT combined.

The Impact of the Next Fatal TTI

Although mortality from established complications of ABT is currently very low (Fig 2-1),[9] a

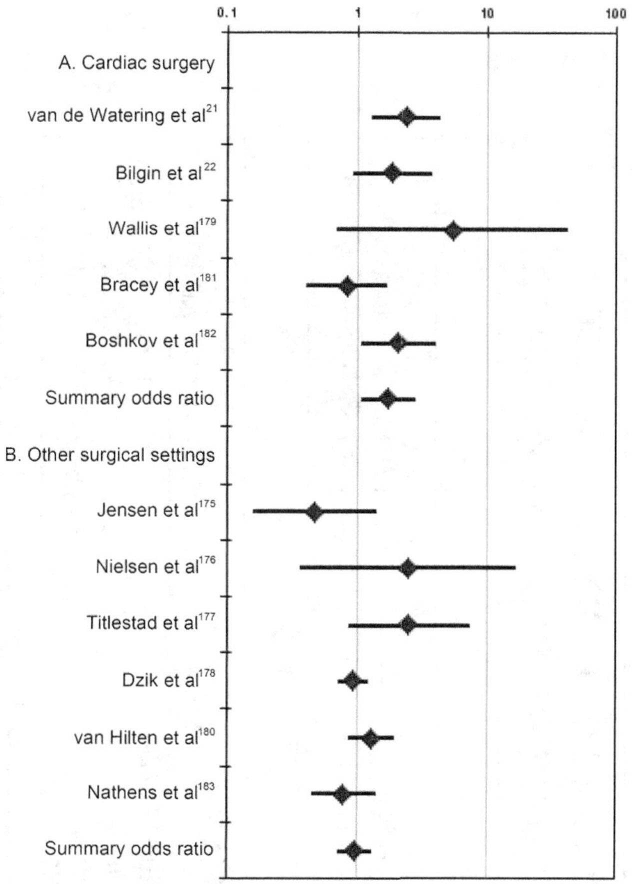

Figure 2-14. Postoperative mortality in cardiac surgery (Part A) compared with other surgical settings (Part B), as calculated from randomized controlled trials (RCTs) investigating the association of non-white-cell (WBC)-reduced allogeneic blood transfusion with short-term (up to 3 months after transfusion) mortality from all causes. The figure shows the odds ratio (OR) of mortality in recipients of non-WBC-reduced vs WBC-reduced allogeneic red cells (RBCs), as calculated from each RCT; across RCTs conducted in the setting of cardiac surgery[21,22,179,181,182] (summary OR = 1.72; 95% CI = 1.05-2.81); and across RCTs conducted in other settings[175-178,180,183] (summary OR = 0.99; 95% CI = 0.73-1.33).[184] An OR of >1 indicates higher mortality in recipients of non-WBC-reduced allogeneic RBCs than in recipients of WBC-reduced allogeneic RBCs, provided that the difference is statistically significant [ie, provided that the corresponding 95% CI (confidence interval) does not contain the null value of 1]. Initially published by Vamvakas and Blajchman in Blood 2009;113:3406-17.[130]

novel and fatal TTI could potentially emerge in the future and reproduce the catastrophe of the transfusion-acquired AIDS epidemic of the 1980s.[1] Three transfusion-transmitted agents have emerged in the past 30 years: HIV, vCJD prions, and WNV. Therefore, it is not mere prudence but simply common sense to assume that what happened in the past can (or will) happen again in the future.

The appearance of HIV has indeed been the most dramatic example of an emerging infection, because it represented a completely new

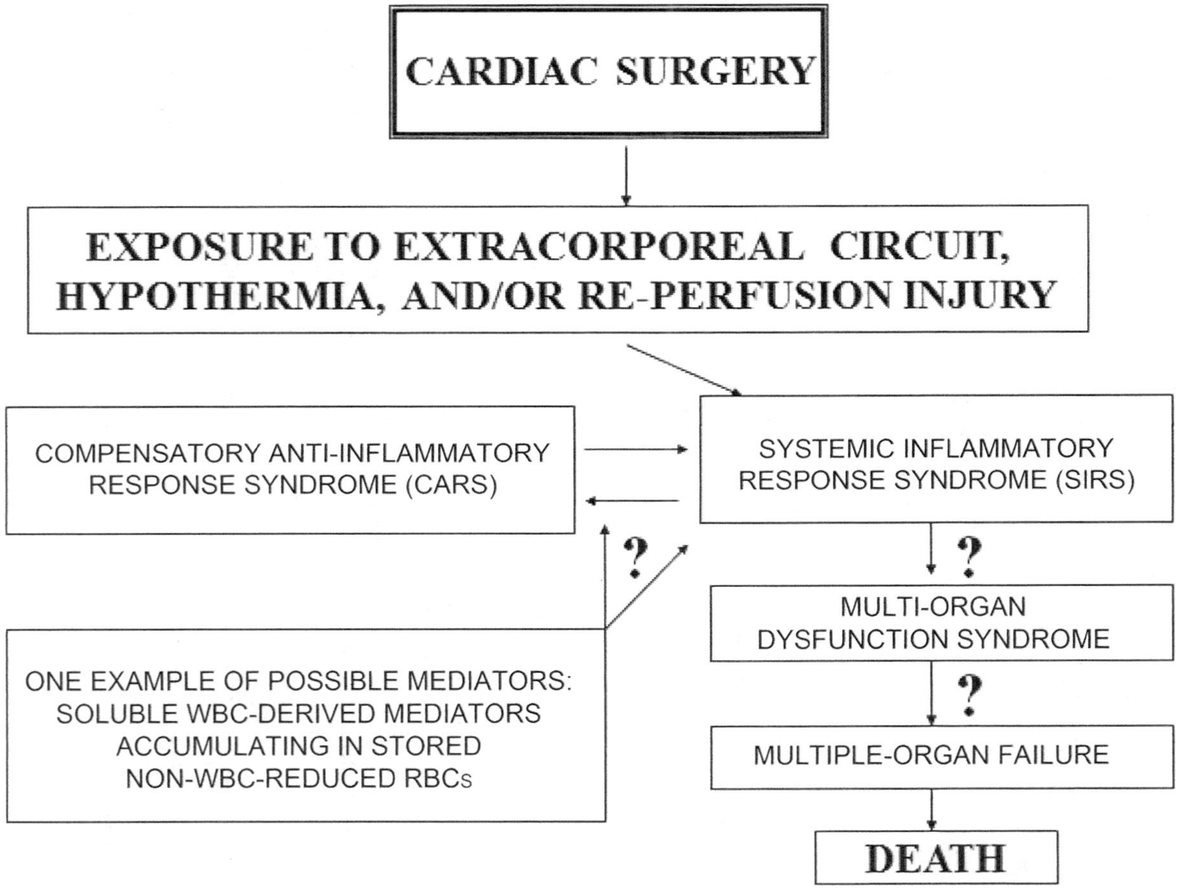

Figure 2-15. White cell (WBC)-dependent mechanism invoked by Bilgin and Brand[185] to explain the increase in all-cause mortality reported by the RCT of van de Watering et al[21] in association with non-WBC-reduced (compared with WBC-reduced) red blood cells (RBCs) (see text). All transfused platelets in that randomized controlled trial (RCT)[21] had been WBC-reduced. Accordingly, the proposed mechanism focuses only on non-WBC-reduced RBCs.

infection. HIV infection of humans probably occurred as a result of a cross-species transmission of simian immunodeficiency viruses from monkeys to great apes and then to humans.[187] The original transmission probably occurred as a result of the preparation of bushmeat derived from apes. Another cause of the emergence of novel agents is the expansion of existing infections into a larger geographic area; a striking example of such expansion was the recent appearance of WNV in the Americas.[188] In a similar manner, dengue fever virus and Chikungunya virus may very well be expanding their current geographic regions.[189-191]

Provided that an agent can survive in blood components and can be transmitted by the intravenous route, any infection with an asymptomatic blood-borne phase has the potential for transmission by ABT (Chapter 3). This possibility exists, whether the infectious phase is prolonged (as is the case with HIV, HBV, or HCV infection) or short (as is the case with WNV or DFV infection). The frequency with which an infection is transmitted to a transfusion recipient depends on the length of the asymptomatic blood-borne phase, the frequency of blood donation during this period, and the immune status of the recipient population.[8] The worst that can happen is the emergence of an HIV-like pathogen with a long incubation period that, owing to its long asymptomatic blood-borne phase, could accumulate to a significant extent in the blood donor population before it becomes recognized, thereby almost reaching the prevalence of the HIV infection in the US blood donor population before testing for HIV antibody was introduced. In 1984, the year before testing of US blood donors for HIV infection commenced, the prevalence of HIV infection in donors exceeded 1 per 1000.[192] Because of the surveillance systems put in place after the 1980s epidemic of transfusion-acquired HIV infection, it is unlikely that a new viral agent causing chronic infection could go undetected for as long as HIV went undetected, and therefore infection with a new viral agent would be most unlikely to reach a similar prevalence of 1 per 1000 US blood donors.

Although a future HIV-like agent would certainly be detected much faster than HIV was recognized, it is still possible that—before measures are implemented to interrupt its transmission through ABT—the future HIV-like agent could reach a prevalence as high as one-tenth the 1984 HIV prevalence.[71] Thus, worst-case scenarios of all strategies to further reduce ABT-related mortality should consistently model the possibility of an HIV-like pathogen reaching a prevalence of 1 per 10,000 US blood donors before measures are introduced to interrupt its transmission through transfusion.[71] It is important that we do not exclude the possibility that the accumulation of such a pathogen in the US blood donor population may have already begun. In addition, a WNV-like agent can change its geographic distribution and emerge in the United States as a transfusion-transmitted pathogen, with the potential to cause 380 transmissions through ABT in its first epidemic, as was the case with WNV in the summer of 2002.[193] The next "HIV-like" major transfusion-transmitted pathogen would cause chronic asymptomatic pathogenemia (like HIV), although it would not have to be a virus or be transmitted sexually like HIV. Similarly, the next "WNV-like" transfusion-transmitted pathogen would cause asymptomatic pathogenemia only during the period of acute infection and would occur in epidemic form (like WNV), although it would have to be neither a virus nor vector-borne like WNV.

If such a novel and fatal TTI emerged in the future, most transmissions (as well as cases of transfusion-transmitted disease and of transfusion-related fatalities) would occur through transfusions of RBCs,[194] because RBCs are the most frequently transfused blood component.[43] An epidemic of such a TTI could be prevented in the future only if an effective PR system(s) targeting all blood components (RBCs, plasma, and platelets) were to be introduced before the next transfusion-transmitted pathogen accumulated in blood donors. Absent such an all-encompassing (as well as effective and safe) PR system, the epidemic of the next major ("HIV-like" or "WNV-like") transfusion-transmitted pathogen to emerge in the future cannot be prevented and can be contained only by ensuring the avoidance of unnecessary transfusions through development and implementation of evidence-based transfusion guidelines for all blood components. Such a strategy must be combined with a "paradigm shift" (Chapter 8) that would regard ABT not as the "default" therapeutic option for nonbleeding patients but as an option to be used only when there is no (safer) alternative. Such interventions for reducing the number of ABTs (and thereby the number of exposures to allogeneic donors) through policies developed and enforced by hospital blood banks and medical staffs are considered in Chapter 4. Blood suppliers could also protect transfusion recipients from the next fatal transfusion-transmitted pathogen if they ceased production and distribution of (nonpathogen-reduced) pooled blood components whenever nonpooled alternatives can be substituted without jeopardizing the availability of the blood components needed for transfusion.

Preventable Risk of TTIs Due to Transfusions of Pooled Blood Components

Simple arithmetic indicates that pooled blood components should not be transfused when nonpooled alternatives are available. However, 12.9% of therapeutic platelet doses are still transfused as platelet pools in the United States,[43] even though apheresis (single-donor) platelets could be used instead.[71] If the prevalence of the next TTI to emerge in blood donors were p, we can assume that 1) a particular transfusion recipient has a negligible probability of receiving >1 infectious unit (ie, each distributed blood component contaminated with the new pathogen will infect a different transfusion recipient and will therefore represent a new case of the TTI); 2) all transfusion recipients are at risk, that is, there is a negligible probability of an infectious component's being given to a transfusion recipient who is already infected; and 3) the probability that at least one donor of the four, five, or six donors to a pool of four to six WBD platelets is infectious approximates 4p to 6p.

In the case of an emerging transfusion-transmitted virus similar to HIV or WNV, infectivity in blood or plasma (number of infectious copies/milliliter) is usually so high that any patient transfused with even a few milliliters of blood or plasma could contract the infection. Thus, if the next TTI to emerge had the characteristics of (chronic) HIV or (acute) WNV infection, pools of four or six platelet concentrates would have four or six times the transmission risk associated with an apheresis (single-donor) platelet concentrate, no matter what manipulations were attempted during the manufacturing process to minimize the plasma contribution of each of the four to six individual donors to the platelet pool. (As discussed in Chapter 3, these manipulations aim at removing plasma-associated infectivity, and thus they usually consist of the removal of as much of the donor plasma from each platelet concentrate as possible, followed by resuspension of the platelets in a platelet additive solution.)

Two studies have examined whether the increase in donor exposures owing to the use of pooled (rather than single-donor) platelets is clinically important in the context of the total number of allogeneic donors to whom a patient is exposed through transfusions of RBC and plasma components in addition to platelets. A recent study[195] that used pools consisting of four WBD platelets considered the total number of allogeneic donors (including donors of RBC and plasma components) to whom recipients of pooled WBD platelets, but not apheresis platelets, had been exposed. Compared with recipients of apheresis platelets, hematology-oncology patients receiving pooled platelets were exposed to 2.6 to 2.8 times as many—and surgical patients to 1.7 to 1.9 times as many—total allogeneic donors. Similarly, when pools of seven WBD platelets were used from 1991 through 1995,[196] the number of total allogeneic donors to whom each platelet transfusion recipient was exposed in association with pooled platelets was three to four times as high for hematology-oncology and 1.5 to 2 times as high for cardiac surgery patients as the exposure for patients receiving apheresis (single-donor) platelets.

For the sake of simplicity, it is presumed here that two assumptions cancel each other out. The first of these assumptions pertains to the potentially lower risk of known TTIs in plateletpheresis donors than in whole-blood donors. The second assumption concerns the possibility that infected plateletpheresis donors may donate more than once during the window period of HBV infection.

The prevalence of HIV, HCV, and HBV infection is 6 to 25 times ($p<0.05$) lower in ARC plateletpheresis donations than in whole-blood donations.[197] Such a lower TTI prevalence would translate into a lower risk of transmission of these TTIs after transfusion of apheresis (single-donor) platelets than of pooled WBD platelets if the lower TTI prevalence correlated with lower TTI incidence in donors, but this author knows of no published evidence of such a correlation.[198] The lack of such a correlation is shown with the ARC data[197] in Figs 8-1 through 8-4 and Table 8-5. When HIV nucleic acid, HCV nucleic acid, and HBc (antibody to the HBV core antigen) testing is performed in addition to testing for HIV and HCV antibody and PRISM (Abbott Laboratories, Abbott Park, IL) HBV surface antigen (HBsAg), the window periods of HIV, HCV, and HBV infection (in days, along with the associated 95% CI) are 9.5 (8.2-10.8), 8.0 (6.8-9.2), and 38.3 (33.0-43.7) days, respectively.[199] It is possible that a donor who has denied all risk factors may develop incident HBV infection during the 38.3-day window period; cases of such multiple transmissions (by an infected plateletpheresis donor who donates more than once during the window period of her or his HBV infection) have been reported,[200] albeit only in settings that do not test for HBc. This author knows of no such case reported from a blood system that performs testing for HBc.

In theory, even in countries using testing for HBc, the possibility of a plateletpheresis donor's donating more than once during the window period of HBV infection remains, as does the possibility that a 25-fold lower prevalence of HBV infection in plateletpheresis donors than in whole-blood donors (see Fig 8-3) may correlate with a lower incidence of HBV infection in donors denying all risk factors and therefore also with a lower risk of HBV transmission to platelet transfusion recipients. As there is no published evidence for either of these possibilities, they were not considered in the calculations discussed in the next section.

Projected Number of Transmissions of TTIs and of Cases of TAS Owing to the Continuing Use of Platelet Pools in the United States

Figure 2-16 shows the derivation of the contemporary risk of TAS secondary to platelet transfusions, as estimated by Vamvakas[71] and Vamvakas and Blajchman.[5] The depicted historical risks are based on empirical data from settings[18,32] in which all febrile reactions to platelet transfusions were monitored and followed by culture of the transfused components.[33,71] More specifically, the depicted historical risks (1 per 3000 platelet pools and 1 per 15,000 single-donor concentrates) are based on the seminal observational study conducted at the Johns Hopkins Hospital when that hospital moved toward transfusing 100% of therapeutic platelet doses as apheresis concentrates.[32] The same historical risk (1 per 3000 platelet pools) was also observed during the initial 2 years of the Quebec hemovigilance program under conditions approaching active surveillance.

In very approximate terms, based on the studies reviewed by McDonald and Blajchman,[39] it is assumed here that the process improvements introduced around 2004 [improved donor-arm disinfection, diversion of the initial flow of donor blood (presumed to contain most skin contaminants) from the collection bag into a pouch, overnight hold of the collected whole blood in the European studies, and/or WBC reduction]—interventions whose precise design and timing of introduction varied between settings[39]—reduced the risk of TAS by 50%. Moreover, it is assumed, also in very approximate terms, that bacterial culture of platelet components introduced in 2004 reduced the risk of TAS by a further 50%. This latter reduction in the magnitude of the risk is supported by a mathematical model,[62] an inoculation experiment,[63] and the ARC passive surveillance study[64] that observed a risk of TAS amounting to 1 per 40,000 transfused apheresis concentrates and 1 per 75,000 transfused apheresis

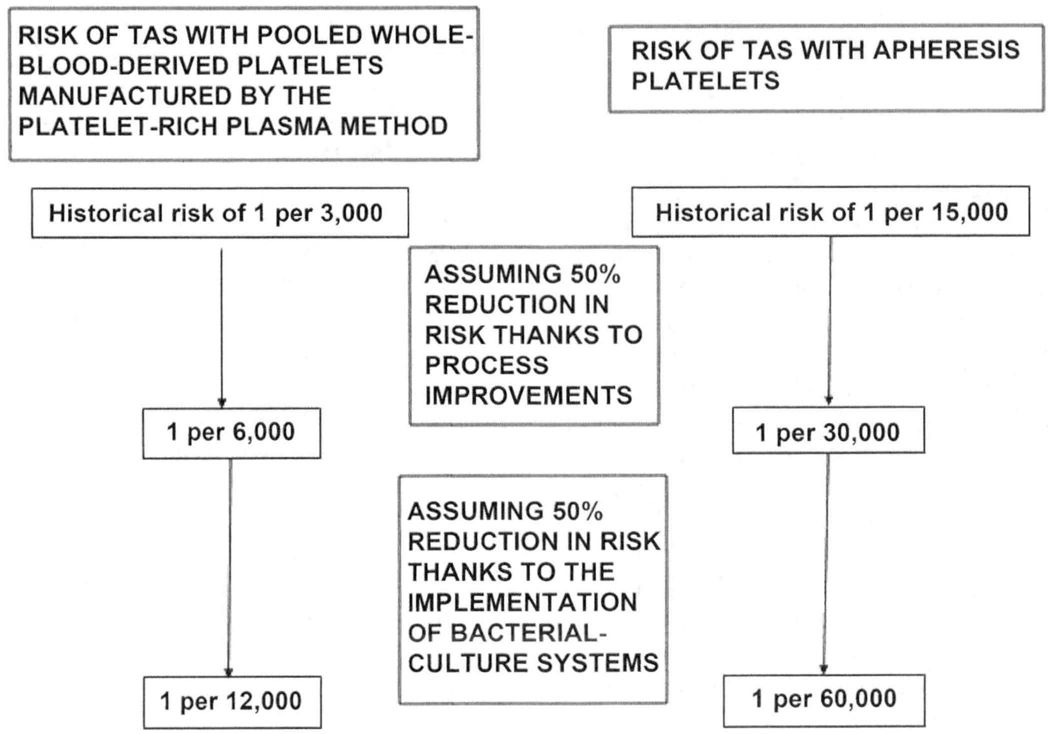

Figure 2-16. Estimation of the risk of transfusion-associated sepsis (TAS) from platelet transfusions in the United States today (see text). Initially published by Vamvakas and Blajchman in Transfus Med 2010;24:77-124.[5]

concentrates before and after, respectively, the implementation of bacterial culture.

The resulting estimate for the contemporary risk of TAS secondary to single-donor concentrates (1 per 60,000) is consistent with the results of passive surveillance studies reported from the ARC,[64,69] which observed–after the implementation of culture of 4 mL of platelet product in 2004-2006–a risk of symptomatic TAS (diagnosed by the local transfusion service as TAS and reported as such passively to the ARC) of 1 per 75,000 single-donor concentrates; and–after the implementation of culture of 8 mL of platelet product in 2007-2008–a risk of 1 per 87,000 single-donor concentrates.

Both the historical[32] and current[64,69] risk of TAS secondary to apheresis platelets shown in the figure is consistent with published empirical observations from observational[32] or passive surveillance[64,69] studies. In the case of platelet pools, only the historical risk is supported by empirical observations from observational[32] or active surveillance studies.[18] Passive surveillance studies[64] have reported a contemporary risk of TAS secondary to platelet pools lower than that shown in Fig 2-16. However, because the estimate of the historical risk of TAS secondary to platelet pools is robust,[18,32] and because both process improvements and bacterial culture similar to the ones implemented for plateletpheresis collections have by now been implemented for whole-blood collections as well, it is reasonable to extrapolate that the fourfold reduction in risk documented for apheresis (single-donor) concentrates because of all these measures[39,62-64,69] (Fig

2-16) should apply to pooled WBD platelets as well.

The reason that passive surveillance studies[64] have reported a contemporary risk of TAS secondary to pooled platelets lower than the risk shown in the figure may be that environments transfusing pooled platelets have a lower awareness of TAS than do environments transfusing apheresis (single-donor) platelets and/or that environments transfusing pooled platelets expend fewer resources on monitoring and working up febrile reactions to platelet transfusions.[130] Although no proof exists for this assertion, the decision to continue to transfuse noncultured platelet pools after bacterial culture had been mandated for apheresis platelets[19] was, in many cases, an economic decision–perhaps made in environments affording less attention and fewer resources to ABT than did environments that moved to a 100% apheresis supply for platelet transfusions in 2004.

Platelets were prepared from 16.9% of allogeneic whole-blood units in 2006, compared with 30.3% in 2004.[43]An even larger reduction in the proportion of platelet pools had been realized between 2002 and 2004, which indicated that–had there been a mandate to do so–blood establishments could probably have replaced the remaining pools with apheresis (single-donor) platelets by 2009. Of 2.021 million apheresis dose-equivalents transfused in the United States in 2008, 0.260 million (12.9%) were transfused as pools.[43] In 2008, pools had been usually made from five WBD platelets (compared with six WBD platelets in 2006).[43] Rather than relying on 1.3 million whole-blood donors in 2008, these platelet doses could have been collected from 260,000 plateletpheresis donors, thereby avoiding 1.04 million exposures of platelet transfusion recipients to allogeneic donors. The risk from continuing to transfuse 12.9% of platelet doses as pooled platelets is the annual number of infectious platelet pools that would no longer be transfused in the United States if all platelet doses were transfused as apheresis (single-donor) platelets. These preventable donor exposures from the continued use of pools result in a small number of HIV, HCV, and HBV transmissions and 86.7 cases of TAS every year (Table 2-1 and Fig 2-17).[199] Perhaps much more important, these preventable donor exposures would generate 104 transmissions in the year preceding the introduction of testing if the next major transfusion-transmitted pathogen to emerge in the United States were "HIV-like"; and 18.7 transmissions in the year in which the first major epidemic occurred before the introduction of testing if the next agent were "WNV-like" (Table 2-1 and Fig 2-17).[71] These latter risks, as well as the small risks of HIV, HCV, and HBV transmissions owing to window-period infections,[199-203] would apply regardless of whether 12.9% of platelet doses continued to be transfused in the United States as platelet pools manufactured by the PRP method or whether the United States converted to using platelet pools manufactured by the buffy-coat method.[204] The only risk secondary to the continued use of platelet pools that could be prevented by a conversion to the buffy-coat method for manufacturing WBD platelets is the risk of TAS (Fig 2-5).[71] Studies from Europe have shown no difference in the risk of bacterial contamination between buffy-coat platelet pools and apheresis platelets.

The preventable transmissions of HIV, HCV, and HBV infection depicted in Fig 2-17 are due to "window-period" infections and are based on published mathematical models of the residual risk of transmission.[71,199,201,202] Observed numbers of known TTIs do not approach these modeled estimates,[203] either because transmissions are underrecognized or underreported with current surveillance, or because the assumptions made in the published models[199,201,202] are overly conservative.[203]

Of the preventable infectious risks owing to the continued use of platelet pools in the United States depicted in Fig 2-17, the one potentially associated with the greatest number of transfusion-related fatalities would be the emergence of the next HIV-like pathogen.[1] Although most transfusion recipients infected with HIV in the 1980s did not live long enough to develop AIDS, the transfusion-acquired AIDS epidemic of the 1980s was still responsible for close to 1000 deaths.[1] Most of the transmissions of the next WNV-like pathogen to emerge in the future

Table 2-1. Expected Reduction in the Annual Number of TTI Transmissions and TAS Cases Occurring in the United States When *All* Platelet Doses Are Transfused as Apheresis (Single-Donor) Platelets

2.021 million apheresis (single-donor) dose equivalents transfused in the US in 2008*:

- 1.761 million (87.1%) transfused as apheresis (single-donor) platelets
- 0.260 million (12.9%) transfused as pooled whole-blood-derived platelets

For therapeutic platelet doses provided as pooled whole-blood-derived platelets:

- 1.3 million whole-blood donors were used
- these patient needs could have been met instead by 260,000 donors of apheresis (single-donor) platelets
- thereby avoiding 1.04 million exposures of transfusion recipients to allogeneic donors

In theory, the 260,000 therapeutic platelet doses provided as platelet pools in 2008 could have been harvested from:

- 13,000 apheresis donors who donate 10 times a year on average and whose *every* plateletpheresis donation is split

OR

- 26,000 apheresis donors who donate 5 times a year on average and whose *every* plateletpheresis donation is split

OR

- 34,667 apheresis donors who donate 5 times a year on average and whose *half* the plateletpheresis donations are split

OR

- 650,000 whole-blood donors who donate twice a year on average and whose 1.3 million donations generate 260,000 platelet pools

OR

- Any other combination of assumptions regarding:1) the number of apheresis (vs whole-blood) donors; 2) the corresponding average number of donations per year by apheresis (vs whole-blood) donors; and 3) the corresponding "split rate" of plateletpheresis components at US blood centers.

If the next HIV-like transfusion-transmitted pathogen attained a prevalence of 1 per 10,000 in US blood donors in the year before testing was introduced, the aforementioned approaches to harvesting 260,000 therapeutic platelet doses would correspondingly result in:

- 13,000 times 10 times 2 divided by 10,000 = 26 recipient infections with the new HIV-like pathogen
- 26,000 times 5 times 2 divided by 10,000 = 26 recipient infections
- 34,667 times 5 (ie, 173,335) plus 86,667 (the one half of the 173,335 collections that are split) divided by 10,000 = 26 recipient infections
- 650,000 times 2 divided by 10,000 = 130 recipient infections

Table 2-1. Expected Reduction in the Annual Number of TTI Transmissions and TAS Cases Occurring in the United States When *All* Platelet Doses Are Transfused as Apheresis (Single-Donor) Platelets (Continued)

Regardless of the number of apheresis (vs whole-blood) donors actually used to harvest 260,000 therapeutic platelet doses [which depends on the average number of donations per year by apheresis (vs whole-blood) donors and the "split rate" of plateletpheresis components at US blood centers], if platelet pools are made from 5 whole-blood-derived platelet concentrates, the total number of resulting recipient infections in the population of all recipients of 260,000 platelet doses will always be 5 times higher if platelet pools rather than apheresis (single-donor) concentrates are used.† Thus:

- 1.04 million preventable allogeneic donor exposures (owing to the use of pools) result in 104 preventable recipient infections with the next "HIV-like" pathogen:
  - 130 (if platelet pools are used) minus 26 (if apheresis platelets are used to provide the 260,000 doses) = 104

  OR SIMPLY

  - 1.04 preventable allogeneic donor exposures divided by 10,000 = 104

Risk of TTI in the US today‡	Expected annual reduction in the number of cases of TTIs if 1.04 million allogeneic donor exposures are prevented by the use of single-donor concentrates rather than platelet pools
HIV: 1 per 2.135 million donations[201]	0.48
HCV: 1 per 1.935 million donations[201]	0.54
HBV: 1 per 0.280 million donations[202,203]	3.7
Next WNV-like pathogen to emerge§	18.7
TAS: 1 per 12,000 platelet pools‖	86.7
Next HIV-like pathogen to emerge¶	104

*According to the *2009 National Blood Collection and Utilization Survey Report*.[43]

†A plateletpheresis donor donating 5 or 10 times a year and whose plateletpheresis donations are split would infect more recipients if s/he were infected with the next major HIV-like transfusion-transmitted pathogen than would a whole-blood donor donating 2 (or fewer) times a year. For example, a plateletpheresis donor donating 10 times in the year before the introduction of testing for a new HIV-like pathogen and whose every plateletpheresis donation is split would infect 20 transfusion recipients, while a whole-blood donor donating 2 times during that year would infect 2 transfusion recipients. However, the number of transmissions attributable to each individual donor would not influence the total number of resulting TTIs in the entire population of platelet transfusion recipients if 260,000 therapeutic platelet doses had to be harvested from a donor population in which the prevalence of the new pathogen was 1 per 10,000 plateletpheresis or whole-blood donors. Thus, when the entire population of all platelet transfusion recipients is considered, if the platelet pools were made from 4, 5, or 6 whole-blood donors, the transfusion of pools would correspondingly result in 4, 5, or 6 times more recipient infections compared with the transfusion of single-donor concentrates.

(Continued)

Table 2-1. Expected Reduction in the Annual Number of TTI Transmissions and TAS Cases Occurring in the United States When *All* Platelet Doses Are Transfused as Apheresis (Single-Donor) Platelets (Continued)

‡Based on published mathematical models of the residual risk of transmission of HIV, HCV, and HBV because of "window-period" infections.[201-203]
§Reproducing the WNV experience from the summer and fall of 2002. For this calculation, it is assumed that 380 infections would be contracted through ABT and that all blood components (RBCs, platelets, and plasma) made from whole blood are equally infectious. Of 23,668,000 blood components transfused in the US in 2008,[43] 1,040,000 component transfusions (4.39%) could be prevented if the platelet pools were replaced by single-donor concentrates (with 4.39% of the 380 transmissions of the new WNV-like pathogen also prevented).
||Risk estimate derived in Fig 2-16.
¶Assuming that, at the peak of the epidemic before measures are introduced to interrupt transmission through ABT, the next HIV-like pathogen to emerge in the future will have reached a prevalence of 1 per 10,000 donations in the population of eligible US blood donors.

would result in asymptomatic disease, with a minority of transmissions progressing to symptomatic disease and only a very small proportion of the transmissions resulting in a transfusion recipient's death. Similarly, the cases of TAS depicted in Fig 2-17 range from febrile reactions to platelet transfusions not suspected of being TAS to transfusion reactions suspected of being TAS, perhaps investigated as being TAS, and sometimes passively reported to the local blood center as TAS. Only a small minority of the cases of TAS depicted in the figure would thus result in a transfusion recipient's death. In the ARC passive surveillance study of 2004-2006,[64] the fatality rate corresponding to a TAS risk of 1 per 75,000 apheresis platelets was 1 per 500,000 transfusions of apheresis (single-donor) platelets; there were three fatalities in the 2004-2006[64] study and no fatalities in the follow-up (2007-2008) study.[69] If 1 per 20 cases of TAS were fatal, the continued transfusion of 0.260 million platelet doses as platelet pools in the United States could be causing, each year, an incremental risk of 4.4 preventable TAS deaths from platelet transfusion.

Conclusions

Despite the uncertainty about the mechanisms and frequency of TAS and TRALI, measures implemented in 2004[19] to limit and detect bacterial contamination in all platelet components and in 2006-2007[20] to collect plasma and apheresis (single-donor) platelets solely from male donors (or from female donors who have not previously been pregnant or who do not have circulating WBC antibodies) have been associated with a reduction in the number of the reported deaths from TAS and TRALI (Fig 2-18). After the implementation of these measures, the total number of transfusion-related deaths reported to the FDA in 2010 was 40, as compared with 62 in 2005.[9] Deaths from TAS were reduced from 8 in 2005 to 1 in 2010 (Fig 2-18)[9]; deaths from TRALI were reduced from 29 in 2005 to 18 in 2010 (Fig 2-18).[9] It is important that the implementation of the use of male-only plasma reduced the number of ABT-related fatalities associated with plasma transfusion by approximately sixfold (see the number of fatalities reported to the FDA in 2010 compared with the number in 2006; Fig 2-4). However, the use of male-only plasma did not completely prevent such deaths; furthermore, when the total number of deaths due to TRALI associated with all blood components is considered, male-only plasma and the reduction in plateletpheresis collections from female donors who have been pregnant or who have circulating WBC antibodies have reduced the total number of TRALI

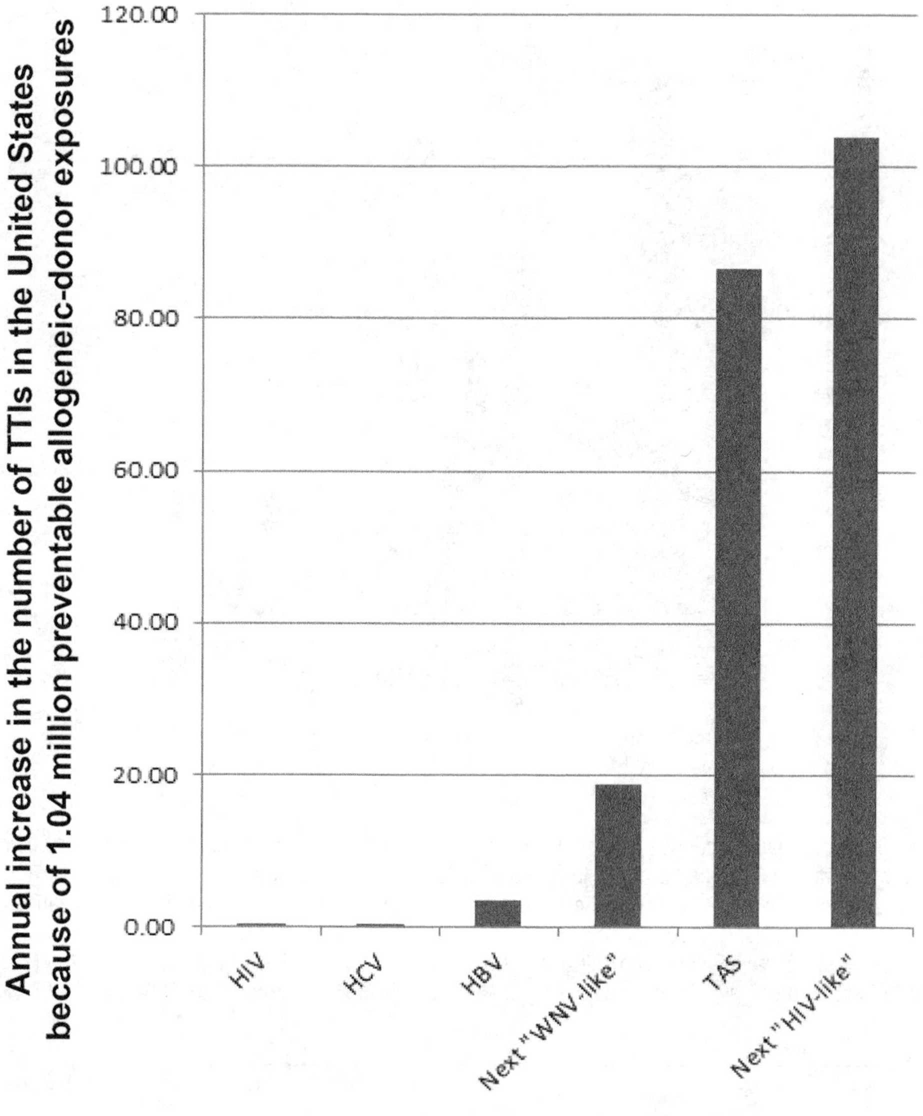

Figure 2-17. Effect of the use of pooled blood components when nonpooled equivalents are available. The figure shows the annual increase in the number of transfusion-transmitted infections (TTIs) contracted in the United States because of the 1.04 million preventable allogeneic-donor exposures that result from the continued transfusion of 12.9% of platelet doses as pooled (rather than apheresis) platelets.[43]
TAS = transfusion-associated sepsis.

deaths by approximately 50% (Fig 2-19). TRALI thus remains the leading cause of ABT-related deaths in the United States (Fig 2-18), and more needs to be done to prevent this fatal complication of ABT.

Deaths due to ABO HTRs—which were slightly fewer than five per year in each of the years from 2005 through 2010 (Fig 2-12)—were also reduced, from the 1990s figure based on New York State data (1 death per 1.8 million

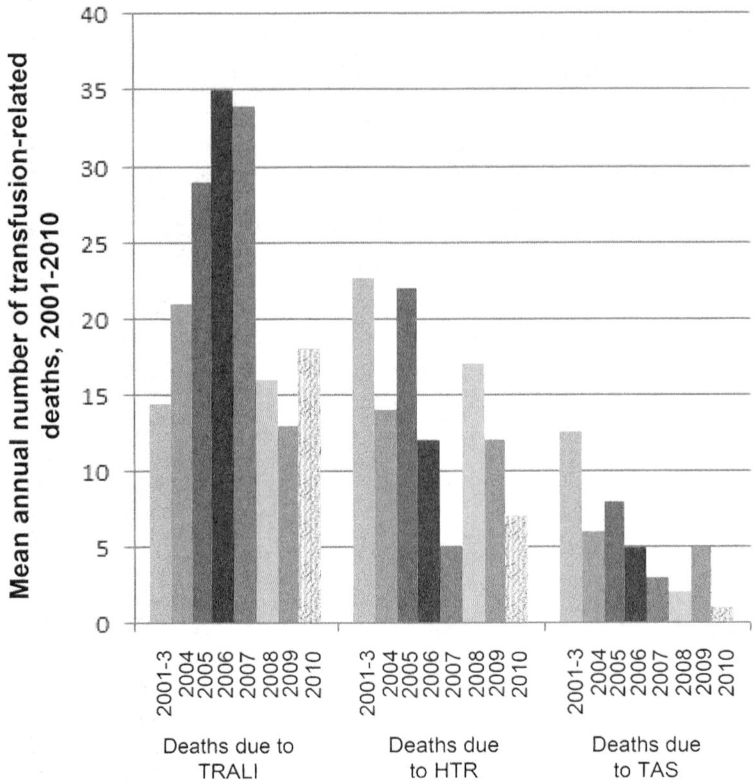

Figure 2-18. The three leading causes of transfusion-related deaths in the first decade of the 21st century (2001-2010) were transfusion-related acute lung injury (TRALI), hemolytic transfusion reaction (HTR), and transfusion-associated sepsis (TAS). Shown here are the mean annual number of deaths from each cause passively reported to the Food and Drug Administration in each year from 2001 through 2010.[9,130] The numbers depicted incorporate both the effect of increasing awareness of the risks of TAS (see Fig 2-3) and TRALI (see Fig 2-4) and the effect of the preventive measures for TAS[19] and TRALI[20] introduced in 2004 and 2006-2007, respectively.

RBC units[133]; Fig 2-11) to 1 per 3 million RBC units (on the basis of the number of deaths passively reported to the FDA[9] and the national data on RBC transfusions[43]). The total (ABO and non-ABO) number of deaths from HTRs (currently 1 death per 1.2 million RBC units[9,43]), however, remains largely unchanged from that in the previous decades; the reason for this lack of progress is the increase in the number of reported deaths due to non-ABO HTRs as awareness is increasing that non-ABO HTRs (Figs 2-12 and 2-18) can indeed contribute to a patient's death. Unlike the risk of TAS[19] and TRALI,[20] the risk of HTRs has not yet been specifically addressed via the implementation of a preventive measure(s) required for all RBC transfusions administered in the United States.

Although TAS, TRALI, and HTRs continue to cause transfusion-related deaths in the United States, the greatest threat to blood transfusion safety is the possible appearance in the future of a novel and fatal TTI that could reach a prevalence as high as 1 per 10,000 US blood donors[71] before measures are introduced to pre-

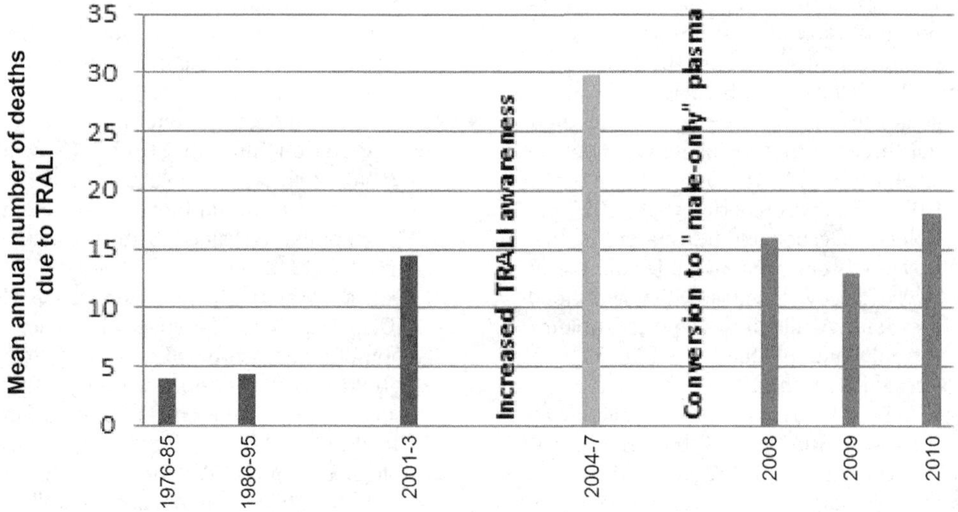

Figure 2-19. Effect of the increasing awareness of the risk of transfusion-related acute lung injury (TRALI) in the first decade of the 21st century and the effect of the preventive measures for TRALI introduced in 2006-2007[20] on the number of TRALI deaths passively reported to the Food and Drug Administration in association with transfusion of all blood components.[9,130] Implementation of the use of "male-only" plasma in 2006-2007 reduced by sixfold the number of TRALI deaths secondary to transfusion of plasma (see Fig 2-4), but it was associated with a reduction of only about 50% in the total number of TRALI deaths secondary to transfusion of all blood components. The greater TRALI awareness in 2004-2007 than in 2001-2003 had an effect of approximately the same magnitude on the total number of passively reported TRALI deaths as did the implementation of "male-only" plasma in 2006-2007.[20]

vent its transmission through ABT. Chapter 3 examines the complexities of investigating whether a new and fatal infectious disease may prove to be a fatal TTI or, worse yet, a TTI amounting to almost an HIV-like risk to blood transfusion safety. Chapter 4 builds upon the estimates of ABT-related mortality presented here to advocate the adoption of specific risk-reduction strategies for further decreasing ABT-related mortality in the United States in the 21st century.

References

1. Peterman TA, Lui K-J, Lawrence DN, Allen JR. Estimating the risks of transfusion-associated acquired immune deficiency syndrome and human immunodeficiency virus infection. Transfusion 1987;27:371-4.
2. Alter HJ. Pathogen reduction: A precautionary principle paradigm. Transfus Med Rev 2008; 22:97-102.
3. Seef LB, Hollinger FB, Alter HJ, et al. Long-term mortality and morbidity of transfusion-associated non-A, non-B, and type C hepatitis: A National Heart, Lung, and Blood Institute Collaborative Study. Hepatology 2001;33:455-63.
4. Vamvakas EC, Taswell HF. Long-term survival after blood transfusion. Transfusion 1994; 34:471-7.
5. Vamvakas EC, Blajchman MA. Blood still kills: Six strategies to further reduce allogeneic blood transfusion-related mortality. Transfus Med Rev 2010;24:77-124.
6. Dodd RY. Germs, gels, and genomes: A personal recollection of 30 years in blood-safety testing.

In: Stramer SL, ed. Blood safety in the new millennium. Bethesda, MD: AABB, 2001:99-121.
7. Murphy W. Managing threats rather than risks in blood transfusion: Robust design for a complex system. Transfusion 2006;46:2011-13.
8. Stramer SL, Hollinger FB, Katz LM, et al. Emerging infectious disease agents and their potential threat to transfusion safety. Transfusion 2009;49(Suppl 2):1S-236S.
9. FDA/CBER. Fatalities reported to the FDA following blood collection and transfusion. Annual summary for fiscal year 2010. [Available at http://www.fda.gov/downloads/BiologicsBlood Vaccines/SafetyAvailability/ReportaProblem/ TransfusionDonationFatalities/UCM254860. htm (accessed May 25, 2011).]
10. Honig CL, Bove JR. Transfusion-associated fatalities: Review of Bureau of Biologics reports, 1976-78. Transfusion 1980;20:653-61.
11. Sazama K. Reports of 355 transfusion-associated deaths: 1976 through 1985. Transfusion 1990;30:583-90.
12. Holness L, Knippen MA, Simmons L, Lachenburch PA. Fatalities caused by TRALI. Transfus Med Rev 2004;18:184-8.
13. Holness L, Knippen M, Simmons L. Characteristics of donors implicated in fatal transfusion-related acute lung injury (TRALI) reactions. [Available at http://www.accessdata.fda.gov/ ScienceForums/forum06/K-34.htm (accessed May 25, 2011).]
14. Holness L, Jones P, Knippen M, et al. 19-year review of fatalities due to contaminated blood and blood components. [Available at http:// www.accessdata.fda.gov/ScienceForums/ forum06/K-35.htm (accessed May 25, 2011).]
15. Andreu G, Morel P, Forester F, et al. Hemovigilance network in France: Organization and analysis of immediate transfusion incident reports from 1994 to 1998. Transfusion 2002;42: 1356-64.
16. Serious Hazards of Transfusion (SHOT). Annual reports. Manchester, UK: SHOT office, 2011. [Available at http://www.shot-uk.org (accessed May 25, 2011).]
17. Stainsby D, Jones H, Asher D, et al. Serious Hazards of Transfusion: A decade of hemovigilance in the UK. Transfus Med Rev 2006;20:237-82.
18. Robillard P, Nawej KI, Jochem K. The Quebec hemovigilance system: Description and results from the first two years. Transfus Apher Sci 2004;31:111-22.
19. Further guidance on methods to detect bacterial contamination of platelet components. AABB Association Bulletin #03-12 (October 1, 2003). Bethesda, MD: AABB, 2003. [Available at http://www.aabb. org/resources/publications/ bulletins/Documents/obsolete/AB%2003-12%20OBSO LETE.pdf (accessed October 12, 2011).]
20. Transfusion-related acute lung injury. AABB Association Bulletin #06-07 (November 3, 2006). Bethesda, MD: AABB, 2006. [Available at http://www. aabb.org/resources/publica tions/bulletins/Pages/ab06-07.aspx (accessed October 12, 2011).]
21. van de Watering LMG, Hermans J, Houbiers JGA, et al. Beneficial effect of leukocyte depletion of transfused blood on post-operative complications in patients undergoing cardiac surgery: A randomized clinical trial. Circulation 1998;97:562-8.
22. Bilgin YM, van de Watering LMG, Eijsman L, et al. Double-blind, randomized controlled trial on the effect of leukocyte-depleted erythrocyte transfusions in cardiac-valve surgery. Circulation 2004;109:2755-60.
23. Hébert PC, Wells G, Blajchman MA, et al. A multicenter randomized controlled trial of transfusion requirements in critical care. N Engl J Med 1999;340:409-17.
24. Centers for Disease Control and Prevention. The National Healthcare Safety Network (NHSN) manual: Biovigilance component. Atlanta, GA: CDC Division of Healthcare Quality Promotions, 2010. [Available at http:// www.cdc.gov/nhsn/PDFs/hemovigModule Protocol_current.pdf (accessed May 25, 2011).]
25. Robillard P, Hyson C, McCombie N. TRALI, possible TRALI and respiratory complications of transfusion reported to the Canadian Transfusion-Transmitted Injuries Surveillance System (abstract). Transfusion 2007;47(Suppl):5A.
26. Silliman CC, Boshkov LK, Mehdizadehkashi Z, et al. Transfusion-related acute lung injury: Epidemiology and a prospective analysis of etiologic factors. Blood 2003;101:454-62.
27. Gajic O, Rana R, Winters JL, et al. Transfusion-related acute lung injury in the critically ill: Prospective nested case-control study. Am J Respir Crit Care Med 2007;176:886-91.
28. Kleinman S, Caulfield T, Chan P, et al. Toward an understanding of transfusion-related acute lung injury: Statement of a consensus panel. Transfusion 2004;44:1774-89.
29. Bux J, Sachs UJ. The pathogenesis of transfusion-related acute lung injury (TRALI). Br J Haematol 2007;136:788-99.

30. Kehler MR, Masumo T, Moore EE, et al. Plasma from stored packed red blood cells and MHC class I antibodies causes acute lung injury in a 2-event in vivo rat model. Blood 2009;113: 2079-87.
31. Silliman CC, Ambruso DR, Boshkov LK. Transfusion-related acute lung injury. Blood 2005; 105:2266-73.
32. Ness P, Braine N, King K, et al. Single-donor platelets reduce the risk of septic platelet transfusion reactions. Transfusion 2001;41:857-61.
33. Ness PM, Campbell-Lee SA. Single-donor versus pooled random-donor platelet concentrates. Curr Opin Hematol 2001;8:392-6.
34. Zoon KC. Transfusion-related acute lung injury letter (October 19, 2001. Rockville, MD: CBER Office of Community Outreach, and Development, 2001. [Available at http://www.fda.gov/BiologicsBloodVaccines/SafetyAvailability/ucm105850.htm (accessed May 25, 2011).]
35. Bernard GR, Artigas A, Brigham KL, et al. The American-European Consensus Conference on ARDS: Definitions, mechanisms, relevant outcomes, and clinical trial co-ordination. Am J Respir Crit Care Med 1994;149:818-24.
36. Abraham E, Matthay MA, Dinarello CA, et al. Consensus conference definitions for sepsis, septic shock, acute lung injury, and acute respiratory distress syndrome: Time for a re-evaluation. Crit Care Med 2000;28:232-5.
37. Meade MO, Guyatt GH, Cook RJ, et al. Agreement between alternative classifications of acute respiratory distress syndrome. Am J Respir Crit Care Med 2001;163:490-3.
38. Toy P, Popovsky MA, Abraham E, et al. Transfusion-related acute lung injury: Definition and review. Crit Care Med 2005;33:721-6.
39. McDonald CP, Blajchman MA. Bacterial contamination in blood and blood components. In: Barbara JSJ, Regan FAM, Contreras MC, eds. Transfusion microbiology. Cambridge, UK: Cambridge University Press, 2008:87-115.
40. Food and Drug Administration. Bacterial Contamination of Platelets Workshop. September 24, 1999. Rockville, MD: CBER Office of Community Outreach, and Development, 1999. [Available at http://www.fda.gov/downloads/BiologicsBloodVaccines/NewsEvents/Workshops/MeetingsConferences/TranscriptsMinutes/UCM055446.pdf (accessed September 19, 2011).]
41. Brecher ME, Hay SN. Bacterial contamination of blood components. Clin Microbiol Rev 2005; 18:195-204.
42. Silva MA, Gregory KR, Carr-Greer MA, et al. Summary of the AABB Interorganizational Task Force on Bacterial Contamination of Platelets: Fall 2004 impact survey. Transfusion 2006;46: 636-41.
43. US Department of Health and Human Services. The 2009 national blood collection and utilization survey report. Washington, DC: DHHS, 2011.
44. Wallis JP, Lubenko A, Wells AW, Chapman CE. Single-hospital experience of TRALI. Transfusion 2003;43:1053-9.
45. Roth VR, Kuehnert MJ, Haley NR, et al. Evaluation of a reporting system for bacterial contamination of blood components in the United States. Transfusion 2001;41:1486-92.
46. Zou S, Wu Y, Cable R, et al. A prospective study of multiple-donor-exposure blood recipients: Surveillance value and limitations for hemovigilance. Transfusion 2010;50:128-38.
47. Tambyah PA, Koay ESC, Poon MLM, et al. Dengue hemorrhagic fever transmitted by blood transfusion. N Engl J Med 2008; 359:1526-7.
48. Seed CR, Kiely P, Hyland CA, Keller AJ. The risk of dengue transmission by blood during a 2004 outbreak in Cairns, Australia. Transfusion 2009;49:1482-7.
49. Gubernot DM, Lucey CT, Leek C, et al. Babesia infection through blood transfusions: Reports received by the US Food and Drug Administration, 1997-2007. Clin Infect Dis 2009;48:25-30.
50. Gubernot DM, Nakhasi HL, Mied PA, et al. Transfusion-transmitted babesiosis in the United States: Summary of a workshop. Transfusion 2009;49:2759-71.
51. Tonelti L, Eder AE, Dy B, et al. Transfusion-transmitted *Babesia microti* identified through hemovigilance. Transfusion 2009;49:2557-63.
52. Goldman M, Blajchman MA. Blood products-associated bacterial sepsis. Transfus Med Rev 1991;5:73-83.
53. Blajchman MA, Ali AM. Bacteria in the blood supply: An overlooked issue in transfusion medicine. In: Nance SJ, ed. Blood safety: Current challenges. Bethesda, MD: AABB, 1992:213-28.
54. Perez P, Sahmi LR, Follea G, et al. Determinants of transfusion-associated bacterial contamination: Results of the French BACTHEM case-control study. Transfusion 2001;41:862-72.
55. Kuehnert MJ, Roth VR, Haley NR, et al. Transfusion-transmitted bacterial infection in the

United States, 1998 through 2000. Transfusion 2001;41:1493-9.
56. Brecher ME, Holland PV, Pineda AA, et al. Growth of bacteria in inoculated platelets: Implications for bacterial detection and the extension of platelet storage. Transfusion 2000;40:1308-12.
57. Wagner SJ, Maroff G, Katz AJ, Friedman LI. Comparison of bacterial growth in single and pooled platelet concentrations after deliberate inoculation and storage. Transfusion 1995;35: 298-303.
58. Heal JM, Jones ME, Forey J, et al. Fatal Salmonella septicemia after platelet transfusion. Transfusion 1987;27:2-5.
59. Kleinman S, Dumont LJ, Tomasulo P, et al. The impact of discontinuation of 7-day storage of apheresis platelets (PASSPORT) on recipient safety: An illustration of the need for proper risk assessments. Transfusion 2009;49:903-12.
60. Hogman CF, Engstrand L. Factors affecting growth of Yersinia enterocolitica in cellular blood platelets. Transfus Med Rev 1996; 10:259-75.
61. Murphy WG, Foley M, Doherty C, et al. Screening platelet concentrates for bacterial contamination: Low numbers of bacteria and slow growth in contaminated units mandate an alternate approach to product safety. Vox Sang 2008;95:13-19.
62. Benjamin RJ, Wagner SJ. The residual risk of sepsis: Modeling the effect of concentration on bacterial detection in two-bottle culture systems and an estimation of false-negative culture rates. Transfusion 2007;47:1381-9.
63. Nussbaumer W, Allesdorfer D, Grabmer C, et al. Prevention of transfusion of platelet components contaminated with low levels of bacteria: A comparison of bacterial culture and pathogen inactivation methods. Transfusion 2007; 47:1125-33.
64. Eder AF, Kennedy JM, Dy BA, et al. Bacterial screening of apheresis platelets and the residual risk of septic transfusion reactions: The American Red Cross experience (2004-2006). Transfusion 2007;47:1134-42.
65. Ramirez-Arcos S, Chin-Yee I, Hume H, et al. Fatal septic shock associated with transfusion-transmitted *Serratia marcescens*. Transfusion 2006;46:679-81.
66. Ramirez-Arcos S, Jenkins C, Dion J, et al. Canadian experience with detection of bacterial contamination in apheresis platelets. Transfusion 2007;47:421-9.
67. de Korte D, Curvers K, de Kort WL, et al. Effects of skin disinfection method, deviation bag, and bacterial screening on clinical safety of platelet transfusions in the Netherlands. Transfusion 2006;46:476-85.
68. Schmidt M. Comparison of different methods of bacterial detection in blood components. ISBT Sci Ser 2009;4:80-6.
69. Eder AF, Kennedy JM, Dy BA, et al. Limiting and detecting bacterial contamination of apheresis platelets: Inlet-line diversion and increased culture volume improve component safety. Transfusion 2009;49:1554-63.
70. Fuller AK, Uglik KM, Savage WM, et al. Bacterial culture reduces but does not eliminate the risk of septic transfusion reactions to single-donor platelets. Transfusion 2009;49:2588-93.
71. Vamvakas EC. Relative safety of pooled whole-blood-derived versus single-donor (apheresis) platelets in the United States: A systematic review of disparate risks. Transfusion 2009;49: 2743-58.
72. Yomtovian RA, Palavecino EL, Dysktra AH, et al. Evolution of surveillance methods for detection of bacterial contamination of platelets in a university hospital, 1991 through 2004. Transfusion 2006;46:719-30.
73. Kleinman SH, Kamel HT, Harpool DR, et al. Two-year experience with aerobic culturing of apheresis and whole-blood-derived platelets. Transfusion 2006;46:1787-94.
74. Benjamin RJ, Kline L, Dy BA, et al. Bacterial contamination of whole-blood-derived platelets: The introduction of sample diversion and prestorage pooling with culture testing in the American Red Cross. Transfusion 2008;48: 2348-55.
75. Larsen CP, Ezligini F, Hermansen NO, Kjeldsen-Kragh J. Six years' experience of using the Bact/ALERT system to screen all platelet concentrates to estimate the frequency of false-negative results. Vox Sang 2005;88:93-7.
76. Schrezenmeier H, Walther-Wenke G, Mullter TH, et al. Bacterial contamination of platelet concentrates: Results of a prospective multicenter study comparing pooled whole-blood-derived platelets and apheresis platelets. Transfusion 2007;47:644-52.
77. Mohr H, Bayer A, Gravemann U, Muller TH. Elimination and multiplication of bacteria during preparation and storage of buffy-coat-derived platelet concentrates. Transfusion 2006;46:949-55.

78. Pearce S, Rowe GP, Field SP. Screening of platelets for bacterial contamination at the Welsh Blood Service. Transfus Med 2010;21:25-32.
79. Walther-Wenke G, Wirsing von Konig CH, Daubener W, et al. Monitoring bacterial contamination of blood components in Germany: Effect of contamination reduction measures. Vox Sang 2011;100:359-66.
80. Jacobs MR, Smith D, Heaton WA, Good CE. Detection of bacterial contamination in prestorage culture-negative apheresis platelets on day of issue with the Pan Genera Detection Test. Transfusion 2011;51:2573-82.
81. Middelberg RA, van Stein D, Briet E, van der Bom JG. The role of donor antibodies in the pathogenesis of transfusion-related acute lung injury: A systematic review. Transfusion 2008; 48:2167-76.
82. Chapman CE, Stainsby D, Jones D, et al. Ten years of hemovigilance reports of transfusion-related acute lung injury in the United Kingdom and the impact of the preferential use of male donor plasma. Transfusion 2009;49:440-52.
83. Eder AF, Herron R, Strupp A, et al. Transfusion-related acute lung injury surveillance (2003-2005) and the potential impact of the selective use of plasma from male donors in the American Red Cross. Transfusion 2007;47:599-607.
84. Keller-Stanislawski B, Reil A, Gunay S, Funk MB. Frequency and severity of transfusion-related acute lung injury: German hemovigilance data (2006-2007). Vox Sang 2010;98: 70-7.
85. Kopko PM, Paglieroni TG, Popovsky MA, et al. TRALI: Correlation of antigen-antibody and monocyte activation in donor-recipient pairs. Transfusion 2003;43:177-84.
86. Popovsky MA, Moore SB. Diagnostic and pathogenetic considerations in transfusion-related acute lung injury. Transfusion 1985;25:573-7.
87. Popovsky MA, Chaplin HC Jr., Moore SB. Transfusion-related acute lung injury: A neglected, serious complication of hemotherapy. Transfusion 1992;32:589-92.
88. Triulzi DJ, Kleinman S, Kakaiya RM, et al. The effect of previous pregnancy and transfusion on HLA alloimmunization in blood donors: Implications for a transfusion-related acute lung injury risk reduction strategy. Transfusion 2009;49:1825-35.
89. Webert MA, Blajchman MA. Transfusion-related acute lung injury. Curr Opin Hematol 2005; 12:480-7.
90. van Stein D, Beckers EA, Sintnicolaas E, et al. Transfusion-related acute lung injury reports in the Netherlands: An observational study. Transfusion 2010;50:213-20.
91. Middelburg RA, Porcelijn L, Lardy N, et al. Prevalence of leukocyte antibodies in the Dutch donor population. Vox Sang 2011;100:327-35.
92. Shaz BH, Stowell SR, Hillyer CD. Transfusion-related acute lung injury: From bedside to bench and back. Blood 2011;117:1463-71.
93. Eastlund T, McGrath PC, Burkart P. Platelet transfusion reaction associated with inter-donor HLA incompatibility. Vox Sang 1988;55:157-60.
94. Bux J, Hoch J, Bindl L, et al. Transfusion-associated acute pulmonary insufficiency. Diagnostic confirmation by the demonstration of granulocytic antibodies. J Dtsch Med Wochenschr 1994;119:19-24.
95. Ramanthan RK, Triulzi DJ, Logan TF. Transfusion-related acute lung injury following random-donor platelet transfusion: A report of two cases. Vox Sang 1997;73:43-5.
96. Lin Y, Kanani N, Naughton F, et al. Case report: Transfusion-related acute lung injury (TRALI)—A clear and present danger. Can J Anesth 2007;J4:1011-16.
97. Salman SS, Fernandez Perez ER, Stubbs JR, Gajic O. The practice of platelet transfusion in the intensive care unit. J Intern Care Med 2007;22:105-10.
98. Win N, Chapman CE, Bowles KM, et al. How much residual plasma may cause TRALI? Transfus Med 2008;18:276-80.
99. Silliman CC, Curtis BR, Kopko PM, et al. Donor antibodies to HNA-3a implicated in TRALI reactions prime neutrophils and cause PMN-mediated damage to human pulmonary microvascular endothelial cells in a two-event in vivo model. Blood 2007;109:1752-5.
100. ISBT Working Party on Granulocyte Immunobiology. Recommendations of the ISBT Working Party on Granulocyte Immunobiology for leukocyte antibody screening in the investigation and prevention of antibody-mediated transfusion-related acute lung injury. Vox Sang 2009;96: 266-9.
101. Reil A, Keller-Stanislawski B, Gunay S, Bux J. Specificities of leukocyte alloantibodies in transfusion-related acute lung injury and results of leukocyte antibody screening of blood donors. Vox Sang 2008;95:313-17.
102. Davoren A, Curtis RJ, Shulman IA, et al. TRALI due to granulocyte-agglutinating human neutro-

phil antigen-3a(5b) alloantibodies in donor plasma: A report of 2 fatalities. Transfusion 2003;43:641-5.
103. Gottschall JL, Triulzi DJ, Curtis B, et al. The frequency and specificity of human neutrophil antigen antibodies in a blood donor population. Transfusion 2011;51:820-7.
104. Triulzi D. Transfusion-related acute lung injury. Current concepts for the clinician. Anesth Analg 2009;108:770-6.
105. Cooling L. Transfusion-related acute lung injury. JAMA 2002;288:315-16.
106. Toy P, Hollis-Perry KM, Jun J, Nakagawa M. Recipients of blood from a donor with multiple HLA antibodies: A lookback study of transfusion-related acute lung injury. Transfusion 2004;44:1683-8.
107. Win N, Ranasinghe E, Lucas G. Transfusion-related acute lung injury: A 5-year look-back study. Transfus Med 2002;12:387-9.
108. Nicolle AL, Chapman CE, Carter V, Wallis JP. Transfusion-related acute lung injury caused by two donors with anti-human leukocyte antigen class II antibodies: A look-back investigation. Transfus Med 2004;64:225-30.
109. Maslanka K, Michur H, Zupanska B, et al. Leucocyte antibodies in blood donors and a look back on recipients of their blood components. Vox Sang 2007;92: 247-9.
110. Fadeyi EA, Adams S, Sheldon S, et al. A preliminary comparison of the prevalence of transfusion reactions in recipients of platelet components from donors with and without human leukocyte antigen antibodies. Vox Sang 2008;94:324-8.
111. Kleinman SH, Triulzi DJ, Murphy EL, et al, for the National Heart, Lung, and Blood Institute Retrovirus Epidemiology Donor Study-II (REDS-II). The Leukocyte Antibody Prevalence Study-II (LAPS-II): A retrospective cohort study of transfusion-related acute lung injury in recipients of high-plasma-volume human-leukocyte-antigen antibody-positive or negative components. Transfusion 2011;51:2078-91.
112. Quillen K, Medrano C, Adams S, et al. Screening plateletpheresis donors for HLA antibodies on two high-throughput platforms and correlation with recipient outcome. Transfusion 2011;51: 504-10.
113. Fung Y, Silliman C. The role of neutrophils in the pathogenesis of transfusion-related acute lung injury. Transfus Med Rev 2009;23:266-83.
114. Seeger W, Schneider U, Kreusler B, et al. Reproduction of transfusion-related acute lung injury in an ex-vivo lung model. Blood 1990;76: 1438-44.
115. Palfi M, Berg S, Berlin G. A randomized controlled trial of transfusion-related acute lung injury: Is plasma from multiparous blood donors dangerous? Transfusion 2001;41:317-22.
116. Wright SE, Snowden CP, Athey SC, et al. Acute lung injury after abdominal aortic aneurysm repair: The effect of excluding donations from females from the production of fresh-frozen plasma. Crit Care Med 2008;36:1796-802.
117. Nakazawa H, Ohnishi H, Okazaki H, et al. Impact of fresh-frozen plasma from male-only donors versus mixed-sex donors on postoperative respiratory function in surgical patients: A prospective case-control study. Transfusion 2009;49:2434-41.
118. Gong MN, Thompson BT, Williams P, et al. Clinical predictors of and mortality in acute respiratory distress syndrome: Potential role of red-cell transfusion. Crit Care Med 2005;33: 1191-8.
119. Vlaar AP, Binnekade JM, Prins D, et al. Risk factors and outcome of transfusion-related acute lung injury in the critically ill: A nested case-control study. Crit Care Med 2010;38:771-8.
120. Wiersum-Osselton JC, Middelburg RA, Beckers EA, et al. Male-only fresh-frozen plasma for transfusion-related acute lung injury prevention: Before-and-after comparative cohort study. Transfusion 2011;51:1278-83.
121. Kopko P, Silva M, Shulman I, Kleinman S. AABB survey of transfusion-related acute lung injury policies and practices in the United States. Transfusion 2007;47:1679-85.
122. Watkins TR, Rubenfeld GD, Martin TR, et al. Effects of leukoreduced blood on acute lung injury after trauma: A randomized controlled trial. Crit Care Med 2008;36:1493-9.
123. Silliman CC. The transfusion of pre-storage leukoreduced packed red blood cells to injured patients. Crit Care Med 2008;36:1661-2.
124. Watkins TR, Nathens AB. TRALI: A new case definition, a new epidemic? Am J Respir Crit Care Med 2007;176:839-42.
125. Davis A, Mandal R, Johnson M, et al. A touch of TRALI. Transfusion 2008;48:541-5.
126. Koch C, Li L, Figueroa P, et al. Transfusion and pulmonary morbidity after cardiac surgery. Ann Thorac Surg 2009;88:1410-18.

127. Silliman C. High volume transfusion from male-only versus female donor plasma and hypoxemia in the critically ill. Crit Care Med 2007; 35:1775.
128. Welsby I, Troughton M, Phillips-Bute B, et al. The relationship of plasma transfusion from female and male donors with outcome after cardiac surgery. J Thorac Cardiovasc Surg 2010; 140:1353-60.
129. Middelburg RA, van Stein D, Zupanska B, et al. Female donors and transfusion related acute lung injury: A case-referent study from the International TRALI Unisex Research Group. Transfusion 2010;50:2447-54.
130. Vamvakas EC, Blajchman MA. Transfusion-related mortality: The on-going risks of allogeneic blood transfusion and the available strategies for their prevention. Blood 2009;113: 3406-17.
131. Tormey C, Stack G. The persistence and evanescence of blood group alloantibodies in men. Transfusion 2009;49:505-12.
132. Pineda AA, Taswell HF, Brzica SJ. Delayed hemolytic transfusion reaction: An immunologic hazard of blood transfusion. Transfusion 1978;18:1-7.
133. Linden JV, Wagner K, Voytovich AE, Sheehan J. Transfusion errors in New York State. Transfusion 2000;40:1207-13.
134. Food and Drug Administration. Bar code label requirement for human drug products and biological products; final rule. (February 26, 2004) Fed Regist 2004;69(38):9120.
135. Callum JL, Kaplan HS, Merkley LL, et al. Reporting of near-miss events for transfusion medicine: Improving transfusion safety. Transfusion 2001;41:1204-11.
136. Mercurilali F, Inghilleri F, Colotti MT, et al. One-year use of the Bloodloc system in an orthopedic institute. Transfus Clin Biol 1994; 1:227-30.
137. Figueroa P, Zinan A, Wheeler C, et al. Nearly two decades using the check-type to prevent ABO-incompatible transfusions: One institution's experience. Am J Clin Pathol 2006; 126:1-5.
138. Lau FY, Wong R, Chui CH, et al. Improvement in transfusion safety using a specially-designed transfusion wristband. Transfus Med 2000;10: 121-4.
139. Sandler S, Langberg A, Dotinalek L. Bar code technology improves positive patient identification and transfusion safety. Dev Biol 2005; 120:19-24.
140. Turner CL, Casbard AC, Murphy MF. Barcode technology: Its role in increasing the safety of blood transfusion. Transfusion 2003;43:1200-9.
141. Wenz B, Burns ER. Improvement in transfusion safety using a new blood-unit and patient identification system as part of safe transfusion practice. Transfusion 1991;31:401-3.
142. Ahrens N, Pruss A, Kiesewetter H, Salama A. Failure of bedside ABO testing is still the most common cause of incorrect blood transfusion in the barcode era. Transfus Apher Sci 2005; 33:25-9.
143. Goodnough LT, Viele M, Fontaine MJ, et al. Implementation of a two-specimen requirement for verification of ABO/Rh for blood transfusion. Transfusion 2009;49:1321-8.
144. Higgins JM, Sloan SR. Stochastic modeling of human RBC alloimmunization: Evidence for a distinct population of immunologic responders. Blood 2008;112:2546-53.
145. Schoneville H, van de Watering LM, Loomans DS, Brand A. Red blood cell alloantibodies after transfusion: Factors influencing incidence and specificity. Transfusion 2006;46:250-6.
146. Schoneville H, van de Watering LMG, Brand A. Additional red-blood-cell alloantibodies after blood transfusion in a non-hematologic alloimmunized cohort: Is it time to take precautionary measures? Transfusion 2006;46:630-5.
147. Schoneville H, de Vries RPR, Brand A. Alloimmune response after additional red-blood-cell antigen challenge in immunized hemato-oncology patients. Transfusion 2009;49:453-7.
148. Pomper G, Simpson M. The prevention of alloimmunization: A balance of precaution, expectation, and outcome. Transfusion 2009;49: 406-8.
149. Young P, Uzieblo A, Trulock E, et al. Autoantibody formation after alloimmunization: Are blood transfusions a risk for autoimmune hemolytic anemia? Transfusion 2004;44:67-72.
150. Heddle N, Soutar R, O'Hoski P, et al. A prospective study to determine the frequency and clinical significance of alloimmunization post-transfusion. Br J Haematol 1995;91:1000-5.
151. Singer ST, Wu V, Mignacca R, et al. Alloimmunization and erythrocyte autoimmunization in transfusion-dependent thalassemia patients of predominantly Asian descent. Blood 2000;96: 3369-73.
152. Osby M, Shulman I. Phenotype matching of donor red blood cell unit for non-alloimmunized sickle-cell disease patients: A survey of

1182 North-American laboratories. Arch Pathol Lab Med 2005;129:190-3.
153. Cox J, Steane E, Cunningham G, et al. Risk of alloimmunization and delayed hemolytic transfusion reactions in patients with sickle-cell disease. Arch Intern Med 1988;148:2485-9.
154. Castro O, Sandler SG, Houston-Yu P, Ranat S. Predicting the effect of transfusing only phenotype-matched RBCs to patients with sickle-cell disease: Theoretical and practical implications. Transfusion 2002;42:684-90.
155. Afenyi-Annan A, Brecher ME. Transfusion phenotype matching for sickle-cell disease patients. Transfusion 2004;44:619-20.
156. Luban NL. Variability in rates of alloimmunization in different groups of children with sickle-cell disease: Effect of ethnic background. Am J Pediatr Hematol Oncol 1989;11:314-19.
157. Vichinsky EP, Earles A, Johnson RA, et al. Alloimmunization in sickle-cell anemia and transfusion of racially unmatched blood. N Engl J Med 1990;322:1617-21.
158. Beiboer SH, Wieringa-Jelsma T, Maaskant-van Wijk PA, et al. Rapid genotyping of blood cohort antigens by multiplex polymerase chain reaction and DNA microarray hybridization. Transfusion 2005;45:667-79.
159. Bugert P, McBride S, Smith G, et al. Microarray-based genotyping for blood cohorts: Comparison of gene array and 5′-nuclease assay techniques with human platelet antigen as a model. Transfusion 2005;45:654-9.
160. Denomme GA, Van OM. High-throughput multiplex single-nucleotide polymorphism analysis for red cell and platelet antigen genotypes. Transfusion 2005;45:660-6.
161. Hashmi G, Shariff T, Seul M, et al. A flexible array format for large-scale, rapid blood cohort DNA typing. Transfusion 2005;45:680-8.
162. Hashmi G, Shariff T, Zhang Y, et al. Determination of 24 minor red blood cell antigens for more than 2,000 blood donors by high-throughput DNA analysis. Transfusion 2007; 47:736-47.
163. Klapper E, Zhang Y, Figueroa P, et al. Toward extended phenotype compatibility: A new operational paradigm for the transfusion service. Transfusion 2010;50:536-46.
164. Silliman CC, Clay KL, Thurman GW, et al. Partial characterization of lipids that develop during the routine storage of blood and prime the neutrophil NADPH oxidase. J Lab Clin Med 1994;124:684-94.
165. Zallen G, Moore EE, Ciesla DJ, et al. Stored red blood cells selectively activate human neutrophils to release IL-8 and secretory PLA2. Shock 2000;13:29-33.
166. Chin-Yee I, Keeney M, Krueger L, et al. Supernatant from stored red cells activates neutrophils. Transfus Med 1998;8:49-56.
167. Hachida M, Hanayama N, Oamura T, et al. The role of leukocyte depletion in reducing injury to myocardium and lung during cardiopulmonary bypass. ASAIO J 1995;41:M291-4.
168. Gu YJ, de Vries AJ, Boonstra PW, van Oeveren W. Leukocyte depletion results in improved lung function and reduced inflammatory response in cardiac surgery. J Thorac Cardiovasc Surg 1996;112:494-500.
169. Pearl JM, Drinkwater DC, Laks H, et al. Leukocyte-depleted reperfusion of transplanted human heart prevents ultrastructural evidence of reperfusion injury. J Surg Res 1992;52:298-308.
170. Forceville X, Plouvier E, Chaise C. The deleterious effect of heminic iron in transfused intensive-care-unit patients. Crit Care Med 2002;30: 1182-3.
171. Zimmerman JJ. Defining the role of oxyradicals in the pathogenesis of sepsis. Crit Care Med 1995;23:616-17.
172. Alayash AI, Ryan BA, Cashon RE. Peroxynitrite-mediated heme oxidation and protein modification of native and chemically modified hemoglobins. Arch Biochem Biophys 1998;349:65-73.
173. McCord JM. Iron, free radicals, and oxidative injury. Semin Hematol 1998;35:5-12.
174. Shander A, Cappellini MD, Goodnough LT. Iron overload and toxicity: The hidden risk of multiple transfusions. Vox Sang 2009;97:185-97.
175. Jensen LS, Kissmeyer-Nielsen P, Wolff B, Quist N. Randomized comparison of leukocyte-depleted versus buffy-coat-poor blood transfusion and complications after colorectal surgery. Lancet 1996;348:841-5.
176. Nielsen HJ, Hammer JH, Kraup AL, et al. Prestorage leukocyte filtration may reduce leukocyte-derived bioactive substance accumulation in patients operated for burn trauma. Burns 1999;25:162-70.
177. Titlestad IL, Ebbesen LS, Ainsworth AP, et al. Leukocyte-depletion of blood components does not significantly reduce the risk of infectious complications: Results of a double-blind, randomized study. Int J Colorectal Dis 2001; 16:147-53.

178. Dzik WH, Anderson JK, O'Neill EM, et al. A prospective, randomized clinical trial of universal WBC reduction. Transfusion 2002;42:1114-22.
179. Wallis JP, Chapman CE, Orr KE, et al. Effect of WBC reduction of transfused RBCs on postoperative infection rates in cardiac surgery. Transfusion 2002;42;1127-34.
180. van Hilten JA, van de Watering LMG, van Bockel JH, et al. Effects of transfusion with red cells filtered to remove leukocytes: Randomized controlled trial in patients undergoing major surgery. Br Med J 2004;328:1281-4.
181. Bracey AW, Radovancevick R, Nussimeier NA, et al. Leukocyte-reduced blood in open-heart surgery patients: Effects on outcome (abstract). Transfusion 2002;42(Suppl):5S.
182. Boshkov LK, Furnary A, Morris C, et al. Prestorage leukoreduction of red cells in elective cardiac surgery: Results of a double-blind randomized controlled trial (abstract). Blood 2004;104:112a.
183. Nathens AB, Nester TA, Rubenfeld GD, et al. The effects of leukoreduced blood transfusion on infection risk following injury: A randomized controlled trial. Shock 2006;26:342-7.
184. Vamvakas EC. White-blood-cell containing allogeneic transfusion and postoperative infection or mortality: An updated meta-analysis. Vox Sang 2007;92:224-32.
185. Bilgin YM, Brand A. Transfusion-related immunomodulation: A second hit in an inflammatory cascade? Vox Sang 2008;95:261-71.
186. Vamvakas EC, Blajchman MA. Transfusion-related immunomodulation (TRIM): An update. Blood Rev 2007;21:327-48.
187. Parrish CR, Holmes EC, Morens DM, et al. Cross-species virus transmission and the emergence of new epidemic disease. Microbiol Mol Biol Rev 2008;72:457-70.
188. Petersen LR, Hayes EB. Westward ho?—The spread of West Nile virus. N Engl J Med 2004; 351:2257-9.
189. Dodd RY. Current risk of transfusion-transmitted infections. Curr Opin Hematol 2007;14: 671-6.
190. Dodd RY, Leiby DA. Emerging infectious threats to the blood supply. Am Rev Med 2004; 55:191-207.
191. Alter HJ, Stramer SL, Dodd RY. Emerging infectious diseases that threaten the blood supply. Semin Hematol 2007;44:32-41.
192. Goodnough LT, Brecher ME, Kanter MH, AuBuchon JP. Transfusion medicine. First of two parts—Blood transfusion. N Engl J Med 1999;340:438-47.
193. Dodd RY. Emerging infections, transfusion safety, and epidemiology. N Engl J Med 2003; 349:1205-6.
194. Kleinman S, Cameron C, Custer B, et al. Modeling the risk of an emerging pathogen entering the Canadian blood supply. Transfusion 2010; 50:2592-606.
195. Heuft HG, Mende W, Blasczyk R. A general change of the platelet transfusion policy from apheresis platelet concentrates to pooled platelet concentrates is associated with a sharp increase in donor exposures and infection rates. Transfus Med Hemother 2008;35:106-13.
196. Lopez-Plaza I, Weissfeld J, Triulzi DJ. The cost-effectiveness of reducing donor exposures with single-donor versus pooled random-donor platelets. Transfusion 1999;39:925-32.
197. Zou S, Musavi F, Notari E, et al. Prevalence, incidence, and residual risk of major blood-borne infections among apheresis collections to the American Red Cross Blood Services, 2004-2008. Transfusion 2010;50:1487-94.
198. Wang B, Schreiber GB, Glynn SA, et al. Does prevalence of transfusion-transmitted viral infection reflect corresponding incidence in United States blood donors? Transfusion 2005;45: 1089-96.
199. Kleinman SH, Busch MP. Assessing the impact of HBV NAT on window-period reduction and residual risk. J Clin Virol 2006;36(Suppl):S523-9.
200. Chudy M, Schmidt M, Czudai V, et al. Hepatitis B virus genotype G monoinfection and its transmission by blood components. Hepatology 2006;44:99-107.
201. Dodd RY, Notari EP IV, Stramer SL. Current prevalence and incidence of infectious disease markers and estimated window-period risk in the American Red Cross blood donor population. Transfusion 2002;42:975-9.
202. Kleinman SH, Busch M. Hepatitis B virus: Amplified and back in the blood safety spotlight. Transfusion 2001;41:1081-5.
203. Anderson SA, Yang H, Gallagher LM, et al. Quantitative estimate of the risks and benefits of possible alternative blood donor deferral strategies for men who have had sex with men. Transfusion 2009;49:1102-14.
204. Vamvakas EC. The relative safety of pooled-whole-blood-derived platelets prepared by the buffy-coat method versus single-donor (apheresis) platelets. Clin Lab 2010;56:263-79.

In: Vamvakas EC.
Decision Making in Transfusion Medicine
Bethesda, MD: AABB Press, 2011

3

Assessment of the Risk of Emerging Transfusion-Transmitted Infections

THREE TRANSFUSION-TRANSMITTED agents have been recognized in the past 30 years: human immunodeficiency virus (HIV), variant Creutzfeldt-Jakob disease (vCJD) prions, and West Nile virus (WNV). Two of these agents (HIV and vCJD prions) were novel, whereas WNV was a known virus that had not previously been reported to be transmitted by transfusion and that "emerged" as a transfusion-transmitted agent when it changed its geographic distribution and arrived in North America to cause a major vector-borne epidemic in the summer and fall of 2002.

It is not prudence, but common sense, to assume that what happened over the past 30 years with the emergence or recognition of three transfusion-transmitted agents can (or will) happen again in the future. The worst that could happen is that a novel HIV-like pathogen causing a fatal disease and having a long incubation period could emerge. Owing to its long asymptomatic blood-borne phase, this novel pathogen could accumulate to a significant extent in the blood donor population before it becomes recognized, reaching a prevalence as high as HIV reached in the United States (US) blood donor population before testing for HIV antibody was introduced in the spring of 1985. In such a scenario, the novel pathogen could cause as many cases of transmission through transfusion as HIV caused in the 1980s.

In 1984—the year before the testing of US blood donors for HIV infection commenced—the prevalence of HIV in donors exceeded 1 per 1000.[1] Thanks to the surveillance systems put in place after the epidemic of transfusion-acquired HIV infection, it is unlikely that a new virus causing chronic infection could go undetected for as long as HIV did, and therefore infection with a new virus would be unlikely to reach a prevalence as high as 1 per 1000 US blood donors.[2,3]

Nonetheless, although a future HIV-like agent would certainly be detected much faster than HIV was recognized, it is possible that—before measures are implemented to interrupt its transmission through allogeneic blood transfusion (ABT)—this future HIV-like agent could reach a prevalence as high as one-tenth the 1984 HIV prevalence. [In fact, as will be discussed in this chapter, 1 per 10,000 blood donors is a likely estimate of the current prevalence of vCJD prions in the United Kingdom (UK) population]. Thus, worst-case scenarios supporting each of the competing paradigm shifts for improving blood safety in the foreseeable future (see Chapter 8 for further discussion) should consistently model the possibility that an HIV-like pathogen could reach a prevalence of 1 per 10,000 US blood donors before measures are introduced to interrupt the transmission of the novel pathogen through ABT.[2,3] It is important to note that we cannot exclude the possibility that the accumulation of such a pathogen with a long blood-borne incubation period in the US blood donor population has already started.

Furthermore, another WNV-like agent could change its geographic distribution and emerge in the United States as a transfusion-transmitted pathogen, causing hundreds of transmissions through ABT in its first epidemic,[4] as was the case with WNV in the summer of 2002.[4-7] Both HIV-like and WNV-like future pathogens could be transmitted equally effectively through transfusion of red cells, platelets, or plasma. Thus, the risk of contracting a transfusion-transmitted infection (TTI) from a transfusion of n blood components (or from exposure to n donors) would equal np, where p is the per-component probability of transmission of the emerging TTI—provided that each component is harvested from a single donor rather than being pooled from the donations of multiple donors, and n is the number of components to whom a recipient is exposed.

In principle, emerging agents achieving a significant prevalence in the general population (and thus also in the blood donor population) can have the potential to be transmitted through transfusion, and their transmissibility through transfusion should be investigated by means of inoculation studies in animal models and by the study of linked donor–recipient pairs. If the agent is capable of causing disease in exposed individuals, new measures to enhance blood safety may be required. All components of this investigation [assessment of the prevalence of subclinical disease, assessment of transmissibility through transfusion, and evaluation of question- or test-based (or other) strategies for preventing transmission by transfusion] have been completed—over the past 15 years (1996 through 2011) of the vCJD epidemic in the United Kingdom—for the vCJD prions. Making use of the experience accumulated with vCJD in the United Kingdom, this chapter reviews the hitherto-adduced evidence of vCJD transmission by transfusion, as well as the estimates of the prevalence of subclinical (asymptomatic) disease in the UK population and the measures already taken (or currently under development) to prevent transfusion transmission of the vCJD prions. This chapter also endeavors to produce an estimate of the current risk of fatal vCJD transmission through transfusion in the United Kingdom, and introduces the possibility of a "second wave" of vCJD cases in the United Kingdom that are primarily transmitted through blood transfusion.

Emerging TTIs

Provided that an agent can survive in blood components and can be transmitted by the intravenous route, any infection with an asymptomatic blood-borne phase has the potential for transmission by ABT. This possibility exists, whether the infectious phase is prolonged [as is the case with HIV, hepatitis B virus (HBV), or hepatitis C virus (HCV) infection] or short [as is the case with WNV or dengue fever virus (DFV) infection]. The frequency with which an infection is transmitted to a transfusion recipient depends on the length of the asymptomatic blood-borne phase, the frequency of blood donation during this period, and the immune status of the recipient population.[8]

An AABB Task Force[8] prioritized 68 potential or known transfusion-transmitted agents on the basis of both the existing scientific and epidemiologic evidence of their transmissibility through ABT and their potential for severe clinical outcomes that could result in public attention and concern. Four priority categories were assigned to convey a particular agent's significance: white, yellow, orange, and red. Agents included in the orange category were *Leishmania* species, *Plasmodium* species, *Trypanosoma cruzi*, Chickungunya virus, and St. Louis encephalitis virus (SLEV).[8] Agents included in the red category were the vCJD prions, DFV, and *Babesia* species. With the exception of the last two orange category agents (Chickungunya virus and SLEV), all other agents prioritized as orange or red have been shown to be transfusion-transmitted.

Because the focus of this report[8] was on the United States, protozoa that represent major transfusion risks in developing countries (*Plasmodium* species and *T. cruzi)* were placed in the same category as SLEV—for which there is no evidence of transmission by transfusion, but which is endemic in the United States. For both Chickungunya virus and SLEV, the Task Force's concern was that these agents have the potential to replicate the 2002 WNV US experience in the future. Concerning the United States, the Task Force judged the medical and scientific evidence for transmission of *Babesia* species to be moderate to high, whereas the evidence for DFV and vCJD prions was judged to be low. Nonetheless, concerning the effect in developing countries, the medical and scientific evidence for transmission of DFV was judged to be moderate.[8]

Known agents that have been shown to be (or have the potential to be) transfusion-transmitted fall into five categories: 1) agents known to cause disease, but for which the epidemiologic evidence for transmission by transfusion is inconclusive; 2) agents known to cause disease and to be transmitted by transfusion, but for which the extent of the problem with regard to any potential threat to the safety of the blood supply cannot be determined with the tools hitherto employed to assess this risk; 3) agents known to cause disease and to be transmitted by transfusion, but whose prevalence in the US volunteer blood donor population is too low to threaten the safety of the blood supply; 4) agents that are transmitted by transfusion, but that cause disease in only a small proportion of transfusion recipients who have specific underlying diseases or other predisposing risk factors; and 5) agents that presently cause disease in only a small proportion of transfusion recipients, but that may reach larger populations of susceptible recipients in the future, because of the introduction of new, pooled blood products.

Classic Creutzfeldt-Jakob disease (CJD) is the most widely publicized example of an agent from the first category. No case of classic CJD has been causally attributed to a transfusion, and a consensus has emerged that classic CJD is probably not transmissible by transfusion.[9,10] However, it is impossible to prove that classic CJD cannot be transmitted by transfusion, because statistical hypothesis testing (reviewed in Chapter 2 of the electronic supplement) is designed to either reject or fail to reject a null hypothesis, as opposed to proving a negative hypothesis. In the context of CJD, the available epidemiologic studies cannot prove that classic CJD is *not* transmitted by transfusion, because the absence of evidence of risk cannot be equated with evidence of the absence of risk.[11,12]

Arguably, transfusion-associated sepsis (TAS) owing to bacterial contamination of blood and blood components is the most important example of an entity from the second category. Cases of TAS, as well as fatalities from TAS, are reported every year, but these cases generally are those in which a clearly symptomatic outcome has been observed (as well as suspected of being and shown to be TAS; see Chapter 2). It is certain that the problem is far greater than it appears to be on the basis of the reported incidents,[2,3] and posttransfusion bacterial sepsis currently is the most significant infectious risk of ABT in the United States.

Malaria,[13-16] babesiosis,[17-22] leishmaniasis,[23] Rocky Mountain spotted fever,[24] and tick-borne viral encephalitis[25] are examples of agents that belong[13-16,23-25] (or at least used to belong[17-22]) to the third category. For example, malaria is restricted to specific parts of the world by climate and by control measures aimed at removing the vector from nonendemic areas. The prevalence and incidence of malaria in populations of prospective blood donors from nonendemic countries are exceedingly low, and thus screening of donated blood for *Plasmodia* may not be justified in Western Europe and North America. There is concern, however, that malaria may re-emerge in previously endemic areas and/or spread into previously low-prevalence areas, because of changing global patterns of climate, increasing global travel, and falling public health standards. For example, it has reappeared in southern and eastern Mediterranean regions and in the Central Asian republics, and that return has created the potential for transmission by blood donated by volunteer blood donors who do not report a history of travel to endemic countries.[26]

Human parvovirus B19[27] and Epstein-Barr virus (EBV)[28] are examples of agents from the fourth category. Human parvovirus B19 may cause hydrops fetalis in fetuses, aplastic crisis in patients with chronic hemolytic anemias, and chronic hypoplastic anemia in immunodeficient patients. However, this agent causes no disease in the vast majority of transfusion recipients. Similarly, EBV has been reported as a cause of posttransfusion disease only very rarely, despite the fact that—in theory—it may cause catastrophic illness in transfusion recipients suffering from an X-linked T-cell defect (Duncan's disease or X-linked lymphoproliferation syndrome), as well as in transplant recipients with compromised T-cell function secondary to the receipt of cyclosporine.

Human parvovirus B19 is also the most widely publicized example[29] of an agent from the fifth category. This nonenveloped virus resists treatment with solvents and detergents, and it is not inactivated by the methods employed to inactivate viruses in plasma pools that are used for the manufacture of solvent/detergent-treated, pooled (S/D-P) plasma. Each lot of S/D-P plasma is derived from up to 2500 volunteer blood donors. The incidence of parvovirus B19 viremia in blood donors has been estimated to range from 1 in 3300 to 1 in 40,000,[27] and thus some lots of S/D-P plasma can be expected to be contaminated with parvovirus B19. Neutralizing antibodies to parvovirus are present in the plasma of approximately one-half of the donors who contribute to a pool of S/D-P plasma in the United States, but this antibody level may not be sufficient to prevent transmission of the virus to plasma recipients. Koenigbauer et al[29] reported a case of an immunocompetent recipient with myasthenia gravis who developed clinical disease (fatigue, rash, and severe polyarthralgia) because of parvovirus B19 infection traced to the infusion of contaminated S/D-P plasma.

Similar to parvovirus B19, hepatitis A virus (HAV) lacks a lipid envelope and is not inactivated by solvent/detergent treatment. HAV may be detected in the circulation of volunteer blood donors for up to 4 weeks before symptoms develop, and isolated cases of hepatitis A have been attributed to the transfusion of cellular blood components. Moreover, a curious outbreak of hepatitis A among recipients of virus-inactivated clotting factor concentrates was reported from Europe in 1993.[30]

In addition to these "known" transfusion-transmitted agents, "novel" infectious agents that are transmissible by transfusion and that also cause clinical disease in transfusion recipients may threaten the safety of the blood supply in the future.[26] If both the transmissibility of an agent by transfusion and its clinical relevance are demonstrated, after recognition of the presence of the agent in the US blood donor population, preventive measures should be introduced to protect the safety of the blood supply. However, the transmissibility and the clinical significance of an agent should be understood before blood services consider screening or other measures that are intended to minimize the risk of transmission of the agent by transfusion. With the tools available today, it is easy to identify novel infectious agents on the basis of nucleic acid sequences, but it is difficult to assign any clinical significance to these agents. The discovery of "new" agents inevitably leads to the finding of these agents in the blood of blood donors and transfusion recipients and thus to the concern that there may be yet another transfusion-transmitted disease. However, agents that are transmissible by transfusion may not necessarily cause clinically significant disease in recipients and thus may not represent a threat to the safety of the blood supply.[26] All of these considerations will be illustrated here by the examination of the threat posed to blood safety by a novel agent causing a fatal disease after a long incubation period that includes a blood-borne phase.

Prevalence of Subclinical vCJD in the United Kingdom

The bovine spongiform encephalopathy (BSE) epidemic in the UK started in 1980, peaked in the period 1989-1992, and has since been contained. UK residents born after January 1, 1996, are considered not to have had any dietary exposure to BSE. Exposure of the UK population to BSE has been widespread, with more than 181,000 cases confirmed in cattle and the estimates of total infections in cattle ranging between 1 and 3 million.[31] Although the number of clinical cases of vCJD has been only 175 in the United Kingdom,[32] the number of infected individuals with subclinical disease remains unknown.[33] A retrospective study of UK appendix samples found that 3 of 11,246 samples (approximately 1 per 4000) were positive for abnormal prion protein (PrP^{Sc}) on Western blot analysis.[34] Further investigations of tonsil samples found that 0 of 32,661 specimens contained PrP^{Sc}. The prevalence of subclinical vCJD estimated from tonsil specimens[35,36] [95% confidence interval (CI) = 0-113 per million] was lower than, but still consistent with, the initial estimate of prevalence[34] (95% CI = 49-692 per million). The major limitation of all these studies is the uncertain capability of either appendix- or tonsil-tissue testing to identify all (as opposed to only a proportion) of the individuals who have contracted food-borne vCJD.[34-36]

The available animal data suggest that accumulation of PrP^{Sc} in the appendix and/or tonsil during the subclinical phase of infection is a common (albeit nonuniform) feature of vCJD pathogenesis.[37] Moreover, PrP^{Sc} was detected in appendix tissue from two asymptomatic individuals who later developed vCJD.[38] However, it is unknown at what stage of the incubation period (following exposure to BSE prions) PrP^{Sc} accumulates at detectable levels in either appendix or tonsil tissue before the onset of clinical disease. Genetic differences between individuals may determine the timing of onset and the extent of accumulation of PrP^{Sc}. Furthermore, although the quantities of PrP^{Sc} deposited in neural tissues are sufficient during the clinical phase of disease for detection by conventional immunoassays [such as the Western blot or enzyme immunoassay (EIA)], the concentrations of PrP^{Sc} at peripheral tissues are substantially lower.

The UK Spongiform Encephalopathy Advisory Committee (SEAC) deemed that the data from the appendix[34] and tonsil[35,36] surveys could not be combined to give a single credible estimate of the prevalence of subclinical vCJD in the UK population for risk-management purposes.[33] There was no reason to suspect that the three PrP^{Sc}-positive appendix samples identified by immunohistochemistry[34] represent false-positive results or that the dual EIA employed in the (ongoing) tonsil survey is failing to identify samples with detectable levels of PrP^{Sc}. The SEAC thus considered it prudent that the estimate based on the appendix survey alone (1 per 4000)[34] be considered to provide a "reasonable, pragmatic, and precautionary working scenario for the prevalence of subclinical infections."[33] The appendix survey[34] provides evidence for the existence of subclinical infections that there is no reason to disregard, although the various uncertainties indicate that this could be an underestimate—or overestimate—of the true prevalence of subclinical infection in the population as a whole.

The three positive samples[34] all were from individuals born between 1961 and 1985 (the 1961-1985 "birth cohort"). This birth cohort is presumed to be the most vulnerable to infection because a large proportion of the vCJD cases to date have been from this cohort and because the BSE epidemic peaked between 1989 and 1992. Although 91% of the samples in the appendix survey[34] were from the 1961-1985 birth cohort, the tonsil survey[35] studied the 1961-1995 combined cohort. No positive tonsil samples had been found in the tonsil survey by March 2010, after testing of 85,000 samples by dual EIAs.[33] However, in a subsample of 10,000 tissues tested by immunohistochemistry, one follicle in a single sample tested positive for two different antibodies.[33] The SEAC deemed that the most effective approach to establish the prevalence of subclinical vCJD is the testing of *spleen* and—when possible—of brain samples collected from coroners' autopsies. Coroners' autopsies provide the only source of a sufficiently large number of spleen and brain samples that can be collected within a reasonable time from appropriate birth cohorts.

The Possibility of Natural Resistance to vCJD

The discrepancy between the high prevalence estimates of subclinical infection (1 per 4000)[34] and the low number of cases of clinical disease hitherto observed (<200)[32] can perhaps be explained by the long incubation periods seen in natural human prion infections[39] and by the existence of subclinical carrier states of prion infection in animal models.[40-42] If the BSE epidemic peaked in 1989-1992, it is possible that an interval equal to the mean incubation period of vCJD has not yet elapsed. Patients with clinical vCJD diagnosed thus far may have been a selected subset from among all patients incubating the agent of vCJD—that is, the subjects with the shortest incubation periods for vCJD. Such a selected subset could include the patients having an unusual combination of alleles at multiple genetic loci that define susceptibility to prion disease and/or the patients who received unusually high doses of BSE prions.[39]

Heterozygosity at codon 129 of the prion-protein gene (*PRNP*) is a major determinant of natural resistance to and prolongation of the incubation period of human prion diseases.[43-46] Most sporadic CJD occurs in individuals homozygous for the codon-129 polymorphism of the *PRNP* gene,[43] whereas most elderly survivors of the kuru epidemic among the Fore people of Papua New Guinea are heterozygous at codon 129.[44,45] Before traditional Fore mortuary practices ceased by 1960, kuru used to be the most common cause of death among Fore women who—as a sign of respect—ate the whole body of deceased family members. There were some 2700 cases of kuru among the Fore people between 1957 and 2004—the only known example of a major human epidemic of a prion disease. The survival advantage vis-à-vis prion disease conferred by codon-129 heterozygosity provided a powerful basis for selection pressure in the Fore.[45] However, the higher-than-expected prevalence of codon-129 heterozygosity is much more geographically widespread. Fifty-one percent of Europeans are codon-129 heterozygous, compared with 11% who are valine homozygous and 38% who are methionine homozygous. If heterozygosity is associated with extended incubation periods and resistance to prion disease,[43-46] cannibalism resulting in several prion-disease epidemics in human prehistory—and thereby giving a survival advantage to codon-129 heterozygotes[45]—could explain the higher-than-expected prevalence of codon-129 heterozygosity in Europe.

The mean incubation period for kuru has been estimated to be around 12 years,[47] with a similar estimate for iatrogenic CJD associated with the use of human-cadaver-derived pituitary growth hormone.[48] In both of these cases of human-to-human transmission, no species barrier is involved. The cattle-to-mouse barrier for BSE transmission results in a 300% to 400% increase in incubation period.[47,49] If the human-to-human transmission of kuru has a mean incubation period of 12 years, cattle-to-human transmission of BSE could have a mean incubation period of >30 years,[47] thereby explaining why—because the epidemic of BSE in cattle peaked in 1989-1992—the peak of the human (food-borne) vCJD epidemic may not have yet been reached.[50]

Between 1996 and 2004, Collinge et al[39] identified 11 patients with kuru among the Fore people of Papua New Guinea. All of these patients had been born before the cessation of cannibalism. Likely incubation periods ranged from 39 to 56 years, with the minimum incubation periods being 34 to 41 years.[39] Ten patients were genotyped for codon-129 polymorphism; eight were methionine-valine heterozygous (as would have been expected for patients manifesting disease after such a prolonged incubation period of 39 to 56 years[39]—compared with the 12-year average for kuru[47]). One patient was methionine homozygous, and one was valine homozygous.[39] If incubation periods of >50 years are possible in the absence of a species barrier in kuru, incubation periods of >100 years (ie, exceeding the human lifespan) could be possible in the presence of a species barrier in vCJD.[39]

Samples previously collected from the Fore people had enabled Lee et al[44] to show that patients dying of kuru at an age younger than that of the 11 patients of Collinge et al[39] were more likely to be methionine homozygous. Patients developing kuru at a younger age likely had developed kuru after a shorter incubation period. The shortest incubation periods for kuru (4 to 5 years) were estimated from the age of the youngest patients, who were 4-5 years old when they developed kuru. Although fewer than 200 Britons have hitherto developed vCJD,[32] the earliest onsets of disease have been at or above age 12 years, which suggests that 12 years might be the minimum incubation period for (food-borne) vCJD.[39]

If that were the case, the vCJD patients hitherto identified would indeed be those who received especially high doses of BSE prions and/or those who were especially vulnerable because they had an unusual combination of alleles at the multiple genetic loci[51-53] defining susceptibility to BSE. Because of the powerful genetic effects on incubation periods in laboratory animals,[51-53] a human BSE (ie, food-borne vCJD) epidemic could be multiphasic. Although a peak has passed,[32] there may be further peaks–perhaps in different genetic groups.

All vCJD patients with histopathologically confirmed clinical disease have been methionine homozygous at codon 129 of the *PRNP* prion-protein gene. As already discussed, however, in other acquired prion diseases, cases have occurred in all genotypes, albeit with different incubation periods.[54] In addition, in animal models of vCJD, different clinicopathologic phenotypes of prion disease occurred with various codon-129 genotypes.[55,56] One possible (not histopathologically confirmed) case of clinical vCJD was reported in a codon-129-heterozygous patient in 2009.[57] An autopsy was not performed. A clinical diagnosis of vCJD was made on the basis of the patient's young age (30 years), a characteristic clinical onset (personality changes, progressive unsteadiness, and intellectual decline), and the magnetic resonance imaging and electroencephalographic findings. Whether this case is the first of several (or even many) cases of clinical vCJD arising in codon-129 heterozygotes (perhaps after a prolonged incubation period) is not known at this time.

Five cases of subclinical vCJD have hitherto been reported: the three positive appendix samples in the retrospective survey of Hilton et al[34]; one recipient of non-white-cell (WBC)-reduced Red Blood Cells (RBCs) from a donor who later developed vCJD[58]; and one recipient of Factor VIII concentrate made from a UK plasma pool to which a donor who later developed vCJD had contributed.[59] Both this recipient of non-WBC-reduced RBCs[58] and the patient with hemophilia[59] died of unrelated causes without any evidence of neurologic disease. At autopsy, however, these two patients were found to have abnormal PrP^{Sc} protein in their spleen. Both the transfusion recipient[58] and the patient with hemophilia[59] were codon-129 heterozygous. Two of the three positive appendix samples identified by Hilton et al[34] were valine homozygous at codon 129[60]; adequate DNA was not available for analysis of the third sample.

The transfusion recipient died 5 years after receiving the implicated transfusion from a donor who later developed vCJD.[58] The patient with hemophilia, however, died 14 years after receiving Factor VIII concentrate manufactured from a UK plasma pool to which a donor who later developed vCJD had contributed. In the case of the transfusion recipient, 5 years may have been too short a period for clinical vCJD to develop. In the case of the patient with hemophilia, 14 years may (or may not) have been a sufficient interval for the infection to progress to clinical disease. It is possible that this patient was protected by his codon-129 heterozygosity and/or by having received a very low dose of infectious prions–owing to the dilution of the plasma unit of the donor who later developed vCJD by the 1000 or 8025 other units of UK plasma contained in the two vCJD-implicated plasma pools.[59]

Projections of the Number of Future Cases of Clinical vCJD in the United Kingdom

In the United Kingdom, 175 cases of vCJD had occurred by March 2011. This total encompassed 172 food-borne cases (including four patients who are still alive) and three secondary (transfusion-transmitted) cases of clinical vCJD.[32] By the end of 2009, 170 cases, including the three transfusion-transmitted cases, had occurred.[61] Of the 167 of these patients who had died by the end of 2009, 153 had been genotyped: 152 were codon-129 methionine homozygous, and 1[57] was heterozygous.[61] The median number of days from the onset of clinical disease to the establishment of a vCJD diagnosis was 326 days, and that from the onset of disease to death was 413 days.[61]

The epidemic peaked in 2000, with 28 deaths, and subsequently declined, with five deaths recorded in each of the years 2006 and 2007 and only one death occurring in 2008, although the number of deaths in 2009 (two) was slightly higher than the number expected by the employed quadratic-trend model for the epidemic, which had predicted 1 death for 2009 (95% CI = 0-2).[61] Nonetheless, with the incidence of the disease thus falling, the most recent mathematical model predicts that only 100 further food-borne cases of disease (95% CI = 11-220) will occur in the United Kingdom.[62]

Fourteen years after the beginning of the epidemic in 1996, however, the median age of death (28 years for the deaths recorded by the end of 2009) has remained the same.[61] This stable age of death is not compatible with what would be expected if a particular cohort of individuals had been exposed to BSE from dietary sources during a specified window of time (eg, 1980-1996). The best-fit mathematical model for explaining both the falling incidence (one death in 2009[61]) and high prevalence (1 in 4000[34]) data, as well as the stable age of death,[61] suggests an age-dependent exposure/susceptibility variation that makes children and adolescents more susceptible to infection than adults. On the basis of such an age-dependent model and the tonsil data,[34] we can expect 3000 (95% CI = 520-6810) future vCJD cases in the United Kingdom, mainly in persons aged 10-30 years—cases that have not yet occurred, perhaps owing to a prolonged asymptomatic phase in codon-129 heterozygotes or valine homozygotes.[63] The model of Clarke and Ghani[63] considers that 93% (95% CI = 60%-97%) of infected individuals do not go on to develop clinical disease.

Only one case of clinical vCJD has yet occurred in a codon-129 heterozygote,[57] and none has occurred in a valine homozygote. Codon-129 heterozygotes and valine homozygotes together represent ≥60% of the UK population, but there is a stark contrast in the codon-129 polymorphism of the *PRNP* gene between patients hitherto diagnosed with clinical versus subclinical vCJD (Table 3-1). The most optimistic scenario holds that such individuals have natural resistance to the disease: they do not develop clinical vCJD and they will live their lives without attaining a level of infectivity in peripheral blood capable of infecting transfusion recipients. The worst-case scenario, however, holds that codon-129 heterozygotes or valine homozygotes enter a long (or even lifelong) asymptomatic phase, during which they have sufficient infectivity in their blood to infect susceptible (methionine-homozygous) transfusion recipients. Susceptible transfusion recipients then develop disease before the infection becomes manifest in the infectious donor, who therefore continues to donate blood and to cause disease in susceptible recipients. This pos-

Table 3-1. Codon-129 Polymorphism of the *PRNP* Gene of Patients Diagnosed with Clinical or Subclinical vCJD in the United Kingdom

	Number (%) of Genotyped Patients*	
Diagnosis	**Methionine Homozygous**	**Heterozygous or Valine Homozygous**
Clinical vCJD	152 (99.3)	1 (0.7)
Subclinical vCJD	0 (0.0)	4 (100.0)

*Through the end of 2009.
vCJD = variant Creutzfeldt-Jakob disease.

sibility is consistent with what we know about the natural history of kuru.[39]

If even a fraction of such asymptomatic carriers accumulate sufficient infectivity in their blood to infect transfusion recipients, secondary transmission from infected individuals via transfusion or tissue transplantation could extend the outbreak of the disease in the United Kingdom.[64] Because no interspecies barrier is involved, transmission through transfusion could be more effective than the dietary route. As evidence is accumulating to suggest that all codon-129 genotypes may be susceptible to vCJD infection,[42,60,65] the presumed number of UK residents infected by a dietary source who can potentially accumulate sufficient infectivity in their peripheral blood to infect transfusion recipients increases. At the same time, transmissibility of vCJD by blood transfusion has been established by the hitherto reported human cases of transmission among a small number of "at-risk" individuals, as well as by effective experimental transmission in sheep.

Transfusion-Transmitted Cases of Clinical vCJD

Eighteen UK vCJD patients had been blood donors, and 66 patients were identified as having received a labile blood component from a donor who later developed vCJD. Thirty-two of these subjects (of whom 13 can be statistically expected to be methionine homozygous) have, at the time of this writing, survived for ≥5 years after the implicated transfusion.[66] Only one deceased recipient underwent post-mortem examination for the presence of abnormal prion protein; as already described, that person was found to have evidence of subclinical infection in the spleen and to be heterozygous at codon 129.[58] Three of the (likely) 13 methionine homozygotes have developed vCJD,[67-69] indicating a 23% probability that methionine homozygotes surviving for ≥5 years will develop clinical vCJD after receiving the non-WBC-reduced RBCs of a donor who later developed vCJD.

This probability most likely underestimates the risk, because the identification of a case of transfusion-transmitted vCJD requires that the vCJD infection be recognized in both the donor and the recipient. Nonetheless, the 23% estimate far exceeds the expected incidence of disease acquired from dietary sources among UK methionine homozygotes. Moreover, two of the four probable transfusion-transmitted cases were contracted from the same donor, with the index donations separated by just 4 months[70]; three of the four recipients were >60 years old, which is an unusual occurrence for patients with vCJD acquired from dietary sources; and the donors developed clinical signs of vCJD between 17 and 42 months after donating, which indicated that they were at an advanced stage of the incubation period when they made the donation that transmitted vCJD.

All four recipients who apparently contracted vCJD from transfusion had received non-WBC-reduced RBCs between 1996 and 1999. They had been exposed to 5, 8-10, 23, and 56 donors, and three of the four developed vCJD between 6 and 8.5 years after the index transfusion—a short incubation period compared with that associated with vCJD acquired from dietary sources.[71] This short incubation period might indicate the effectiveness of human-to-human transmission of vCJD through transfusion (a situation in which no species barrier is involved).[71]

Recently, circumstances raised the possibility of an additional two cases of transfusion-transmitted vCJD.[66] These vCJD cases were linked by a possible common donor of non-WBC-reduced RBCs who had not developed vCJD by the time of the report.[66] The codon-129 genotype of this donor is unknown. Between 1989 and 2005, blood components from this donor were transfused to 27 additional recipients who have not been traced because the donor has not developed vCJD. Nevertheless, except for the aforementioned two patients who developed vCJD at 18 or 41 years of age—after possibly contracting the infection from the identified common donor, in 1989 or 1993, respectively—no other vCJD patient has been linked to this donor by the UK's comprehensive vCJD surveillance system.[66]

Cholan et al[66] showed that this pattern of events (two patients with vCJD being associated by means of a possible common donor) would not be unexpected in the absence of any causal link between the two cases. The first patient received non-WBC-reduced RBCs from (probably) four different donors when he or she was a premature neonate in 1989. Although blood from the common donor would have been at the hospital's inventory at that time, the donor blood would have been 13 days old on the day of the transfusion and thus unlikely to have been used for transfusion to a neonate. Had the patient contracted vCJD from that transfusion, however, the incubation period of transfusion-transmitted vCJD would have been extraordinarily long compared with that seen in the previously reported cases.[67-69] Experimental exposure of neonatal mice to scrapie can be associated with extension of the incubation period owing to inefficient infection of the premature spleen. The second patient was exposed to 103 donors and could have been exposed to the identified common donor in 1993—a possibility that cannot be confirmed, because, in 1989-1993, systems were not in place in the United Kingdom to ensure full traceability of the components issued for transfusion.[66] It is due to the fact that this second recipient was exposed to so many donors that a possible common donor could be identified by coincidence for these two vCJD cases.

Cholan et al thus concluded that the circumstances did not support the interpretation that one (or perhaps two) additional vCJD transmissions by transfusion had occurred.[66] Transfusion remains just as likely a source of infection as the dietary route, however, because of the extremely low probability that each of these patients would have contracted vCJD from dietary sources: 0.39 and 0.08 per million for the 18- and 41-year-old patients, respectively.[66] This latter interpretation of transfusion transmission would have significant implications for the length of the period during which an asymptomatic blood donor can transmit infection—implications that reproduce the pessimistic scenario discussed above because the donor in question is alive and well more than 20 years after having made the first implicated donation.

Moreover, this potential link between two clinical vCJD cases and a donor who remains alive and well 20 years after donation[66] highlights the possibility that—if indeed the proportion of subclinical infections is high[63] and subclinically infected Britons are infectious during the latter part of the natural history of their infection (no matter whether they end up developing clinical vCJD during their lifetime)—only a small proportion of the transfusion-transmitted cases of vCJD would be identified as transfusion-transmitted. That would be the case because blood transfusion transmissions in which the donor or recipient(s) remain subclinically infected cannot be detected. At least in theory, some of the cases that are currently presumed to have been food-borne[61] could have been contracted through blood transfusion.[62]

In this spirit, the latest model of Garske and Ghani[62] anticipates 277 additional transfusion-transmitted cases to arise in the United Kingdom, although it anticipates only 100 (95% CI = 11-220) further food-borne cases. Of the 277 transfusion-transmitted cases, 17 (95% CI = 1-220) would be "identifiable through blood"—that is, attributable to a blood transfusion because both the donor and the recipient would have developed vCJD. The large majority of the transfusion-transmitted cases (260; 95% CI = 30-2700), though, would not be identifiable through blood, because they would not be linked to a donor who had developed vCJD as the (likely methionine-homozygous) transfusion recipient would have developed vCJD before the (likely codon-129 heterozygous or valine-homozygous) donor. Ninety-one (91%) of the 100 food-borne cases are expected to arise in codon-129 heterozygotes or valine homozygotes (who were exposed to BSE prions before January 1, 1996, but who have had a prolonged incubation period because of natural resistance to vCJD owing to these genotypes). In contrast, 202 (72.9%) of the 277 transfusion-transmitted cases are expected to arise in the most susceptible genetic group (ie, the methionine homozygotes).

Transmission of vCJD Through Plasma

No individuals with hemophilia have developed vCJD, and a previous retrospective study of autopsy samples from individuals with hemophilia had shown no evidence of subclinical infection.[72] Recently, however, it was reported that a hemophilia patient who died of non-vCJD causes (after having twice received Factor VIII clotting factor concentrate prepared from pools manufactured from UK plasma to which a donor who later developed vCJD had contributed) had been found at postmortem examination to have abnormal prion protein in his spleen.[59] Although this patient had also been exposed to vCJD from dietary sources and through blood transfusions, it was more likely that the infection had occurred from the administration of clotting factors prepared from the plasma of a donor who went on to develop vCJD 4.5 years after making the first implicated plasma donation.[59]

This patient was the only 1 of 17 UK patients with hemophilia who were studied histologically for accumulation of abnormal prion protein because they had been exposed to clotting factor concentrates manufactured from plasma of UK donors between 1980 and 2001.[59] Eleven of the 17 patients in this study had died by the time of the report, and six of those 11 had received vCJD-implicated pools of Factor VIII concentrates. Only the patient discussed above was found at autopsy to have deposition of abnormal prion protein in his spleen.[59]

Another study prospectively followed 604 UK patients with inherited bleeding disorders for ≥13 years to assess their risk of developing vCJD after receiving "implicated" clotting factor concentrates made from plasma pools to which a donor(s) who subsequently developed clinical vCJD had contributed.[73] Total potential vCJD infectivity incurred by each patient was estimated by adding the possible plasma-fraction infectivity contained in all doses received during each patient's lifetime. The estimated vCJD risk from exposure to potentially contaminated plasma was ≥1% in 595, ≥50% in 164, and 100% in 51 patients. By January 2009, none of these patients had developed clinical vCJD.[73] Further follow-up of this patient cohort is planned because—owing to the dilution of the plasma unit(s) of the donor(s) who later developed vCJD by the thousands of other units of UK plasma pooled to manufacture the "implicated" clotting factor concentrates—the incubation period of vCJD after receipt of clotting factor concentrates may be longer than that after receipt of non-WBC-reduced RBCs.[73]

Alternatively, the estimates of plasma-fraction infectivity used in the calculations of Zaman et al[73] may have been overly precautionary. Data from different experiments consistently show that conventional bioseparation processes used in the manufacturing of clotting factor concentrates are capable of removing prion agents to a significant extent. Accordingly, the infectivity of clotting factors concentrates should not be considered equal to that of plasma.

Experimental vCJD Transmission by Transfusion in Sheep

With the testing methods used until recently, infectivity had remained undetectable in the peripheral blood of patients with vCJD, although clinical transmission of the disease through human blood had clearly occurred. This apparent contradiction was explained by the technical challenge of developing a test capable of detecting the presence of abnormal prion protein in peripheral blood. Infection-associated forms of the prion protein constitute only a minuscule proportion of the total prion protein in blood, which represents a formidable obstacle to detecting infectivity in blood, even in patients with clinical disease. In rodent models employed to detect infectivity in human blood, the contradiction was further explained by the presence of a species barrier between humans and mice and the limited volumes of blood that could be inoculated into such small animals.

The relative closeness in size of sheep and humans means that volumes of blood comparable to those transfused in humans can be collected from and transfused into sheep. Houston et al[74] took 9 years to complete a blood transfusion experiment in sheep, concluding that blood transfusion represents an effective route of vCJD transmission. Two different transmissible spongiform encephalopathy (TSE) agents (scrapie and BSE) could be effectively transmitted between sheep by transfusion.[74] The overall transmission rates (percentage of all recipients who became infected) were 36% for BSE and 43% for scrapie. More specifically, 22 sheep received blood from BSE-exposed donor sheep; five recipient sheep developed clinical disease and three showed histopathologic evidence of infection—when they were sacrificed 7 years after exposure—without having developed any symptoms or signs of disease. Moreover, nine of 21 recipients of blood from scrapie-exposed sheep developed clinical scrapie. The incubation period of the five sheep who developed clinical disease after they had received blood from BSE-exposed donor sheep varied between 531 and 610 days (ie, it was <2 years). The incubation period of the nine sheep who developed clinical disease after they had received blood from scrapie-exposed donor sheep varied between 575 and 1138 days (ie, it was <3.2 years). Two of the five BSE-exposed recipient sheep that developed clinical disease had received blood from donor sheep with preclinical disease. All but one scrapie-exposed recipient sheep that developed clinical disease had received blood from donor sheep with preclinical disease.

The effect of the stage of the incubation period in the donor animal when each donation was made could best be deduced from the results of the scrapie experiment, because the *PRNP* genotype of the sheep used made them almost 100% susceptible to natural and experimental infection.[74] These results were consistent with a gradual increase in infectivity in peripheral blood as the incubation period progressed (Fig 3-1). Moreover, when blood was collected early (at 20%-50% of the estimated incubation period in the donor animals), the incubation period of scrapie in the recipient animals was longer.

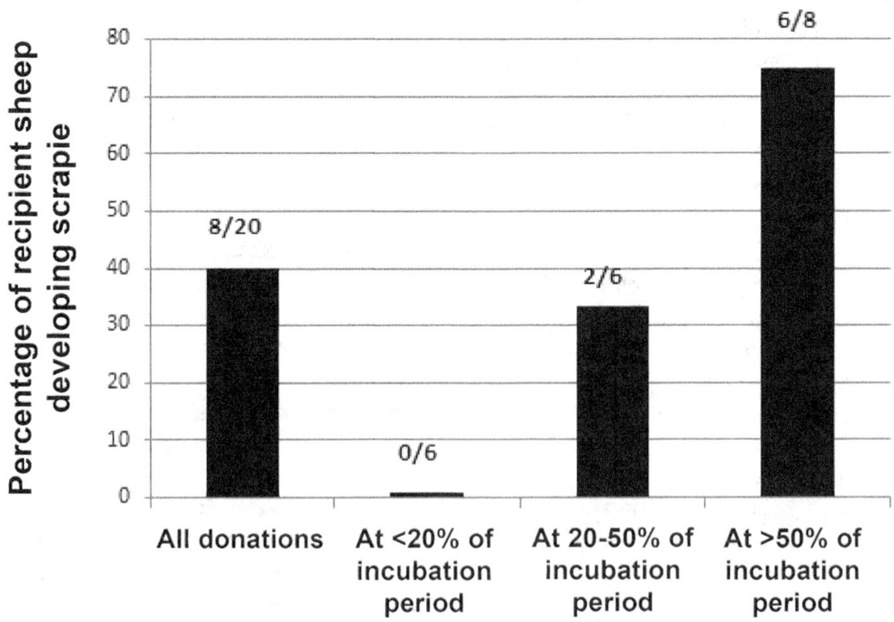

Figure 3-1. Proportion of recipient sheep developing scrapie after receiving whole-blood transfusion from donor sheep exposed to scrapie and assumed to be at various stages (from <20% to >50%) of the estimated incubation period.[75] The number of sheep developing scrapie among all transfused sheep is shown above each column. A donation made by a donor sheep during the clinical phase of scrapie[75] is not included. One recipient sheep suspected of clinically having scrapie, but showing no evidence of infection on postmortem examination,[75] is counted as not having the disease.

Risk of vCJD Transmission by Transfusion in the United Kingdom

Although vCJD is transmissible by transfusion, the magnitude of the risk of transmission is hard to estimate.[75] The scenarios that the United Kingdom currently uses for risk management employ combinations of "high" and "low" values for three determinants of the risk: the prevalence of subclinical disease in the blood donor population, the infectivity of blood components, and the susceptibility of blood recipients to clinical disease. Because several of these scenarios have overestimated the number of cases recorded, the SEAC requested at its March 2010 meeting that the scenarios used be calibrated against the observed data or that the assumptions made be refined to better approximate the observed data.[33]

As already discussed, the SEAC deemed that the appendix[34] and tonsil[35,36] data should not be combined to provide a single estimate of the prevalence of subclinical vCJD in the UK population on the basis of all available data, and it opted to continue using the initial 1 per 4000 prevalence estimate[34] for risk-management purposes.[33] If the data for both the appendix[34] and the tonsil[35,36] samples were to be combined, however, an approximate estimate of the prevalence of subclinical disease in the UK population would be in the range of 1 per 10,000,[59] because—among 32,661 tonsil samples[35,36] and 11,246 appendix samples[34]—four samples[33-36] have tested positive. Although further examinations of the tonsils and spleens of UK patients are under way or planned, the interpretation of their results—in terms of both the true prevalence of abnormal prion protein accumulation in the UK population and the frequency of infectious blood donors—is uncertain.[75]

Despite this uncertainty, codon-129 methionine homozygotes born after the containment of the BSE epidemic (ie, after January 1, 1996) may have a risk as high as 1 per 100,000[76] of developing a fatal disease after exposure to vCJD through transfusion if they survive for ≥ 5 years after a transfusion. Such would be the risk of transfusion-acquired clinical disease if 1) ordinary WBC reduction (as practiced in the United Kingdom today) did not prevent transmission of vCJD; 2) the probability of developing clinical disease after receiving blood from a donor who later developed vCJD were 23% (as derived above); 3) the prevalence of subclinical disease in the UK population were approximately 1 per 10,000[59]; and 4) 40% of donors with subclinical disease were infectious, as was the case in the completed sheep scrapie experiment[74] (Fig 3-1). A risk of this magnitude warrants preventive measures to protect recipients from a fatal transfusion-acquired disease.

Blood-Based Assays for the Detection of Clinical vCJD

Recently, Edgeworth et al[77] published the first report of an assay capable of discriminating vCJD-infected blood (drawn from individuals with clinical vCJD) from the blood of individuals who—at the time of sampling—were either healthy or affected by non-vCJD neurodegenerative disorders.[78] The investigators tested whole-blood samples from 21 patients with clinical vCJD, 27 patients with sporadic CJD, 42 patients with other neurologic disease, and 100 healthy controls. Each sample was tested twice and blindly in independent assay runs; only samples that were reactive in both runs were scored as positive.[77] The assay performance (approximately 70% sensitivity and >97% specificity; Table 3-2) is acceptable for a diagnostic test, which is intended for use in patients with neurodegenerative disease and a clinical presentation consistent with vCJD.[77,78] A lot more work is needed before such an assay can develop into a practical blood screening test.[77,78]

The technical challenges of developing a test for vCJD have been formidable.[79] Prions are composed principally, if not entirely, of a misfolded form of host cellular prion protein (PrP^C). Blood assays to detect an infectious agent use either a host humoral immune response or agent-specific nucleic acid, neither of which applies in vCJD. PrP^C is expressed ubiquitously, albeit at highest concentrations in the central nervous system (CNS) and cells of the immune system. During prion propagation after infection with vCJD, PrP^C is remodeled to aggregated,

Table 3-2. Diagnostic Accuracy of the First Blood-Based Assay for vCJD Infectivity

Study Subjects	Number (%) of Patients Tested*	
	Positive	Negative
21 patients with vCJD	15 (71.4)†	6 (28.6)
27 patients with sporadic CJD 42 patients with other neurologic disease 100 normal controls	0 (0.0)	169 (100.0)‡

*According to the first published study of the assay.[77]
†Sensitivity of 71.4% (95% CI = 47.8%-88.7%).
‡Specificity of 100.0% (95% CI = 97.8%-100.0%).
CJD = Creutzfeldt-Jakob disease; vCJD = variant Creutzfeldt-Jakob disease.

detergent-insoluble isoforms designated as PrP^{Sc}, which is chemically identical, but conformationally distinct from PrP^{C}. To successfully identify infection in blood, an assay has to be able to detect PrP^{Sc} at a concentration that is several orders of magnitude lower than the sensitivity of conventionally used immunoassays (Western blots or EIAs). Furthermore, the ratio of background PrP^{C} (which is chemically identical to PrP^{Sc}) to PrP^{Sc} is higher in blood than in any other tissue.[80]

Conventionally, immunoassays for PrP^{Sc} have depended on protease pretreatment of tissues to degrade PrP^{C} and thus to reduce the cross-reactivity between PrP^{C} and PrP^{Sc}. Rather than using preassay treatment with protease, Edgeworth et al[77] relied on the avid binding of prions to some surfaces, including metals such as stainless steel.[81,82] Stainless steel had previously been shown to absorb brain-derived prion-disease infectivity, but the properties of steel had not previously been studied with vCJD-infected peripheral blood. Moreover, steel had not previously been shown to selectively absorb abnormal PrP^{Sc} (as opposed to PrP^{C}).

In the assay of Edgeworth et al,[77] stainless steel selectively captured minute amounts of abnormal PrP^{Sc} in the presence of a large excess of normal prion protein in blood. Then, the disease-associated prion protein concentrated on the surface of metal was detected with an antibody to prion protein. The antibody was not specific for abnormal PrP^{Sc}, and thus the reported exquisite specificity must have been conferred exclusively by the selective absorption of abnormal PrP^{Sc} onto the stainless-steel particles.[78] This possibility is a remarkable discovery that–if confirmed–opens up a host of potential new studies. For example, it will be interesting to inoculate the stainless-steel particles exposed to vCJD agents into brains of vCJD-susceptible mice to establish whether infectivity is indeed bound to the particles.[78] The results of Edgeworth et al[77] further suggest that concentrations of abnormal prion protein in the blood of patients with vCJD may be higher[78] than the few picograms (or even femtograms) of abnormal PrP^{Sc} previously estimated to circulate in 1 mL of infected human blood.[83-85]

Prion-Reduction Filters

The term "infectious dose" refers to the minimal dose capable of transmitting infection to an animal in a particular animal model.[71] Studies in rodents with TSE showed infectivity of 1-10 infectious doses per mL of whole blood.[86-88]

About 40% of this infectivity was distributed in the WBCs and the remainder in the plasma.[88] The latter form of infectivity probably predominated, because the majority of the cell-associated infectivity was loosely bound and could be washed off.[88] Infectious prions, however, may partition between the cellular and acellular fractions of human blood differently from the manner in which they partitioned in these rodent models.

On the basis of the findings from the animal models, it can expected that ordinary WBC reduction through filtration (as implemented in the United Kingdom in 1999) would remove 40% to 70% of the total infectivity present in a whole-blood unit[88] but would have little impact on the plasma-borne infectivity. Under optimal conditions, only 10 mL of donor plasma can be left in an RBC unit prepared in an additive solution, although—under the usual conditions of manufacturing RBCs by the buffy-coat method in the United Kingdom—20 mL of plasma usually remains in the supernatant fluid. If 1) 40% of the infectivity resides in the WBCs and 60% in the plasma; 2) the starting whole-blood infectivity is 10 infectious doses/mL; 3) the whole-blood unit is WBC reduced; and 4) the residual plasma volume at the completion of all manufacturing steps is 10 mL, then >100 infectious doses would be left in the RBC unit distributed for transfusion[75] (Fig 3-2).

To achieve <1 infectious dose/transfused RBC component, a further 3-log reduction would be required (to successively reduce the total infectivity of the unit, for each successive log, to 11, 1.1, and ≥0.1 infectious doses). Uncertainty about the starting level of whole-blood infectivity (1 vs 10 infectious doses/mL or more in published rodent models) and the volume of plasma left in an RBC unit distributed in the United Kingdom (10 vs ≥20 mL) can each affect the extent of the necessary reduction to remove plasma-borne infectivity by approximately 1 log.[75]

Published studies of the efficacy of prion-reduction filters in rodent models[88-93] show a >3-log reduction in infectivity on brain homogenate spikes and a reduction in the limit of detection (>1 log) in endogenous infectivity studies. No data show the removal of infectivity from the blood of infected humans, however, and fundamental questions relating to the relevance of brain-homogenate-spike material to the clinical setting remain unanswered.[75] Exogenous infectivity models generally use 10% homogenized infected brain tissue. This approach achieves extremely high infectivity levels, but that does not imply that the spike behaves in blood in the same manner as endogenous abnormal prions (which would have naturally found their way to the peripheral blood of donors). The form in which infectivity circulates in the blood of infectious donors is unknown, so that the behavior of spiked infectivity across a filter may not reflect the behavior of true endogenous infectivity across the same filter. Therefore, the assessment of the efficacy of prion-reduction filters in removing human peripheral-blood infectivity continues to represent a formidable challenge.

The potential for deleterious effects on the RBC concentrate itself is also a matter of concern, both in terms of the possibility of alterations to the rheological or antigenic profile of the red cells and the red cell loss in the volume of the additional filter.[75] Nonetheless, in-vitro studies by the manufacturers did not raise concerns other than the high volume of blood retained by the filters, which is approximately 50 mL.[91] In the evaluations of the MacoPharma (Tourcoing, France) filter—which were performed by the UK[94] and Irish[95] blood services under the conditions in which prion reduction filters would likely be put into use in the United Kingdom and Ireland—up to 7-8 g of donor hemoglobin was retained by the filter.[94] As a result, WBC-reduced RBCs prepared by the buffy-coat-reduced ("bottom-and-top") manufacturing method could not meet the European Union (EU) minimum standard for a therapeutic adult RBC dose as applied in the United Kingdom (where ≥75% of the RBC units must contain ≥40 g of donor hemoglobin): only 58% of the units prepared by this method contained the minimum amount of red cells. When the whole-blood-filtration ("top-and-top") manufacturing method was used, however, the minimum hemoglobin requirement was met.[94]

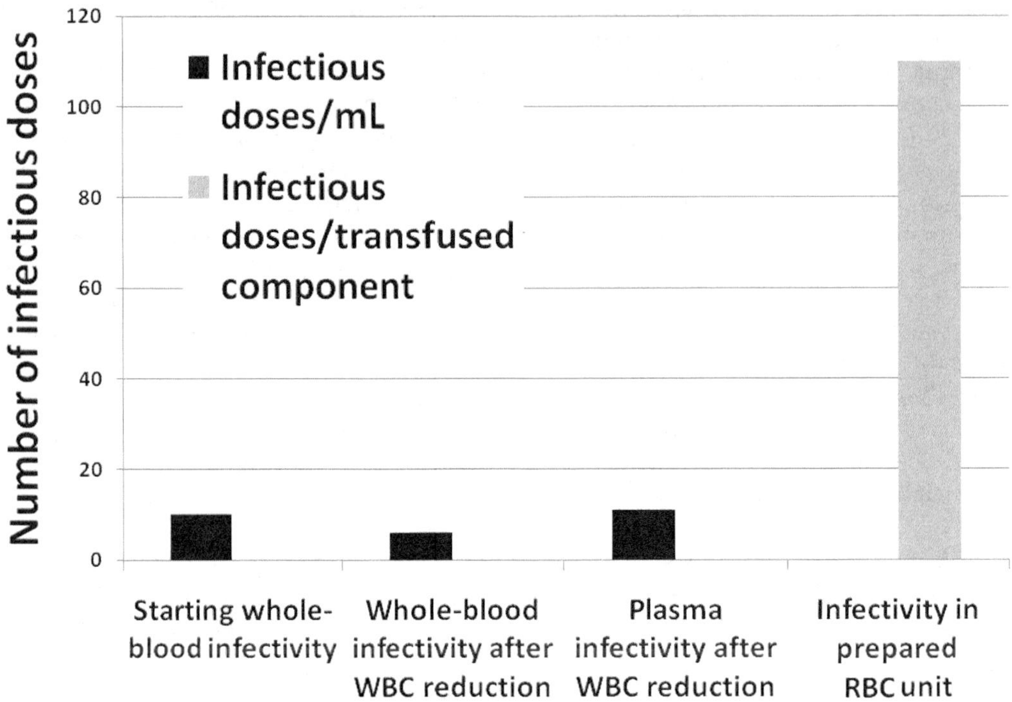

Figure 3-2. Infectivity residing in the plasma of a red blood cell (RBC) unit manufactured in the United Kingdom under ideal conditions.[75] If the starting infectivity in whole blood is 10 infectious doses/mL, six infectious doses/mL are left in the whole-blood unit after white blood cell (WBC) reduction, and all this infectivity resides in the unit's plasma. Assuming a 45% hematocrit for the donor, the concentration of infectivity in the unit's plasma is ≥10 infectious doses/mL. If only 10 mL of plasma is left in the component after the donor's plasma is replaced with additive solution, the total infectivity of the RBC unit distributed for transfusion is ≥100 infectious doses (≥10 infectious doses/mL × 10 mL of residual plasma). Initially published by Vamvakas in Transfus Med Rev 2011;25:133-44.[76]

The authors of the UK study[94] concluded that filtration had no detrimental effect on the expression of red cell antigens after they had passed through the filter, but another researcher stated that the employed methods likely would not have detected the generation of neoantigens.[96] Moreover, although appropriate adjustments to the filter sets could overcome the problem, 5.9% of the RBC units failed to filter properly. The response of treated cells to gamma-irradiation and freezing was essentially unaffected, and routine quality measures (extracellular potassium, 2,3-disphosphoglycerate, and adenosine triphosphate) were satisfactory.[94]

A safety (Phase I/II) clinical trial of the MacoPharma filter in volunteer allogeneic RBC recipients raised no safety concerns.[95] Twenty patients uneventfully received the transfusion of one RBC unit that had undergone prion filtration, and six of them received further prion-reduced units without adverse effects. Clinical events and laboratory test results (liver function tests and red cell antibody screen and antiglobulin test) were recorded during the transfusion, during the first 24 hours, and at a 6-week follow-up visit. The posttransfusion hemoglobin increment (mean ± SD) was 0.70 ± 0.50 g/unit (compared to 0.98 ± 0.30 g/unit in historical controls). Although the controls were not matched to the cases, both cases and controls were multitransfused hematology patients, and the minimum EU standard for hemoglobin content (40 g/unit) had been met in all of the transfused units. Further studies of the safety of prion-reduction filters are warranted for extending these safety data to other adult (and especially pediatric) populations.

At least three manufacturers have pursued the development of prion-reduction filters. Pall (Port Washington, NY) extended the original use of WBC-reduction filters to prion adsorption through a modification of the filter that rendered it capable of adsorbing infectious prions with a practicable degree of specificity and efficacy. Other manufacturers (PRDT, Cambridge, UK; and MacoPharma in collaboration with Pathogen Removal and Diagnostic Technologies, Inc., Edinburgh, UK) incorporated in a prion filter, separate from the WBC-reduction filter, ligands developed with combinatorial chemistry to specifically bind to the abnormal prion protein. The reported capability of these two types of filters is the same.[88-93] The devices remove infectivity from plasma, or at least from the amount of plasma present in RBCs manufactured in additive solution. An excess of plasma–such as can be present in a unit of whole blood or fresh frozen plasma (FFP)–may interfere with the efficacy of the filter.[97]

At the March 2010 meeting of the SEAC, it was reported that the Advisory Committee on the Safety of Blood, Tissues, and Organs had recommended that blood prion filtration be used for transfusion recipients with no prior evidence of dietary exposure to BSE.[33] The UK Department of Health is presently considering this recommendation.

Has Ordinary WBC Reduction Prevented Transfusion Transmission of vCJD?

No case of transfusion-transmitted vCJD has been reported from the United Kingdom in a patient who received blood after the implementation of universal WBC reduction in October 1999.[76] For blood donors acquiring vCJD from dietary sources, clinical disease would appear after a long incubation period. Therefore, such donors (infected during the years of the BSE epidemic in the 1980s) would have been in the preclinical phase of disease (with sufficient infectivity in their peripheral blood to infect transfusion recipients) in the late 1990s and/or in the first decade of the 21st century. If 1) vCJD transmission by transfusion continued to occur after the implementation of universal WBC reduction, and 2) three recipients who contracted vCJD infection from transfusions given between 1996 and 1999 manifested clinical disease by 2006, which would make the incubation period of transfusion-acquired vCJD 6 to 8.5 years,[67-69] then, by the end of 2010, there should have been a few more cases of clinical vCJD contracted from transfusions given in the period 1999-2002.

Although the current WBC reduction would not be expected, according to the prevailing infectivity assumptions based on the findings from rodent models, to sufficiently reduce infectivity to prevent infection of a transfusion recipient,[75] it remains possible that WBC reduction does afford protection. Four sources of uncertainty make this possible: 1) the starting level of infectivity in human whole blood (which may be lower than the 1to 10 infectious doses/mL level observed in animal models); 2) the distribution of the infectivity between human plasma and WBCs (which may differ from the 60:40 ratio indicated by rodent models); 3) the effectiveness of human-to-human transmission; and 4) the susceptibility of transfused patients to infection from any given inoculum.

Until a case of transfusion-transmitted vCJD is reported to have been contracted through transfusion of a WBC-reduced component, one cannot conclude that the ordinary WBC reduction currently taking place in the United Kingdom and several other European countries does not protect from transfusion transmission of vCJD. Any measure of safety (including complete protection) that such ordinary WBC reduction affords vis-à-vis vCJD transmission remains unknown. Therefore, the current universal WBC reduction for the prevention of vCJD in Europe should continue.

The effect of WBC reduction was being addressed in a follow-up study of the completed sheep scrapie experiment. In the completed sheep scrapie experiment,[74] transmission rates were the same in recipient sheep transfused with whole blood (4 of 10) and recipient sheep transfused with buffy coat (4 of 10). In the follow-up study, all clinically-relevant blood components prepared by methods similar to those used by blood services transmitted BSE from asymptomatic donor sheep to recipient sheep and WBC reduction did not prevent transmission.[98] In fact, a single transfusion of WBC-reduced RBCs, platelets, or plasma transmitted BSE in several cases. Although the transmission efficiencies of WBC-reduced components were lower than those of non-WBC-reduced equivalent components, the data reported in August 2011[98] represent only interim transmission efficiencies (at approximately 1200 days following transfusion of a blood component collected from an asymptomatic donor sheep), and they may well change over time as follow-up continues. It is thus possible that–in sheep as well as in humans–WBC reduction, by removing the WBC-associated fraction of infectivity, protracts the asymptomatic phase of disease in transfusion recipients infected with a low inoculum.[76] If this were the case, 1200 days–although exceeding the incubation periods of BSE observed in the completed experiment[74]–may be too short a period for BSE contracted through a WBC-reduced blood transfusion in sheep to manifest itself.

Such a reduction in infectivity because of WBC reduction also could explain why no transfusion-transmitted cases (contracted in 1999-2002) were reported by the end of 2009. In other words, just as the reference to the risk of transmission of vCJD through transfusion moved from "theoretical" to "possible," "probable," and "definite" with the reporting of the four cases of transfusion-transmitted vCJD from non-WBC-reduced RBCs between 2003 and 2007,[67-70] the same scenario could unfold in the coming years as cases of transfusion-transmitted vCJD from WBC-reduced RBCs appear after a protracted incubation period. The reporting of cases of vCJD transmission through transfusion of WBC-reduced RBCs will change the prevailing estimates of the risk of vCJD transmission by transfusion both inside and outside the United Kingdom. Such cases (contracted after 1999–that is, after the United Kingdom implemented universal WBC reduction to prevent transmission of vCJD and after the BSE epidemic in the United Kingdom had been contained) would confirm the prediction of a UK vCJD epidemic sustained by blood transfusion.[99] It is for this reason that–on a precautionary basis–all transfusion recipients have already been deferred from donating blood in the United Kingdom, France, and The Netherlands.

Are Further Measures Needed to Prevent Transfusion Transmission of vCJD?

To protect recipients with no dietary exposure to BSE, the United Kingdom implemented extraordinary measures for transfused plasma (Table 3-3) in the absence of a vCJD case linked to vCJD infectivity residing in human plasma. Thus, even without a reported case of vCJD contracted through transfusion of WBC-reduced RBCs, the endorsement of prion-reduction filters for recipients without evidence of dietary exposure to BSE would be consistent with the measures already adopted to prevent transmission of vCJD through plasma. The only caveat pertaining to this endorsement is that the UK blood services employ a manufacturing method ensuring that prion-reduced RBC units meet the EU minimum standard for hemoglobin content (40 g/unit). Like the importation of plasma from low-risk countries (Table 3-3), until a case of transmission of vCJD through WBC-reduced RBCs is reported, the initiative to introduce prion-reduction filters represents a precautionary measure (Chapter 1). As such, it can be deemed appropriate according to the existing precedent: if the measure for plasma intended for transfusion to UK patients born after January 1, 1996, is appropriate, provision to these same patients of WBC-reduced RBCs that have undergone the

Table 3-3. Measures Already Adopted in the United Kingdom to Reduce the Risk of Transmission of vCJD by Transfusion

- Universal WBC reduction of all cellular blood components.
- Reduction in allogeneic-donor exposures through the use of apheresis (as opposed to pooled whole-blood-derived) platelets.
- Deferral from donating blood of all persons with a history of blood transfusion since 1980.
- Cessation of use of indigenous plasma for the manufacturing of plasma derivatives.
- Specifically for patients born after January 1, 1996 and considered not to have had any dietary exposure to BSE: Importation for transfusion of methylene-blue-treated plasma donated by donors in low-risk countries.*
- Optimization of blood component use:
  - Assurance that blood components are transfused only when needed.
  - Communication of the uncertainties about the risks of allogeneic blood transfusion to patients and the public.

*Imported plasma for transfusion is subjected to a pathogen reduction procedure because the risk of transfusion-transmitted human immunodeficiency virus, hepatitis C virus, and hepatitis B virus infection in some of the countries from which plasma is imported (eg, the United States) is higher than that in the United Kingdom.
BSE = bovine spongiform encephalopathy; vCJD = variant Creutzfeldt-Jakob disease; WBC = white cell.

further step of prion filtration can be deemed appropriate as well.

An alternative could be to provide washed WBC-reduced RBCs to these young UK patients,[97] although–as the number of patients with no dietary exposure to BSE increases with each passing year–washing may prove just as disruptive to safeguarding an adequate blood supply as may the use of prion-reduction filters. Nonetheless, the possibility of washing RBCs–which surely is a safe alternative with respect to any untoward effects of prion filtration and which also may offer some protection from transfusion-related acute lung injury (TRALI)[100]–should not be forgotten amid the effort to validate and implement the new technology of prion filtration.

Elsewhere in Europe, there were 41 cases of vCJD by the end of 2009 (Table 3-4). No new cases were recorded between the end of 2009 and March 2011. Nonetheless, the description in other countries–such as Spain and Saudi Arabia–of vCJD patients who had been blood donors in the past suggests that the problem has already taken on an international dimension[71] and that it warrants proportional responses from outside the United Kingdom as well. If we accept the prevalence of subclinical vCJD in the United Kingdom to be 1 per 10,000,[59] then–from the relative incidence of clinical disease between each particular country and the United Kingdom–we can expect the prevalence of subclinical vCJD in Europe to be as shown in Table 3-4.

The prevalence in each country cannot be inferred simply from the relative incidence of clinical disease, because the epidemics in these other countries have lagged behind the UK epidemic and there has not yet been a sufficient number of cases to characterize each epidemiologic curve. Nonetheless, at least in the interim, decisions in these countries could be proportional to the relative incidence of clinical disease between each other country and the United Kingdom. Outside the United Kingdom and Ireland, the risk from transfusion of plasma has not been deemed worthy of the precautionary measures implemented in the United Kingdom and Ireland for patients born after January 1, 1996 (Table 3-3). Accordingly, at this point, neither should the vCJD infectivity residing in the resid-

Table 3-4. Estimated Prevalence of Subclinical Variant Creutzfeldt-Jakob Disease (vCJD) in Europe as of March 2011

Country	Number of Clinical vCJD Cases*	Presumed Prevalence	
		% of UK Cases†	Estimate‡
UK	175	100	1 per 10,000
Ireland	2 (4)*	17	1 per 60,000
France	25	14	1 per 70,000§
The Netherlands	3	6.5	1 per 150,000
Portugal	2	6.5	1 per 150,000
Spain	5	4	1 per 250,000
Italy	2	1	1 per 1,000,000

*When cases had resided in the United Kingdom for longer than 6 months between 1980 and 1996, they are presumed to have been exposed to bovine spongiform encephalopathy in the United Kingdom. The total number of vCJD cases in Ireland (including the two cases probably exposed in the United Kingdom) is shown within parentheses.[32]
†Based on the relative incidence of clinical disease between each country and the United Kingdom. The population of cases in each country was obtained from http://en.wikipedia.org/wiki/Demographics_of_the_European_Union.
‡Approximation that does not take into account the differences in the epidemiologic curve of each country vs that of the United Kingdom. Based on the "average" UK estimate of prevalence[59] (1 per 10,000) derived when the tonsil[35,36] and appendix[34] data are combined (4/43,907[33-36]).
§Compared to the estimate of 1 per 120,000 generated from data on the French vCJD epidemic.[71]

ual plasma of WBC-reduced RBCs be deemed worthy of prion filtration.

Platelets[101] and RBCs[102] appear to contain no vCJD infectivity. The current opinion held by the SEAC is that—while there may be interspecies differences in the distribution of TSE infectivity in the blood—according to data from animal models, vCJD infectivity in human blood is likely to be partitioned between plasma and WBCs[102,103] and to be only minimally associated with RBCs and platelets.[104] With regard to platelet concentrates—whether pooled whole-blood-derived platelets prepared by the buffy-coat method or apheresis platelets—minimization of plasma pooling and resuspension in additive solutions rather than plasma would reduce the amount of residual plasma to 80 to 90 mL.[75] That amount of plasma would contain more than enough infectivity to transmit infection to the recipient, under even optimistic infectivity assumptions.[75] Thus, efforts to minimize the plasma volume of platelets through replacement with additive solutions are likely to be ineffectual,[75] and the United Kingdom is in the process of converting its platelet supply from pooled whole-blood-derived to single-donor platelets (Table 3-3). Prion-reduction filters are not currently applicable to either platelets or FFP. They may become available for S/D-P plasma in the near future, which would make S/D-P plasma perhaps superior to male-only FFP—at least in Europe—for the prevention of both TRALI[105] and transfusion transmission of vCJD.[106]

Summary

One interpretation of the progression of the 1996-2010 UK vCJD epidemic (with <5 cases having occurred annually over the past several years[32]) is that the epidemic is nearly over. Another interpretation is that, although the *food-borne* epidemic may be nearly over (with only 100 future cases expected, primarily in codon-129 heterozygotes and valine homozygotes exposed to BSE prions before 1996), there maybe a "second wave" of the vCJD epidemic, primarily propagated through blood transfusion (with 277 future cases expected, primarily in methionine homozygotes).[62] Although the assumed prevalence of subclinical vCJD in UK blood donors (1 per 10,000[59]; Table 3-4) might lead one to expect more transfusion-transmitted vCJD cases in the future, the median life expectancy of transfusion recipients[107] is shorter than the mean incubation period of vCJD, even in codon-129 methionine homozygotes. Therefore, many transfusion recipients infected with vCJD prions through ABT will die before they develop vCJD (and will not be included in the UK statistics as either food-borne or transfusion-transmitted vCJD cases). Nonetheless, the upper 95% CI of the prediction interval of Garske and Ghani[62] anticipates as many as 2700 transfusion-transmitted cases of vCJD. The expectation of such a second wave of vCJD cases in the United Kingdom (which may be primarily transfusion-transmitted) must be carefully considered in future decisions to adopt (or to withdraw) further proposed blood safety measures.

Variant CJD is a fatal infection that can be contracted from blood donated by an asymptomatic blood donor during an exceedingly long incubation period that includes a long blood-borne phase. Therefore, vCJD shares all the characteristics of HIV infection in the 1980s, highlighting the fact that the next major HIV-like transfusion-transmitted pathogen to emerge may well have a primary mode of transmission all together different from that of HIV. The recognition of such an HIV infection-like transfusion-transmitted new disease led to unprecedented efforts to protect the safety of the UK blood supply (Table 3-3). The transmissibility of vCJD through ABT is considered proven, and the prevalence of subclinical vCJD in the UK general population (and thus the population of UK blood donors as well) may be as high as 1 per 10,000[59] (Table 3-4). Thus, the present situation in the United Kingdom reproduces the worst-case scenario described in the introduction to this chapter: that is, the possibility of a novel HIV-like pathogen reaching a prevalence of 1 per 10,000 in the US blood donor population.

Although the UK vCJD situation illustrates how realistic the worst-case scenario described in the introduction to this chapter is, careful consideration of the research data on transmission through transfusion for other emerging agents has supported the opposite conclusion (ie, that transmission through transfusion most likely does not occur). An example of an emerging and potentially TTI for which the aggregate data are most consistent with the interpretation of lack of transmission through transfusion[108] is infection with the human herpesvirus-8 (HHV-8). The literature on transfusion transmission of HHV-8 is presented as part of Chapter 6.

References

1. Goodnough LT, Brecher ME, Kanter MH, AuBuchon JP. Transfusion medicine. First of two parts—blood transfusion. N Engl J Med 1999;340:438-47.
2. Vamvakas EC. Relative safety of pooled whole-blood-derived versus single-donor (apheresis) platelets in the United States: A systematic review of disparate risks. Transfusion 2009;49: 2743-58.
3. Vamvakas EC, Blajchman MA. Blood still kills: Six strategies to further reduce allogeneic blood transfusion-related mortality. Transfus Med Rev 2010;24:77-124.
4. Dodd RY. Emerging infections, transfusion safety, and epidemiology. N Engl J Med 2003; 349:1205-6.
5. Pealer LN, Martin AA, Petersen LR, et al. Transmission of West Nile virus through blood transfusion in the United States in 2002. N Engl J Med 2003;349:1236-45.
6. Macedo de Oliveira A, Beecham BD, Montgomery SP, et al. West Nile virus blood transfusion-

related infection despite nucleic acid testing. Transfusion 2004;44:1695-9.
7. Biggerstaff BJ, Petersen LR. Estimated risk of transmission of West Nile virus through blood transfusion in the US, 2002. Transfusion 2003; 43:1007-17.
8. Stramer SL, Hollinger FB, Katz LM, et al. Emerging infectious disease agents and their potential threat to transfusion safety. Transfusion 2009(Suppl 2):49:1S-236S.
9. Variant Creutzfeldt-Jakob disease (vCJD). Association Bulletin #00-6. December 8, 2000. Bethesda, MD: AABB, 2000.
10. Dodd RY, Sullivan MT. Creutzfeldt-Jakob disease and transfusion safety: Tilting at icebergs? Transfusion 1998;38:221-3.
11. Richetts MN, Cashman NR, Stratton EE, Elsaadany S. Is Creutzfeldt-Jakob disease transmitted by blood? Emerg Infect Dis 1997;3:155-63.
12. Richetts MN. Is Creutzfeldt-Jakob disease transmitted by blood? Is the absence of evidence of risk evidence of the absence of risk? Can Med Assoc J 1997;157:1367-70.
13. Bruce-Chwatt LJ. Transfusion-transmitted malaria revisited. Trop Dis Bull 1982;79:827-40.
14. Turc JM. Malaria and blood transfusion. In: Westphal RG, Carlson KB, Turc JM, eds. Emerging global patterns in transfusion-transmitted infections. Arlington, VA: AABB, 1990:31-43.
15. Mungai M, Tegtmeier G, Chamberland M, Parisel M. Transfusion-transmitted malaria in the United States from 1963 through 1999. N Engl J Med 2001;344:1973-8.
16. Slinger R, Giulivi A, Bodie-Collins M, et al. Transfusion-transmitted malaria in Canada. CMAJ 2001;164:377-9.
17. Gerber MA, Shapiro ED, Krause PJ, et al. The risk of acquiring Lyme disease or babesiosis from a blood transfusion. J Infect Dis 1994; 170:231-4.
18. Gubernot DM, Lucey CT, Lee KC, et al. Babesia infection through blood transfusions: Reports received by the US Food and Drug Administration, 1997-2007. Clin Infect Dis 2009;48:25-30.
19. Tonnetti L, Eder AF, Dy B, et al. Transfusion-transmitted Babesia microti identified through hemovigilance. Transfusion 2009;49:2557-63.
20. Gubernot DM, Nakhasi HL, Mied PA, et al. Transfusion-transmitted babesiosis in the United States: Summary of a workshop. Transfusion 2009;49:2759-71.
21. Johnson ST, Cable RG, Leiby DA. Lookback investigations of *Babesia microti*-seropositive blood donors: Seven-year experience in a Babesia-endemic area. Transfusion 2012 (in press).
22. Herwaldt BL, Linden JV, Bosserman E, et al. Transfusion-associated babesiosis in the United States: A description of cases. Ann Intern Med 2011;155:509-19.
23. Cardo LJ. Leishmania: Risk to the blood supply. Transfusion 2006;46:1641-5.
24. Wells GM, Woodward TE, Fiset P, Hornick RB. Rocky Mountain spotted fever caused by blood transfusion. JAMA 1978;239:2763-5.
25. Wahlberg P, Saikku P, Brummer-Korvenkontio M. Tick-borne viral encephalitis in Finland. The clinical features of Kumlinge disease during 1959-1987. J Intern Med 1989;225:173-7.
26. Kitchen AD, Barbara JA. Which agents threaten blood safety in the future? Baillieres Clin Haematol 2000;13:601-14.
27. Prowse C, Ludlam CA, Yap PL. Human parvovirus B19 and blood products. Vox Sang 1997; 72:1-10.
28. Gunter K, Luban N. Transfusion-transmitted cytomegalovirus and Epstein-Barr virus diseases. In: Rossi EC, Simon TL, Moss GL, Gould SA, eds. Principles of transfusion medicine. 2nd ed. Baltimore, MD: William & Wilkins, 1996: 717-32.
29. Koenigbauer UF, Eastlund T, Day JW. Clinical illness due to parvovirus B19 infection after infusion of solvent/detergent-treated pooled plasma. Transfusion 2000;40:1203-6.
30. Dodd R. Hepatitis. In: Petz LD, Swisher SN, Kleinman S, et al, eds. Clinical practice of transfusion medicine. 3rd ed. New York: Churchill Livingstone, 1996:847-73.
31. Ghani AC, Donnelly CA, Ferguson NM, Anderson RM. The transmission dynamics of BSE and vCJD. C R Biol 2002;325:37-47.
32. The National Creutzfeldt-Jakob Disease Surveillance Unit. Information on variant CJD. Edinburgh, UK: University of Edinburgh, 2011. [Available at: http://www.cjd.ed.ac.uk (accessed September 20, 2011).]
33. SEAC. Minutes of the 104th meeting of the Spongiform Encephalopathy Advisory Committee, London, UK, March 5, 2010. [Available at: http://www.seac.gov.uk/summaries/seac104-summary.pdf (accessed March 19, 2011).]
34. Hilton DA, Ghani AC, Conyers L, et al. Prevalence of lymphoreticular prion protein accumulation in UK tissue samples. J Pathol 2004; 203:733-9.

35. Crewly JP, Kelly CM, Andrews N, et al. Prevalence of disease-related prion protein in anonymous tonsil specimens in Britain: Cross-sectional opportunistic survey. Br Med J 2009; 338:b1442.
36. deMarco MF, Linehan J, Gill ON, et al. Large-scale immunohistochemical examination for lymphoreticular prion protein in tonsil specimens collected in Britain. J Pathol 2010;222: 380-7.
37. Mabbott N, Turner M. Prion and the blood immune systems. Haematologica 2005;90: 542-8.
38. Hilton DA, Fathers E, Edwards P, et al. Prion immunoreactivity in appendix before clinical onset of variant Creutzfeldt-Jakob disease. Lancet 1998;352:703-4.
39. Collinge J, Whitfield J, Mckintosh E, et al. Kuru in the 21st century—an acquired human prion disease with very long incubation periods. Lancet 2006;367:2068-74.
40. Hill AF, Joiner S, Lineman J, et al. Species-barrier independent prion replication in apparently resistant species. Proc Natl Acad Sci U S A 2000;97:10248-53.
41. Race R, Raines A, Raymond GJ, et al. Long-term subclinical carrier state precedes scrapie replication and adaptation in a resistant species: Analogies to bovine spongiform encephalopathy and variant Creutzfeldt-Jakob disease. J Virol 2001; 75:10106-12.
42. Bishop MT, Hart P, Aitchison L, et al. Predicting susceptibility and incubation time of human-to-human transmission of vCJD. Lancet Neurol 2006;5:393-8.
43. Palmer MS, Dryden AJ, Hughes JT, Collinge J. Homozygous prion protein genotype predisposes to sporadic Creutzfeldt-Jakob disease. Nature 1991;352:340-2.
44. Lee HS, Brown P, Cervenakova L, et al. Increased susceptibility of Kuru carriers to the *PRNP* 129 methionine/methionine genotype. J Infect Dis 2001;183:192-6.
45. Mead S, Stumpf MP, Whitfield J, et al. Balancing selection at the prion protein gene consistent with prehistoric kurulike epidemics. Science 2003;300:640-3.
46. Collinge J, Palmer S, Dryden AJ. Genetic predisposition to iatrogenic Creutzfeldt-Jakob disease. Lancet 1991;337:1441-2.
47. Collinge J. Variant Creutzfeldt-Jakob disease. Lancet 1999;354:317-23.
48. Brown P, Preece M, Brandel JP, et al. Iatrogenic Creutzfeldt-Jakob disease at the millennium. Neurology 2000;55:1075-81.
49. Barlow RM, Middleton DJ. Dietary transmission of bovine spongiform encephalopathy to mice. Vet Res 1990;126:111-12.
50. Lessons from kuru (editorial). Lancet 2006; 367:2034.
51. Lloyd SE, Onwuazor ON, Beck JA, et al. Identification of multiple quantitative trait loci linked to prion disease incubation period in mice. Proc Natl Acad Sci U S A 2001;98:6279-83.
52. Lloyd SE, Uphill JB, Targonski PV, et al. Identification of genetic loci affecting mouse-adapted bovine spongiform encephalopathy incubation time in mice. Neurogenetics 2002;4:77-81.
53. Stephenson DA, Chiotti K, Ebeling C, et al. Quantitative trait loci affecting prion incubation time in mice. Genomics 2000;69:47-53.
54. Collinge J. Prion diseases of humans and animals: Their causes and molecular basis. Annu Rev Neurosci 2001;24:519-50.
55. Asante E, Linehan J, Gowland I, et al. Dissociation of pathological and molecular phenotype of variant Creutzfeldt-Jakob disease in transgenic human prion protein 129 heterozygous mice. Proc Natl Acad Sci U S A 2006;103:10759-64.
56. Wadsworth JD, Asante E, Desbruslais M, et al. Human prion protein with valine 129 prevents expression of variant CJD phenotype. Science 2004;306:1793-6.
57. Kaski D, Mead S, Hyare H, et al. Variant CJD in an individual heterozygous for *PRNP* codon 129. Lancet 2009;374:2128.
58. Peden AH, Head MW, Ritchie DL, et al. Preclinical vCJD after blood transfusion in a *PRNP* codon-129 heterozygous patient. Lancet 2004; 364:527-9.
59. Peden A, McCardle L, Head MW, et al. Variant CJD infection in the spleen of a neurologically asymptomatic UK adult patient with haemophilia. Haemophilia 2010;16:296-304.
60. Ironside JW, Bishop MT, Connolly K, et al. Variant Creutzfeldt-Jakob disease: Prion protein genotype analysis of positive appendix tissue samples from a retrospective prevalence study. Br Med J 2006;332:1186-8.
61. Andrews NJ. Incidence of variant Creutzfeldt-Jakob disease diagnoses and deaths in the UK: January 1994-December 2009 (updated June 22, 2010). London, UK: Statistics Unit, Center for Infections, Health Protection Agency, 2010. [Available at http://www.cjd.ed.ac.uk/cjdq64 jun10.pdf (accessed Mar 23, 2011).]

62. Garske T, Ghani AC. Uncertainty in the tail of variant Creutzfeldt-Jakob disease epidemic in the UK. PLoS ONE 2010;5:e15626.doi.10.1371/journal.pone.0015626.
63. Clarke P, Ghani AC. Projections of future course of the primary vCJD epidemic in the UK: Inclusion of subclinical infection and the possibility of wider genetic susceptibility. J R Soc Interface 2005;2:19-31.
64. Clarke P, Will RG, Ghani AC. Is there a potential for an epidemic of variant Creutzfeldt-Jakob disease via blood transfusion in the UK? J R Soc Interface 2007;4:675-84.
65. Mead S, Joiner S, Desbruslais M, et al. Creutzfeldt-Jakob disease, prion-protein gene codon 129 VV, and a novel PrPSc type in a young British woman. Arch Neurol 2007;64:1780-4.
66. Cholan G, Llewelyn C, Mackenzie J, et al. Variant Creutzfeldt-Jakob disease in a transfusion recipient. Coincidence or cause? Transfusion 2010;50:1003-6.
67. Pincock S. Patient's death from vCJD may be linked to blood transfusion. Committee to discuss need for further precautions to prevent possible vCJD transmission through blood. Lancet 2004;363:43.
68. Llewelyn CA, Hewitt PE, Knight RS, et al. Possible transmission of variant Creutzfeldt-Jakob disease by blood transfusion. Lancet 2004;363:417-21.
69. Hewitt PE, Llewelyn CA, Mackenzie J, Will RG. Creutzfeldt-Jakob disease and blood transfusion: Results of the UK Transfusion Epidemiology Review Study. Vox Sang 2006;91:221-30.
70. Health Protection Agency. Fourth case of transfusion-associated variant CJD. Health Prot Rep 2007;1:3.
71. Lefrère JJ, Hewitt P. From cows to sensible blood transfusion: The risk of prion transmission from labile blood components in the United Kingdom and France. Transfusion 2009;49:797-812.
72. Lee CA, Ironside JW, Bell JE, et al. Retrospective neuropathological review of prion disease in UK hemophilia patients. Thromb Haemost 1998;80:909-11.
73. Zaman SM, Hill FG, Palmer B, et al. The risk of variant Creutzfeldt-Jakob disease among UK patients with bleeding disorders known to have received potentially contaminated plasma products. Haemophilia 2011;17:931-7.
74. Houston F, McCutcheon S, Goldmann W, et al. Prion diseases are efficiently transmitted by blood transfusion in sheep. Blood 2008;112:4739-45.
75. Turner ML, Ludlam CA. An update on the assessment and management of the risk of transmission of variant Creutzfeldt-Jakob disease by blood and plasma products. Br J Haematol 2009;144:14-23.
76. Vamvakas EC. Universal white-blood-cell reduction in Europe: Has transmission of vCJD been prevented? Transfus Med Rev 2011;25:133-44.
77. Edgeworth JA, Farmer M, Sicilia A, et al. Detection of prion infection in variant Creutzfeldt-Jakob disease: A blood-based assay. Lancet 2011;377:487-93.
78. Gregori L. A prototype assay to detect vCJD-infected blood. Lancet 2011;377:444-6.
79. Brown P. Blood infectivity, processing, and screening tests in transmissible spongiform encephalopathy. Vox Sang 2005;89:63-70.
80. Tattum MH, Jones S, Pal S, et al. A highly sensitive immunoassay for the detection of prion-infected material in whole human blood without the use of proteinase K. Transfusion 2010;50:2619-27.
81. Zobeley E, Flechsig E, Cozzio A, et al. Infectivity of scrapie prions bound to a stainless steel surface. Mol Med 1999;5:240-3.
82. Edgeworth JA, Jackson GS, Clarke AR, et al. Highly sensitive, quantitative cell-based assay for prions absorbed to solid surfaces. Proc Natl Acad Sci U S A 2009;106:3479-83.
83. Brown P, Cervenakova L, Diringer H. Blood infectivity and the prospects for a diagnostic screening test in Creutzfeldt-Jakob disease. J Lab Clin Med 2001;137:5-13.
84. Gregori L, Gray BN, Rose E, et al. A sensitive and quantitative assay for normal PrP in plasma. J Virol Methods 2008;149:251-9.
85. Chen B, Morales R, Barria MA, Soto C. Estimating prion concentration in fluids and tissues by quantitative PMCA. Nat Methods 2010;7:519-20.
86. Brown P, Rohwer RG, Dunstan BC, et al. The distribution of infectivity in blood components and plasma derivatives in experimental models of transmissible spongiform encephalopathy. Transfusion 1998;38:810-16.
87. Cervenakova L, Yakovleva O, McKenzie C, et al. Similar levels of infectivity in the blood of mice infected with human-derived vCJD and GSS strains of transmissible spongiform encephalopathy. Transfusion 2003;43:1687-94.
88. Gregori L, Grugel PV, Lathorp JT, et al. Reduction in infectivity of endogenous transmissible

spongiform encephalopathies present in blood by adsorption to selective affinity resins. Lancet 2006;368:2226-30.
89. Gregori L, McCombie N, Palmer D, et al. Effectiveness of leukoreduction for removal of infectivity of transmissible spongiform encephalopathies from blood. Lancet 2004;364:529-31.
90. Gregori L, Lambert BC, Gurgel PV, et al. Reduction of transmissible spongiform encephalopathy infectivity from human red cells with prion protein affinity ligands. Transfusion 2006;46: 1152-61.
91. Saunders C, Herbert P, Rowe M, et al. In-vitro evaluation of the Pall Leukotrap® affinity prion reduction filter as a secondary device following primary leukoreduction. Vox Sang 2007;89: 220-8.
92. Sowenimo-Coker SO, Kascsak R, Kim A, et al. Removal of exogenous (spiked) and endogenous prion infectivity from red cells with a new prototype of leukocyte filtration filer. Transfusion 2005;45:1839-44.
93. Sowemimo-Coker SO, Pesci S, Andrade F, et al. Pall leukotrap affinity prion-reduction filter removes exogenous infectious prions and endogenous infectivity from red cell concentrates. Vox Sang 2006;90:265-75.
94. Wiltshire M, Thomas S, Scott J, et al. Prion reduction of red blood cells: Impact on component quality. Transfusion 2010;50:970-9.
95. Cahill MR, Murphy T, Khan M, et al. Phase I/II safety study of transfusion of prion-filtered red-cell concentrates in transfusion-dependent patients. Vox Sang 2010;99:174-6.
96. Dodd RY. Prions and precautions: Be careful for what you ask. Transfusion 2010;50:956-8.
97. Eglin RP, Murphy WG. Beyond leukodepletion: Removing infectious prions by filtration. Transfusion 2005;45:1836-8.
98. McCutcheon S, Blanco ARA, Houston EF, et al. All clinically-relevant blood components transmit prion disease following a single blood transfusion: A sheep model of vCJD. PLoS One 2011;6:e23169.
99. Farrugia A, Ironside JW, Giagrande P. Variant Creutzfeldt-Jakob disease transmission by plasma products: Assessing and communicating risk in an era of scientific uncertainty. Vox Sang 2005;89:186-92.
100. Benson AB, Moss M, Silliman CC. Transfusion-related acute lung injury (TRALI): A clinical review with emphasis on the critically ill. Br J Haematol 2009;147:431-43.
101. Holada K, Vostal JG, Theisen PW, et al. Scrapie infectivity in hamster blood is not associated with platelets. J Virol 2002;76:4649-50.
102. Barclay GR, Hope J, Brickett CR. Turner ML. Distribution of cell-associated prion protein in normal adult blood determined by flow cytometry. Br J Haematol 1999;107:804-14.
103. Sivakumaran M. Infectivity of buffy coat in variant CJD. Transfusion 2000;40:754-5.
104. SEAC. Position statement on TSE infectivity in blood. London, UK: Spongiform Encephalopathy Advisory Committee, 2006. [Available at: http://www.seac.gov.uk/statements/statement0806.htm.]
105. Prowse C. Properties of pathogen-inactivation plasma components. Transfus Med Rev 2009; 23:124-33.
106. MacLennan S, Barbara JA. Risks and side-effects of therapy with plasma and plasma fractions. Best Pract Res Clin Haematol 2006;19:169-89.
107. Vamvakas EC, Taswell HF. Long-term survival after blood transfusion. Transfusion 1994;34: 471-7.
108. Vamvakas EC. Is human herpesvirus-8 (HHV-8) transmitted by blood transfusion? Transfus Med Rev 2010;24:1-14.

In: Vamvakas EC.
Decision Making in Transfusion Medicine
Bethesda, MD: AABB Press, 2011

4

Strategies to Further Reduce Allogeneic-Blood-Transfusion-Related Mortality

ALLOGENEIC BLOOD TRANSFUSION (ABT) can be life-saving for bleeding patients but, if a patient is not bleeding, positive evidence of benefit should be required before that patient is exposed to the risks of transfusion. Transfusion should never be considered inherently "safe" nor should it be administered prophylactically without evidence of its efficacy to improve oxygen consumption by tissues [in the case of red cells (RBCs)] or its efficacy to prevent hemorrhage (in the case of plasma and platelets). Although one can acknowledge that "zero" risk is not an attainable goal, discussions of recent progress in blood safety should not detract from the fact that more needs to be done to reduce the risks of ABT.

As discussed in Chapter 2, transfusion-related acute lung injury (TRALI), hemolytic transfusion reactions (HTRs), and transfusion-associated sepsis (TAS) have been the three leading causes of transfusion-related fatalities in the 21st century; recently, transfusion-associated circulatory overload (TACO) displaced TAS as the third leading cause of ABT-related deaths.[1] While TRALI, HTRs, TACO, and TAS caused 34 of the 40 transfusion-related deaths passively reported to the FDA in 2010,[1] and mortality from ABT is currently low in the US,[1] a novel and fatal transfusion-transmitted infection (TTI) might appear in the future and reproduce the epidemic of transfusion-acquired AIDS of the 1980s.

Such a future TTI is the greatest potential threat to blood transfusion safety, and Chapter 3 reviews the complexities inherent in assessing whether a novel infectious disease represents a novel TTI that could pose a significant threat to transfusion safety. Both human immunodeficiency virus (HIV) and variant Creutzfeldt-Jakob disease (vCJD) prions have been novel infectious agents. The vCJD prions had many of the characteristics of HIV, including a very long incubation period before causing detectable clinical disease, so that this infectious agent reached a prevalence in United Kingdom (UK) blood donors that was reported to be as high as 1 per 4000 donors.[2] Despite these similarities between HIV and vCJD prions, vCJD did not reproduce the epidemic of transfusion-acquired AIDS of the 1980s. Nevertheless it is still possible that a novel "HIV-like" transfusion-transmitted agent could appear in the future.

This chapter builds on the conclusions reached in Chapter 2 (on the causes of transfusion-related fatalities and the threat of the next major transfusion-transmitted pathogen) to advocate the adoption of preventive strategies that can further reduce ABT-related mortality.

Preventive strategies are discussed here in ascending order of their impact on mortality: from the strategy expected to prevent the least number of transfusion-related deaths to the strategy expected to prevent the greatest number of deaths. Pathogen reduction (PR) of blood components is ranked as having the least impact among the strategies considered in this chapter, because no novel "HIV-like" pathogen is currently on the horizon, PR systems for RBCs are not yet available, and questions regarding the safety of the PR systems made available for platelets remain to be addressed. Limiting the number of allogeneic-donor exposures through development and implementation of evidence-based transfusion indications for the administration of all blood components and through the management of the patient's own blood as a precious and unique resource that should not be wasted is the strategy ranked in this chapter as having the greatest impact.

The reason for this ranking is that avoidance of unnecessary transfusions reduces the risk of *all* complications of ABT, including infectious complications (TTIs as well as TAS), immunologic complications (TRALI and non-ABO HTRs), complications secondary to clerical (ABO HTRs) or medical (TACO) errors, as well as complications attributed to *any* [non-white-cell (WBC)-reduced or WBC-reduced] ABT. Avoidance of unnecessary transfusions encompasses timely diagnosis and management of reversible anemia, meticulous surgical hemostasis, minimization of the blood losses incurred for the purpose of laboratory testing, and tolerance of anemia in hemodynamically stable patients, as well as consideration of all alternatives to ABT when appropriate and administration of ABT only as a last resort when evidence-based criteria indicate that benefit from the ABT can be expected. Additional strategies that can further reduce ABT-related mortality (Table 4-1) include, in ascending order of effect, interventions for: 1) preventing poorly understood adverse effects of non-WBC-reduced ABT in cardiac surgery; 2) decreasing the risk of TTIs and TAS secondary to transfusion of pooled blood components such as pooled whole-blood-derived (WBD) platelets; 3) preventing ABO and non-ABO HTRs; and 4) reducing the risk of TRALI by limiting the number of *immunologic* exposures to allogeneic blood donors by reserving the RBCs and/or platelets and plasma from the same multicomponent apheresis collection for transfusion to the same recipient.

Four strategies proposed in this chapter (WBC reduction of cellular blood components administered in cardiac surgery, avoidance of pooled blood components such as pooled WBD platelets, avoidance of female plasma and female platelet donors with a history of pregnancy who have not been shown not to have circulating WBC antibodies, and development and implementation of evidence-based transfusion guidelines) have already been—at least partly—implemented in the United States. Strategies that have already been introduced, however, have not been adopted universally or uniformly, and the benefit that they can confer in preventing ABT-related deaths has not yet been fully realized. For example, 12.9% of therapeutic platelet doses continue to be transfused as pooled WBD platelets; also, female platelet donors with a history of pregnancy who have not been tested for WBC antibodies continue to donate at many US blood centers, while platelets and plasma (and/or RBCs) harvested from the same multicomponent apheresis collection are not generally reserved for transfusion to the same patient.

Three of the strategies presented in this chapter—PR of platelets and plasma components; transitioning from the whole-blood collections of the 20th century to the multicomponent apheresis collections of the 21st century, which includes reserving all components harvested from the same multicomponent apheresis collection for transfusion to the same recipient; and considering ABT only when the evidence indicates that actual (as opposed to postulated) benefit can be expected for a particular patient and only when ABT cannot be avoided by substituting other interventions—likely amount to "paradigm shifts" in transfusion medicine. These (perhaps competing) paradigm shifts receive greater coverage in this chapter than do the other interventions; and they are considered again in Chapter 8.

Table 4-1. Preventive Strategies to Further Reduce Mortality Related to Allogeneic Blood Transfusion (ABT) in Ascending Order of Their Impact in Preventing ABT-Related Deaths[3,4]

Strategy	Cause(s) of ABT-Related Deaths Targeted by the Strategy
Pathogen reduction (PR) of platelet and plasma components	All TTIs secondary to infectious agents susceptible to PR technologies, including: • (Residual risk of) TTIs for which blood donors are tested (HIV, HCV, HBV, HTLV, WNV, *Trypanosoma cruzi* infection) • TTIs for which blood donors are not currently tested (eg, malaria, babesiosis) • Transfusion-associated sepsis (TAS) • Novel TTIs to appear in the future
WBC reduction of RBCs transfused in cardiac surgery	Poorly understood adverse effects of non-WBC-reduced RBC transfusion associated with increased mortality in cardiac surgery
Replacement of pooled blood components by apheresis (single-donor) blood components	• All infectious risks of ABT* • TRALI†
Augmentation of patient identification procedures to prevent transfusion of an RBC unit to a recipient other than the intended recipient	ABO HTRs
Extended donor-recipient red cell antigen matching to prevent formation of additional red cell alloantibodies	Non-ABO HTRs
Collection of apheresis (single-donor) platelets, plasma, and/or RBCs by means of multicomponent apheresis; and transfusion of all components harvested from the same multicomponent apheresis collection to the same recipient to reduce the number of *immunologic* exposures to donors	• TRALI • All infectious risks of ABT*
Development and implementation of evidence-based indications for transfusion of all blood components; consideration of ABT only when actual (rather than postulated) benefit can be expected and only when no other intervention(s) can be substituted	• Poorly understood adverse effects of both non-WBC-reduced and WBC-reduced RBC transfusion • All infectious risks of ABT* • ABO and non-ABO HTRs • TRALI • All other ABT complications/adverse effects

*Including TAS, novel TTIs to appear in the future, and TTIs for which blood donors are (or are not) currently tested, and regardless of whether the infectious agents are (or are not) susceptible to the available PR technologies.

†Prevention through reduction in the number of immunologic exposures to donors (see 6th row in the Table).

HBV = hepatitis B virus; HCV = hepatitis C virus; HIV = human immunodeficiency virus; HTR = hemolytic transfusion reaction; HTLV = human T-cell lymphotropic virus; RBC = Red Blood Cell; TRALI = transfusion-related acute lung injury; TTI = transfusion-transmitted infection; WBC = white blood cell; WNV = West Nile virus.

Reduction in the Risk of TTIs Through PR of Platelet and Plasma Components

So many agents can potentially threaten blood safety[5] that blood establishments cannot easily keep up with implementing safety measures in response to each one of them. Rather than this "agent-by-agent" approach, it makes sense to adopt an all-encompassing "proactive" approach to blood safety that would address most transfusion-transmitted pathogens by means of PR accomplished by systems targeting nucleic acids or constituents peculiar to viral envelopes.[5-8] Systems targeting nucleic acids inactivate the nucleic acids of pathogens, while permitting the nucleic-acid-free constituents of donor blood (plasma proteins, platelets, and RBCs) to continue to function; systems targeting constituents of viral envelopes specifically inactivate enveloped viruses, such as HIV, hepatitis B virus (HBV), hepatitis C virus (HCV), and West Nile virus (WNV). In this way, systems targeting nucleic acids or viral envelopes (and made available, respectively, for platelets or plasma) can eliminate most of the residual risks of bacterial contamination of platelets (and therefore most of the residual risk of TAS), as well as the risks associated with a long list of transfusion-transmitted pathogens for which blood donors are not currently screened (eg, *Plasmodium* sp, *Babesia* sp, and so on).

Perhaps more important, these technologies offer potential, pre-emptive protection against the next potentially fatal transfusion-transmitted agent that may emerge in the future and replicate the experience with HIV or WNV.[9] Nucleic-acid intercalating agents used in the PR systems developed for platelets that target nucleic acids should be effective against novel viruses that contain nucleic acids and against all bacteria except for some rare spore-forming bacteria. Nucleic-acid intercalating agents, however, cannot be assumed to be effective against novel pathogens whose biologic properties are unpredictable—such as the vCJD prions, which are devoid of nucleic acids and invulnerable to the platelet PR systems hitherto developed. Thus, when it comes to the prevention of the next potentially fatal TTI, we should remember that PR systems are validated against pathogens that are already known; therefore, they may (or may not) be effective against a novel pathogen whose properties cannot be predicted before its appearance.[10] Of two infections shown to be transmissible through ABT in the 21st century and for which safety measures for the protection of transfusion recipients were implemented,[5] one (WNV infection) would have been prevented and one (vCJD infection) would not have been prevented had PR been implemented before the emergence of each TTI.

Although the safety improvement that PR technologies would confer is widely acknowledged, there are three arguments that reduce the enthusiasm for implementing the currently available PR technologies. Firstly, there is debate as to whether PR for all platelets and plasma should be introduced before suitable PR technologies also become available for RBCs. Although a system utilizing riboflavin and ultraviolet light for PR of RBCs is currently undergoing Phase III clinical trials, and such trials are pending for a system utilizing S-303 (amustaline hydrochloride) and ultraviolet-A light, licensed systems for PR of RBCs will likely not be available in the foreseeable future in either Europe or North America. The contribution of PR to safety can only be suboptimal if PR technology cannot simultaneously also be applied to RBCs. RBCs are the most frequently transfused blood components and thus most transmissions of the next major TTI will still occur through transfusions of RBCs even if PR is implemented for platelets and plasma. Furthermore, until there is a comprehensive system of PR that also encompasses RBCs, which would permit various cost-savings from the possible discontinuation of other safety measures, the cost of PR is bound to be incremental and substantial.[11] Along these lines, if an ideal PR system is eventually developed and licensed, it would probably pertain to treatment of whole-blood (prior to component manufacturing); however, such a system will not be available in the foreseeable future.

Secondly, PR causes cellular and functional protein losses, thus reducing the therapeutic efficacy of blood components, necessitating the transfusion of greater volumes of plasma and platelets and exposing patients to more donors, which in turn increases the risk of transmission of agents (such as pathologic prions or spore-forming bacteria) that are not inactivated by PR. Despite this plausible prediction, however, RBC and platelet usage has been reported to remain the same before and after the introduction of the amotosalen-HCl/ultraviolet-A light (Intercept) PR system (Cerus Corp., Concord, CA) for platelets in several Western European countries.[12-15] It is possible that blood components had previously been overutilized or that an increase in mild and moderate bleeding complications went unnoticed in these studies, which were conducted outside the framework of a randomized controlled trial (RCT).

Thirdly, there is concern about potential toxic effects of the candidate PR systems that have been examined in many dimensions—including acute, subacute, and chronic toxicity, blood component incompatibility, genotoxicity, carcinogenicity, and impact on reproduction and development. Although no evidence of such adverse effects has hitherto been adduced,[12-19] the clinical events of interest are rare and may have very long latent periods before they become recognized, especially as regards mutagenicity and carcinogenicity.[5] These concerns about possible long-term toxicities of PR technologies are more relevant when compounds (such as amotosalen) rather than riboflavin (vitamin B2) are used, and they cannot be alleviated until *long-term* outcomes are reported from the Western European countries in which systems for PR have been already (at least partly) introduced into clinical practice.[5] Perhaps more importantly, at least for the available PR systems of platelets, there is concern about the possibility of an increase in bleeding complications in recipients of pathogen-reduced (vs non-pathogen-reduced) components. This concern is briefly reviewed here with the specific evidence from RCTs presented in Chapter 5.

The concerns about short-term toxicity of PR must be considered, however, in the context of possible additional short-term benefits from the PR technologies. Unlike WBC reduction filters that leave up to 5×10^6 residual WBCs behind in each WBC-reduced blood component, PR technologies eliminate *all* allogeneic WBCs. In this way, they can prevent the rare deaths from transfusion-associated graft-vs-host disease (TA-GVHD) that can occur in patients given unirradiated components by mistake or because they do not have a recognized indication for irradiation.[7] Furthermore, an RCT of the efficacy and safety of platelets that had undergone PR with the amotosalen-HCl/ultraviolet-A light (Intercept) system demonstrated a trend toward reduced mortality in the patients supported with pathogen-reduced platelets, concerning especially the mortality from acute lung injury (ALI).[20] ALI is a significant cause of morbidity and mortality in recipients of allogeneic marrow transplants—a setting in which ALI may account for up to 25% to 50% of all deaths. If PR truly rendered platelets less apt to cause ALI in transfusion recipients, plausible explanations for this effect would include reduction in cytokine synthesis and/or antigen presentation, owing to the absence of WBCs in the treated components.[20]

Pathogen-Reduced Plasma

PR processes can be applied to either single-unit plasma units or plasma pools. Thus, there are now four licensed technologies for PR of plasma in Europe[19] including amotosalen and ultraviolet A light, riboflavin and ultraviolet (predominantly ultraviolet-B) light, methylene blue, and solvent-detergent (S-D) treatment. All methods improve blood safety by eliminating microorganisms from plasma, albeit at the expense of some reduction in the function of the plasma (especially coagulation) proteins. Most clinical experience (>6 million units transfused) has hitherto been accrued with *pooled* plasma subjected to S-D treatment.[19] Pooling of 500 to 2500 plasma donations has the disadvantage that one single plasma unit can contaminate the whole pool. However, this drawback can be offset by several advantages, including the virtual elimination of TRALI attributable to WBC antibodies, a significant reduction in the incidence of allergic reactions owing to dilution of allergens, and standardization of the product for therapeutic use in terms of its coagulation-factor content (because individual plasma donors contributing to the pool have a wide range of coagulation-factor levels, varying between 50% and 200%).[19,21,22]

In terms of TRALI reduction, solvent/detergent treated pooled (S/D-P) plasma—which is currently used to meet virtually all the plasma needs of Norway and Ireland and which has contributed 464,582 transfused units of plasma [compared with 650,781 for fresh frozen plasma (FFP)] in France between 2003 and 2006[19]—needs to be compared with the "male-only" FFP currently being used in North America. S/D-P plasma should be at least as effective as "male-only" FFP in reducing the risk of TRALI, because the manufacturing process dilutes, and possibly neutralizes, WBC antibodies.[22] Furthermore, S/D-P plasma could be more effective than "male-only" FFP in preventing TRALI, because the manufacturing process would also dilute any other mediators causing TRALI in recipients of "male-only" plasma (Chapter 2).

Figure 2-4 in Chapter 2 shows that, although the number of deaths has greatly declined, TRALI deaths associated with plasma transfusion have continued to be reported to the Food and Drug Administration (FDA) in 2008-2010 (after the United States converted to the use of "male-only" FFP). In contrast, no reports of TRALI have appeared from Western European countries using S/D-P plasma. In particular, during the aforementioned period (2003-2006),[19] after the French hemovigilance system started appropriate monitoring for TRALI, there were 14 (nine probable or certain and five possible) cases of TRALI in association with transfusion of FFP (1 per 25,346 units), as compared with no case of TRALI in association with transfusion of S/D-P plasma.[23,24] It is not known whether this observation is due to the fact that TRALI does not occur secondary to transfusion of S/D-P plasma or to the fact that cases of TRALI owing to plasma transfusion go unrecorded by the passive surveillance systems of these European countries.

Implementation of S/D-P plasma protects recipients of plasma transfusions from any HIV-like or WNV-like enveloped virus that might appear in the future. If the next fatal transfusion-transmitted pathogen is an enveloped virus, transmissions (and fatalities) secondary to plasma transfusions will be prevented—although transmissions (and fatalities) secondary to transfusions of RBCs and platelets would still occur. The principal reservation concerning adoption of S/D-P plasma derives from the possibility that the next fatal transfusion-transmitted pathogen may be an *unenveloped* virus (like hepatitis A virus or parvovirus B19) and thus not susceptible to solvent-detergent treatment. In that case, because S/D-P plasma entails pooling 500 to 2500 donations, a unit of S/D-P plasma will have up to 500 to 2500 times as high a risk of transmitting the new pathogen as would a unit of FFP. If the new pathogen attains a prevalence of 1 per 10,000 US blood donors before measures are implemented to prevent its transmission through ABT,[10] transfusion of a single unit of S/D-P plasma will have a probability of up to 5% to 25% of transmitting the new pathogen. Thus, if the next major pathogen to emerge in the future is an *unenveloped* virus, transfusions of S/D-P plasma will have the potential to replicate—in the population of *all* transfusion recipients—a catastrophe similar to the 1980s AIDS epidemic in hemophiliacs who had received pooled clotting-factor concentrates before systems for pathogen inactivation were introduced. Nonetheless, recently systems have been developed that permit S-D treatment of units of plasma collected from individual donors.

For most TTIs that might occur secondary to receipt of S/D-P plasma, a single contaminated unit might indeed contaminate the entire plasma pool. However, at least in theory, there can be situations in which pooling offers advantages in terms of preventing TTIs.[25] Although no data exist on the risk of vCJD infectivity in S/D-P plasma, the low titer of prion infectivity in the blood of infected individuals (approximately 10 infectious units/mL; Chapter 3) would, if anything, be greatly diluted by the thousands of units of plasma in the plasma pool. Subsequent manufacturing processes should also remove prions from the final product.[25] If this were the case, the choice of a plasma product ("male-only" FFP or S/D-P plasma) in each European country would likely be based in the future on an assessment of the relative threat posed by vCJD rather than that posed by a novel pathogen not inactivated by solvent/detergent treatment. Such an assessment has not yet been possible, however, because there are still no data on the actual risk of vCJD infectivity in S/D-P plasma. In the United States—where no bloodborne vCJD epidemic is on the horizon—adoption of S/D-P plasma to reduce the risk of TTIs would probably be hard to justify, although prior introduction of S/D-P plasma would, admittedly, have prevented the transmissions of WNV infection through plasma transfusions that occurred in the summer of 2002.

The major reason that S/D-P plasma fell out of favor in North America has been a cluster of deaths in patients undergoing liver transplantation at a hospital using S/D-P plasma.[26] Solvent-detergent treatment of pooled plasma results in appreciable losses of protein S, antitrypsin, and antiplasmin.[19] These losses have generated concern when the product is used in patients with hyperfibrinolysis (such as occurs during the reperfusion stage of liver transplantation). The current manufacturing process used in Europe is different, resulting in reduced—albeit still appreciable—losses of these three proteins. Nonetheless, the Irish—who almost exclusively use S/D-P plasma for the plasma needs of their transfusion recipients—do not use this product for patients undergoing liver transplantation.[27]

Pathogen-Reduced Platelets

Because it cannot be predicted when the next major transfusion-transmitted pathogen will emerge, it has been advocated[3,4,8] that PR technologies for platelets and plasma be implemented by the transfusion medicine community when they are licensed, rather than after PR technologies for RBCs have also been developed. The latter will hopefully be developed over the next 5 to 10 years.[8] The rationale for this recommendation[3,4,8] is that, if the next major transfusion-transmitted agent to emerge in the future is an enveloped virus (like HIV or WNV), a significant number of future transmissions (and fatalities) through plasma and platelet transfusions can be averted. Several safety measures (including bacteria detection in platelets and screening for antibody to *Trypanosoma cruzi*) could also eventually be discontinued if PR were universally introduced for all blood components. At the same time, it was recognized[3,4] that anticipating an imminent introduction of PR can have a negative effect on blood safety. Such an expectation could result in continued inaction vis-à-vis addressing the (residual) risk of bacteria in platelets and the risk of other known (or emerging) TTIs through adoption of interventions that are already available.

Two technologies for PR of platelets have undergone clinical trials. The amotosalen-HCl/ultraviolet-A-light (Intercept) technology uses a psoralen compound (amotosalen) that targets nucleic acid and is activated by ultraviolet-A (UVA) light. In the dose delivered by the Intercept system, UVA light does not result in nucleic acid modification in the absence of amotosalen. In the presence of UVA light, amotosalen forms adducts in double-stranded regions of DNA or RNA—on average every 80 base-pairs.[28,29] The Mirasol technology (CaridianBCT, Lakewood, CO) utilizes riboflavin and ultraviolet light (predominantly ultraviolet-B [UVB] light).[30] Platelets treated with the Intercept system have been licensed in Europe for up to 7 days of storage, while platelets treated with the Mirasol technology have been licensed for up to 5 days of storage (the same as for platelets that have not undergone PR).[30] Proponents of the Intercept technology have claimed that the mechanism of action of the Intercept system is largely independent of reactive oxygen species, as treatment with Intercept results in only limited generation of reactive oxygen species,[28,29] and that the Mirasol technology depends more on the generation of reactive oxygen species for achieving pathogen inactivation.[30] A third technology using ultraviolet-C light alone (MacoPharma, Tourcoing, France) is presently at the stage of Phase III clinical trials.

Bleeding Complications of Pathogen-Reduced Platelets

The prevailing opinion that favored the adoption of PR technologies for platelets prior to the development of PR technologies for RBCs[3,4,8] was called into question when the findings of the RCT of Kerkhoffs et al[31] were reported. These investigators found a statistically significant (as well as clinically important) increase in the risk of bleeding complications secondary to treatment of platelets with the Intercept technology.[31] All RCTs of PR of platelets have enrolled patients with hypoproliferative thrombocytopenia (ie, with hematologic malignancies) and they have transfused platelets prophylactically for platelet counts falling under 10,000/µL. Kerkhoffs et al[31] reported on *all* bleeding complications [grades 1 through 4 on the Common Toxicity Criteria (CTC) scale] as well as on "clinically significant" bleeding complications (grades 2 through 4 on the CTC scale). Whether the CTC or the World Health Organization (WHO) scale is used, grade 1 bleeding is minor bleeding not requiring intervention; grade 2 bleeding necessitates intervention, but not RBC transfusion; grade 3 bleeding necessitates RBC transfusion; and grade 4 bleeding is catastrophic.

Before the RCT of Kerkhoffs et al[31] was reported, small RCTs of the Intercept technology[32,33] had not reported a difference in all (or in severe) bleeding complications between recipients of pathogen-reduced versus non-pathogen-reduced platelets. The initial report of the large SPRINT trial[34]—which enrolled the majority (n=645) of the patients hitherto studied within the framework of RCTs—had compared recipients of pathogen-reduced platelets to those who received non-pathogen-reduced platelets in terms of WHO grade 2 bleeding complications (primary outcome). That report also presented a separate comparison between the arms in terms of WHO grade 3 and grade 4 bleeding complications (one of several secondary outcomes). The subsequent expanded safety analysis of the SPRINT trial[35] *separately* compared each grade of bleeding complications (grade 1 vs grade 2 vs grade 3 vs grade 4) between the recipients of pathogen-reduced and non-pathogen-reduced platelets. The initial report of the SPRINT trial[34] made per-protocol daily assessments of bleeding complications by blinded assessors during the period of platelet transfusion support for hypoproliferative thrombocytopenia, using the WHO scale. The expanded safety analysis of that study[35] relied on reports filed spontaneously by blinded on-site personnel during both the period of platelet transfusion support and an ensuing 1-week surveillance period, using the (similar) Common Terminology Criteria for Adverse Events/Common Toxicity Criteria (CTCAE/CTC) scale (http://ctep.cancer.gov/protocolDevelopment/electronic_applications/ctc.htm). There was no significant difference in the risk of bleeding complications in any of these published comparisons of the SPRINT trial[34,35] between patients receiving pathogen-reduced platelets and those receiving non-pathogen-reduced platelets.

After the findings of the RCT of Kerkhoffs et al[31] were reported, the SPRINT trial results were re-examined by considering *all* bleeding complications together (grades 1 through 4 on the CTCAE/CTC scale[35]), as well as the "clinically significant" bleeding complications (grades 2 through 4 on the WHO[34] or CTCAE/CTC[35] scale).[36-39] There was a statistically significant ($p<0.05$) increase in clinically significant bleeding complications associated with transfusion of pathogen-reduced (compared to non-pathogen-reduced) platelets when the data on grade 2 through 4 bleeding complications from the expanded safety analysis of the SPRINT trial[35] were combined.[37,39] All bleeding complications are a more reproducible endpoint compared with the grade 2 bleeding on which the initial report of the SPRINT RCT[34] had concentrated. At the same time, "clinically significant" bleeding complications are a more meaningful endpoint than grade 2 bleeding. This is because grade 2 bleeding is hard to distinguish from grade 1 bleeding, so that grade 2 bleeding depends greatly on inter-observer variation even when trained and blinded assessors are used.[40]

A meta-analysis[41] integrated the results of the SPRINT trial on all and on "clinically significant" bleeding complications (as reported in the expanded safety analysis[35] rather than the initial report[34] of that study) with the findings of the other RCTs[31-33,42] of PR of platelets (Chapter 5). When the results of RCTs using either the Intercept[31-33,35] or the Mirasol technology[42] were combined,[41] there was a significant ($p<0.05$) increase in all bleeding complications and in "clinically significant" bleeding complications in association with PR.[41]

The RCT of Lozano et al[43] was published in full after the meta-analysis[41] had been completed. This RCT[43] was available only in summary form at the time of the meta-analysis,[41] and it was excluded from the overview[41] because it had a different design from the other RCTs. The other RCTs had allocated hemato-oncology patients undergoing induction chemotherapy to receive pathogen-reduced or non-pathogen-reduced platelets throughout the period of platelet transfusion support. Lozano et al[43] studied a single "on-protocol" transfusion of pathogen-reduced or non-pathogen-reduced platelets stored past the allowed storage time (ie, platelets stored for 6 or 7 days). The rest of the platelet transfusions given to the enrolled patients had been stored for ≤5 days. Bleeding was evaluated within 24 hours of the single "on-protocol" transfusion. After the overview was completed, the RCT of Lozano et al[43] was published in full. It reported that 25 (23.8%) of the 105 recipients of pathogen-reduced platelets and 31 (29.2%) of the 106 recipients of non-pathogen-reduced platelets had suffered at least one hemorrhagic event within 24 hours of a study ("on-protocol") transfusion.

When the eligibility criteria for the RCTs included in the earlier meta-analysis[41] were modified to permit inclusion of the RCT of Lozano et al,[43] five RCTs that had compared *all* bleeding complications between recipients of platelets pathogen-reduced with the Intercept technology and recipients of non-pathogen-reduced platelets[31-33,35,43] were eligible for analysis.[44] Because of the claimed difference in mechanism of action between the Intercept and Mirasol technologies,[28-30] the RCT of the Mirasol technology[42] was excluded from the subsequent meta-analysis.[44] In the updated report,[44] clinically significant bleeding complications increased in association with Intercept treatment when the intergrated results of the SPRINT RCT were extracted from the expanded safety analysis[35] (summary OR = 1.52; 95% CI, 1.09-2.12)—but not the initial report[34] (summary OR = 1.30; 95% CI, 0.54-3.14)—of that study. When all bleeding complications (the only outcome reported by Lozano et al[43]) were considered, treatment with Intercept was not associated with an increase in the risk of bleeding (summary OR = 1.24; 95% CI, 0.79-1.93), although there was a significant increase in bleeding in association with PR across the four RCTs[31-33,35] meeting the eligibility criteria for meta-analysis as initially specified[41] (summary OR = 1.53; 95% CI, 1.06-2.22; $p<0.05$). At the same time, when the RCT of Kerkhoffs et al[31] was excluded from the analysis and the other studies[32,33,35,43] were integrated, the OR of all bleeding complications in recipients of pathogen-reduced vs non-pathogen-reduced platelets approached unity (summary OR = 1.07; 95% CI, 0.70-1.65). Thus, with regard to clinically significant bleeding complications, the conclusions of the meta-analysis[44] depended on whether the data on bleeding complications recorded by blinded observers in the SPRINT RCT were based on the initial report[34] or the expanded safety analysis[35] of that study. With regard to all bleeding complications, the conclusions[44] depended on whether the RCT of Lozano et al[43]—or, alternatively, the RCT of Kerkhoffs et al[31]—was excluded from the analysis.

The meta-analysis concluded that the totality of the evidence (Fig 4-1) indicates that clinical equipoise (Chapter 7) still exists vis-à-vis the undertaking of RCTs of the hemostatic efficacy and capacity of platelets treated with Intercept.[44] The concerns that the Intercept system would alleviate (vis-à-vis emerging TTIs and platelet TAS) are balanced by the concern about possibly increased bleeding complications in association with Intercept treatment. Even if individual clinicians are sufficiently convinced about the benefit-to-risk ratio of Intercept to prescribe treated platelets for their own patients, policy-makers (Chapter 7) must demand more definitive evidence than that depicted in Fig 4-1 about the lack of toxicity of a new treatment

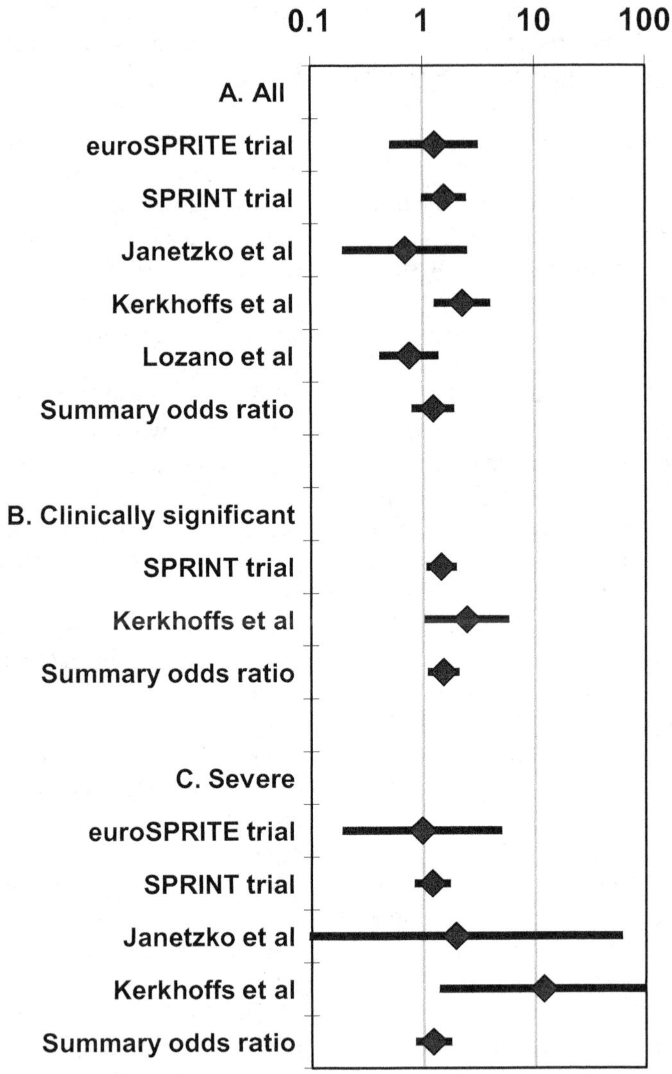

Figure 4-1. Odds ratios (ORs) and associated 95% confidence intervals (CIs) for all (WHO or CTCAE/CTC grades 1 through 4), clinically significant (WHO or CTCAE/CTC grades 2 through 4), and severe (WHO or CTCAE/CTC grades 3 and 4) bleeding complications across five,[31-33,35,43] two,[31,35] and four[31-33,35] RCTs that reported such findings in patients receiving either platelets that were pathogen-reduced with the Intercept system or untreated platelets.[44] For each study, the figure shows the OR of bleeding complications in recipients of treated and untreated platelets. Each OR is surrounded by its 95% CI. When the 95% CI does not include the null value of 1, the difference in bleeding complications between recipients of pathogen-reduced and non-pathogen-reduced platelets is statistically significant ($p<0.05$). An OR >1 indicates a greater risk of bleeding complications in recipients of pathogen-reduced (compared with non-pathogen-reduced) platelets provided that the difference is statistically significant. Compare with Fig 5-1. Initially published by Vamvakas in Vox Sang 2011 (Epub ahead of print, Sep 30).[44]

before they can approve an expensive technology for routine clinical use.

PR and Platelet Function

Although PR results in a predictable (quantitative) loss of platelets, it was believed that this platelet loss could be compensated for by an increase in platelet transfusions. In recipients of pathogen-reduced platelets as compared with recipients of non-pathogen-reduced platelets, RCTs had demonstrated reduced 1-hour and 24-hour corrected count increments (CCIs), along with an increased number of platelet transfusions and a shorter interval between platelet transfusions. An increase in bleeding complications in association with PR was not expected, however, because: 1) subjects enrolled in RCTs had received prophylactic platelet transfusions when their platelet count fell below 10,000/µL; 2) the (quantitative) platelet losses secondary to PR do not exceed 50% of the treated platelets; and 3) the Platelet Dose RCT showed that half-the-standard-dose platelet transfusions prevent bleeding as effectively as standard-dose platelet transfusions.[45] Despite this theoretical prediction that PR should not result in increased bleeding complications, the already-discussed meta-analysis[41] found that all and "clinically significant" bleeding complications increased in association with PR. If PR increases the risk of bleeding complications despite receipt of an increased number of platelet transfusions,[31,41] PR may cause functional impairment of *all* the treated platelets, in addition to causing cellular loss of a proportion of the treated platelets.[31,41]

Previously, the question of functional impairment of PR-treated platelets had been considered in the context of any effect that the damage to the platelet mitochondrial DNA might have exercised on platelet function. Recently reported findings, however, have raised an altogether novel concern, because they showed that platelets contain microRNAs that may regulate platelet protein translation and expression, thereby affecting hemostasis.[46,47] Osman and Falker[46] identified 281 microRNA species in human platelets—a number corresponding to approximately 40% of all microRNAs listed in miRBase v14 (http://www.mirbase.org), which is a relatively high number compared with the number of microRNA species found in nucleated cells. Nagalla et al[47] demonstrated that these platelet microRNA profiles are associated with, and may predict, platelet reactivity. They showed that platelets express 284 different microRNAs, 74 of which were differentially expressed between 19 healthy subjects (such as blood donors) and spontaneously clustered into two groups according to platelet aggregation to epinephrine. A subset of these differentially expressed microRNAs predicted the platelet aggregation response. Moreover, platelet microRNAs were able to repress expression of platelet proteins.

The double-stranded precursors of such platelet microRNAs might be vulnerable to PR, in which case PR could alter the proteome of platelets stored following treatment with amotosalen or riboflavin by prohibiting protein synthesis during storage.[48] If proteins synthesized by platelets during storage in the blood bank affected platelet function, PR could then cause functional impairment of all the treated platelets,[31,41] thereby accounting for the difference in bleeding complications in the RCT of Kerkhoffs et al. Although this thesis is plausible,[48] it rests on the following assumptions: 1) that platelet microRNAs significantly regulate platelet protein synthesis; 2) that significant platelet protein synthesis occurs during platelet storage; and 3) that proteins synthesized by platelets during storage significantly affect platelet function and the platelets' ability to effect hemostasis. If all of these assumptions are corroborated, degradation by PR of the newly discovered (over the last 2 years) platelet microRNAs may be responsible for impairment of the function of pathogen-reduced platelets.

An argument as to why this may not in fact be the case is that amotosalen forms adducts in double-stranded regions of DNA or RNA at every 80 base-pairs on average.[28] The probability of amotosalen's binding to nucleic acid upon activation by UVA light depends on the size of the target, with larger nucleic acid molecules (oligonucleotides of 80 base-pairs or more) being more likely to be modified by such treatment than smaller molecules. MicroRNAs (including their double-stranded precursors) are smaller than 80 base-pairs and thus less likely to be modified by amotosalen in the presence of UVA light. Nonetheless this assertion remains to be empirically proven as there have been no direct comparisons of the microRNA profiles and/or proteome of pathogen-reduced vs non-pathogen-reduced platelets, over 1 to 5 days of platelet storage following PR.[48]

Alternatives to PR of Platelets

PR of platelets could prevent both emerging TTIs and TAS, but its *immediate* benefit–in the absence of a known emerging pathogen–would be the prevention of virtually all cases of TAS (except for rare cases secondary to spore-forming bacteria). Because platelet TAS is a major cause of transfusion-related morbidity and mortality (Chapter 2), a policy direction of introducing PR of platelets in the United States as soon as possible would have considerable merit, despite the preceding discussion concerning a possible impairment of platelet function secondary to PR that could account for the increase in bleeding complications recorded in association with PR in RCTs. When it comes specifically to the prevention of TAS (as opposed to TTIs), however, there is an alternative strategy available that–albeit less effective than PR–is free of the possible risk of increased bleeding complications associated with PR. This strategy is the implementation of a second bacteria detection test on a sample taken from the unit at the time of issue of the platelet component.[49]

As discussed in Chapter 2, a qualitative immunoassay for the detection of bacterial membrane constituents (Pan Genera Detection, Verax, Worcester, MA) has been licensed in the United States as an *adjunct* quality control test for WBC-reduced apheresis platelets that have already tested negative by a different method. In a recent evaluation of the test on 27,620 platelet units,[49] nine of 12 units known in that study to be contaminated with bacteria were detected by the test, while three (25%) contaminated units were missed. Of the three missed units, two were not clinically significant but one resulted in a septic transfusion reaction. Although not a panacea for the prevention of platelet TAS (and of deaths from TAS), such a second bacteria detection test performed at time of issue could significantly reduce platelet transfusion-associated morbidity and mortality in the United States without introducing any risk for the transfusion recipient.[49]

Reduction in Ill-Defined ABT-Associated Adverse Effects Through WBC Reduction of RBCs Transfused in Cardiac Surgery

The greater part of transfusion-associated mortality may not derive from the established noninfectious and infectious complications of ABT. If corroborated by future research, the deaths attributed to transfusion of non-WBC-reduced (rather than WBC-reduced) allogeneic RBCs by the RCTs conducted in cardiac surgery[50-52] will represent a far greater number of deaths than the fatalities caused by the many well-recognized ABT complications. Although 60-day mortality was only a secondary outcome in the cardiac surgery RCT of van de Watering et al,[50] receipt of non-WBC-reduced (compared with WBC-reduced) ABT increased the absolute risk of death by 4.3% (7.8% and 3.5%, respectively), which indicates that for every 23.3 patients receiving non-WBC-reduced (rather than WBC-reduced) ABT, one might have died because of the non-WBC-reduced (rather than WBC-reduced) ABT itself. All platelets transfused in these RCTs[50-52] had been WBC-reduced, and therefore no inference can be made from these studies about any adverse effect of transfusions of non-WBC-reduced platelets in cardiac surgery.

ABT has not been associated with a specific cause(s) of death in these RCTs[50-52] and the mechanism(s) by which ABT might cause such an increase in all-cause mortality is not yet understood (Chapter 2). Although there is a need for further research to elucidate the mechanism of the apparent increase in mortality in recipients of non-WBC-reduced (compared with

WBC-reduced) ABT, where excess mortality has been attributed to non-WBC-reduced (compared with WBC-reduced) ABT by RCTs, WBC reduction of cellular blood components should be implemented to prevent such excess deaths. This situation has been reported only in cardiac surgery—a setting apart from other surgical (or medical) settings, in which idiosyncratic effects of ABT could be expected and would not necessarily be generalizable to other settings.[53,54]

Seventeen million cellular blood components were WBC-reduced in the US in 2008.[55] These included 13.8 million WBC-reduced RBCs (80.4% of all manufactured RBCs), 2.3 million apheresis (single-donor) platelets (100% of all manufactured apheresis platelets), and 0.9 million WBD platelets (47% of all manufactured WBD platelets). From 2006 through 2008, the number of cellular blood components that were WBC-reduced before storage increased by 21%.[55] Approximately 69% of all RBCs transfused in the US in 2008 were reported by the surveyed hospitals to be WBC-reduced compared to 55% of all RBCs transfused in 2006.[55]

US hospitals use WBC-reduced components either universally or selectively, depending primarily on their geographic location and the practices of the local blood center (which may manufacture only WBC-reduced or both WBC-reduced and non-WBC-reduced cellular blood components). The arguments for and against implementing universal WBC reduction are reviewed in Chapter 1. When selective WBC reduction is used, administration of WBC-reduced components to cardiac surgery patients is usually not included among the established indications for WBC reduction. Thus, in some US hospitals, WBC-reduced RBCs are administered routinely to patients whose mortality has not been shown to be affected by WBC reduction, whereas elsewhere, cardiac surgery patients whose mortality has been shown to be improved by WBC reduction may not always receive WBC-reduced components.

To ensure that all cardiac surgery patients receive WBC-reduced cellular blood components, one could redistribute some of the already manufactured WBC-reduced cellular blood components from US hospitals using universal WBC reduction to the cardiac surgery setting of US hospitals not using universal WBC reduction. Alternatively, one could increase the overall proportion of the cellular blood components WBC-reduced in the United States. Whether the goal is accomplished through a redistribution or a net increase in manufactured WBC-reduced components, all cellular blood components transfused in cardiac surgery in the United States should, according to the existing evidence, be WBC-reduced.[53,54] For US hospitals using selective WBC reduction, this safety enhancement can be accomplished by adding cardiac surgery to the three established indications for WBC reduction: prevention of HLA-alloimmunization and refractoriness to WBD platelet transfusions, prevention of transmission of cytomegalovirus, and prevention of febrile, non-hemolytic transfusion reactions.

Reduction in the Risk of TTIs Through Replacement of Pooled Blood Components by Apheresis (Single-Donor) Components

As already discussed, and as judged from the experience with HIV,[56] an HIV-like pathogen that might emerge in the future remains the greatest threat to blood safety,[3,4] as long as the PR methods under development cannot protect the blood supply from all the emerging agents prioritized by the AABB Task Force.[5] For example, of the agents listed in that report,[5] pathologic prions, human parvovirus B19, and hepatitis A virus would not be inactivated or would probably be inactivated only inadequately by PR. Furthermore, the very concept of emerging TTIs is that their evolution and manifestations, as well as the properties of the associated pathogen, are intrinsically unpredictable.[57] Thus, emerging TTIs may be neither inactivated by PR nor associated with specific high-risk groups whose deferral from blood donation could prevent transmission of the pathogens to transfusion recipients. The latter would be the case if the next major transfusion-transmitted pathogen to emerge were food-borne (like vCJD), vector-borne (like WNV), or even airborne (like severe acute respiratory syndrome).[58]

Therefore, reducing the number of donors to whom a patient is exposed is the *only* strategy that can reduce the risk of transmission of *any* TTI that might emerge in the future.[3,4,10] Most of the success of this approach (Table 4-1) depends on the prevention of unnecessary transfusions through the enforcement of evidence-based transfusion guidelines on the hospital side—a strategy discussed later in the this chapter. Much can be accomplished on the blood center side as well, however, by avoiding the production and distribution of pooled blood components, especially pooled WBD platelets.[3,4,10,57]

The Continued Use of Platelet Pools in the United States

In 2006, 87.5% of therapeutic platelet doses administered to US patients were transfused as apheresis (single-donor) platelets; the remainder (12.5% of platelet doses) were transfused as pooled WBD platelets.[55] The total number of platelet doses transfused to US patients increased from 1.731 million in 2006 to 2.021 million in 2008.[55] In 2008, 87.1% of platelet doses were transfused as apheresis (single-donor) platelets; the remainder (12.9%) were administered as pooled WBD platelets. Between 1997 and 2006, the proportion of platelet doses transfused as pooled WBD platelets had progressively declined from 37.6% to 12.5%. Furthermore, the actual *number* of platelet doses transfused as pooled WBD platelets had decreased from 0.566 million in 1997 to 0.216 million in 2006.[55] This downward trend was reversed between 2006 and 2008, with 0.260 million platelet doses transfused as pooled WBD platelets in 2008.

As in the case of WBC-reduced components, US hospitals generally use *either* apheresis (single-donor) *or* pooled WBD platelets depending primarily on their geographic location and the practices of the local blood center [which may manufacture only apheresis (single-donor) or both apheresis (single-donor) and pooled WBD platelets]. In some cases, blood centers that endeavored to convert to an apheresis (single-donor) platelet supply for the purpose of complying with the AABB standard to limit and detect bacteria in *all* platelet components[59] continued to manufacture a small proportion of pooled WBD platelets to accommodate hospitals in their area that were either unable or unwilling to pay the additional cost of apheresis (single-donor) platelets.

Between March 2004 and January 2010, methods used to limit and detect bacteria in apheresis (single-donor) platelets were 4.6 times as sensitive as methods used to limit and detect bacteria in pooled platelets.[60] As of January 31, 2010, the AABB required that all AABB-accredited facilities transfusing platelet pools employ culture to detect bacteria in these pooled components by using methods of sensitivity equivalent to that of the methods used for culturing apheresis (single-donor) platelets.[61,62] Thus, the difference in the sensitivity of the methods used to detect bacteria in apheresis (single-donor) and pooled WBD platelets is no longer a cause of a greater risk of TAS secondary to the use of pooled than of apheresis (single-donor) platelets. Accordingly, this cause of an increased risk of TAS secondary to the use of platelet pools (compared with apheresis platelets) is not included in the risk calculations presented in this chapter.

Platelet Pools and Risk of TRALI

To provide the same therapeutic benefit to a recipient that could be obtained from the transfusion of an apheresis (single-donor) platelet concentrate, pooled WBD platelets expose a patient to four to six times as many allogeneic donors as an apheresis component. Despite this fact, as the increased number of platelet doses transfused as pooled WBD platelets in 2008 compared to 2006[55] indicates, there has recently been a debate in the United States on whether it is appropriate to revert to providing prepooled and cultured (and eventually perhaps pathogen-reduced) WBD platelets, as an alternative to providing apheresis (single-donor) platelets collected exclusively from male donors, female donors without a history of pregnancy, or female donors shown not to have WBC antibodies, in accordance with the 2006 AABB recommendations for TRALI prevention.[63]

Historically,[64,65] apheresis (single-donor) platelets were considered by many to be associated with a higher risk of TRALI compared with pooled WBD platelets, because they contain four to six times as much plasma from a single donor, which can potentially be collected from a female donor who has previously been pregnant and has circulating WBC antibodies directed against a recipient's antigens. Yet there have been reports[66-70] of TRALI associated with pooled WBD platelets, and TRALI has been documented to occur in association with the transfusion of blood components containing as little as ≤20 mL of plasma.[71] A higher risk of TRALI in association with apheresis (single-donor) compared with pooled WBD platelets has not been documented by an observational study or an RCT comparing the two types of platelet components in a setting where both types of platelet concentrates are transfused to the same patient population under the same conditions and at the same time.

A systematic review of the literature[10] through December 31, 2008 retrieved only three studies[72-74] that had diagnosed TRALI based on the Canadian consensus criteria[75]—in "real time" and in settings where *both* apheresis (single-donor) and pooled WBD platelets were transfused—and had reported the risk of TRALI separately for apheresis (single-donor) platelets and for either WBD platelets or platelet pools. All three studies[72-74] observed that the risk of TRALI was approximately equal per apheresis (single-donor) concentrate or per pool of WBD platelets (Table 4-2).

The absence of any TRALI deaths attributed to pooled WBD platelets and reported passively to the FDA between 2005 and 2009[1] had featured in the debate over whether the United States should increase its reliance on prepooled and cultured whole-blood-derived [rather than apheresis (single-donor)] platelets. Some observers reasoned that, because 12.5% of therapeutic platelet doses had continued to be provided as pooled WBD platelets in 2006 in the United States,[55] a few TRALI fatalities ascribed to pooled WBD platelets should have been passively reported to the FDA between 2004 and 2009 if transfusion of platelet pools was indeed associated with a risk of fatal TRALI equal to that attributed to apheresis (single-donor) platelets. Alternative explanations for the absence of such fatalities[1] include: 1) chance, since such reported deaths represent exceedingly rare events; and 2) reduced TRALI awareness and recognition in environments where pooled WBD platelets are administered. The latter certainly is a possibility, because TRALI is known to be grossly underrecognized and underreported.[76]

Notwithstanding the lack of empirical support for a difference in the risk of TRALI between pooled WBD and apheresis (single-donor) platelets,[72-74] as recently as August to September 2009, 22% of US blood centers responding to a questionnaire from an AABB-appointed TRALI Working Group stated that they endeavored to increase production of pooled WBD platelets in an effort to mitigate the risk of TRALI from apheresis (single-donor) platelets.[77] Eight of 10 blood centers proffering this response as a TRALI risk-reduction strategy were increasing production of pooled WBD platelets regardless of the gender of the donor contributing to a platelet pool.[77] This tendency to produce more pooled platelets in an effort to reduce the risk of TRALI[77] was eventually reflected in an increased number of platelet doses transfused as platelet pools in 2008 (0.260 million, compared to 0.216 million in 2006).[55]

In 2010, there was *no* death from TRALI secondary to apheresis (single-donor) platelets passively reported to the US FDA, although one TRALI death was ascribed to transfusion of pooled whole-blood-derived platelets. The reversal of the 2005-2009 trend (of no passively reported TRALI fatalities associated with platelet pools[1]) showed that the "passive surveillance artifact" clouding the interpretation of such passive surveillance data (Chapter 2) can operate in either direction. Future decisions by blood centers[77] should be based on observational studies directly comparing the risk of TRALI in patients who receive *either* pooled *or* apheresis (single-donor) platelets at the same time and under the same conditions,[72-74] as opposed to

Table 4-2. Systematic Review of Studies Diagnosing TRALI Based on the Canadian Consensus Criteria[75] in Settings with Transfusion of Both Apheresis (Single-Donor) and Pooled Whole-Blood-Derived (WBD) Platelets[10]

Study (Study Design)	Risk of TRALI in Association with Transfused Pooled WBD or Apheresis (Single-Donor) Platelets
Robillard et al[72] (passive surveillance; Public Health Agency of Canada; cases of TRALI)	1 per 8847 (2004) or 1 per 40,452 (2005) pools of five WBD concentrates compared with 1 per 11,354 (2004) or 1 per 46,996 (2005) apheresis (single-donor) platelet concentrates
Gajic et al[73] (nested case-control study of 74 TRALI cases and 74 controls, conducted as part of a prospective observational study of 901 patients sequentially admitted to a medical ICU)	The cases received 10 apheresis (single-donor) concentrates and six platelet pools The controls received three apheresis (single-donor) concentrates and three platelet pools Although the cases received more platelet transfusions than the controls (p=0.06), the type of transfused platelet component did not differ from what would be expected by the composition of the local blood-bank inventory at the time of the study†
Eder et al[74] (passive surveillance; American Red Cross; deaths from TRALI)	1 per 2,157,883 distributed individual WBD platelet concentrates; or 1 per 359,647 pools of six[55] WBD platelet concentrates; or 1 per 279,805 transfused pools of WBD platelets* compared with 1 per 320,752 distributed apheresis (single-donor) platelets; or 1 per 285,630 transfused apheresis (single-donor) platelets*

*Given that 22.2% of distributed individual WBD platelet concentrates outdated in 2006, compared with 10.9% of distributed apheresis (single-donor) platelet concentrates.[55]
†Approximately 50% apheresis (single-donor) and 50% pooled WBD platelets.
ICU = intensive care unit; TRALI = transfusion-related acute lung injury.

being based on passive surveillance data reported from environments where, for the most part, one or the other component is being transfused. Even more important, decisions by blood centers should take into account all the disparate risks associated with platelet transfusion,[10] including the risk of TTIs, rather than focusing exclusively on the risk of TRALI.

The Incremental Risk of TTIs from Platelet Pools

Figure 2-17 in Chapter 2 presented the annual increase in the number of TTIs in the United States because of the 1.04 million *preventable* allogeneic donor exposures that result from the continued transfusion of 260,000 platelet doses as pooled WBD [rather than apheresis (single-donor)] platelets. Table 2-1 in Chapter 2 showed the calculations on which the risk estimates depicted in Fig 2-17 (of Chapter 2) were based.[10,55,78-81]

Because 1.04 million *preventable* allogeneic donor exposures still occur in the United States owing to the continued use of platelet pools for 12.9% of the transfused platelet doses,[55] there is a significant opportunity to prevent transmissions of pathogens, as well as cases of TAS, by converting to a 100% apheresis platelet supply.[10] In the short term, as discussed later in this chapter, the greatest benefit from the reduction in allogeneic-donor exposures thanks to an all-apheresis platelet supply will likely be derived from the ensuing reduction in the risk of TRALI. In the longer term, however, should a novel "HIV-like" pathogen appear, the greatest benefit from an all-apheresis platelet supply will be derived from a reduction in the risk of transmission of the next "HIV-like" pathogen, since as many as 104 transmissions of a fatal TTI could be prevented annually.

Prevention of HTRs

Augmentation of Patient Identification Procedures

The continued occurrence of fatalities from ABO HTRs—an ABT hazard whose root cause is virtually always human error and a logistical problem that has remained unsolved since the 1970s—are both deplorable and inexcusable. It is hard to understand why the implementation of information technologies that would *supplement* (rather than replace) the proper patient identification procedures at the time of collection of the pretransfusion sample and—even more important—at the time of transfusion of the donor unit to the recipient has not yet been mandated by US regulatory agencies (such as the FDA) or accrediting organizations (such as the Joint Commission).

Four decades of fatalities secondary to ABO HTRs have demonstrated that relying solely on medical professionals to prevent this hazard by *always* following proper procedure is inadequate. In-depth training of the transfusionists and strict adherence to proper procedure should be supplemented by robust information technologies—barrier systems that will physically prevent transfusion of an RBC unit to the wrong recipient. Such systems are needed both at the time of collection of the pretransfusion sample and at the time of transfusion of the donor unit to the recipient.

Extended Donor-Recipient Red Cell Antigen Matching

The prevention of fatalities from non-ABO HTRs may require a more far-reaching change in blood banking practices for their prevention, and the appropriateness of this change continues to be debated.[82] The data of Schoneville et al[83,84] would argue for the introduction of extended antigen matching for the purpose of preventing the formation of additional red cell alloantibodies in all patients who have already formed their first red cell alloantibody. The probability of forming *additional* red cell antibodies with further RBC transfusions is 20% to 25% in such patients.[83,84] The formation of such additional alloantibodies can be associated with complex serologic work-ups, delay in the provision of compatible blood, as well as delayed and acute HTRs. Preventing the formation of additional red cell alloantibodies would be a significant move toward optimal transfusion safety.

According to Schoneville et al,[83] if extended antigen matching between donor and recipient were restricted to the antigens with the highest immunization risk (ie, C, c, E, K, Fy^a, and Jk^a), finding compatible blood donors would be routinely feasible in The Netherlands. Finding compatible donors would be problematic, although possible, if the extended matching of donor and recipient were to also include the Jk^b and S antigens. It can be debated how extensive the extended antigen matching between donor and recipient ought to be, and whether it should be offered to all transfusion recipients who have made their first red cell alloantibody or reserved for selected categories of alloimmunized patients. It may be, however, that the time has come for the principle of extended antigen matching between donor and recipient to be widely endorsed and implemented. At a minimum, extended antigen matching should include the C, E, and K antigens, and it should be extended to hemato-oncology patients in addition to patients with hemoglobinopathies.

Because the prevalence of red cell alloantibodies in hemato-oncology patients ranges between 9% and 13%,[85,86] and these patients have a 20% to 25% chance of forming *additional* red cell alloantibodies once they have formed their first antibody, already-alloimmunized hemato-oncology patients should perhaps be offered the same standard of care as patients with sickle cell disease in whom the prevalence of alloimmunization ranges between 19% and 43%.[87] When a blood bank uses genotyping (rather than phenotyping) of donors and recipients, as well as an electronic inventory management system for doing the extended antigen matching between the two, it should be possible to expand extended matching beyond the C, E, and K antigens, and beyond the hemato-oncology patients and patients with hemoglobinopathies, without an insurmountable rise in the workload.[88]

Clearly, avoiding red cell alloimmunization will be of benefit to any patient, and the technology is rapidly advancing to support an extended donor genotype repository and routine extended antigen matching between donor and recipient. The counter-argument relates to the magnitude of the expected benefit, and consequently to the cost-benefit ratio associated with genotype technology versus other technologies discussed in this chapter, and other necessary functions presently vying for limited resources.[82] For patients with sickle-cell disease, the higher standard of care can be justified because the inflammatory response associated with the transfusion reaction can provoke sickle cell crisis, stroke, or other severe complications. This considerable benefit does not apply to the alloimmunized hemato-oncology patients (or other alloimmunized transfusion recipients) for whom extended antigen matching is intended to prevent the morbidity and mortality associated with acute and delayed HTRs. Yet, although deaths from delayed HTRs are exceedingly rare,[89] the passively reported deaths from non-ABO HTRs make extended antigen matching between donor and recipient a safety measure very worthy of implementation.

Prevention of TRALI Through Reduction in the Number of Immunologic Exposures to Blood Donors

Apheresis (single-donor) and pooled WBD platelets (collected without regard to donor gender or the presence of WBC antibodies in the donor) are probably associated with an approximately equal risk of TRALI in the transfusion recipient.[10] Although a WBD concentrate contains one-fourth to one-sixth as much plasma from any *individual* donor (who may be a female multiparous donor with WBC antibodies matching a recipient's antigens) as do apheresis platelets, a recipient of a platelet *pool* in the United States has a four to six times greater risk of receiving a 50-mL concentrate from a female multiparous donor with WBC antibodies matching the recipient's antigens, and 50 mL of donor plasma are sufficient to cause TRALI.[71] When all transfused patients are considered, the higher probability of exposure to 50 mL of plasma from such a donor probably carries as much risk on average as the receipt of four to six times as much plasma from an individual donor of apheresis (single-donor) platelets (who may similarly have antibodies matching a recipient's antigens).[10] The case would be the same if US pooled WBD platelets were manufactured in the future in the manner discussed in Chapter 3 for the prevention of vCJD—that is, by minimizing the volume of residual plasma from each donor through the use of platelet additive solutions—because ≤20 mL of donor plasma from a female donor with circulating WBC antibodies are sufficient to cause TRALI.[71]

Moreover, the limited available data[72-74] comparing the risk of TRALI from pooled WBD and apheresis (single-donor) platelets (Table 4-2) do not indicate any difference in risk between the two types of components.[10] It is important to note that no empirical evidence has been adduced to support the opposite opinion that, compared with pooled WBD platelets, apheresis (single-donor) platelets carry a greater risk of TRALI.[90] The latter view continues to represent a theoretical prediction made in 1992[65] based on the antibody hypothesis of TRALI pathogenesis—a prediction that has been continuously carried forward based on case-reports and small case-series, but no controlled studies.

Data from observational[73] (as opposed to passive surveillance) studies—directly comparing all consecutive recipients of apheresis (single-donor) and pooled WBD platelets in the same setting—are needed to calculate any relative risk of TRALI from apheresis (single-donor) and pooled WBD platelets. In the absence of such reports, active surveillance studies[91] conducted at sentinel sites with transfusion of *both* apheresis (single-donor) and pooled WBD platelets to the same patients and under the same conditions can be informative. However, until such data based on current experience and from settings employing the Canadian consensus criteria are reported,[75] it is impossible to reach any definitive conclusion about the risk of TRALI in association with apheresis (single-donor) and pooled WBD platelets from the available conflicting databases.[10]

If our current apheresis (single-donor) and pooled WBD platelets are associated with an approximately equal risk of TRALI (Table 4-2),[10,72-74] and if apheresis (single-donor) platelets in the future are collected *solely* from male donors or female donors without a history of pregnancy or shown not to have WBC antibodies, these future apheresis (single-donor) platelets should be associated with a *lower* risk of TRALI than the current pooled WBD platelets. A mathematical model[90] considered that the TRALI risk associated with future apheresis (single-donor) platelets (collected from male donors or appropriately screened female donors) would be 40% to 80% lower than the risk of TRALI associated with the current apheresis (single-donor) or pooled WBD platelets.

Because TRALI is the leading cause of transfusion-related mortality in the United States today (Chapter 2), moving to an all-apheresis platelet supply that would rely exclusively on male donors or female donors without a history of pregnancy or shown not to have WBC antibodies would, by itself, be a major improvement in transfusion safety, replicating to some extent the success story realized by the conversion to "male-only" plasma. The full potential in terms of TRALI prevention, however, will be realized only when multicomponent apheresis[92,93] is used to collect platelets along with plasma and/or RBCs from the same donation, with all the components (platelets and/or plasma and/or RBCs) collected at the same time from the same donor reserved for transfusion to the same recipient.[94,95]

Multicomponent Apheresis Collections

Modern apheresis technology permits blood operators to collect *large-size* units of plasma, as well as "*double*" RBCs, in addition to apheresis (single-donor) platelets. Furthermore, it allows blood operators to collect RBCs *along with* platelets and/or plasma. Thus, modern apheresis technology could enable blood services to provide for all of a country's RBC, platelet, and plasma needs by subjecting to the rare risks of donation a number of donors that would not exceed the number of donors bled today by the same blood services to produce components from whole-blood collections. More important, with co-ordinated inventory management between blood centers and hospitals, modern apheresis technology could permit us to meet all of a multitransfused patient's transfusion needs for *various* blood components (RBCs, platelets, and/or plasma) with exposure to fewer donors.

By obtaining *all* the components needed by a multitransfused patient from fewer apheresis donors—who will be male donors, or female donors without a history of pregnancy or shown not to have WBC antibodies because they will be eligible to donate plasma and/or apheresis platelets per the 2006 AABB criteria[63]—multicomponent apheresis would 1) limit the *total* number of immunologic exposures of multitransfused patients to allogeneic donors and 2) restrict a multitransfused patient's allogeneic-donor exposures to male donors and/or female donors without a history of pregnancy or shown not to have WBC antibodies. Thus, to the extent that TRALI is caused by donor WBC antibodies,[63-65] multicomponent apheresis, combined with co-ordinated inventory management between blood centers and hospitals to reserve all components from the same donation for transfusion to the same recipient, offers the most effective approach to TRALI prevention.[94,95]

TRALI usually develops in multitransfused patients simultaneously receiving RBCs, platelets, and plasma (5.3 units on average in the study of van Stein et al[96]). The 49 TRALI cases in that study[96] had received 129 RBCs, 66 WBD platelet concentrates in platelet pools, and 64 units of plasma. Of 10 deaths associated with TRALI, two could have been prevented by "male-only" plasma and one by "male-only" platelets. Seven deaths, however, were associated with European RBCs manufactured by the buffy-coat method. Such "buffy-coat RBCs" are already plasma-reduced, containing ≤20 mL of plasma; their association with the majority of TRALI fatalities occurring over 2.5 years in The Netherlands[96] shows that efforts to reduce the plasma content of either RBCs or platelets by replacing the donor plasma with additive solutions are unlikely to prevent TRALI.

If that is the case, instead of trying to prevent TRALI by removing as much plasma as possible from the RBC and platelet components, one could strive to prevent TRALI by removing the immunologic exposures to the allogeneic donors themselves[94,95] by means of multicomponent apheresis.[92,93] Multicomponent apheresis and coordinated inventory management between blood centers and hospitals constitute part of the "patient-centric" approach envisioned to replace, in the 21st century, the whole-blood collections and the "component-centric" approach of the 20th century (Chapter 8). Multicomponent apheresis would thus meet all of a multitransfused patient's transfusion needs with exposure to fewer donors. This paradigm shift in the procurement of allogeneic blood components for multitransfused patients would serve in the short-term to reduce the risk of TRALI, while also reducing the risks of TAS and TTIs; in the longterm it would serve to mitigate the risk of the next "HIV-like" pathogen that may appear in the future.

Objections to the use of apheresis (single-donor) platelets for reducing the risk of TRALI have been presented from Canada[97] and Germany,[98] where a higher risk of bacterial contamination secondary to pooled WBD [rather than apheresis (single-donor)] platelets has not been observed,[10] because buffy-coat (rather than platelet-rich-plasma) WBD platelets are used. Devine et al[97] hypothesized that the production of buffy-coat platelets may reduce the risk of TRALI secondary to the associated RBC units manufactured by this same process, because "buffy-coat" RBCs are plasma-reduced. However, seven of 10 TRALI deaths over 2.5 years in The Netherlands[96] were associated with precisely such "plasma-reduced" buffy-coat RBCs and the mechanism of TRALI secondary to RBC transfusion may differ from the antibody-mediated mechanism postulated for the "plasma-rich" components.[99]

Schrezenmeier and Seifried[98] proposed that—because all platelet transfusion needs of patients who are not alloimmunized to human leukocyte antigens can be met by pooling already-available buffy coats—any donor reactions to plateletpheresis collections represent an "additional" and thus hard to justify risk. As already discussed, however, multicomponent apheresis could meet all transfusion needs of US patients by subjecting to the rare risks of donation a number of donors that will not exceed the number of donors bled today to produce the same number of components from whole-blood donations.[95] This is because any country with a North American/Western European health-care system requires several times more therapeutic doses of RBCs than of platelets or plasma to meet the needs of all its transfusion recipients.[55] Furthermore, and in contrast to what the literature on donor reactions reviewed by Schrezenmeier and Seifried had indicated,[98] this modern approach to meeting all of a country's needs should not be associated with any increase in donor reactions. In the largest reported multivariate analysis of moderate and severe donor reactions, Kamel et al[100] observed no increase in donor reactions after each of three types of apheresis collections compared with whole-blood donation. In fact, donors who self-select for plateletpheresis (as well as plasmapheresis or "double" RBC apheresis) donation have fewer ($p<0.05$) reactions than whole-blood donors (Figs 4-2 and 4-3).[100]

Other Inventory Practices to Reduce Immunologic Exposures to Donors

Even before multicomponent apheresis is implemented in the United States in the manner envisioned here, exposures to donors can be reduced through judicious use of apheresis (single-donor) platelets. The Prophylatic Platelet Dose on Transfusion Outcomes (PLADO) RCT[45] demonstrated no difference in bleeding complications between patients receiving half-the-standard dose and those receiving the standard dose of platelets, yet it showed a small but significant ($p<0.05$) difference in the total number of transfused platelets between these subjects who received half-the-standard dose and those who received the standard dose of platelets during the period of platelet transfusion support for hypoproliferative thrombocytopenia (Fig 4-4). Because patients receiving half-the-standard dose needed prophylactic platelet transfusion every 1.1 days, they could have received half of an apheresis (single-donor) concentrate the first time that they needed prophylactic platelet transfusion and the other half of the same apheresis (single-donor) concentrate the next time that they needed platelet transfusion.

Thus, although patients would need transfusion more often if they received half-the-stan-

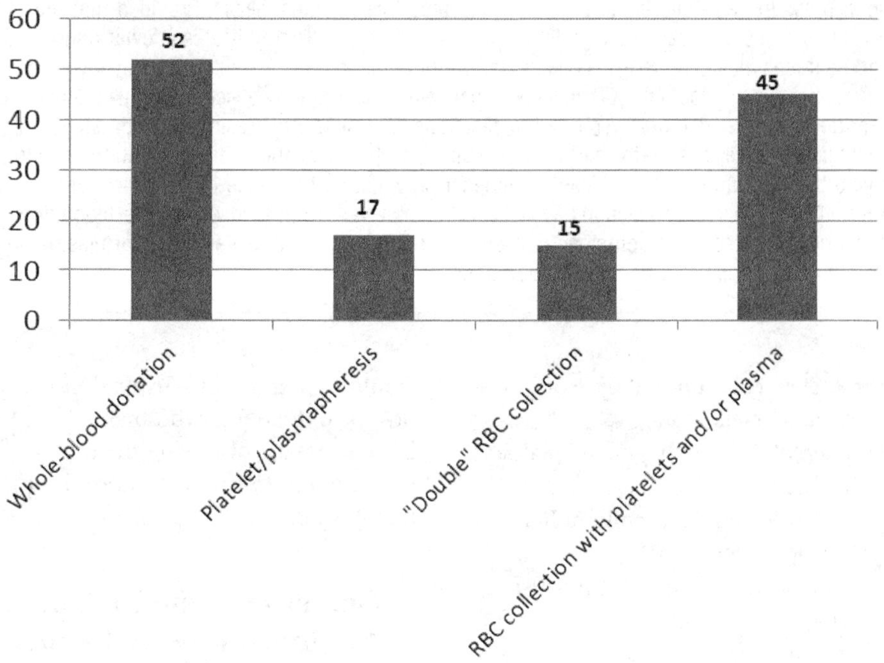

Figure 4-2. Rate of moderate or severe donor reactions per 10,000 donations made at the blood centers of one US blood provider (Blood Systems) in 2007.[100] These data are based on 793,293 allogeneic collections, including 552,183 whole-blood, 54,841 platelet/plasmapheresis, and 164,179 "double" RBC collections, and 18,790 Red Blood Cell collections combined with collections of plasma and/or platelets.

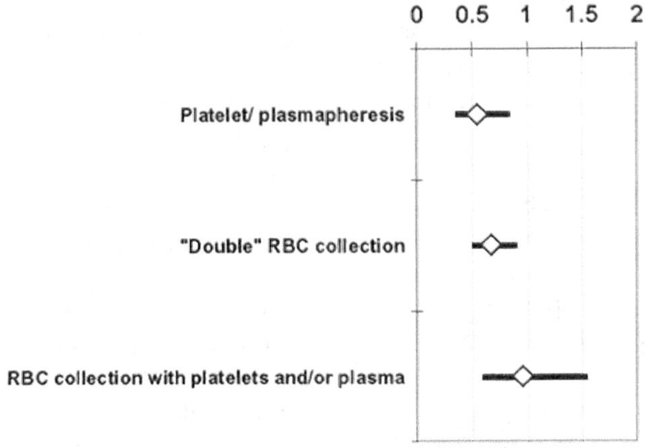

Figure 4-3. OR of moderate or severe donor reactions with platelet/plasmapheresis or "double" Red Blood Cell (RBC) collection, or RBC collection with concomitant collection of plasma and/or platelets, compared with whole-blood collection.[100] These data are based on 793,293 allogeneic collections made at the blood centers of one US blood provider (Blood Systems) in 2007, and on a multivariate model into which (in addition to collection type) the following variables were eligible for entry: donation site (fixed or mobile), association type (high school or college or other), age, gender, race, donation history, blood volume, weight, body mass index, pulse, systolic blood pressure, diastolic blood pressure, and blood center identifier.[100] Provided that the 95% confidence interval (CI) of the OR does not include the null value of 1, an OR<1 indicates a lower donor reaction rate with each of the three types of apheresis collections. Donor reaction rates were significantly lower ($p<0.05$) with platelet/plasmapheresis or "double" RBC collection than with whole-blood collection. Unlike the historical literature that reported a greater risk of adverse donor reactions with plateletpheresis than with whole-blood collections,[98] when plateletpheresis is performed with the cell separators available today—and in the hands of trained personnel who have accumulated significant experience with the performance of the procedure—donors who self-select for a plateletpheresis collection have a lower reaction rate compared with whole-blood donors. Moreover, donors who self-select for a combined collection of RBCs along with platelets and/or plasma do not have a higher reaction rate compared with whole-blood donors.

dard dose of platelets each time, they would be exposed to *one* allogeneic donor of apheresis (single-donor) platelets for each *pair* of platelet transfusions that they received. Overall, compared with patients receiving an entire apheresis (single-donor) concentrate each time they needed a prophylactic platelet transfusion, patients receiving half-the-standard dose of platelets [with the two halves of each apheresis (single-donor) concentrate reserved for them by the blood bank] would be exposed to a significantly ($p<0.05$) lower number of allogeneic donors during the period of platelet transfusion support. According to many clinicians, this approach would be beneficial for inpatients who would be exposed to fewer donors; but perhaps not for outpatients who might want to avoid the inconvenience of having to come to the hospital more often to receive more frequent platelet transfusions.

Decrease in the Risk of all ABT Complications by Reducing the Number of Donor Exposures Through Avoidance of Unnecessary Transfusions

Transfusion of blood to bleeding patients rests on solid principles of resuscitation, tissue oxy-

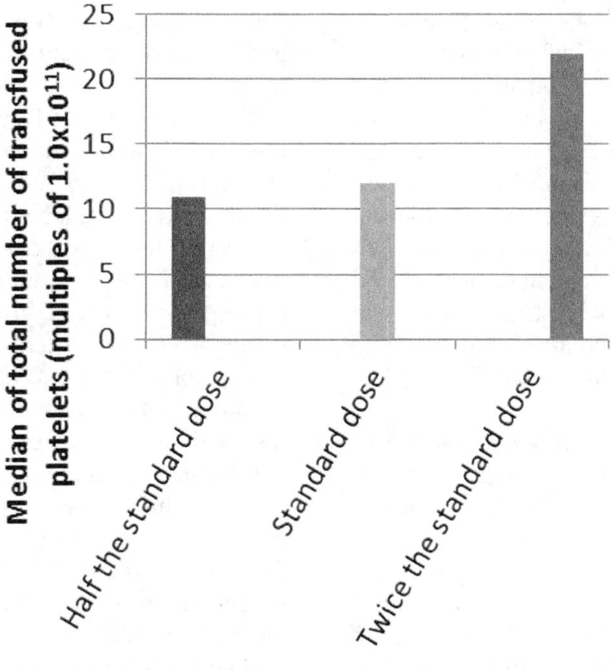

Figure 4-4. Median total number of transfused platelets (in multiples of 1.0×10^{11}) given to patients allocated to each of the three arms of the Prophylactic Platelet Dose on Transfusion Outcomes randomized controlled trial[45] that is, patients allocated to receive half-the-standard dose, the standard dose, or twice-the-standard dose of platelets each time that they needed a prophylactic platelet transfusion. The total number of transfused platelets pertains to the period of platelet transfusion support for hypoproliferative thrombocytopenia. The patients receiving half-the-standard dose [three WBD platelets or half an apheresis (single-donor) concentrate] received fewer total platelets ($p=0.02$) than did the subjects receiving the standard dose (six WBD platelets or one apheresis concentrate) each time that they needed to be transfused.[45]

genation, and the repletion of the vital elements of hemostasis. Many lives are saved by ABT given to bleeding patients, and, in many more cases, ABT serves as an exquisite life-support measure while other interventions are used concurrently to stop hemorrhage. In contrast, ABT given as prophylaxis because of abnormal screening test results for coagulation is associated with unfavorable risk-to-benefit ratios.[101] Each unnecessary ABT avoided through the use of evidence-based transfusion guidelines is potentially tantamount to avoidance of one (or several) of the infectious and noninfectious causes of ABT-related mortality discussed in Chapter 2, including those deaths attributed to ABT by observational studies and RCTs through pathophysiologic mechanisms that we do not yet understand.

There is probably no other preventive strategy that can be employed if ABT per se—rather than allogeneic WBCs or soluble WBC-derived mediators that accumulate in the supernatant fluid of RBCs during storage (Chapter 2) or the senescence of the red cells themselves (Chapter 7)—is indeed related to all-cause mortality through such ill-defined mechanisms. If the association of any ABT (as opposed to non-WBC-reduced or WBC-reduced ABT or transfusion of "old" rather than "fresh" RBCs) with mortality were confirmed, ABT would emerge as a considerably hazardous medical intervention. Thus evidence-based transfusion guidelines preventing unnecessary transfusions could save more lives than a combination of all the other strategies aimed toward a safer blood supply and discussed in this chapter. Even if such an association between ABT and mortality through ill-defined pathophysiologic mechanisms is not confirmed by future RCTs, the use of evidence-based transfusion guidelines for all transfused blood components (RBCs, platelets, plasma, and cryoprecipitate) is the only strategy that can reduce the risk of—and the associated mortality from—all currently established ABT complications.

Transfusion of blood components has never undergone prospective randomized testing in the manner that a new drug would be expected to undergo.[102] Although the "10/30 rule" (of transfusing patients for a hemoglobin level decreasing to 10 g/dL or for a hematocrit decreasing to or below 30%) had been a belief for five decades,[103] the 1999 Transfusion Requirements in Critical Care (TRICC) RCT[104] documented the fallacy of the previous indoctrination.

The delivery of oxygen and its utilization by tissues is only partly understood. In theory, RBCs are transfused to improve tissue oxygen delivery, although it is not always clear that such potentally increased oxygen delivery translates into increased local availability of oxygen at the tissue level, or increased intracellular consumption of oxygen,[105] nor is it always clear that all microcirculatory beds respond equally to ABT.[106] These are basic clinical questions that still warrant study.[103,107] How do we decide which patients need RBC transfusion? Which variables should we assess to identify patients who might benefit from ABT? What are the outcomes of patients who receive one, some, or many RBC transfusions? How do we determine if a RBC transfusion is effective? Is a low hemoglobin detrimental to the critically ill patient? If a higher hemoglobin could be achieved without risk, would it benefit the critically ill patient?

Thus, there is now considerable interest in formulating evidence-based transfusion guidelines for nonbleeding patients. Of the 24 concept proposals for RCTs in transfusion medicine presented at the September 2009 State-of-the-Science Symposium on Transfusion Medicine and Hemostasis held at the National Heart, Lung, and Blood Institute (NHLBI) of the National Institutes of Health,[108] 11 pertained to the formulation of appropriate indications for the transfusion of the various blood components. Of these, five were aimed at the development of criteria for the appropriate transfusions of RBCs, two at the development of criteria for the appropriate transfusions of platelets, and five at the development of criteria for the appropriate transfusions of plasma. Eight concept proposals proposed to investigate the safety of *lower* transfusion thresholds or the safety of withholding prophylactic transfusions of platelets and plasma, whereas only three presentations proposed to investigate possible benefits obtained from higher transfusion thresholds or from the liberal administration of prophylactic platelet or plasma transfusions.

The current interest in formulating evidence-based transfusion guidelines for nonbleeding patients is complemented by a growing appreciation of the need to differentiate between therapeutic and prophylactic transfusions when making a decision to transfuse and by a growing awareness of the fact that *prophylactic* transfusions greatly outnumber *therapeutic* transfusions for *all* blood components.[109-111] Because most transfusions are prophylactic, and therefore giving them is optional, physicians should always consider the risks of ABT, ask whether outcomes after ABT are better, and consider adopting a "nontransfusion default position" when there is no empirical evidence for potential benefit.[110] Proponents of patient blood management (Chapter 8) hold that the role of RBC transfusions should be reassessed, especially in the perioperative setting and for the management of anemia in hemodynamically stable patients without co-morbidities. In this group of patients, little evidence can be found to support improvement in clinical outcomes after ABT, and efforts should be directed at correcting defects in the hematopoietic system so as to correct anemia without RBC transfusions.[111] In this spirit, correction of reversible anemias before surgery and the use of blood conservation techniques have made "bloodless" surgery possible in most uncomplicated elective settings.[112]

Several alternatives to RBC transfusions exist[112] and their use (in lieu of ABT) could perhaps become the "default" position.[113] Nonetheless, use of such transfusion alternatives demands the same attention to balancing risks and benefits as the use of ABT itself.[113-115] Proponents of patient blood management advocate that all options (ie, both ABT and its alternatives) should be evaluated on a "level playing field" when the options available to a patient are being considered and that RBC transfusion should no longer be considered as the default or "safe" option when there is clinical uncertainty about the benefit that a specific patient will derive from ABT or about the risks of ABT.[109-111,113,116-118]

Evidence for the appropriate indications for transfusion of RBCs in clinically-stable adult or neonatal patients has been produced by RCTs. Such evidence is also available for the prophylactic platelet transfusions given to hemato-oncology patients with hypoproliferative thrombocytopenia, but it has not hitherto become available for prophylactic platelet or plasma transfusions administered in other settings.

The TRICC RCT

In the TRICC RCT,[104] although the difference did not attain significance in the comparison of the primary outcome (30-day mortality; $p = 0.11$), allocation to a liberal (rather than restrictive) transfusion-strategy arm—which resulted on average in the transfusion of 3.0 more RBC units in the Intensive Care Unit (ICU)—was marginally associated with a 5.8% increase ($p \geq 0.05$) in the absolute risk of death in the hospital. This finding has not been confirmed by another RCT and—in the interim—it can be attributed to the effect of multiple comparisons, that is, the reporting of several mortality and morbidity outcomes by the authors of the TRICC RCT. If it is confirmed by future RCTs, it would suggest that, for every 16.9 patients receiving ABT per liberal criteria (for a hemoglobin level falling to or below 10 g/dL, as opposed to falling to or below 7 g/dL), one patient might die during her/his hospitalization because of the excess RBC transfusions received. Although such a figure is far from having been established, it would represent a staggering number of deaths secondary to ABT even if it were off by two orders of magnitude.

Further RCTs would clearly be needed to produce an unambiguously significant ($p<0.05$) result with respect to a difference in a primary mortality outcome, as well as to determine whether the findings of the TRICC RCT[104] pertain to clinical settings outside the ICU. However, based on the existing findings,[104] physicians should endeavor to limit their patients' exposure to ABT by administering RBC transfusions to raise the hemoglobin level only when a patient's hemoglobin falls to or below 7 g/dL (provided that the patient is not actively bleeding and does not have ischemic heart disease). Once a hemoglobin level of >7 g/dL (with a maintenance hemoglobin level of 7 to 9 g/dL as shown in the TRICC RCT[104]) has been reached through ABT, further RBC transfusion(s) should be withheld unless a patient has symptoms or signs relating to the anemia.[119,120]

The reason for withholding such transfusions is that, as the TRICC RCT[104] unambiguously demonstrated, transfusion for a hemoglobin target of ≤7 g/dL is as good as transfusion for a hemoglobin target of ≤10 g/dL (with a maintenance hemoglobin level of 10-12 g/dL) in the absence of symptoms or signs of anemia. In the analysis of all patients, there were no statistically significant ($p<0.05$) differences between the arms other than for the adjusted multiple-organ dysfunction score (and difference from the baseline score), as well as the development of myocardial infarction and pulmonary edema. All four significant differences in outcome between the two arms favored the restrictive-strategy arm.[104] Moreover, with the sole exception of septic shock, all observed trends in outcome favored the restrictive-strategy arm as well. Compared with the liberal-strategy arm, the patients in the restrictive-strategy arm consistently demonstrated better clinical outcomes in terms of mortality, multiple-organ failure, length of stay in the hospital or the ICU, organ-specific complications, or any studied complication.[104]

Admittedly, the TRICC RCT[104] left open the possibility that both trial arms might have had a worse outcome than would have been the case had a third, "standard-of-care" arm (Fig 4-5) also been included–that is, an arm in which physicians would have been allowed to use their own judgment to transfuse for a hemoglobin target of between ≤7 g/dL and ≤10 g/dL based on their assessment of each patient's clinical presentation. More specifically, before the TRICC RCT[104] was reported, only 3% of Canadian doctors would have let the hemoglobin decrease to 7 g/dL before transfusing patients with ischemic heart disease. Only 12% of doctors would have transfused relatively healthy patients [ie, patients under 55 years of age or patients with an Acute Physiology and Chronic Health Evaluation (APACHE) II score of under 20] for a hemoglobin of ≤10 g/dL.[121,122] The TRICC RCT randomly assigned patients with ischemic heart disease to the restrictive arm and relatively healthy patients (<55 years of age and/or with an APACHE II score of <20) to the liberal arm. The former patients enrolled in the trial were to

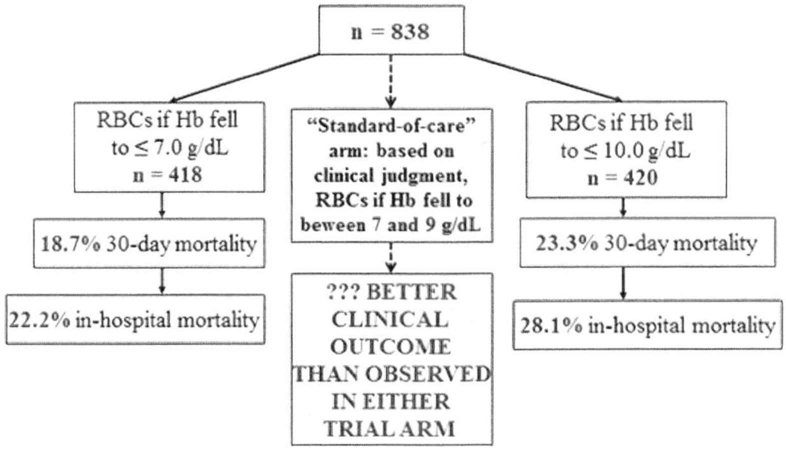

Figure 4-5. Actual (limited to the outer two arms) compared with optimal (including the middle arm) design for the Transfusion Requirement in Critical Care (TRICC) randomized controlled trial (RCT).[104] When all clinically stable adult patients admitted to the intensive care unit were transfused—regardless of their illness severity—per the transfusion threshold (≤7.0 g/dL compared with ≤10.0 g/dL) required by the arm to which they had been randomly assigned, there was no difference between the arms in the primary outcome (30-day mortality). However, one of the mortality outcomes (in-hospital mortality) reported by the authors approached statistical significance ($p \geq 0.05$). It was subsequently proposed[121,122] that the randomization scheme used in the TRICC RCT[104] resulted in worse clinical outcomes in both trial arms compared with the outcome that would have been expected in a third, "standard-of-care" arm, which was not part of the trial. For patients randomly assigned to such a third arm, clinicians would have been allowed to make individual decisions about whether to transfuse a patient whose hemoglobin decreased to a level between the transfusion thresholds employed in the liberal compared with the restrictive arms of the trial. Thus, patients with ischemic heart disease in this third arm would have been transfused before their hemoglobin levels decreased to ≤7 g/dL and relatively healthy subjects (under 55 years of age or with an Acute Physiology and Chronic Health Evaluation (APACHE) II score under 20) would *not* have been transfused if their hemoglobin level decreased to ≤10 g/dL. Practice misalignments would have been prevented in this third arm between the treatment that patients received in the trial[104] and the treatment that they would have received outside the trial if their physicians had been allowed to make their own decisions about whether (or not) to transfuse their patients.
RBCs = Red Blood Cells.

be transfused only when their hemoglobin levels fell to ≤7 g/dL; the latter subjects were to be transfused when their hemoglobin levels dropped to 10 g/dL. Thus, the TRICC RCT created practice misalignments between the treatment that these patients received in the trial and the treatment that they would have received outside the trial. Subgroup analyses further demonstrated that it was only these relatively healthy subjects (<55 years of age or with an APACHE II score of <20) who derived benefit—that is, experienced a significant ($p<0.05$) reduction in mortality—from being given fewer RBC transfusions because of the trial design (Fig 4-5).[121]

Other RCTs of Transfusion Thresholds in Stable Adult Patients

The Functional Outcomes in Cardiovascular Patients Undergoing Surgical Hip Fracture Repair (FOCUS) transfusion RCT[123] showed no difference in mortality between the liberal and restrictive transfusion strategy arms and another recent RCT from Brazil[124] further bolstered this conclusion. Prior to the publication of the FOCUS RCT[123] and the Transfusion Requirements After Cardiac Surgery (TRACS) RCT from Brazil,[124] a meta-analysis had integrated all RCTs that had compared liberal to restrictive transfusion.[125] Based on all the evidence hitherto adduced,[104,123-125] and particularly for clinically stable adult patients, there is no indication from RCTs that a "liberal" transfusion strategy (administration of blood transfusion for a hemoglobin level falling below any target value greater than 7 g/dL in the absence, or greater than 8 g/dL in the presence, of cardiovascular disease) confers any benefit to patients beyond that obtained with a "restrictive" transfusion strategy (administration of RBC transfusion for a target hemoglobin level of ≤7 g/dL in the absence of cardiovascular disease or a target hemoglobin level of ≤8 g/dL in its presence.

In contrast to the *overall* results of the TRICC RCT[104] (which showed a trend toward reduced mortality in patients randomly assigned to the restrictive-strategy arm), the subgroup analysis of 257 patients with ischemic heart disease showed a trend toward reduced mortality in the liberal-strategy arm.[126] For this reason, the FOCUS RCT[123] enrolled 2016 patients with a mean age of 81 years to investigate whether subjects with cardiovascular disease or cardiovascular risk factors undergoing surgical repair of hip fracture benefit from a higher (≤10 g/dL) or a lower (≤8 g/dL) transfusion threshold. The risks of in-hospital acute coronary syndrome or death (5.2% in the restrictive arm and 4.3% in the liberal arm), 60-day mortality, and various morbidity and functional endpoints did not differ between the arms. However, unlike the TRICC RCT,[104] the FOCUS RCT[123] did not find an increase in the risk of adverse outcomes (ie, myocardial infection and pulmonary edema) in subjects allocated to the liberal (compared with the restrictive) transfusion arm. Observed trends operated in either direction, as would have been expected by chance.

The TRACS RCT[124] from Brazil enrolled 502 patients admitted to the ICU after undergoing cardiac surgery. The liberal and restrictive randomization arm criteria (hemoglobin level of ≤10 g/dL and ≤8 g/dL respectively) were the same as those used in the FOCUS trial.[123] The main outcome measure was a composite endpoint of 30-day all-cause mortality and severe morbidity (cardiogenic shock, acute respiratory distress syndrome, or acute renal failure) occurring during the hospital stay. This primary endpoint occurred in 10% of patients allocated to the liberal transfusion arm and in 11% of patients allocated to the restrictive transfusion arm ($p=0.85$). The authors concluded that a restrictive transfusion strategy is not inferior to a liberal transfusion strategy in patients undergoing cardiac surgery vis-à-vis their combined outcome of mortality and severe morbidity.

A meta-analysis[125] undertaken before publication of the FOCUS[123] and TRACS[124] RCTs integrated 17 heterogeneous RCTs enrolling 3746 patients. The authors concluded that the totality of the evidence supports the use of restrictive transfusion thresholds in patients who are free of serious cardiac disease.[125] However, unlike the TRICC RCT,[104] the meta-analysis of all 17 available studies comparing the clinical outcome of restrictive and liberal transfusion thresholds did not find an increase in adverse clinical outcomes in patients allocated to receive RBC transfusions under liberal criteria compared with those transfused under restrictive criteria. Mortality, cardiac events, myocardial infarction, stroke, pneumonia, and thromboembolism were all similar in patients transfused under liberal or restrictive criteria. Restrictive transfusion strategies were associated only with a statistically significant reduction in the risk of infection [odds ratio (OR) = 0.76; 95% CI, 0.60-0.97]. The use of restrictive decision-making strategies did not reduce the length of stay either at the hospital or in the ICU. Restrictive strategies did, however, reduce the number of allogeneic donor exposures. The risk of receiving a RBC transfusion was reduced by 37% (OR = 0.63; 95% CI, 0.54-0.74; $p<0.05$), and the mean number of RBC units received was reduced by 0.75 unit (95% CI, 0.20-1.30; $p<0.05$).

The 17 RCTs[104,127-142] included in the meta-analysis[125] varied greatly with respect to the restrictive and liberal transfusion thresholds used: the former ranged between 7 g/dL and 9 g/dL, the latter between 9 and 12 g/dL. Enrolled patients included surgical patients, ICU patients, hemato-oncology patients, or trauma patients and/or patients having acute blood loss. With five exceptions,[129,134,139-141] the individual RCTs had found a statistically significant reduction in the risk of receiving a RBC transfusion for patients allocated to the restrictive rather than the liberal transfusion strategy arm. When the transfusion thresholds differed by ≥2.0 g/dL between the liberal and restrictive strategy arms, the amount of RBC use documented by these RCTs in the arm using a restrictive transfusion threshold was much lower than that seen in other trials. Accordingly, adoption of a ≤7.0 g/dL transfusion threshold for clinically stable patients should have an effect (in terms of ABT avoidance or reduction in the number of RBC units transfused) greater than that observed by the meta-analysis.

As far as the association of a liberal (compared with restrictive) transfusion threshold with adverse clinical outcomes is concerned, however, neither the meta-analysis[125] of 17 RCTs[104,127-142] nor the recent FOCUS[123] and TRACS[124] studies corroborated the TRICC trial[104] finding of an association between non-WBC-reduced ABT and mortality or major morbidity. Both the meta-analysis[125] and the subsequently presented evidence,[123,124] however, corroborate the TRICC finding[104] that a restrictive transfusion strategy is not inferior to a liberal transfusion strategy in terms of its effect on mortality and major morbidity. Moreover, a restrictive transfusion strategy is safe even in the case of patients with high cardiovascular risk. Finally, a restrictive transfusion strategy does reduce the number of allogeneic-donor exposures, both by altogether preventing ABT and by reducing the number of RBC units transfused.[123-125] Perhaps the recent publication of the FOCUS[123] and TRACS[124] RCTs will end the debate about whether the recommendation[143] to use RBC transfusion to maintain hemoglobin levels greater than 10 g/dL in high-risk patients should be adhered to. The rationale for transfusing patients with impaired ventricular function to a hemoglobin of ≥10 g/dL[143] has been that the lack of compensatory increase in cardiac output leaves ABT as the only means to increase postoperative oxygen delivery.

RBC Transfusions for Stable Adult Patients

Recent practice guidelines for RBC transfusion promulgated by professional societies,[144,145] such as the guidelines published in 2009 by the American College of Critical Care Medicine,[145] have incorporated the restrictive (≤7.0 g/dL) RBC transfusion threshold as the most appropriate hemoglobin level that can justify RBC transfusion in hemodynamically stable patients. More specifically, there is no evidence of greater benefit from a liberal transfusion strategy (≤ 10 g/dL), than from a restrictive transfusion strategy (≤7 g/dL), in critically ill patients requiring mechanical ventilation, resuscitated critically ill trauma patients, or critically ill patients with stable cardiac disease, although there is insufficient evidence for making recommendations for patients with sepsis, patients with ALI or acute respiratory distress syndrome, and patients with neurologic injury or neurologic diseases.[145] Otherwise, RBC transfusion is indicated for patients with hemorrhagic shock, and it may be indicated for bleeding patients with hemodynamic instability or inadequate oxygen delivery.[145] However, the exclusive use of a hemoglobin level as a threshold for RBC transfusion should be avoided. The decision for RBC transfusion should be based on an individual patient's intravascular volume status, evidence of shock, duration and extent of anemia, and cardiopulmonary physiologic parameters. In the absence of acute hemorrhage, RBC transfusions should be given as single units.[145] AABB expects to publish RBC transfusion guidelines in the near future.

The guidelines promulgated by the Society of Thoracic Surgeons and the Society of Cardiovascular Anesthesiologists in 2007[146] placed the emphasis on a multimodality approach to blood conservation combining all of the following: 1) drugs that increase preoperative blood volume (eg, erythropoietin) or decrease postoperative bleeding (eg, antifibrinolytics); 2) devices that conserve blood (eg, intraoperative blood recovery and blood-sparing interventions); 3) interventions that protect the patient's own blood from the stress of the operation (eg, preoperative autologous donation and normovolemic hemodilution); and 4) point-of-care testing to guide rational decision making vis-à-vis blood component therapy, depending on what is needed by the individual patient. In this regard, the 2009 guidelines of the American College of Critical Care Medicine[145] stated that there are insufficient data to support definitive recommendations regarding alternatives to RBC transfusion (such as erythropoietin) or strategies to reduce RBC transfusion (such as intraoperative or postoperative blood recovery), although both erythropoietin and perioperative blood conservation techniques may lead to a significant reduction in allogeneic RBC use.

The safety and benefit of these patient blood management approaches indeed need to be assessed with the same rigor as do the safety and benefit of ABT.[113-115] Use of erythropoietin for the purpose of avoiding the risks of ABT may create new risks of deep vein thrombosis[147] and related adverse events, especially in patients with cancer[148] and renal[149] (albeit not heart[150]) disease. Erythropoietin and perioperative autologous blood recovery or conservation techniques are widely used in many countries, but the extent to which these modalities prevent or reduce ABT in settings where restrictive transfusion guidelines have already been implemented is disputed. A meta-analysis of available studies found that–although perioperative blood recovery produced a significant reduction in the likelihood of exposure to allogeneic RBCs–the mean difference (ie, reduction) in the number of allogeneic-donor exposures achieved per patient was only 0.67 (95% CI, 0.49-0.89; $p<0.05$).[151] Indeed, British guidelines no longer support preoperative autologous blood donation as a RBC transfusion alternative.[152] Although the safety and benefit of these patient blood management approaches needs to be further assessed, many unnecessary RBC transfusions can be avoided through a *combination* of restrictive transfusion guidelines and a multimodal approach to patient blood management developed and endorsed locally at each hospital (as discussed in Chapter 8).

RBC Transfusions for Stable Low-Birthweight Neonates

The benefit from a liberal or restrictive transfusion strategy (compared with the clinical equivalence of the two) needs to be further elucidated in low-birthweight preterm infants. The Canadian Premature Infants in Need of Transfusion (PINT) RCT that enrolled 451 neonates with a birthweight of <1 kg recorded composite outcomes of 74.0% in the restrictive-strategy arm and 69.7% in the liberal-strategy arm ($p=0.25$).[153] The composite outcome consisted of death before discharge from the hospital, survival with severe retinopathy, bronchopulmonary dysplasia, and/or brain injury identified on cranial ultrasound.[153]

Owing to multiple exclusion criteria, the neonates enrolled in the PINT trial[153] may have had a "better-than-average" prognosis. The neurodevelopmental outcomes of these same infants were assessed at 18 to 21 months of age.[154] There was no statistical difference in the primary outcome (death or presence of cerebral palsy, cognitive delay, or severe visual or hearing impairment), which was found in 45% of the infants from the restrictive arm and 38% of the infants from the liberal arm. There was also no difference in any of the planned secondary outcomes. However, the difference in cognitive delay (Mental Development Index score of <70) approached statistical significance (Fig 4-6). A post-hoc analysis, with the Mental Development Index score redefined as <85, showed a statistically significant difference favoring the liberal-strategy arm.[154] A small US RCT enrolling 100 infants with a birthweight of between 0.5 and 1.3 kg concluded that infants in the restrictive-strategy arm were more likely to have intraparenchymal brain hemorrhage or periventricular leukomalacia, and they also had more frequent episodes of both mild and severe apnea.[155] These conclusions, however, were based on a very small number of events (with zero versus four and zero versus six infants, respectively, having grade IV brain hemorrhage or grade IV brain hemorrhage and/or periventricular leukomalacia), and any benefit from a liberal transfusion strategy needs to be investigated further in future RCTs.

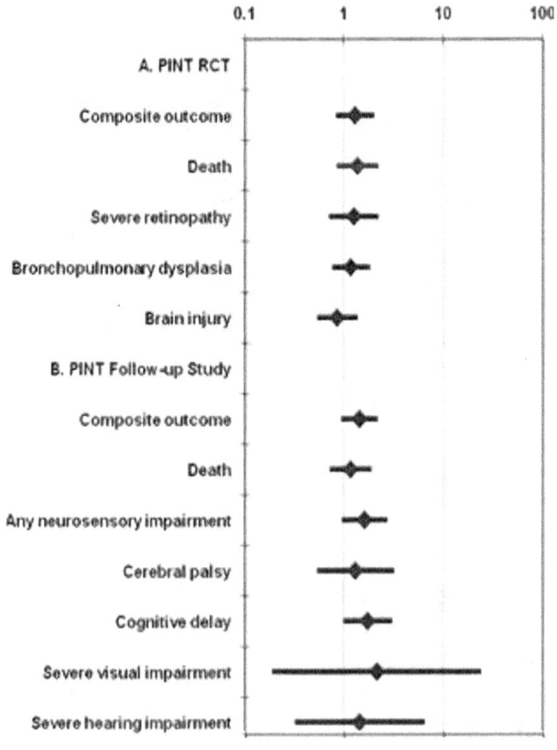

Figure 4-6. Clinical outcomes analyzed as categorical variables in the Premature Infants in Need of Transfusion (PINT) RCT[153] (Section A) and in the follow-up study to the PINT RCT[154] (Section B). For each comparison, the figure shows the odds ratio (OR) of an adverse outcome in patients from the restrictive (compared with the liberal) transfusion strategy arm. Each OR is surrounded by its 95% CI. When the 95% CI includes the null value of 1, the corresponding OR is not statistically significant (ie, p>0.05). Of all the comparisons reported by the authors,[153,154] only the difference in cognitive delay in the follow-up study[154] approached significance. However, with the sole exception of brain injury in the initial RCT,[153] all observed trends favored the liberal (rather than the restrictive) transfusion arm.

Prophylactic Platelet Transfusions for Patients with Hypoproliferative Thrombocytopenia

The dose of platelets transfused was originally based upon the perceived need to raise the patient's platelet count above a certain "safe" threshold. However, this threshold that defined the "standard" platelet dose was not based on data, and we should examine whether low-dose or high-dose platelet transfusions might be better for patients than the standard dose. If low-dose platelet transfusions were clinically as effective as standard-dose platelet transfusions in preventing bleeding, the risks of ABT to which a given patient is exposed could decrease. Alternatively, if high-dose platelet transfusions prolonged the interval between platelet transfusions or provided more effective hemostasis compared with standard-dose transfusions, high-dose transfusions could be preferred to standard-dose transfusions.

The PLADO RCT[45] concluded that it is safe to transfuse platelets prophylactically to hemato-oncology patients with hypoproliferative thrombocytopenia—when the 10,000 platelets/μL threshold is reached—at a dose half the standard dose. Data were analyzed on 1272 patients hospitalized at 26 trial sites who received at least one platelet transfusion. Patients were transfused prophylactically for monitoring platelet counts of ≤10,000/μL or at a different transfusion threshold (or dose) if therapeutically indicated.

The primary endpoint was bleeding of WHO grade 2 or greater. Whether the analysis targeted bleeding of WHO grade 2 or greater or only bleeding greater than grade 2, the same proportion of patients developed bleeding (Fig 4-7), whether they were assigned to receive half the standard dose, the standard dose, or twice the standard dose—that is, respectively, 1.1×10^{11} platelets/m^2, 2.2×10^{11} platelets/m^2, or 4.4×10^{11} platelets/m^2 doses that correspond, respectively, to half of an apheresis (single-donor) concentrate, one apheresis (single-donor) concentrate, or two apheresis (single-donor) concentrates; or an equivalent dose of pooled WBD platelets. The most common bleeding sites were the gastrointestinal tract and the genitourinary tract. There was no difference in bleeding sites among the three trial arms, with the exception of oral bleeding, which was more common in the half-the-standard-dose arm than in the standard-dose and twice-the-standard-dose arms. Regardless of randomization arm, subjects with a monitoring platelet count of <5000/μL had the highest bleeding risk. Equivalent bleeding risk was observed for platelet counts between 6000/μL and 80,000/μL. More specifically, bleeding occurred on 25% of study days when the platelet count was <5000/μL, compared with 17% of study days when the platelet count was between 6000/μL and 80,000/μL. There was no difference between the three trial arms in the number of RBC units transfused.[45]

The median number of days with greater than grade 2 bleeding was one in all three arms. Patients were stratified by cause of hypoproliferative thrombocytopenia (chemotherapy for hematologic malignancy or for solid tumor compared with autologous or allogeneic marrow transplant), and platelet dose did not affect bleeding in any patient stratum. Patients receiving half the standard dose had more transfusion episodes than patients from the other two arms (five, three, and three episodes, respectively; $p<0.001$), but they were also transfused a lower total number of platelets (median of $11 \times 10,^{11}$ $12 \times 10,^{11}$ and $22 \times 10,^{11}$ respectively). Although the difference in the total transfused dose of platelets received by the half-the-standard-dose arm and that received by the standard-dose arm was small (9%), it was statistically significant (Fig 4-4).

Nonetheless, the Strategies for the Transfusion of Platelets (SToP) RCT[156]—which similarly compared low-dose and standard-dose prophylactic platelet transfusions—was terminated early by the Data Safety Monitoring Board because a 5% difference (a specified stopping rule for that trial) in WHO grade 4 bleeding was reached. At that time, three of 58 (5.2%) patients in the low-dose arm, and none of 61 (0%) patients in the standard-dose arm, had suffered grade 4 bleeding. The same proportion of patients (30 of 58 in the low-dose arm and 30 of 61 in the standard-dose arm) had experienced grade 2 or greater bleeding, which was the trial's primary endpoint (Fig 4-8). However, there was no dif-

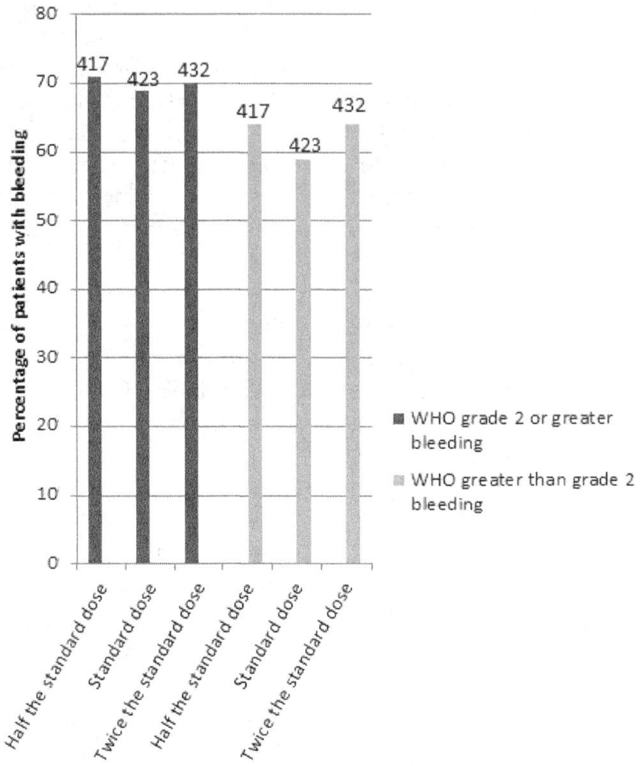

Figure 4-7. Comparison of the proportion of patients having at least one episode of grade 2, grade 3, and/or grade 4 bleeding on the WHO scale, and of the proportion of patients having at least one episode of grade 3 or grade 4 bleeding on the WHO scale, following random assignment to the half-the-standard-dose, standard-dose, and twice-the-standard-dose arm of the Prophylactic Platelet Dose on Transfusion Outcomes (PLADO) RCT.[45] The number of subjects assigned to each arm is shown above each column. All randomly assigned subjects received at least one platelet transfusion. There was no difference among the three arms in the primary endpoint of "clinically significant" bleeding (ie, WHO grade 2 or greater bleeding) or the secondary endpoint (WHO grade 3 or 4 bleeding), regardless of the dose of platelets received. Initially published by Vamvakas in Clin Lab 2010;56:263-79.

ference in the number of donor exposures between the two arms (mean ± SD of 26.3 ± 28.2 in the low-dose and 22.2 ± 15.6 in the standard-dose arm, $p = 0.34$), with the mean ± SD interval between transfusions (in days) being 1.8 ± 1.1 and 2.8 ± 1.8, respectively.

Of the three patients who developed "catastrophic" (ie, WHO grade 4) bleeding in the half-the-standard dose arm, two suffered retinal hemorrhage with visual impairment that slowly improved over time. The third patient developed a subdural hemorrhage with associated neurologic signs. In the discussion section of their paper, Heddle et al queried whether it was appropriate to categorize retinal hemorrhages as "catastrophic," which in turn, led them to question the clinical relevance of the WHO bleeding assessment.[156]

In interpreting the results of the half-the-standard dose versus standard dose of platelets RCTs,[45,156] it is important to consider that different doses are regarded as "standard" in different countries. For example, in the United Kingdom—where pools of four WBD platelets are consid-

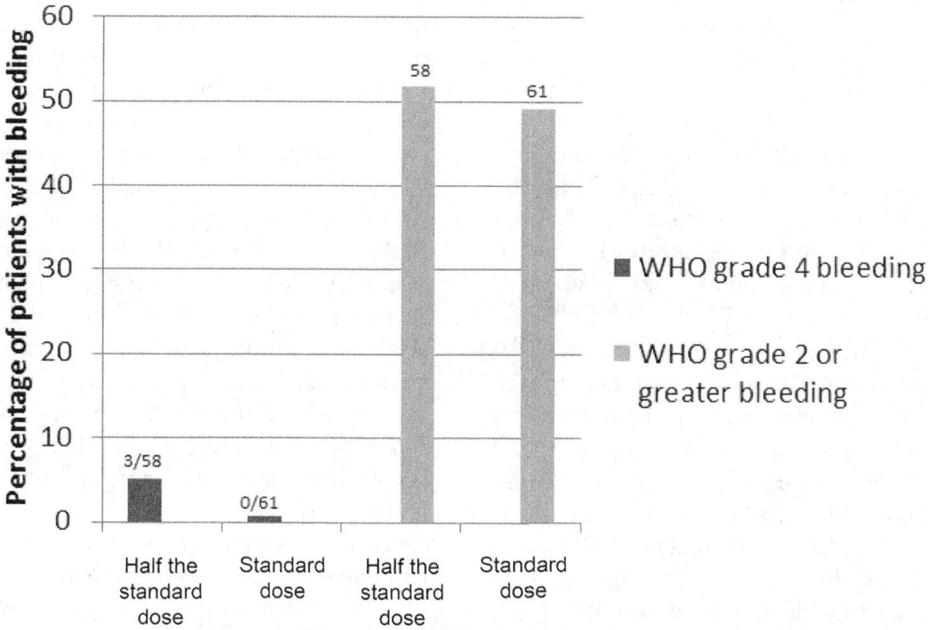

Figure 4-8. Comparison of the proportion of patients having at least one episode of grade 2, grade 3, or grade 4 bleeding on the WHO scale following random allocation to the half-the-standard dose or the standard-dose arm of the Strategies for the Transfusion of Platelets (SToP) RCT.[156] The number of subjects allocated to each arm is shown above each column. The results shown reflect the patients' bleeding status at the time that the trial was interrupted early, because three of 58 patients receiving half-the-standard dose (compared with none of 61 patients receiving the standard dose) of platelets had developed catastrophic (WHO grade 4) bleeding ($p = 0.05$). At the time that the trial was interrupted, there was no difference between the arms in the trial's primary endpoint of "clinically-significant" bleeding (ie, WHO grade 2 or greater bleeding).

ered to represent a "standard" adult dose—the standard adult dose is $>2.4\times10^{11}$ platelets per transfused component. In the United States—where an apheresis (single-donor) concentrate represents the "standard" adult dose—the standard adult dose is $>3.0\times10^{11}$ platelets per transfused component. Thus, the standard UK dose for platelet transfusions would be nearer to the half-the-standard dose than the standard dose used in the PLADO RCT,[45] and it would fall within the half-the-standard dose range of the SToP trial.[156] Blood systems or countries transfusing pools of four WBD platelets may thus have already de facto implemented a policy of nearly low-dose platelet transfusions.

Prophylactic Compared with Therapeutic Platelet Transfusions

After the PLADO RCT[45] had demonstrated no difference in WHO grade 2 or greater bleeding complications, as well as no difference in WHO grade 3 and grade 4 bleeding complications (Fig 4-7), UK and Australian investigators undertook the Trial of Platelet Prophylaxis (TOPP) RCT.[157] In this currently ongoing trial, hemato-oncology patients with hypoproliferative thrombocytopenia are randomly allocated to receive *prophylactic* platelet transfusion for a platelet count falling below 10,000/µL or *therapeutic* platelet transfusion for documented signs or symptoms of bleeding. The premise of the study is that all previous RCTs evaluating the threshold level for prophylactic platelet transfusion or the optimal dose for platelet transfusion were making an assumption that a patient derives benefit from prophylactic platelet transfusion. However, it is now uncommon for patients undergoing induction chemotherapy or hematopoietic stem-cell transplantation to die of hemorrhage. Thus, the benefit that an individual patient derives from prophylactic platelet transfusion must be considered in relation to the definite risks (Chapter 2) of ABT.[157]

As in the case of the PLADO[45] and SToP[156] RCTs, the primary outcome measure in the TOPP RCT[157] is the proportion of patients who have at least one clinically significant (WHO grade 2 or greater) bleeding complication during the trial period (defined for the TOPP trial[157] as 30 days from randomization). The WHO scale, however, was developed to monitor adverse events in cancer patients several decades ago,[158] at a time when the standard for supportive care for hemato-oncology patients was very different.[156] The TOPP investigators[157] modified the WHO scale[158] to designate as clinically significant some bleeding complications categorized as grade 1 by the WHO scale: namely, spreading or generalized petechiae and nose bleeds lasting for more than 30 minutes.[159] These "grade 1" bleeding complications are now regarded by many hematologists as a threshold for therapeutic platelet transfusion. In the TOPP RCT,[157] patients with *modified* WHO grade 2 bleeding complications are given one apheresis (single-donor) concentrate (or a pool of four WBD platelets), in accordance with standard clinical practice. Patients with WHO grade 3 and grade 4 bleeding complications may receive further doses of platelets at their own physician's discretion.

The TOPP investigators[157] deemed that–with the aforementioned modification–WHO grade 2, grade 3, and/or grade 4 bleeding complications represent the most relevant clinical outcome, because they encompass clinically significant bleeding (such as prolonged epistaxis and/or pharyngeal bleeding, melena, hematemesis, hemoptysis, and vaginal bleeding) with or without RBC transfusion requirement. WHO grade 1 bleeding complications were not included as an endpoint for the trial because they are very common in severely thrombocytopenic patients and are considered clinically less relevant.[157] Reduction in the frequency of such minor bleeding episodes may not necessarily equate with survival benefit, depending on whether they are a predictor of more severe subsequent bleeding. As was the case in the PLADO RCT,[45] the TOPP investigators are also considering grade 3 and grade 4 bleeding as a secondary endpoint. This is because the customarily used primary endpoint[45,156] (bleeding of WHO grade 2, 3, and/or 4) may fail to capture all clinically important information needed for ruling out any difference in efficacy between a prophylactic and therapeutic approach to platelet transfusion.

To some extent, all outcome measures that are based on the frequency and description of bleeding events require a subjective assessment by the trialists, which makes systematic recording and standardization difficult (if not problematic).[157] Even in RCTs, there can be potential for bias if clinicians are making subjective judgments about the severity of bleeding that a patient has suffered and about the decision to transfuse. If blinding cannot be adequately incorporated in the study design, other measures have been proposed to help minimize the potential for bias.[160] Along these lines,[160] in lieu of blinding the assessors, the TOPP investigators[157] have opted to rely on several other measures: namely, educational meetings, widely distributed and common definitions for bleeding, as well as the undertaking of duplicate assessments.

Interim results from another RCT[161] of prophylactic and therapeutic platelet transfusions in patients with acute myelogenous leukemia have been equivocal. The duration of thrombocytopenia was significantly longer in the therapeutic arm yet the patients in that study arm received significantly fewer platelet transfusions than those in the control arm. As was anticipated, clinically significant bleeding complications (defined in this study as "more than petechiae") occurred more frequently ($p<0.05$) in the therapeutic arm. Yet, the majority of these hemorrhages were effectively treated by platelet transfusion and there was no difference in the number of RBC units received or the length of stay at the hospital. Nonetheless, two fatal cerebral hemorrhages occurred in the therapeutic arm, compared with none in the prophylactic arm. One of these two cerebral hemorrhages could have been prevented had the subject been assigned to the prophylactic arm, because his or her platelet count was <5000/μL and he or she would have received prophylactic platelets. This patient should have been moved to the prophylactic arm because he or she had developed invasive aspergillosis–an indication for moving the patient from the therapeutic to the prophylactic arm. As the results have hitherto been reported only in abstract form,[161] it is unclear why this patient had not been moved to the prophylactic arm of the trial. Moreover, an autopsy was not performed and it is unknown whether the reason for the fatal cerebral hemorrhage was fungal involvement of the brain.

Other Prophylactic Platelet and Plasma Transfusions

An extensive body of evidence from observational studies indicates that patients with moderately decreased platelet counts (>20,000/μL) or moderately elevated international normalized ratios (INRs) (<3) who underwent a variety of invasive procedures (central venous catheter insertion, liver biopsy, thoracocentesis or paracentesis, gastrointestinal endoscopy and biopsy, tracheotomy, bronchoscopy and transbronchial biopsy, renal biopsy, diagnostic lumbar puncture, epidural anesthesia, neurologic procedures, or angiography) without receiving a transfusion of platelets or plasma did not bleed more often than did patients who received prophylactic platelet or plasma transfusion before the procedure.[101] In the absence of coagulopathy, the available observational studies suggest that a platelet count of ≥20,000/μL is adequate for performing these procedures without a prophylactic platelet transfusion. Conversely, with a platelet count of ≥50,000/μL, the available observational studies suggest that an INR of <3 is adequate for performing these procedures without the need for a prophylactic plasma transfusion.[101]

There are no data from RCTs, however, to support the safety of such conservative transfusion thresholds, and thus liberal transfusion guidelines for prophylactic platelet and plasma transfusions are used at many US institutions, in accordance with available (published) transfusion guidelines.[162-170] The safety of these thresholds (platelets of ≤20,000/μL in the absence of coagulopathy, and INR of >3 when the platelet count is ≥50,000/μL) is unlikely to be demonstrated by RCTs in the foreseeable future, because an RCT using clinical bleeding as the primary endpoint would have to enroll a prohibitively large number of patients to establish any difference between the arms. Such an enrollment would be required because a very small proportion of subjects from either the conservative- or the liberal-strategy transfusion arm are expected to bleed.

The College of American Pathologists' 1994 guidelines[163] recommend transfusion of FFP when the coagulation times are greater than 1.5 times the midpoint of the normal range in the laboratory performing the tests. The Canadian Medical Association 1997 guidelines[164] state that "plasma may be administered to prepare for surgery or liver biopsy when the results of coagulation assays are deemed sufficiently abnormal. Prophylactic plasma transfusion is *not* indicated for certain invasive procedures (eg, percutaneous liver biopsy, paracentesis, thoracentesis) in patients with liver disease if their INR is 2.0 or less."

Following a review of data from observational studies in which procedures were performed on patients with platelet counts <100,000/μL, <50,000/μL, or even <20,000/μL without prophylactic platelet transfusions, the American Society of Clinical Oncology's 2001 panel[166] concluded that a platelet count of 40,000/μL to 50,000/μL suffices for performing lumbar puncture, liver biopsy, gastrointestinal endoscopy, fiberoptic bronchoscopy and bronchoalveolar lavage, transbronchial biopsy, central venous catheter insertion, and tooth extraction. The panel further observed that "there are sparse data about the safety of invasive procedures at much lower count levels." However, with the exception of marrow aspiration and biopsy (which the panel said can "clearly be performed safely at counts of <20,000/µL), the panel stopped short of making a recommendation, because it was "difficult to draw firm data-driven conclusions as to the lower level of platelet count that is safe for these various procedures." The panel accordingly concluded that "more systematic research in this area is clearly needed."

The British Committee for Standards in Hematology (BCSH) guidelines for the use of platelets and FFP in massive transfusion anticipate coagulation times of >1.5 times the mean normal values after replacement of 1 to 1.5 times the patient's blood volume; and a platelet count of <50,000/µL after replacement of twice the patient's blood volume.[167,168] According to the 2003 BCSH guidelines, transfusion of FFP and platelets is indicated when these thresholds are reached. The 2006 guidelines, however, recommended that a "margin of safety" be allowed to ensure that the platelet count remains at >50,000/µL. Toward this end, a platelet transfusion threshold of <75,000/µL is recommended for a patient with ongoing bleeding, with the threshold increased to <100,000/µL for a patient with multiple or central nervous system (CNS) trauma.[169]

Even in a prophylactic setting, a platelet transfusion threshold of ≤50,000/µL is recommended before lumbar puncture, epidural anesthesia, gastroscopy and biopsy, insertion of indwelling lines, transbronchial biopsy, liver biopsy, and laparatomy or similar procedures. For operations in critical sites–such as the brain or the eyes–the platelet transfusion threshold is set at ≤100,000/µL. Nonetheless, marrow aspiration and biopsy can be performed without platelet transfusion support even in patients with severe thrombocytopenia.[169]

AABB Guidelines for Plasma Transfusion

In 2010, the AABB published evidence-based guidelines for plasma transfusion,[171] based on a systematic review and meta-analysis of both RCTs and observational studies reporting on the risks and benefits of plasma transfusion in common clinical scenarios.[172] On the basis of evidence ranging from moderate to very low in quality, the AABB panel suggested that plasma be transfused to patients requiring massive transfusion, but could not recommend for or against transfusion of plasma at a plasma-to-RBCs ratio of ≥1:3 during massive transfusion.[171] Neither could the panel recommend for or against transfusion of plasma to patients undergoing surgery in the absence of massive transfusion.[171] Furthermore, the panel suggested that plasma be transfused to patients with warfarin-therapy-related intracranial hemorrhage, but could not recommend for or against transfusion of plasma to reverse warfarin anticoagulation in patients without intracranial hemorrhage.[171] Finally, the panel recommended against plasma transfusion for other selected groups of patients.[171]

The panel underscored that available literature addressing plasma transfusion is sparse, typically of low quality, and often does not address common clinical situations (eg, plasma transfusion for nonsurgical invasive procedures). Given the low quality of the published data, only relatively weak recommendations (such as a *suggestion* that plasma be transfused to trauma patients requiring massive transfusion) could be issued by the panel regarding many of the common clinical scenarios considered. In the Grading of Recommendations, Assessment, Development, and Evaluation (GRADE) system,[173,174] weak recommendations of this sort indicate that while many well-informed people would make the same choice, a substantial minority would not. To appreciate the extent of uncertainty that still exists about appropriate indications for plasma transfusion, the controversy on whether a higher plasma-to-RBCs ratio improves survival during massive transfusion for trauma is briefly reviewed here and in Chapter 8.

In the span of 3 years (2007-2009), 13 observational studies[175-187] reported on the purported benefit of using a higher plasma-to-RBCs ratio during massive transfusion for trauma. Endorsing this approach to the management of severely injured trauma victims would be akin to reverting to the historical practice of transfusing whole blood. Among the 10 nonoverlapping observational studies[175-184] that permitted extraction of ORs at the time of the meta-analysis,[172] the reported ORs had varied 30-fold (from 0.05 to 1.5—Fig 4-9). The likelihood of this situation's arising by chance was smaller than 1% ($p<0.01$ for the Q test statistic). This statistical heterogeneity reflected extreme clinical heterogeneity of the studies,[175-184] which could arguably preclude the undertaking of a synthesis of the findings of the 10 reports (Chapter 5). Nonetheless, while pointing out the very-low quality of the studies, the meta-analysis[172] integrated the results of the 10 reports, observing that a higher plasma-to-RBCs ratio reduced mortality by 62% (95% CI, 40% to 76%) and that the benefit was statistically highly significant.

Yet, there are three alternative explanations for why all but two[183,184] of the observational studies shown in Fig 4-9 demonstrated a significant ($p<0.05$) reduction in mortality in association with the transfusion of a higher plasma-to-

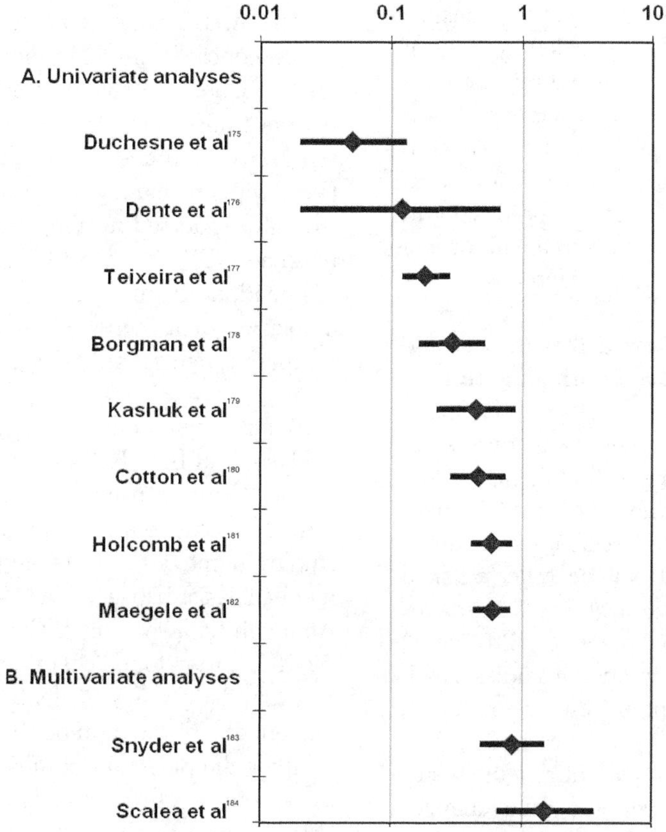

Figure 4-9. Observational studies[175-184] of the reduction in mortality following massive transfusion to trauma patients if a higher (closer to 1:1) than lower (closer to 1:4) plasma-to-RBCs ratio is used for the administered blood components. For each of the eight studies[175-182] of the upper panel, the *unadjusted* odds ratio (OR) of mortality is given, surrounded by its 95% CI. For the two studies[183,184] of the lower panel, an *adjusted* OR calculated from a multivariate analysis is shown, also surrounded by its 95% CI. When the 95% CI does not include the null value of 1, the effect of an increased plasma-to-RBCs ratio is statistically significant ($p<0.05$).

RBCs ratio. All three alternative explanations represent different forms of selection bias. First, the clinicians might have opted to expend the most resources (including plasma transfusions) on the patients deemed most likely to survive. (This is especially relevant in a military setting in which such patients might have been triaged to the lowest priority category for surgery, thereby not receiving transfusions before dying.) Second, patients with the worst prognosis might have died too rapidly to receive multiple plasma transfusions. Third, studies with positive results may have been selectively submitted for publication by the investigators or published. Thus, at this time, it is impossible to know if the conspicuous reduction in mortality recorded by eight of the 10 observational studies is entirely attributable to selection bias or whether some part of it is real. At the 2009 NHLBI conference convened to prioritize research questions for transfusion-medicine RCTs,[108] the proposal to randomly assign trauma victims to a high or low plasma-to-RBCs ratio received a favorable reception.

Snyder et al[183] emphasized that the plasma-to-RBCs ratio is not constant during the resuscitation period. Instead, when historical databases are retrospectively analyzed—as was the case in the studies depicted in Fig 4-9—this ratio starts out low and increases with time, as the patient survives long enough to receive the multiple plasma transfusions that will be reflected in a high plasma-to-RBCs ratio if he or she survives up to an arbitrary cutoff point (eg, 24 hours) used in the available observational studies. Analyses finding a significant benefit from a high plasma-to-RBCs ratio[175-182] were carried out as though this ratio were constant during the resuscitation period.[183] However, the ratio changes constantly, and it becomes fixed only at the time of a patient's death.[183] Therefore, to investigate the effect of a high plasma-to-RBCs ratio outside the setting of an RCT administering a predetermined plasma-to-RBCs ratio to each randomization arm, a statistical analysis that takes into account the time of administration of each blood product must be employed. Such detailed information on the timing of the transfusions is usually unavailable to the authors of observational studies.

Across these same observational studies, the meta-analysis[172] also found that increasing the plasma-to-RBCs ratio was associated with a reduction in the risk of multiorgan failure by 60% (95% CI, 40% to 74%; $p<0.05$). In patients undergoing surgery without massive transfusion, however, plasma transfusion was associated with a trend toward increased mortality (OR = 1.22; 95% CI, 0.73-2.03; $p>0.05$).[172] In particular, plasma transfusion was associated with a significantly ($p<0.05$) increased risk of ALI (OR = 2.92; 95% CI, 1.99-4.29).[172]

The AABB panel[171] noted the contradiction in the conclusions of the meta-analysis[172] vis-à-vis the benefit (versus the harm) associated with plasma transfusion in patients undergoing massive transfusion and in patients undergoing surgery without massive transfusion. The panel strongly endorsed further testing of a higher plasma-to-RBCs ratio in RCTs, but could not recommend, at this time, for or against transfusion of plasma at a higher plasma-to-RBCs ratio to trauma patients undergoing massive transfusion.

Before the undertaking of the meta-analysis[172] of both RCTs and observational studies of plasma transfusion commissioned by the AABB,[171] only one systematic review of such studies (limited to RCTs and not including a meta-analysis) had appeared in the literature.[188] Although Stanworth et al[188] were able to locate 57 RCTs, they found that many published trials had enrolled too few patients and had provided inadequate information on the ability of the trial to allow the detection of meaningful differences in outcomes between the two comparison arms. Other concerns about the design of the trials included the dose of plasma used (which might have been inadequate) and the comparison of different types of plasma (eg, pathogen-reduced or non-pathogen-reduced), in lieu of the desired comparison between a plasma-transfusion and a non-plasma-transfusion strategy. The authors concluded that there is little evidence supporting the efficacy of prophylactic use of plasma.[188]

Conclusions

Like most therapies, ABT is associated with significant risks. Minimizing the risks and optimizing the benefits of ABT depend on close collaboration throughout the transfusion chain from blood centers to hospitals. The two main elements for safe and effective transfusion are a sufficient supply of safe blood and good clinical transfusion practice.[189]

Good clinical transfusion practice encompasses avoidance of errors leading to "wrong" blood transfusions; and appropriate decision-making based on assessment of the patients' clinical status and laboratory parameters about the optimal use of all blood components. The objective of ABT is to prevent or treat a clinical problem caused by a deficiency of blood cells or a plasma constituent. Alternative ways of treating the deficiency without transfusion should always be considered and should be preferred if they are deemed to be safer than ABT. The combination of using alternatives to ABT and resorting to ABT only when these alternatives are ineffective or less safe than ABT is known as patient blood management. Clinically important deficiencies in blood cells or coagulation factors should be documented so that transfusion therapy can be guided by objective measurements as well by observation of its clinical effects.[189]

A major paradigm shift in clinical transfusion practice that is currently being promoted or adopted on the hospital side consists of the administration of ABT only when empirical evidence supports actual (as opposed to postulated) benefit from the transfusion in terms of either improvement of oxygen delivery to tissues or prevention of hemorrhage; and/or administration of ABT only when alternatives to ABT are ineffective or less safe compared with ABT. A sufficient supply of safe blood is also being provided by blood centers, as major causes of ABT-related mortality (such as TAS and TRALI) have finally been addressed, and continue to be addressed, in the beginning of the 21st century. More needs to be done to reduce the residual risks of TAS and TRALI, and also to protect the blood supply from the next transfusion-transmitted pathogen that will likely emerge in the future. Plasma and platelets should be collected solely from male donors or female donors without a history of pregnancy or shown not to have WBC antibodies; and use of non-pathogen-reduced pooled components (such as pooled WBD platelets) should, in the author's opinion, be discontinued when apheresis (single-donor) alternatives are available. Furthermore, two major paradigm shifts remain to be realized in the future: the move from whole-blood collections to multicomponent apheresis collections (with administration of the various blood components harvested from the same collection to the same multitransfused patient) as well as the implementation of PR technologies once the efficacy and safety of these systems have been sufficiently tested to allow licensure of the systems by the FDA.

Although extended antigen matching for RBC transfusions has also been discussed as a paradigm shift[190] the prevention of HTRs has inexplicably received less emphasis in the early 21st century than the aforementioned causes of ABT-related mortality. HTRs need to be addressed at the same time that we are striving to reduce the residual risks of TAS and TRALI and to protect the blood supply from the next major transfusion-transmitted pathogen to emerge in the future. A further potential paradigm shift (the move toward transfusion of "fresh" RBCs, depending on the results of the currently ongoing RCTs) is examined in Chapter 7, and Chapter 8 considers all the candidate paradigm shifts and their relation to a "patient-centric" versus "component-centric" practice of transfusion medicine.

References

1. Food and Drug Administration. Fatalities reported to the FDA following blood collection and transfusion. Annual summary for fiscal year 2010. Rockville, MD: CBER Office of Community Outreach and Development, 2010. [Available at: http://www.fda.gov/downloads/BiologicsBloodVaccines/SafetyAvailability/ReportaProblem/TransfusionDonationFatalities/UCM254860.htm (accessed May 25, 2011).]

2. Hilton DA, Ghani AC, Conyers L, et al. Prevalence of lymphoreticular prion protein accumulation in UK tissue samples. J Pathol 2004; 203:733-9.
3. Vamvakas EC, Blajchman MA. Transfusion-related mortality: The on-going risks of allogeneic blood transfusion and the available strategies for their prevention. Blood 2009;113: 3406-17.
4. Vamvakas E, Blajchman MA. Blood still kills: Six strategies to further reduce allogeneic blood transfusion-related mortality. Transfus Med Rev 2010;24:77-124.
5. Stramer SL, Hollinger FB, Katz LM, et al. Emerging infectious disease agents and their potential threat to transfusion safety. Transfusion 2009;49(Suppl 2):1S-236S.
6. Allain JP, Bianco C, Blajchman MA, et al. Protecting the blood supply from emerging pathogens: The role of pathogen inactivation. Transfus Med Rev 2005;19:110-26.
7. McCullough J. Pathogen inactivation: A new paradigm for blood safety. Transfusion 2007; 47:2180-4.
8. Klein HG, Anderson D, Bernardi MJ, et al. Pathogen inactivation: Making decisions about new technologies. Report of a consensus conference. Transfusion 2007;47:2338-47.
9. Alter HJ. Pathogen reduction: A precautionary-principle paradigm. Transfus Med Rev 2008; 22:97-102.
10. Vamvakas EC. Relative safety of pooled whole-blood-derived versus single-donor (apheresis) platelets in the United States: A systematic review of disparate risks. Transfusion 2009; 49:2743-58.
11. Custer B, Hochs JS. Cost-effectiveness analysis: What it really means for transfusion-medicine decision making. Transfus Med Rev 2009;23:1-12.
12. Osselaer JC, Messe N, Hervig T, et al. A prospective observational cohort safety study of 5106 platelet transfusions with components prepared with photochemical pathogen inactivation treatment. Transfusion 2008;48:1061-71.
13. Osselaer JC, Cazenave JP, Lambermont M, et al. An active haemovigilance programme characterizing the safety profile of 7437 platelet transfusions prepared with amotosalen photochemical treatment. Vox Sang 2008;94:315-23.
14. Osselaer JC, Doyen C, Defoin L, et al. Universal adoption of pathogen inactivation of platelet components: Impact on platelet and red-blood-cell component use. Transfusion 2009;49: 1412-22.
15. Cazenave JP, Isola H, Waller C, et al. Use of additive solutions and pathogen inactivation treatment of platelet components in a regional blood center: Impact on patient outcomes and component utilization during a 3-year period. Transfusion 2011;51:622-9.
16. Politis C, Kavalierou L, Hantziara S, et al. Quality and safety of fresh frozen plasma inactivated and leukoreduced with the Theraflex methylene blue system including the Blueflex filter: 5 years' experience. Vox Sang 2007;92:319-26.
17. Larrea L, Calaburg M, Solves MA, et al. Our nine years' experience in plasma inactivation. Vox Sang 2007;93(Suppl 1):167.
18. Reddy HL, Dayan AD, Cavagnaro J, et al. Toxicity-testing of a novel riboflavin-based technology for pathogen reduction and white-blood-cell inactivation. Transfus Med Rev 2008;22:133-53.
19. Prowse C. Properties of pathogen-inactivated plasma components. Transfus Med Rev 2009; 23:124-33.
20. Corash L, Lin JS, Sherman CD, Eiden J. Determination of acute lung injury following repeated platelet transfusions. Blood 2011;117:1014-20.
21. Solheim BG. Pathogen reduction of blood components. Transfus Apher Sci 2008;39:75-82.
22. Solheim BG, Seghatchian J. Update on pathogen reduction technology for therapeutic plasma: An overview. Transfus Apher Sci 2006;35:83-90.
23. Flesland O. A comparison of complication rates based on published hemovigilance data. Int Care Med 2007;33(Suppl 1):S17-S21.
24. Renaudier P, Schlanger S, Mai MPV, et al. Epidemiology of transfusion-related acute lung injury in France: Preliminary results. Transfus Med Hemother 2009;35:89-91.
25. MacLennan S, Barbara JA. Risks and side-effects of therapy with plasma and plasma fractions. Best Pract Res Clin Haematol 2006;19:169-89.
26. Coignard BP, Colquhoun SD, Nguyen GT, et al. Intraoperative deaths in liver transplant recipients associated with the use of solvent/detergent plasma. Hepatology 2002;36:A209.
27. Salge-Bartels U, Breitner-Ruddock S, Hunfeld A, et al. Are quality differences responsible for different adverse reactions reported for SD-plasma from USA and Europe? Transfus Med 2006; 16:266-75.
28. Wollowitz S. Fundamentals of the psoralen-based Helinx technology for inactivation of

infectious pathogens and leukocytes in platelets and plasma. Semin Hematol 2001;38(Suppl 11):4S-11S.
29. Bruchmuller I, Janetzko K, Bugert P, et al. Polymerase chain reaction inhibition assay documenting the amotosalen-based photochemical pathogen inactivation process of platelet concentrates. Transfusion 2005;45:1464-72.
30. Kumar V, Lockerbie O, Keil SD, et al. Riboflavin and UV-light based pathogen reduction: Extent and consequence of DNA damage at the molecular level. Photochem Photobiol 2004; 80:15-21.
31. Kerkhoffs JLH, van Putten WLJ, Novotny VMJ, et al. Clinical effectiveness of leukoreduced, pooled donor platelet concentrates, stored in plasma or additive solution with and without pathogen reduction. Br J Haematol 2010;150: 209-17.
32. van Rhenen D, Gulliksson H, Cazenave JP, et al. Transfusion of pooled buffy-coat platelet components prepared with a photochemical pathogen inactivation treatment: The euroSPRITE trial. Blood 2003;101:2426-33.
33. Janetzko K, Cazenave JP, Kluter H, et al. Therapeutic efficacy and safety of photochemically-treated apheresis platelets processed with an optimized integrated set. Transfusion 2005;45: 1443-52.
34. McCullough J, Vesole DH, Benjamin RJ, et al. Therapeutic efficacy and safety of platelets treated with a photochemical process for pathogen inactivation: The SPRINT trial. Blood 2004;104:1534-41.
35. Snyder E, McCullough J, Slichter SJ, et al. Clinical safety of platelets photochemically-treated with amotosalen HCl and ultraviolet A light for pathogen inactivation: The SPRINT trial. Transfusion 2005;45:1864-75.
36. Corash L, Sherman CD. Evaluation of platelet transfusion clinical trial (letter). Br J Haematol 2011;153:529-31.
37. Kerkhoffs JLH. Evaluation of platelet transfusion clinical trials—Response to Corash and Sherman (letter). Br J Haematol 2011;153:531-2.
38. Corash L. The hemostatic efficacy of platelet components prepared with pathogen inactivation (letter). Transfusion 2011;51:1355-6.
39. Vamvakas EC. The hemostatic efficacy of platelet components prepared with pathogen inactivation—In reply (letter). Transfusion 2011;51: 1356-9.
40. Heddle NM. Optimal timing and dosing of platelet transfusions. ISBT Science Series 2010;5: 88-94.
41. Vamvakas EC. Meta-analysis of the randomized controlled trials of the hemostatic efficacy and capacity of pathogen-reduced platelets. Transfusion 2011;51:1058-71.
42. The Mirasol Clinical Evaluation Study Group. A randomized controlled clinical trial evaluating the performance and safety of platelets treated with MIRASOL pathogen reduction technology. Transfusion 2010;50:2363-75.
43. Lozano M, Knutson F, Tardivel R, et al. A multicenter study of the therapeutic efficacy and safety of platelet components treated with amotosalen and ultraviolet-A pathogen inactivation stored for 6 or 7 days prior to transfusion. Br J Haematol 2011;153:393-401.
44. Vamvakas EC. Meta-analysis of studies of the bleeding complications of platelets pathogen-reduced with the Intercept system. Vox Sang 2012 (in press).
45. Slichter SJ, Kaufman RM, Assmann SF, et al. Dose of prophylactic platelet transfusions and prevention of hemorrhage. N Engl J Med 2010; 362:600-13.
46. Osman A, Falker K. Characterization of human platelet microRNA by quantitative PCR coupled with an annotation network for predicted target genes. Platelets 2011;22:433-41.
47. Nagalla S, Shaw C, Kong X, et al. Platelet microRNA-mRNA co-expression profiles correlate with platelet reactivity. Blood 2011;117: 5189-97.
48. Hitzler W, Vamvakas EC. Platelet microRNA profiles and the effect of pathogen reduction on platelet function. Clin Lab 2011;57:451-4.
49. Jacobs MR, Smith D, Heaton WA, Good CE. Detection of bacterial contamination in prestorage culture-negative apheresis platelets on day of issue with the Pan Genera Detection Test. Transfusion 2011;51:2573-82.
50. van de Watering LMG, Hermans J, Houbiers JGA, et al. Beneficial effect of leukocyte depletion of transfused blood on post-operative complications in patients undergoing cardiac surgery: A randomized clinical trial. Circulation 1998;97:562-8.
51. Bilgin YM, van de Watering LMG, Eijsman L, et al. Double-blind, randomized controlled trial on the effect of leukocyte-depleted erythrocyte transfusions in cardiac-valve surgery. Circulation 2004;109:2755-60.

52. Boshkov LK, Furnary A, Morris C, et al. Prestorage leukoreduction of red cells in elective cardiac surgery: Results of a double-blind randomized controlled trial (abstract). Blood 2004; 104:112a.
53. Bilgin YM, Brand A. Transfusion-related immunomodulation: A second hit in an inflammatory cascade? Vox Sang 2008;95:261-71.
54. Vamvakas E, Blajchman MA. Transfusion-related immunomodulation (TRIM): An update. Blood Rev 2007;21:327-48.
55. Department of Health and Human Services. The 2009 National Blood Collection and Utilization Survey Report. Washington, DC: DHHS, 2011.
56. Peterman TA, Lui K-J, Lawrence DN, Allen JR. Estimating the risks of transfusion-associated acquired immune deficiency syndrome and human immunodeficiency virus infection. Transfusion 1987;27:371-4.
57. Heuft HG, Mende W, Blasczyk R. A general change of the platelet transfusion policy from apheresis platelet concentrates to pooled platelet concentrates is associated with a sharp increase in donor exposures and infection rates. Transfus Med Hemother 2008;35:106-13.
58. Vamvakas EC. Why are all men who have had sex with men even once since 1977 indefinitely deferred from donating blood? Transfusion 2009;49:1037-42.
59. Further guidance on methods to detect bacterial contamination of platelet components. AABB Association Bulletin #03-12. Bethesda, MD: AABB, 2003. [Available at http://www.aabb.org/resources/publications/bulletins/Documents/obsolete/AB%2003-12% 20OBSOLETE.pdf (accessed May 25, 2011).]
60. Silva MA, Gregory KR, Carr-Greer MA, et al. Summary of the AABB Interorganizational Task Force on Bacterial Contamination of Platelets: Fall 2004 impact survey. Transfusion 2006;46:636-41.
61. Developments in bacterial testing and BBTS Standard 5.1.5.1. Association Bulletin #09-04. Bethesda, MD: AABB, 2009. [Available at http://www.aabb.org/resources/publications/bulletins/Documents/obsolete/AB%2009-04%20OBSOLETE.pdf (accessed October 14, 2011).]
62. Interim Standard 5.1.5.1.1. Association Bulletin #10-02. Bethesda, MD: AABB, 2010. [Available at http://www.aabb.org/resources/publications/bulletins/Pages/ab10-02.aspx (accessed October 14, 2011).]
63. Transfusion-related acute lung injury. AABB Association Bulletin #06-07. Bethesda, MD: AABB, 2006. [Available at http://www.aabb.org/resources/publications/bulletins/Pages/ab06-07.aspx (accessed October 14, 2011).]
64. Popovsky MA, Moore SB. Diagnostic and pathogenetic considerations in transfusion-related acute lung injury. Transfusion 1985;25:573-7.
65. Popovsky MA, Chaplin HC Jr., Moore SB. Transfusion-related acute lung injury: A neglected, serious complication of hemotherapy. Transfusion 1992;32:589-92.
66. Eastlund T, McGrath PC, Burkart P. Platelet transfusion reaction associated with inter-donor HLA incompatibility. Vox Sang 1988;55:157-60.
67. Bux J, Hoch J, Bindl L, et al. Transfusion-associated acute pulmonary insufficiency. Diagnostic confirmation by the demonstration of granulocytic antibodies. J Dtsch Med Wochenschr 1994;119:19-24.
68. Ramanthan RK, Triulzi DJ, Logan TF. Transfusion-related acute lung injury following random-donor platelet transfusion: A report of two cases. Vox Sang 1997;73:43-5.
69. Lin Y, Kanani N, Naughton F, et al. Case report: Transfusion-related acute lung injury (TRALI)—A clear and present danger. Can J Anesth 2007; J4:1011-16.
70. Salman SS, Fernandez Perez ER, Stubbs JR, Gajic O. The practice of platelet transfusion in the intensive care unit. J Intern Care Med 2007; 22:105-10.
71. Win N, Chapman CE, Bowles KM, et al. How much residual plasma may cause TRALI? Transfus Med 2008;18:276-80.
72. Robillard P, Hyson C, McCombie N. TRALI, possible TRALI and respiratory complications of transfusion reported to the Canadian Transfusion-Transmitted Injuries Surveillance System (abstract). Transfusion 2007;47(Suppl):5A.
73. Gajic O, Rana R, Winters JL, et al. Transfusion-related acute lung injury in the critically ill: Prospective nested case-control study. Am J Respir Crit Care Med 2007;176:886-91.
74. Eder AF, Herron R, Strupp A, et al. Transfusion-related acute lung injury surveillance (2003-2005) and the potential impact of the selective use of plasma from male donors in the American Red Cross. Transfusion 2007;47:599-607.
75. Kleinman S, Caulfield T, Chan P, et al. Toward an understanding of transfusion-related acute lung injury: Statement of a consensus panel. Transfusion 2004;44:1774-89.

76. Kopko PM, Marshall CS, Mackenzie MR, et al. Transfusion-related acute lung injury: Report of a look-back investigation. JAMA 2002;287:1968-71.
77. Kleinman S, Grossman B, Kopko P. A national survey of transfusion-related acute lung injury reduction policies for platelets and plasma in the United States. Transfusion 2010;50:1312-21.
78. Dodd RY, Notari EP 4th, Stramer SL. Current prevalence and incidence of infectious disease markers and estimated window-period risk in the American Red Cross blood donor population. Transfusion 2002;42:975-9.
79. Kleinman SH, Busch MP. Assessing the impact of HBV NAT on window-period reduction and residual risk. J Clin Virol 2006;36(Suppl):S523-9.
80. Kleinman SH, Busch M. Hepatitis B virus: Amplified and back in the blood safety spotlight. Transfusion 2001;41:1081-5.
81. Dodd RY. Emerging infections, transfusion safety, and epidemiology. N Engl J Med 2003;349:1205-6.
82. Pomper G, Simpson M. The prevention of alloimmunization: A balance of precaution, expectation, and outcome. Transfusion 2009;49:406-8.
83. Schoneville H, van de Watering LMG, Brand A. Additional red-blood-cell alloantibodies after blood transfusion in a non-hematologic alloimmunized cohort: Is it time to take precautionary measures? Transfusion 2006;46:630-5.
84. Schoneville H, de Vries RPR, Brand A. Alloimmune response after additional red-blood-cell antigen challenge in immunized hemato-oncology patients. Transfusion 2009;49:453-7.
85. Fluit CR, Kunst DA, Drenthe-Schonk AM. Incidence of red-cell antibodies after multiple transfusion. Transfusion 1990;30:532-5.
86. Schoneville H, Haak HL, van Zijl AM. Alloimmunization after blood transfusion in patients with hematologic and oncologic diseases. Transfusion 1999;39:763-71.
87. Shaz BH, Zimring JC, Demmons DG, Hillyer CD. Blood donation and blood transfusion: Special considerations for African Americans. Transfus Med Rev 2008;22:202-14.
88. Klapper E, Zhang Y, Figueroa P, et al. Toward extended phenotype compatibility: A new operational paradigm for the transfusion service. Transfusion 2010;50:536-46.
89. Hillman NM. Fatal delayed hemolytic transfusion reaction due to anti-c + E. Transfusion 1979;19:548-51.
90. Kleinman S, Dumont LJ, Tomasulo P, et al. The impact of discontinuation of 7-day storage of apheresis platelets (PASSPORT) on recipient safety: An illustration of the need for proper risk assessments. Transfusion 2009;49:903-12.
91. Silliman CC, Boshkov LK, Mehdizadehkashi Z, et al. Transfusion-related acute lung injury: Epidemiology and a prospective analysis of etiologic factors. Blood 2003;101:454-62.
92. Popovsky MA. Multicomponent apheresis blood collections in the United States: Current status and future directions. Transfus Apher Sci 2010;3:299-304.
93. Zingsem J. Multicomponent apheresis. ISBT Science Series 2010;5:83-7.
94. Popovsky MA. Transfusion-related acute lung injury: Incidence, pathogenesis, and the role of multicomponent apheresis in its prevention. Transfus Med Hemother 2008;35:76-9.
95. Vamvakas EC. The ethics of wasting the donor's gift of buffy coat. Vox Sang 2010;100:256-7.
96. van Stein D, Beckers EA, Sintnicolaas K, et al. Transfusion-related acute lung injury in the Netherlands: An observational study. Transfusion 2010;50:213-20.
97. Devine D, Jenkins G, Howe D, Goldman M. Relative safety of buffy-coat platelet pools. Transfusion 2010;50:1591-2.
98. Schrezenmeier H, Seifried E. Buffy-coat-derived pooled platelet concentrates and apheresis platelet concentrates: Which product type should be preferred? Vox Sang 2010;99:1-15.
99. Middelburg RA, van Stein D, Zupanska B, et al. Female donors and transfusion-related acute lung injury. Transfusion 2010;50:2447-54.
100. Kamel H, Tomasulo P, Bravo M, et al. Delayed adverse reactions to blood donation. Transfusion 2010;50:556-65.
101. Dzik WH. Blood components to achieve hemostasis for surgery and invasive procedures. In: Simon TL, Snyder EL, Solheim BG, et al, eds. Rossi's principles of transfusion medicine. 4th ed. Bethesda, MD: AABB, 2009:575-88.
102. Spiess B. Red cell transfusions and guidelines: A work in progress. Hematol Clin North Am 2007;21:185-200.
103. Surgenor SD, Hampers MJ, Corwin HL. Is blood transfusion good for the heart? Crit Care Med 2001;29:442-4.
104. Hébert PC, Wells G, Blajchman MA, et al. A multicenter randomized controlled trial of trans-

fusion requirements in critical care. N Engl Med 1999;340:409-17.
105. Fernandez CJ Jr, Akamine N, DeMarco FVC, et al. Red blood cell transfusion does not increase oxygen consumption in critically ill septic patients. Crit Care 2001;5:362-7.
106. den Uil CA, Klijn E, Lagrand WK, et al. The microcirculation in health and critical disease. Prog Cardiovasc Dis 2008;51:161-70.
107. Steiner ME, Stowell C. Does red-blood-cell storage affect clinical outcome? When in doubt, do the experiment. Transfusion 2009;49:1286-90.
108. Josephson CD, Glynn SA, Kleinman SH, Blajchman MA. A multidisciplinary "think tank": The top 10 clinical trial opportunities in transfusion medicine from the National Heart, Lung, and Blood Institute-sponsored 2009 State-of-the-Art Symposium. Transfusion 2011;51:328-41.
109. Isbister JP. Decision making in perioperative transfusion. Transfus Apher Sci 2002;27:19-28.
110. Isbister JP. Clinicians as gatekeepers: What is the best route to optimal blood use? Dev Biol 2007;127:9-14.
111. Goodnough LT, Shander A. Blood management. Arch Pathol Lab Med 2007;131:695-701.
112. Pape A, Habler O. Alternatives to allogeneic blood transfusions. Best Pract Res Clin Anaesthesiol 2007;21:221-39.
113. Isbister JP, Shander A, Spahn DR, et al. Adverse transfusion outcomes: Establishing causation. Transfus Med Rev 2011;25:89-101.
114. Vamvakas EC. Establishing causation in transfusion medicine and related tribulations. Transfus Med Rev 2011;25:81-8.
115. Fergusson DA, Hebert PC, Mazer CD, et al. A comparison of aprotinin and lysine analogues in high-risk cardiac surgery. N Engl J Med 2008; 358:2319-31.
116. Beale R. The rational use of blood. A N Z J Surg 1976;46:309-13.
117. Jackson GN, Snowden CA, Indrikovs AJ. A prospective audit program to determine blood component transfusion appropriateness at a large university hospital: A 5-year experience. Transfus Med Rev 2008;22:154-61.
118. Gombotz H, Rehak P, Shander A, Hofmann A. Blood use in elective surgery: The Austrian benchmark study. Transfusion 2007;47:1468-80.
119. Consensus conference. Perioperative red blood cell transfusion. JAMA 1988;260:2700-3.
120. Practice strategies for elective blood cell transfusion. Ann Intern Med 1992;116:403-6.
121. Deans KJ, Minneci PC, Suffredini AF, et al. Randomization in clinical trials of titrated therapies: Unintended consequences of using fixed treatment protocols. Crit Care Med 2007;35:1509-16.
122. Deans KJ, Minneci PC, Danner RL, et al. Practice misalignments in randomized controlled trials: Identification, impact, and potential solutions. Anesth Analg 2010;111:444-50.
123. Carson JL, Terrin ML, Noveck H, et al. Liberal or restrictive transfusion in high-risk patients after hip surgery. N Engl J Med 2012 (in press).
124. Hajjar LA, Vincent JL, Galas FR, et al. Transfusion requirements after cardiac surgery: The TRACS randomized controlled trial. JAMA 2010;304:1559-67.
125. Carless PA, Henry DA, Carson JL, et al. Transfusion thresholds and other strategies for guiding allogeneic red blood cell transfusions. Cochrane Database Sys Rev 2010;(10):CD002042.
126. Hébert PC, Yetisir E, Martin C, et al. Is a low transfusion threshold safe in critically-ill patients with cardiovascular diseases? Crit Care Med 2001;29:227-34.
127. Blair SD, Janvrin SB, McCollum CN, Greenhalgh RM. Effect of early blood transfusion on gastrointestinal hemorrhage. Br J Surg 1986; 73:783-5.
128. Bracey AW, Radovancevic R, Riggs SA, et al. Lowering the hemoglobin threshold for transfusion in coronary artery bypass procedures: Effect on patient outcome. Transfusion 1999; 39:1070-7.
129. Bush RL, Pevec WC, Holcroft JW. A prospective, randomized trial limiting perioperative red blood cell transfusions in vascular patients. Am J Surg 1997;174:143-8.
130. Carson JL, Terrin ML, Barton FB, et al. A pilot randomized trial comparing symptomatic vs. hemoglobin-level-driven red blood cell transfusions following hip fracture. Transfusion 1998; 38:522-9.
131. Colomo A, Hernandez-Gea V, Muniz-Diaz E, et al. Transfusion strategies in patients with cirrhosis and acute gastrointestinal bleeding. Hepatology 2008;48(Suppl):413A.
132. Fortune JB, Feustel PJ, Saifi J, et al. Influence of hematocrit on cardiopulmonary function after acute hemorrhage. J Trauma 1987;27: 243-9.

133. Foss NB, Kristensen MT, Jensen PS, et al. The effects of liberal versus restrictive transfusion thresholds on ambulation after hip fracture surgery. Transfusion 2009;49:227-34.
134. Grover M, Talwalker S, Csbard A, et al. Silent myocardial ischemia and haemoglobin concentration: A randomized controlled trial of transfusion strategy in lower limb arthroplasty. Vox Sang 2006;90:105-12.
135. Hébert PC, Wells G, Marshall J, et al. Transfusion requirements in critical care. A pilot study. JAMA 1995;273:1439-44.
136. Johnson RG, Thurer RL, Kruskall MS, et al. Comparison of two transfusion strategies after elective operations for myocardial revascularization. J Thorac Cardiovasc Surg 1992;104:307-14.
137. Lacroix J, Hébert PC, Hutchison JS, et al. Transfusion strategies for patients in pediatric intensive care units. N Engl Med 2007;356:1609-19.
138. Lotke PA, Barth P, Garino JP, Cook EF. Predonated autologous blood transfusions after total knee arthroplasty: Immediate versus delayed administration. J Arthroplasty 1999;14:647-50.
139. So-Osman C, Nelissen R, Te Slaa R, et al. A randomized comparison of transfusion triggers in elective orthopedic surgery using leukocyte-depleted red blood cells. Vox Sang 2010;98:56-64.
140. Topley ET, Fisher MR. The illness of trauma. Br J Clin Pract 1956;10:770-6.
141. Webert KE, Cook RJ, Couban S, et al. A multicenter pilot-randomized controlled trial of the feasibility of an augmented red blood cell transfusion strategy for patients treated with induction chemotherapy for acute leukemia or stem cell transplantation. Transfusion 2008;48:81-91.
142. Zygun DA, Nortje J, Hutchinson PJ, et al. The effect of red blood cell transfusion on cerebral oxygenation and metabolism after severe traumatic brain injury. Crit Care Med 2009;37:1074-8.
143. Baxter BT, Minion DJ, McCance CL, et al. Rational approach to postoperative transfusion in high-risk patients. Am J Surg 1993;166:720-5.
144. West MA, Shapiro MB, Nathens AB, et al. Guidelines for transfusion in the trauma patient. J Trauma 2006;61:463-9.
145. Napolitano LM, Kurek S, Luchette FA, et al. Clinical practice guidelines: Red blood cell transfusion in adult trauma and critical care. Crit Care Med 2009;37:3124-49.
146. Ferraris VA, Ferraris SP, Saha SP, et al. Perioperative blood transfusion and blood conservation in cardiac surgery: The Society of Thoracic Surgeons and the Society of Cardiovascular Anesthesiologists Clinical Practice Guidelines. Ann Thorac Surg 2007;83:S27-86.
147. Stowell CP, Jones SC, Enny C, et al. An open-label randomized parallel-group study of perioperative epoetin alfa versus standard of care for blood conservation in major elective spinal surgery: Safety analysis. Spine 2009;34:2479-85.
148. Hershman DL, Buono DL, Malin J, et al. Patterns of use and risks associated with erythropoiesis-stimulating agents among Medicare patients with cancer. J Natl Cancer Inst 2009;101:1633-41.
149. Lipp G, Franchini M, Favaloro EJ. Thrombotic complications of erythropoiesis-stimulating agents. Semin Thromb Hemost 2010;36:537-49.
150. van der Meer P, Groenveld HF, Januzzi JL Jr., et al. Erythropoietin treatment in patients with chronic heart failure: A meta-analysis. Heart 2009;95:1309-14.
151. Carless PA, Henry DA, Moxey AJ, et al. Cell-salvage for minimizing perioperative allogeneic blood transfusion. Cochrane Database Syst Rev 2010;(4):CD001888.
152. Boulton FE, James V. Guidelines for policies on alternatives to allogeneic blood transfusion. 1. Predeposit autologous blood donation and transfusion. Transfus Med 2007;17:354-65.
153. Kirpalani H, Whyte RK, Andersen C, et al. The Premature Infants in Need of Transfusion (PINT) study: A randomized, controlled trial of a restrictive (low) versus liberal (high) transfusion threshold for extremely low-birth-weight infants. J Pediatr 2006;149:301-7.
154. Whyte RK, Kirpalani H, Asztalos EV, et al. Neurodevelopmental outcome of extremely low-birth-weight infants randomly assigned to restrictive or liberal hemoglobin thresholds for blood transfusion. Pediatrics 2009;123:207-13.
155. Bell EF, Strauss RG, Widness JA, et al. Randomized trial of liberal versus restrictive guidelines for red blood cell transfusion in preterm infants. Pediatrics 2005;115:1685-91.
156. Heddle NM, Cook RJ, Timmouth A, et al. A randomized controlled trial comparing standard and low-dose strategies for transfusion of platelets (SToP) to patients with thrombocytopenia. Blood 2009;113:1564-73.
157. Stanworth SJ, Dyer C, Choo L, et al. Do all patients with hematologic malignancies and

severe thrombocytopenia need prophylactic platelet transfusions? Background, rationale, and design of a clinical trial (Trial of Platelet Prophylaxis) to assess the effectiveness of prophylactic platelet transfusions. Transfus Med Rev 2010;24:163-71.
158. Miller AB, Hoogsraten B, Staquet M, et al. Reporting results of cancer treatment. Cancer 1981;47:207-9.
159. Stanworth SJ, Dyer C, Casbard A, et al. Feasibility and usefulness of self-assessment of bleeding in patients with hematologic malignancies, and the association between platelet count and bleeding. Vox Sang 2006;91:63-9.
160. Heddle NM, Cook RJ, Webert KE, et al. Methodologic issues in the use of bleeding as an outcome in transfusion medicine studies. Transfusion 2003;43:742-52.
161. Wandt H, Schaefer-Eckart K, Pilz B, et al. Experience with a therapeutic platelet transfusion strategy in acute myeloid leukemia: Preliminary results of a randomized multicenter study after enrollment of 175 patients (abstract). Blood 2009;113:289a-90a.
162. Platelet transfusion therapy. National Institutes of Health Consensus Conference. Transfus Med Rev 1986;1:195-200.
163. College of American Pathologists: Practice parameter for the use of fresh frozen plasma, cryoprecipitate, and platelets. JAMA 1994;271:777-81.
164. Canadian Medical Association Expert Working Group: Guidelines for red blood cell and plasma transfusion for adults and children. Can Med Assoc J 1997;156(Suppl 11):S1-S29.
165. Norfolk DR, Ancliffe PJ, Contreras M, et al. Consensus conference on platelet transfusion. Br J Haematol 1998;101:609-17.
166. Schiffer CA, Anderson KC, Bennett CL, et al. Platelet transfusion for patients with cancer: Clinical practice guidelines of the American Society of Clinical Oncology. J Clin Oncol 2001;19:1519-38.
167. British Committee for Standards in Hematology. Guidelines for the use of platelet transfusions. Br J Haematol 2003;122:10-23.
168. O'Shaughnessy DF, Attenbury C, Bolton Maggs P, et al for the British Committee for Standards in Haematology, Blood Transfusion Task Force. Guidelines for the use of fresh-frozen plasma, cryoprecipitate, and cryosupernatant. Br J Haematol 2004;126:11-28.
169. Stainsby D, MacLeman S, Thomas D, et al for the British Committee for Standards in Haematology Writing Group. Guidelines on the management of massive blood loss. Br J Haematol 2006;135:634-41.
170. Malloy PC, Grassi CJ, Kundu S, et al. Consensus guidelines for periprocedural management of coagulation status and hemostasis risk in percutaneous image-guided interventions. J Vasc Interv Radiol 2009;20(Suppl):S240-9.
171. Roback JD, Caldwell S, Carson J, et al. Evidence-based practice guidelines for plasma transfusion. Transfusion 2010;50:1227-39.
172. Murad MH, Stubbs JR, Gandhi MJ, et al. The effect of plasma transfusion on morbidity and mortality: A systematic review and meta-analysis. Transfusion 2010;50:1370-83.
173. Guyatt GH, Oxman AD, Vist GE, et al. GRADE: An emerging consensus on rating quality of evidence and strength of recommendations. Br Med J 2008;336:924-6.
174. Guyatt GH, Oxman AD, Kunz R, et al. Going from evidence to recommendations. Br Med J 2008;336:1049-51.
175. Duchesne JC, Hunt JP, Wahl G, et al. Review of current blood transfusion strategies in a mature level I trauma center: Were we wrong for the last 60 years? J Trauma 2008;65:272-6.
176. Dente CJ, Shaz BH, Nicholas JM, et al. Improvements in early mortality and coagulopathy are sustained better in patients with blunt trauma after institution of a massive transfusion protocol in a civilian level I trauma center. J Trauma 2009;66:1616-24.
177. Teixeira PGR, Inaba K, Shulman I, et al. Impact of plasma transfusion in massively transfused trauma patients. J Trauma 2009;66:693-7.
178. Borgman MA, Spinella PC, Perkins JG, et al. The ratio of blood products transfused affects mortality in patients receiving massive transfusions at a combat support hospital. J Trauma 2007;63:805-13.
179. Kashuk J. Post-injury life-threatening coagulopathy: Is 1:1 FFP:RBCs the answer? J Trauma 2008;65:261-71.
180. Cotton B, Au B, Nunez T, Gunter O, et al. Predefined massive transfusion protocols are associated with a reduction in organ failure and post-injury complications. J Trauma 2009;66:41-8.
181. Holcomb JB, Wade C, Michalek J, et al. Increased plasma and platelet to RBC ratios improves outcome in 466 massively transfused civilian trauma patients. Ann Surg 2008;248:447-58.

182. Maegele M, Lefering R, Paffrath T, et al. Red-blood-cell to plasma ratios transfused during massive transfusion are associated with mortality in severe multiple injury: A retrospective analysis from the Trauma Registry of the Deutsche Gesellschaft fur Unfallchirurgie. Vox Sang 2008;95:112-19.
183. Snyder CW, Weinberg JA, McGwin G Jr., et al. The relationship of blood product ratio to mortality: Survival benefit or survival bias? J Trauma 2009;66:358-62.
184. Scalea TM, Bochicchio KM, Lumpkins K, et al. Early aggressive use of fresh frozen plasma does not improve outcome in critically-injured trauma patients. Ann Surg 2008;248:578-84.
185. Gonzalez EA, Moore FA, Holcomb JB, et al. Fresh frozen plasma should be given earlier to patients requiring massive transfusion. J Trauma 2007;62:112-19.
186. Cotton BA, Gunter OL, Isbell J, et al. Damage control hematology: The impact of a trauma exsanguination protocol on survival and blood product utilization. J Trauma 2008;64:1177-82.
187. Gunter O. Optimizing outcomes in damage control resuscitation: Identifying blood product ratios associated with improved survival. J Trauma 2008;65:527-34.
188. Stanworth SJ, Brunskill SJ, Hyde CJ, et al. Is fresh frozen plasma clinically effective? A systematic review of randomized controlled trials. Br J Haematol 2004;126:139-52.
189. Murphy MF, Stanworth SJ, Yazer M. Transfusion practice and safety: Current status and possibilities for improvement. Vox Sang 2011;100:46-59.
190. Westhoff C, Anstee DJ. A new paradigm for pretransfusion testing with the same perennial limitations. Transfusion 2010;50:520-1.

In: Vamvakas EC.
Decision Making in Transfusion Medicine
Bethesda, MD: AABB Press, 2011

5

Applications of Meta-Analysis in Transfusion Medicine

META-ANALYSIS IS POSSIBLY THE most important health policy research method that has been developed since the early 1980s.[1] It is the structured and systematic integration of information from different studies of a given problem,[2] and the term refers to a disciplined synthesis of previous research findings, in which the results of multiple reports on the efficacy of an intervention are compared, contrasted, and re-analyzed. When the results are discrepant, the purpose of the meta-analysis is to investigate the reasons for disagreements among the studies. When the results are concordant, the goal of the meta-analysis is to derive, through the application of a number of quantitative techniques, a measure of the effect of the intervention across the combined investigations. This measure is referred to as the "average" or "summary" effect of the treatment under study.[2-6]

Meta-analysis differs from the traditional narrative reviews of the literature in that 1) all completed investigations on the efficacy of the intervention that meet specific eligibility criteria are retrieved and included in the analysis; 2) the quality of the retrieved studies is assessed systematically; 3) the degree of agreement among the studies is evaluated, both conceptually and on the basis of statistical criteria, and the synthesis of the findings proceeds only if the variation in reported results is sufficiently modest to be attributed to chance; and, 4) providing that this prerequisite is met, quantitative methods are used to calculate the "average" effect of the intervention across the available studies and to test that effect for statistical significance.[1-6] If a meta-analysis is conducted in accordance with these guidelines, it can provide the reader with what Goodman described as "an objective view of the research literature, unaffected by the sometimes distorting lens of individual experience and personal preference that can affect a less structured review."[7]

The term "meta-analysis" was coined by Glass,[8] and it is used synonymously with the term "statistical overview." Glass defined it, in the psychology literature, as "the statistical analysis of a large collection of results from individual studies for the purpose of integrating the findings."[8] Meta-analysis has two generally accepted applications and one controversial use. It can serve to integrate the findings of studies that report a treatment effect operating in the same direction but varying substantially in size between the reports. The purpose of the synthesis is to provide a more precise estimate of the most likely magnitude of the treatment effect, so that a definitive randomized controlled trial (RCT) can be designed, enrolling as many patients as are needed to establish the existence of this effect.[9] Alternatively, meta-analysis can be used to investigate reasons for disagreements among studies that report treatment effects operating in opposite directions or differing markedly in size when they all point in the same direction. The aim of the analysis is to explain discrepancies among published results, according to relevant characteristics of the patients who were included in the available studies, or the treatments that were administered, or differences in the quality of study design and analysis.

The third, and still controversial, application of meta-analysis is to integrate the findings of studies that report a treatment effect operating in the same direction but not attaining statistical significance in any study, presumably because of the small sample size and inadequate statistical power of each report.[10] The purpose of the synthesis is to establish the existence of a treatment effect, by means of a combination of patient populations enrolled in separate studies. This use of meta-analysis makes meta-analysis appear to be a possible alternative to an RCT undertaken to establish the efficacy of a therapeutic intervention. However, a meta-analysis is observational and retrospective even when the combined studies are experimental. As an observational study, a meta-analysis is subject to all sources of bias (see Chapter 2 in the electronic supplement) that afflict traditional observational investigations. Therefore, a treatment effect, associated with a particular treatment by a meta-analysis, may be due either to the treatment itself or to some undetected error or uncontrolled factor that escaped the analysts. Because it is an observational study, a meta-analysis cannot be undertaken to resolve a hypothesis. A hypothesis formulated by a meta-analysis may—or may not—be corroborated when a definitive RCT is eventually conducted.[11,12]

Overviews should thus be considered a supplement (as opposed to an alternative) to RCTs. Even if a definitive RCT for establishing the efficacy of a therapeutic intervention is—eventually—conducted, its findings may not necessarily apply to all patients. Trialists use highly restrictive inclusion/exclusion criteria for patient enrollment, because they strive to include a patient population as homogeneous as possible, to make it easier to detect a treatment effect untainted by confounding factors. The results of an RCT thus may not apply to patients who do not meet the eligibility criteria of that trial. RCTs constitute the gold standard for evaluating the efficacy of therapeutic interventions, but they need to be supplemented by meta-analyses in order to broaden the applicability of the findings. A meta-analysis integrates the findings of separate studies, which usually differ in many aspects of their design. This variation in the design attributes of reports included in a meta-analysis leads to greater generalizability of the findings of a statistical overview, as compared to the results of an RCT, because—by combining studies with disparate design characteristics—a meta-analysis permits examination of the effect of an intervention in many different situations. If the treatment effect is consistent in all studies, this consistency favors a true treatment effect, rather than one due to chance or some systematic error or uncontrolled factor that may have compromised the results of all completed investigations.

To appreciate the value of meta-analyses in the medical literature, it is appropriate to think of an overview as an original report consisting of two parts: a qualitative component and a quantitative component.[1,2,7,13] According to Jenicek,[2] the first phase of a statistical overview should be a "qualitative" meta-analysis, which should precede the "quantitative" phase of the report. An assessment of the quality of all retrieved studies should be made, and studies of unacceptable quality should be excluded from the overview. In Goodman's opinion, a meta-analysis should "raise research and editorial standards, by calling attention to the strengths and weaknesses of the body of research in an area."[7] O'Rourke and Detsky asserted that the major contribution of a meta-analysis lies in the attention that it draws to flaws in the design and conduct of previous studies.[13] When all published studies are subjected to a detailed review of the methods—with a focus on the impact of the methods on the validity of the results—inadequacies can be identified and their resolution encouraged. Recognized shortcomings can be avoided in future individual research efforts, so that more valid results are produced. According to this view,[2,7,13] the assessment of the quality of the completed studies should be one of the main reasons—if not the primary reason—for conducting a meta-analysis.

There is consensus among epidemiologists that meta-analyses should be limited to RCTs[14-16] or that, if both RCTs and observational studies are to be included in an overview, the findings of observational studies should be integrated separately from the results of RCTs. However, having agreed on the criterion of nonrandomized treatment assignment for excluding a study from a meta-analysis, the experts disagree on other quality criteria to be used for disqualifying studies. Indeed, they disagree whether any randomized trial, no matter how poorly designed or conducted, should ever be excluded from an overview.[17]

Whether all available studies should be included in a meta-analysis or whether studies should be selected for inclusion in an overview on the basis of explicit quality criteria depends on our conceptions of the proper role, scope, and meaning of meta-analysis. If the purpose of an overview is to reach a conclusion about the existence of a treatment effect, on the basis of a combination of data on patient populations enrolled in separate studies, the quality of the studies to be included in the overview should be explicitly addressed in the report of the meta-analysis. An overview can only be as good as its component parts, and—if bias and confounding compromise the results of the studies included in the overview—the findings of the meta-analysis will be similarly flawed. Therefore, if the issue of study quality is not addressed in the report of the meta-analysis, the overview can be criticized[18,19] as an "exercise in megasilliness," in which "a mass of reports—good, bad, and indifferent—are fed into the computer in the hope that people will cease caring about the quality of the material on which the conclusions are based," and in which "[the phrase] 'garbage in–garbage out,' a well-known axiom of computer specialists, applies with equal force."[18]

On the basis of all of these considerations, a meta-analysis proceeds in a strict sequence:

- Retrieval of eligible studies from the literature.
- Assessment of the quality of each study.
- Data extraction.
- Assessment of the extent of concordance among the reports.
- Either examination of the reasons for disagreements among the studies or combination of the results of the individual investigations when indicated (Table 5-1).[3]

The purpose of this chapter is to provide readers with the necessary background for reading and evaluating published reports of meta-analyses. The rationale for quantitative research synthesis is presented, and the component parts of a meta-analysis are described. A recommended approach to the medical interpretation of overviews and the reasons for promulgating guidelines for conducting and reporting meta-analyses[3,20-22] are discussed. All concepts are illustrated by using as an example the meta-anal-

Table 5-1. Sequence of Steps to Be Followed in Conducting a Meta-Analysis

1. Retrieval of all completed studies on the effect of the intervention of interest.
2. Determination of the eligibility of the retrieved studies for inclusion in the analysis, on the basis of criteria specified in advance and relating to
   a. the scope of the hypothesis under study.
   b. the quality of the retrieved studies.
3. Extraction of data from each study on the effect of the intervention of interest.
4. Assessment of the degree of concordance among the studies (both conceptually and using statistical criteria).
5. If the studies are concordant, calculation of a "summary" or "average" estimate of the effect of the intervention across the combined investigations.
6. If the studies are discordant, examination of the reasons for disagreement among the studies.

ysis RCTs of the noninferiority of pathogen-reduced (as compared with non-pathogen-reduced) platelets in raising the posttransfusion platelet count and/or preventing bleeding in patients with hypoproliferative thrombocytopenia.[23]

To eliminate the residual risk of transfusion-associated sepsis (TAS) and of known transfusion-transmitted infections (TTIs), as well as to prevent an epidemic of transfusion-associated cases when the next major transfusion-transmitted pathogen emerges (Chapter 3), three pathogen-reduction (PR) systems for platelets have reached or are approaching clinical application.[24-28] All three are photoinactivation methods sharing the use of ultraviolet (UV) light, and two of them [amotosalen-HCl/UVA light (Intercept, Cerus Corp., Concord, CA) and riboflavin/UVB light (Mirasol, CaridianBCT, Lakewood, CO)] have undergone testing of their effects on the hemostatic efficacy and capacity of pathogen-reduced platelets. Hemostatic efficacy refers to the 1- and/or 24-hour posttransfusion corrected count increments (CCIs) of the transfused platelets (Table 5-2); hemostatic capacity refers to the ability of the transfused platelets to prevent bleeding. Treatment of platelets with UV light alone (MacoPharma, Tourcoing, France) is only presently undergoing testing in clinical trials.

PR of platelets results in a predictable loss of platelets.[29,30] Because fewer platelets are transfused, there is an expected 1) decrease in posttransfusion platelet recovery and/or survival (ie, respectively, a decrease in 1- and/or 24-hour posttransfusion CCIs; Table 5-2); 2) increase in the total number of platelet concentrates transfused to hemato-oncology patients during a period of hypoproliferative thrombocytopenia; and 3) reduction in the interval between the platelet transfusions required during the period of hypoproliferative thrombocytopenia.[24-28] However, if the reduction in effective platelet dose owing to PR can be overcome by increasing the number of transfused platelet concentrates, because these platelets are pathogen-reduced, prevailing opinion[24-28] has held that the advantages of PR (ie, the elimination of the residual risk of TAS and the prevention of most emerging TTIs; Chapter 2) more than compensate for any disadvantages. In this spirit, to derive the benefits of PR, transfusion medicine professionals are willing to accept a margin of inferiority in the hemostatic efficacy (or perhaps even capacity) of pathogen-reduced platelets.[24-28]

A recent independently funded RCT[31] questioned the prevailing assumption[24-28] that a reduction in effective platelet dose owing to PR can be overcome by simply increasing the number of transfused platelet concentrates. Accordingly, a meta-analysis[23] of all available RCTs[31-36] of the efficacy of pathogen-reduced platelet concentrates was undertaken to 1) produce an estimate of any inferiority of pathogen-reduced platelets in hemostatic efficacy and capacity that is based on all available data and 2) investigate possible reasons for the variation in the findings of the reported studies.

Table 5-2. 1-Hour Corrected Count Increment (CCI)*

The 1-hour CCI is the observed 1-hour posttransfusion platelet count increment following adjustment for the individual patient's blood volume and the actually-transfused dose of platelets:

$$\text{1-hour CCI} = \frac{\text{(1-hour posttransfusion platelet count increment)} \times \text{(BSA)}}{\text{Number of transfused platelets expressed as multiples of } 1 \times 10^{11}}$$

Abbreviation: BSA = body surface area (1.7 m^2 for the average adult; used here as a surrogate for the patient's blood volume).

*CCIs can be similarly calculated at 24, 4, 6 (etc) hours after transfusion (by using the corresponding 24-, 4-, 6- (etc) hour posttransfusion platelet count increment.

The Unit of Observation in Meta-Analysis

Meta-analysis is the epidemiology of study results. Clinical studies use the individual patient as the unit of observation. In contrast, the unit of observation in meta-analysis is the effect of an intervention, as calculated from each individual original report. For example, the RCTs of the noninferiority of pathogen-reduced (compared with non-pathogen-reduced) platelets in raising the posttransfusion platelet count and preventing bleeding[31-36] used the individual patient as the unit of observation.[24-28] In contrast, the meta-analysis of these reports[23] used as a unit of observation one or more measures of the hemostatic efficacy and capacity of pathogen-reduced platelets calculated from each study. More specifically, the outcomes considered in the meta-analysis[23] were 1) the odds ratio (OR) of bleeding complications in patients receiving pathogen-reduced platelets versus controls (Table 5-3 and Fig 5-1); 2) the mean difference between controls and patients receiving pathogen-reduced platelets in 1- and 24-hour CCIs (Fig 5-2), as well as in the interval between platelet transfusions (Fig 5-3); and 3) the mean difference between patients receiving pathogen-reduced platelets and controls in the total number of

Table 5-3. 2 × 2 Contingency Table Counts: RCTs Reporting on the Bleeding Complications of Patients Receiving Pathogen-Reduced (versus Non-Pathogen-Reduced) Platelets*

Study Arm	Bleeding Patients	Nonbleeding Patients	Totals
Treatment arm (patients randomly assigned to receive pathogen-reduced platelets)	a	b	a+b
Control arm (patients randomly assigned to receive non-pathogen-reduced platelets	c	d	c+d
Total	a+c	b+d	n

*Calculations for the odds of bleeding in each arm and the OR are as follows:

$$\text{Odds of bleeding in patients receiving pathogen-reduced platelets} = \frac{\frac{a}{a+b}}{\frac{b}{a+b}} = \frac{a}{b} \quad (1)$$

$$\text{Odds of bleeding in patients receiving non-pathogen-reduced platelets} = \frac{\frac{c}{c+d}}{\frac{d}{c+d}} = \frac{c}{d} \quad (2)$$

$$\text{Odds ratio (OR)} = \frac{\text{Odds of bleeding in patients receiving pathogen-reduced platelets}}{\text{Odds of bleeding in patients receiving non-pathogen-reduced platelets}} = \frac{\frac{a}{b}}{\frac{c}{d}} = \frac{ad}{bc} \quad (3)$$

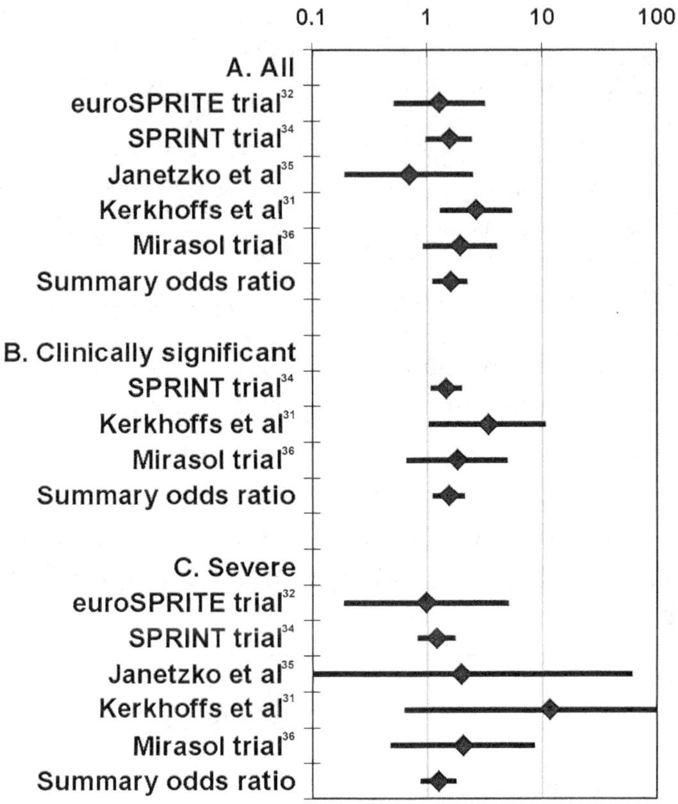

Figure 5-1. Odds ratios (ORs) of all bleeding complications, clinically significant bleeding complications, and severe bleeding complications in patients receiving pathogen-reduced or untreated platelets in the randomized controlled trials (RCTs)[31,32,34-36] included in the meta-analysis of studies of the hemostatic capacity of pathogen-reduced platelets.[23] "Severe" bleeding was bleeding categorized as such by the investigators[32,35] or bleeding of grade 3 or greater on the Common Toxicity Criteria (CTC) scale[31,34] or bleeding of grade 3 or greater on the World Health Organization (WHO) scale[36] if bleeding had not been categorized as severe by the investigators and grading on the CTC scale had not been performed (see text and Table 5-4). The figure also shows the summary OR across the studies that had presented each of these outcomes. All studies[31,32,34-36] had reported on all bleeding and on severe bleeding complications. Only studies that had graded bleeding on the CTC or WHO scale had differentiated between grade 1 and grade 2 bleeding, with bleeding of grade 2 or higher being clinically significant (see text). Accordingly, only the SPRINT trial,[34] the study of Kerkhoffs et al,[31] and the Mirasol trial[36] are included in the meta-analysis of RCTs reporting on clinically significant bleeding. Kerkhoffs et al[31] had presented a comparison among three randomization arms: recipients of platelets that had been pathogen-reduced with Intercept, recipients of untreated platelets suspended in a platelet additive solution (PAS-III), and recipients of untreated platelets stored in plasma (treatment, control, and "reference" arms, respectively). To reduce the impact of the results of Kerkhoffs et al[31] on its conclusions, the meta-analysis[23] included only 179 of the 278 enrolled patients (ie, the subjects included in the treatment arm and in the control arm). In all analyses, when the 95% confidence interval (CI) for the OR does not include the null value of 1, the increase in bleeding complications recorded in patients receiving pathogen-reduced platelets compared with controls is statistically significant ($p<0.05$).[23]

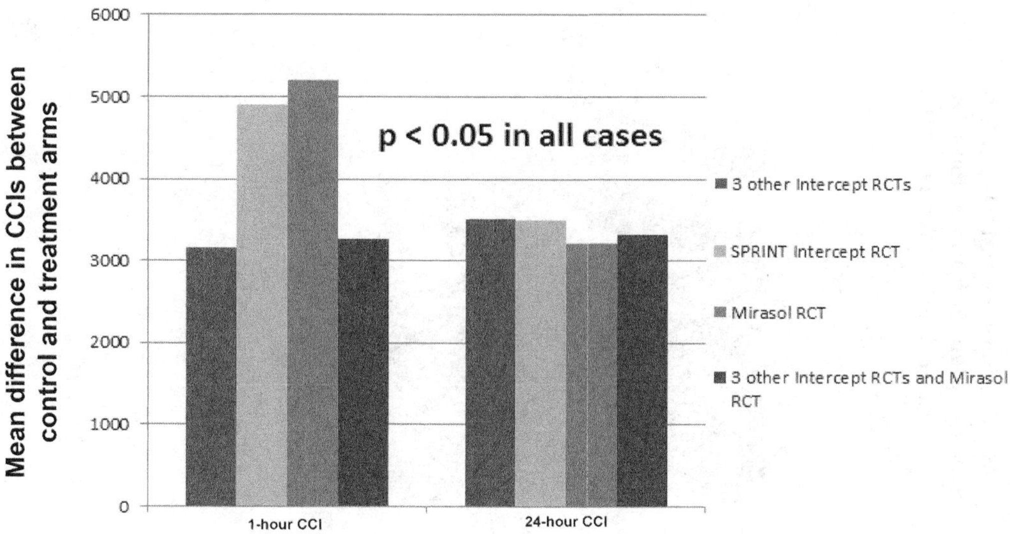

Figure 5-2. The mean difference in the 1- and 24-hour corrected count increments (CCIs) between recipients of non-pathogen-reduced platelets and recipients of pathogen-reduced platelets across the three other randomized controlled trials (RCTs) of the Intercept technology,[31,32,35] in the (individual) SPRINT RCT of the Intercept technology,[33] in the (individual) RCT of the Mirasol technology,[36] and across the three other RCTs of the Intercept technology[31,32,35] and the RCT of the Mirasol technology.[36] Four[31,32,35,36] of the five RCTs had used the 1-hour CCI as their primary endpoint. This primary endpoint differed significantly ($p<0.05$) between the randomization arms, always favoring the control arm, in all but two[32,35] RCTs. This outcome (1-hour CCI) also differed significantly ($p<0.001$) between the control and treatment arms of the SPRINT RCT,[33] which used grade 2 bleeding complications as its primary endpoint. Across the four[31,32,35,36] or three[31,32,35] RCTs that had reported the standard deviation (SD) for the difference between the randomization arms in the 1-hour CCI (and the three[26,31,32] or two[31,32] RCTs that had reported the SD for the difference between the randomization arms in the 24-hour CCI; Janetzko et al[35] did not report 24-hour CCIs), the figure shows the summary mean difference in these quantitative outcomes between the control and treatment arms. The SPRINT RCT[33] had not reported the SD for the difference in the 1- and 24-hour CCIs and could not be included in these meta-analyses. Both the SPRINT RCT[33] and the meta-analyses of the other studies found a statistically significant ($p<0.05$) decrease in the 1- and 24-hour CCIs in association with the receipt of pathogen-reduced (rather than non-pathogen-reduced) platelets. Initially published by Vamvakas in The Scientific World Journal 2011;11:624-40.

platelet transfusions received during the period of hypoproliferative thrombocytopenia (Fig 5-4).

Each study[31-36] thus contributed to the meta-analysis[23] one or more estimates of the effect of PR in potentially reducing the ability of treated (ie, pathogen-reduced) platelets to raise the recipient's posttransfusion platelet count and/or prevent bleeding. The OR of bleeding complications in patients receiving pathogen-reduced platelets versus controls (Fig 5-1) was calculated from each study if the authors had reported the four counts of a 2 × 2 contingency table (Table 5-3). The mean difference in the 1- and 24-hour CCIs, the interval between platelet transfusions, and the total number of platelet transfusions (Figs 5-2 through 5-4) were calculated from each study if the authors had reported 1) the mean ± standard deviation (SD) 1- and 24-hour CCIs, the interval between platelet transfusions, and the total number of platelet transfusions in controls; 2) the mean ± SD of these three outcomes in patients receiving pathogen-reduced

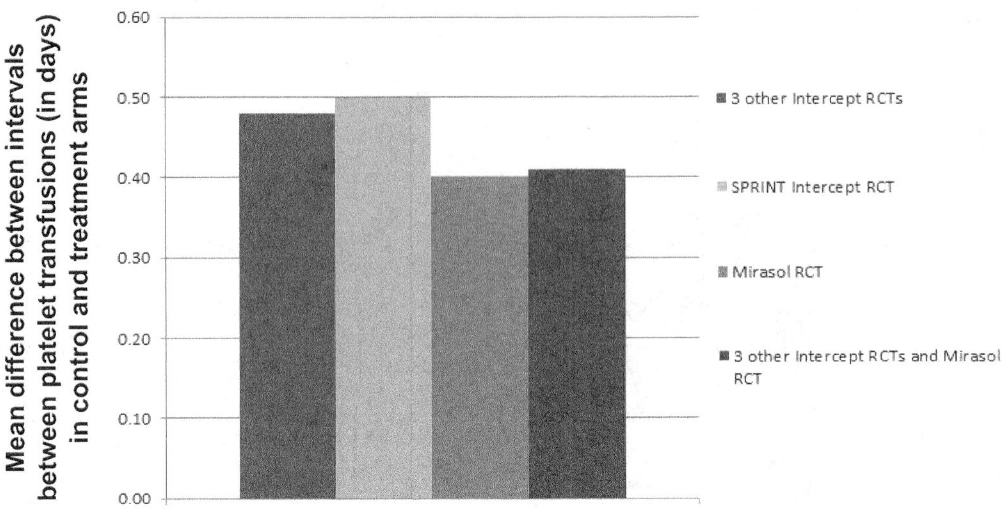

Figure 5-3. The mean difference between recipients of non-pathogen-reduced and recipients of pathogen-reduced platelets in the interval between platelet transfusions (in days) across the three other randomized controlled trials (RCTs) of the Intercept technology,[31,32,35] in the (individual) SPRINT RCT of the Intercept technology,[33] in the (individual) RCT of the Mirasol technology,[36] and across the three other RCTs of the Intercept technology[31,32,35] and the RCT of the Mirasol technology.[36] Across the four[31,32,35,36] or three[31,32,35] RCTs that had reported the standard deviation (SD) for the difference between the randomization arms in the interval between platelet transfusions, the figure shows the summary mean difference between the control and treatment arms. The SPRINT RCT[33] had not reported the SD for the difference and could not be included in this meta-analysis. Both the SPRINT RCT[33] and the meta-analyses of the other studies found a statistically significant ($p<0.05$) reduction in the interval between platelet transfusions received during the period of hypoproliferative thrombocytopenia in association with the receipt of pathogen-reduced (rather than non-pathogen-reduced) platelets.

platelets; and 3) the number of patients included in the treatment and control arms. One[33] of the five studies had not reported the SD of the 1- and 24-hour CCIs, the interval between platelet transfusions, or the total number of platelet transfusions (Figs 5-2 through 5-4). Moreover, the bleeding complications recorded in this RCT[33] were presented in two reports.[33,34] A meta-analysis integrates treatment effects calculated from separate studies, such as the treatment effects shown in Figs 5-1 through 5-4. It is important to appreciate that a meta-analysis "pools" the treatment effects calculated from the individual studies and not the data on the individual patients enrolled in each report. The treatment effect from each trial, as included in the analysis of an overview, is based exclusively on the outcomes of the treated patients and controls who were enrolled in that particular study.

Controls from one study cannot serve as controls for patients receiving the intervention (eg, PR of platelets) in another study. Such a comparison would be invalid, because the studies included in a meta-analysis differ from one another in various aspects of the characteristics of the enrolled patients, the treatments received, and attributes relating to study design and analysis. These differences among the studies are often likely to affect the outcome of interest [eg, the likelihood of bleeding complications after platelet transfusion (Fig 5-1), the difference in 1- and 24-hour CCIs (Fig 5-2), the difference in the interval between platelet transfusions (Fig 5-3), and the difference in the total number of platelet

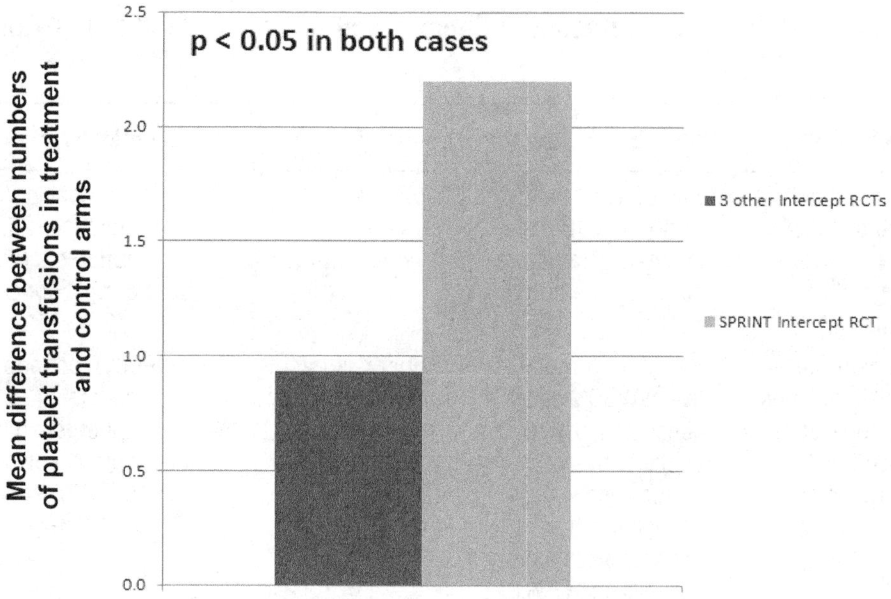

Figure 5-4. The mean difference between recipients of pathogen-reduced and recipients of non-pathogen-reduced platelets in the total number of platelet transfusions received during the period of hypoproliferative thrombocytopenia across the three other randomized controlled trials (RCTs) of the Intercept technology[31,32,35] and in the SPRINT RCT of the Intercept technology.[33] Across the three RCTs of the Intercept technology that had reported the SD for the difference between the randomization arms in the total number of platelet transfusions received,[31,32,35] the figure shows the summary mean difference in the total number of platelet transfusions between the treatment and control arms. The SPRINT RCT[33] had not reported the standard deviation (SD) for the difference and could not be included in this meta-analysis. The RCT of the Mirasol technology[36] had reported the mean ± SD of platelet transfusions per patient-day during the transfusion period (as opposed to the mean ± SD of transfusions during the entire period of hypoproliferative thrombocytopenia). The mean ± SD per patient-day was 0.24 ± 0.16 for the treatment arm and 0.20 ± 0.19 for the control arm.[36] Both the SPRINT RCT[33] and the meta-analysis of the three other studies[31,32,35] found a statistically significant ($p<0.05$) increase in platelet transfusions received during the period of hypoproliferative thrombocytopenia in association with the receipt of pathogen-reduced (rather than non-pathogen-reduced) platelets.

transfusions (Fig 5-4)]. Therefore, because of multiple differences among the available studies, it is invalid to directly compare the experience of individual patients from one study to that of subjects from another report. An overview compares the effect of an intervention in one study with the effect of the intervention in other investigations.

Sources of Variation in the Findings of the RCTs of the Hemostatic Efficacy and/or Capacity of Pathogen-Reduced Platelets

Table 5-4 lists some of the differences between the five available RCTs of the hemostatic efficacy and capacity of pathogen-reduced platelets.[31-36] Eight of the 10 listed sources of

Table 5-4. Possible Sources of Variation in the Five Randomized Controlled Trials (RCTs)[31-36] Reporting on the Hemostatic Efficacy and Capacity of Pathogen-Reduced Platelets*

Source of Variation	Category 1	Category 2	Category 3
Platelet concentrate transfused to patients receiving pathogen-reduced platelets (treatment arm)	Pools of five[31] (or five or six[32]) WBD platelet concentrates prepared by the buffy-coat method	Apheresis (single-donor) concentrates[33,35]	Buffy-coat-pooled WBD platelets (26.1%) or apheresis (single-donor) concentrates (73.9%)[36]
Platelet concentrate transfused to patients receiving non-pathogen-reduced platelets (control arm)	Pools of 5[31] (or four or five[32]) WBD platelet concentrates prepared by the buffy-coat method and suspended in either 1)100% plasma or 35% plasma/65% PAS II[32]; or 2) 100% plasma or 35% plasma/65% PAS III[31]	Apheresis (single-donor) concentrates suspended in 100% plasma[33,35]	Buffy-coat pooled WBD platelets (25.2%) or apheresis (single-donor) concentrates (74.8%) suspended in 100% plasma[36]
Mean ± SD length of storage of platelet concentrates given to the treatment arm (days)	≤3.5[32,33,35,36] (range: 2.7[36] to 3.5[32])	>3.5[31†] (4.0[31])	
Mean ± SD number of platelets contained in the platelet concentrate given to the treatment arm ($\times 10^{11}$)	>5.0[36] (5.2[36])[‡]	3.5-5.0 (range: 3.7[33] to 4.1[35])	<3.5[31†] (3.4[31])
Enrolled population of hemato-oncology patients with hypoproliferative thrombocytopenia	Unselected[31]	Moderately selected[32,33]: patients with clinical factors that could potentially interfere with the assessment of the study endpoint and patients with acute promyelocytic leukemia excluded; splenomegaly, DIC, and/or infection or fever not listed among the exclusion criteria	Selected[35,36]: splenomegaly, DIC, and/or infection or fever also listed among the exclusion criteria

Table 5-4. Possible Sources of Variation in the Five Randomized Controlled Trials (RCTs)[31-36] Reporting on the Hemostatic Efficacy and Capacity of Pathogen-Reduced Platelets* (Continued)

Source of Variation	Category 1	Category 2	Category 3
Threshold for prophylactic platelet transfusion during the period of hypoproliferative thrombocytopenia	≤10,000/μL[31,33,36]	≤20,000/μL[32,35]	
Ascertainment of bleeding complications	Patients evaluated daily by blinded[33] or unblinded[31] assessors	Assessments performed before and after platelet transfusion by blinded[32] or unblinded[36] observers	No bleeding assessments other than safety monitoring for adverse events[35]
Definition of bleeding severity	All bleeding versus severe bleeding§[32,35]	CTC‖ Version 2.0[34] or 3.0[31] scale	WHO scale[33,36]
Frequency of bleeding complications	<30%[31] (21.6%[31])	≥50%[32,35,36] (range: 50.9%[36] to 87.1%[34])	
Proportion of platelet transfusions administered in violation of study protocol	<10%[33] (8.0%[33])	10% - 25%[32,35,36]	>25%[31] (26.7%[31])

*The bleeding complications recorded in the SPRINT trial[33,34] were presented in 2 reports: initially graded on the WHO scale[33] and subsequently graded on the CTC‖ Version 2.0 scale.[34] In both cases, the grading was performed by blinded personnel.

†Extended storage for up to 7 days was permitted in all arms of the study of Kerkhoffs et al.[31] Twenty-six percent of the platelets transfused to the treatment arm and 21% of the platelets transfused to the control arm had been stored for 6 or 7 days. The mean ± SD number of platelets per pooled concentrate transfused to the treatment arm was 3.4 ± 0.8×10^{11}.

‡The Mirasol study[36] exclusively transfused pathogen-reduced platelet components meeting French blood bank standards (ie, containing $\geq 3.0 \times 10^{11}$ platelets per transfused component).

§"Severe" bleeding in the euroSPRINT trial[32] corresponded to bleeding events that "required treatment intervention and change in patient activity status." In the RCT of Janetzko et al,[35] only one episode of hemoptysis was categorized as "severe."

‖Common Terminology Criteria for Adverse Events (CTCAE) and CTC (as used by the US National Cancer Institute). [Available at http://ctep.cancer.gov/protocolDevelopment/electronic_applications/ctc.htm.]

CTC = Common toxicity criteria; DIC = disseminated intravascular coagulation; PAS = platelet additive solution; WBD = whole-blood-derived; WHO = World Health Organization.

variation in the results of the RCTs[31-36] could render some of the available RCTs more likely than others to reduce, or even conceal, a true difference between the hemostatic efficacy (and, potentially, also the capacity) of the pathogen-reduced and the non-pathogen-reduced platelets. Sources of variation that could reduce a difference between the randomization arms include the storage medium of platelets transfused to the control arm, the mean ± SD length of storage of the platelets given to the control (compared with the treatment) arm, the mean ± SD number of platelets contained in the component given to the control (compared with the treatment) arm, the enrollment of selected (rather than unselected) patients, the use of a less stringent platelet transfusion threshold, a more frequent ascertainment (and a higher recorded frequency) of bleeding complications, as well as a higher proportion of platelet transfusions administered in violation of the study protocol. An equally important source of variation that could affect the findings of the available RCTs[31-36] is the reporting of the bleeding events by an RCT as "all" and "severe" bleeding complications as compared with "clinically significant" bleeding complications. As will be discussed below, the recording of clinically significant bleeding complications depends greatly on interobserver variation, whereas bleeding complications classed as "all" or "severe" can be regarded as "hard" endpoints recorded in the same manner by all trained observers.

The Biologic Basis of the Sources of Variation in the Results of the RCTs

PR systems for platelets (Intercept or Mirasol) have been tested on apheresis (single-donor) platelets in both Europe[35,36] and the United States[33,34] and on pooled whole-blood-derived (WBD) platelets prepared by the buffy-coat method in Europe.[31,32] Because buffy-coat pooled WBD and apheresis platelets differ in many quality-control measures,[37] it is possible that one or the other component may incur a greater reduction in hemostatic efficacy and/or capacity after PR. Pooled WBD platelet concentrates transfused to the control arm of the RCTs conducted in Europe had been stored in 1) either 100% plasma or a mixture of platelet additive solution (PAS) III and plasma (depending on the study arm in the latest trial that used two control arms receiving different non-pathogen-reduced platelet components[31]) or 2) either 100% plasma or a mixture of PAS II and plasma (depending on the participating blood center[32]). PAS III has been shown to perform equally as well as plasma.[31] However, there have been significant differences in metabolic, functional, and flow cytometric variables between platelets stored in PAS II and those stored in plasma.[38-40] Platelets stored in PAS II rather than in plasma showed significant decreases in both platelet recovery and survival.[41-43] The use of platelets stored in PAS II in the control arm of some European RCTs[32] could thus conceal a reduction in hemostatic efficacy (and, potentially, also the capacity) associated with the pathogen-reduced platelets transfused to the treatment arm of these studies.

Greater storage time of platelet concentrates similarly correlates with reduced platelet recovery and survival (ie, reduced 1- and 24-hour CCIs) in at least some studies.[31,41-44] Extended storage of platelets for 6 or 7 days has been reported to result in modestly lower 1- and 24-hour CCIs when platelets are stored in plasma[45,46] and in significantly lower CCIs and a shorter interval between platelet transfusions when platelets are stored in PAS II.[47] Greater storage time of platelets transfused to the control than to the treatment arm of the RCTs thus could similarly conceal a reduction in hemostatic efficacy (and, potentially, also in capacity) associated with the pathogen-reduced platelets transfused to the treatment arm of these studies. Such would also be the case if—owing to suboptimal component preparation methods—a smaller number of platelets were transfused to the control arm of the studies. (In the latter case, the smaller number of platelets given to the control arm would mask the effect of the smaller number of platelets given to the treatment arm because of the platelet losses that occur secondary to the PR process itself.[29,30])

More than 80% of platelet transfusions are given to prevent bleeding complications. The cohort of patients with hypoproliferative thrombocytopenia enrolled in the available RCTs of PR of platelet components may have consisted of unselected hemato-oncology patients needing prophylactic platelet transfusions at a given threshold (either 20,000/µL or 10,000/µL) or before invasive procedures, or needing platelet transfusions to treat bleeding. Alternatively, the cohort may have consisted of hemato-oncology patients selected in a manner that excludes patients with factors predisposing the subjects to platelet consumption. Such factors include a history of immune thrombocytopenia, a history of alloimmunization or refractoriness to platelet transfusion, an acute surgical condition, and (as shown in Table 5-4) also splenomegaly, disseminated intravascular coagulation (DIC), or infection/fever. Such factors predispose to platelet transfusion failure.[48-51] Exclusion from RCTs of the thrombocytopenic subjects with these clinical factors (ie, those most likely to bleed or to need increased platelet transfusions while receiving platelet transfusion support) could reduce or conceal any decrease in the hemostatic capacity of platelets treated with PR.

An RCT could have recorded more frequent bleeding complications if it had ascertained the occurrence of bleeding complications more frequently than other RCTs. An RCT also could have recorded bleeding differentially between its arms if it had used unblinded assessors with a preconceived bias concerning the likelihood of bleeding complications in recipients of pathogen-reduced (or, alternatively, non-pathogen-reduced) platelets. Bleeding is a complex outcome because it is a composite: whether the Common Toxicity Criteria (CTC)[52] or the World Health Organization (WHO)[53] scale is used to grade the severity of bleeding, on any given day (or before and after a platelet transfusion) a patient may have one or several grade 1, grade 2, grade 3, and/or grade 4 bleeding events at one (or more than one) of several sites. When more than one bleeding event occurs on the same day (or in the same assessment period), the highest observed bleeding grade is recorded for that day (or period).

Grading bleeding is difficult, and observers often disagree about it. The distinction between grade 1 and grade 2 bleeding is especially subtle, yet grade 2 or greater bleeding has been considered to represent clinically significant bleeding.[54,55] Two recent RCTs of platelet dose[56,57] defined their primary outcome as grade 2 or greater bleeding, which was considered to represent clinically significant bleeding. Nonetheless, the WHO bleeding scale has not been validated by using measurement methodology, and its reproducibility, accuracy, and face validity remain to be established.[55] Results from RCTs pertaining to clinically significant bleeding complications (grade 2 or greater on either the CTC[52] or the WHO[53] scale) greatly depend on interobserver variation, owing to the difficulty in distinguishing between grade 1 and grade 2 bleeding. [For example, "mild" rectal bleeding is grade 1, whereas "persistent" rectal bleeding requiring medication (eg, steroid suppositories) is grade 2; vaginal bleeding is grade 1 if it requires <2 pads per day, but it is grade 2 if it requires ≥ 2 pads per day, and so on].

In contrast, results from RCTs pertaining to all or severe bleeding complications could be considered reliable–that is, not dependent on interobserver variation. Grade 3 or greater bleeding complications on either the CTC[52] or the WHO[53] scale would be considered severe, as would be bleeding complications categorized as severe by the investigators themselves (Table 5-4). Grade 3 bleeding requires Red Blood Cell (RBC) transfusion or other intervention; it also includes generalized petechiae and/or retinal bleeding with visual impairment. Grade 4 bleeding is catastrophic bleeding, such as intracranial bleeding that causes neurologic deficit or disability.

Protocol violations could have occurred in the available RCTs because of errors or because a platelet transfusion was needed when the specially prepared component required by the protocol was not available in the inventory. Violations occurring equally in both arms would reduce, and possibly conceal, any adverse effect of PR on hemostatic efficacy and/or capacity. Violations occurring selectively in the treatment arm (because pathogen-reduced platelets were unavailable when needed) would have the same effect, provided that the component given to the control arm did not have reduced hemostatic efficacy (as would be the case for platelets stored in PAS II).

Assessment of the Eligibility of Original Reports for Inclusion in a Meta-Analysis

Meta-analysis is based on the assumption that all studies evaluating the effect of an intervention of interest are retrieved. Some of these reports are then selected for inclusion in the analysis, on the basis of eligibility criteria specified in advance. Exclusions are initially determined by the medical scope of the overview. If the medical question asked is a general one, broad selection criteria may be used; if it is a more specific one, the criteria must be stricter. The hypothesis under investigation must be defined in precise terms, so that the selection of studies for analysis can be made in an objective and reproducible manner. Additional criteria for exclusion may include the date of publication (because a study's results may no longer be clinically relevant), the language of publication (if reports not published in English cannot be properly evaluated), the length of follow-up (if the length is considered too short for a reliable assessment of the outcome under study), and the completeness of the presented information [if the four counts of a contingency table (Table 5-3) cannot be extracted from an abstract, letter to the editor, or other summary report of a study]. Excluded studies should be catalogued, and the reasons for exclusion should be explicitly stated.

For example, Vamvakas[23] conducted a computerized search of the English literature to identify RCTs comparing the hemostatic efficacy and/or capacity of pathogen-reduced and non-pathogen-reduced platelets that were published between January 1, 2001, and June 30, 2010, and that had reported on at least one of five outcomes. These outcomes were

1. The 1-hour CCI (mean ± SD).
2. The 24-hour CCI (mean ± SD).
3. The platelet transfusion interval (days; mean ± SD).
4. The number of platelet transfusions (number of therapeutic platelet doses; mean ± SE).
5. The proportion of patients having bleeding complications [regardless of bleeding severity; number (%)].

The electronic search was supplemented by a manual search for abstracts published in the supplements of transfusion medicine and hematology journals between January 1, 2008, and June 30, 2010. The reference lists of the retrieved articles were also reviewed for pertinent citations.[23]

To be eligible for inclusion in the meta-analysis, retrieved RCTs had to have assigned patients to receive routine platelet transfusions with either treated (ie, pathogen-reduced) or untreated (ie, non-pathogen-reduced) platelets. Platelet transfusions were regarded as "routine" if 1) transfusion decisions had been made by the patients' treating physicians on the basis of the standard criteria used at each participating institution and 2) transfused components had not been manipulated in ways other than PR.

Table 5-5 presents the employed electronic-search strategy that identified six RCTs (four studies included in the overview[31-33,35] and two excluded studies[58,59]) that were potentially eligible for inclusion in the meta-analysis. An additional RCT was identified through the manual search of abstracts; it has since become available in complete form,[36] and it was included in the meta-analysis. One more RCT identified through the manual search of abstracts[60] was excluded. The other reports located by the last step of the electronic search (Table 5-5) were observational studies,[61] further analyses of the SPRINT trial,[29,34] experimental studies in normal volunteers,[62] or studies unrelated to the purpose of the search. Review of the abstracts of all studies located in the penultimate step of the search (Table 5-5) did not identify any other RCT meeting the eligibility criteria of the meta-analysis.

Two RCTs[58,59] (n = 20 and n = 10, respectively) retrieved electronically were excluded because they were crossover studies in which patients had received both pathogen-reduced

Table 5-5. PUBMED Search Strategy in the Meta-Analysis[23] of RCTs of the Hemostatic Efficacy and Capacity of Pathogen-Reduced Platelets

Search Statement	Search Terms	Number of Citations
#1	Platelet AND transfusion	12,764
#2	Pathogen reduction OR pathogen inactivation	411
#3	Amotosalen OR "S 59" OR S59	902
#4	Riboflavin	12,919
#5	"Ultraviolet-A light" OR "UVA light"	547
#6	Intercept OR Mirasol	5,264
#7	#2 OR #3 OR #4 OR #5 OR #6	19,817
#8	#1 AND #7	191
#9	#1 AND #7 Limits: English; Publication Date from 2001/01/01 to 2010/06/30	159
#10	#1 AND #9	13

and untreated platelets in different periods. A significant treatment-by-period interaction had been observed in one study,[58] while, in the other study,[59] the investigators had transfused RBCs to maintain a hematocrit of ≥25% (because hematocrit affects bleeding time—the study's primary outcome). Two RCTs[58,60] (n = 20 and n = 201, respectively) retrieved electronically[58] or through the manual search of abstracts[60] were excluded because they had transfused only platelets stored for 6 (20%) or 7 (80%) days[60] or 7 days[58]—that is, past the allowed storage period of platelets. Rather than evaluating efficacy, these studies[58,60] targeted cost-effectiveness and aimed to show that the introduction of PR with the Intercept technology could permit the extension of the platelet storage period to 7 days (so as to offset the cost of PR by reducing platelet outdating). As already discussed, a greater length of storage reduced platelet efficacy, which made the intervention evaluated in these studies[58,60] different from that in the other studies.[31-36]

Equally important, the RCT of Lozano et al[60] (available only in abstract form at the time of the meta-analysis) had employed a study design different from that of the other RCTs.[31-36] Rather than allocating patients with hypoproliferative thrombocytopenia to receive pathogen-reduced or non-pathogen-reduced platelets throughout the study period (ie, for all their platelet transfusion needs during the study), this RCT randomly assigned patients to receive one pathogen-reduced or one non-pathogen-reduced platelet transfusion of a component stored past the allowed storage period (ie, for 6 or 7 days). All other platelet transfusion needs of these patients enrolled in either the treatment or the control arm of this study were met with routine components (ie, non-pathogen-reduced concentrates stored for ≤5 days). Each enrolled patient could thus be observed for the occurrence of relevant outcome measures (1- and 24-hour CCIs and bleeding complications) only during the period immediately following the single experimental platelet transfusion of the (expired) pathogen-reduced or non-pathogen-reduced platelet concentrate. For the 24 hours after the experimental transfusion, Lozano et al[60] reported on all bleeding complications, without making a distinction between bleeding complications of different severity.

Five RCTs[31-36] enrolling a total of 1080 subjects thus were eligible for analysis. One large study[33,34] had enrolled 645 of these 1080 patients. The most recent RCT of Kerkhoffs et al[31] had enrolled 278 patients in three study arms: recipients of pathogen-reduced platelets, recipients of buffy-coat pools suspended in a mixture of PAS III and plasma like the pathogen-reduced platelets (n = 94; control arm used in the meta-analysis), and recipients of buffy-coat pools suspended in 100% plasma (n = 99; reference arm not used in the meta-analysis). There were also two RCTs of modest size (n = 103[32] and n = 110[36]) and one small RCT (n = 43[35]).

In all five RCTs,[31-36] patients with hypoproliferative thrombocytopenia were randomly assigned to receive either pathogen-reduced or non-pathogen-reduced platelets, and all randomly assigned patients receiving at least one platelet transfusion were included in the reported analyses. When subjects with hypoproliferative thrombocytopenia are randomly assigned to receive pathogen-reduced or non-pathogen-reduced platelets, patients from either arm of an RCT should have the same baseline probability of responding with an adequate or inadequate posttransfusion CCI (Table 5-2) and of developing or not developing bleeding complications. Provided that the number of enrolled subjects is very large, the play of chance will distribute equally between the treatment and control arms all prognostic factors for a patient's response to a platelet transfusion and development of bleeding complications (see Chapter 2 in the electronic supplement). Therefore, in the absence of any intervention (such as PR of the transfused platelets), the same proportion of subjects from either randomization arm should be expected to respond inadequately to platelet transfusion or to develop bleeding complications. For this reason, any significant difference in posttransfusion CCI or frequency of bleeding complications between the two randomization arms can be ascribed to the receipt of pathogen-reduced (or non-pathogen-reduced) platelets.

The intent to investigate the existence of a causal relationship (see Chapter 2 in the electronic supplement) is the reason that, when meta-analyses were initially introduced in medicine, only RCTs were eligible for inclusion in an overview. When results from observational studies are also available, the findings of observational studies either are not considered at all or are integrated separately from the results of RCTs. When findings from observational studies are integrated (as shown in Chapter 7), only adjusted results from multivariate analyses of these studies should be considered eligible for inclusion in an overview. In a correctly designed and analyzed observational study, such findings from multivariate analyses should be free of the effects of known and measurable confounding factors (see Chapter 2 in the electronic supplement), although the effects of unknown and poorly quantifiable confounding factors persist.

Assessment of the Quality of RCTs Included in a Meta-Analysis

The assessment of the quality of studies meeting the eligibility criteria for inclusion in a meta-analysis was listed as a necessary part of any statistical overview in the early guidelines for meta-analysis in clinical research.[2,3,7,63] This position was also endorsed by Moher and Olkin[20] in their call for standards for reports of meta-analyses published in the medical literature. Formal instruments for assessing the quality of RCTs are now available.[64-68] Chalmers et al[64] developed a detailed list of items to be used for scoring the quality of published RCTs on a scale from 0 to 1. A simplified scaling technique was presented by Detsky et al,[65] and a third instrument was proposed by Zelen.[66] Guidelines for evaluating observational studies were presented by Lichenstein et al[69] and Feinstein.[70]

A simple instrument was developed by Jadad et al[71] for use by all readers of RCTs. The maximum quality score that can be given to a study based on this instrument is 5. Two points are given to a report for random assignment of subjects to treatment and control groups, two points are granted for blinding both investigators and patients, and one point is added if the number of patients excluded from the analysis, along with the reasons for all dropouts and withdrawals, is presented in the report of the RCT. With regard to the randomization procedure, one point is given if a study is designated as "randomized" but the randomization procedure is not described; zero points are given if the randomization procedure is described but is judged to be inappropriate, and two points are given if the randomization procedure is described and is appropriate. With regard to the blinding technique, one point is given if a study is designated as "double-blind" but the procedure for blinding investigators and patients is not described, zero points are given if the blinding procedure is described but is judged to be inappropriate, and two points are given if the blinding procedure is described and is appropriate.

Moher et al[72] used the instrument of Jadad et al[71] to measure the quality of 127 RCTs from the medical literature. Few RCTs had reported either the method used to generate the randomization sequence (15%) or the method used to conceal this sequence until the point of randomization occurred (14%). RCTs that had not adequately described the measures taken to conceal the treatment allocations exaggerated the effect of the intervention under study by 37% ($p<0.01$), compared to RCTs that had adequately reported the method(s) used for concealment. Furthermore, RCTs receiving a low total quality score (≤ 2) exaggerated the estimate of the effect of the intervention by 34%, compared with trials receiving a high quality score (>2) ($p<0.001$). Moher et al[72] concluded that the pooling of the findings of low-quality RCTs resulted in a clinically important and statistically significant exaggeration of the efficacy of an intervention under study.

Therefore, after a quality score has been assigned to each study that is eligible for inclusion in a meta-analysis, meta-analysts must confront the contentious issue of whether studies of inferior quality are to be included in the calculation of the "average" treatment effect. The main argument for including studies that are not of the best quality is that using a larger number of studies permits examination of the effect of the intervention in more situations. However, this advantage must be balanced against the disadvantage of including questionable results. There is a general consensus that, if studies of poor quality are to be included, the differences in quality must be taken into account in the analysis.[63,73,74] Computational methods used in meta-analysis assign weights to each study that are proportional to a study's sample size.[75,76] In theory, the quality scores could also be incorporated into the weights assigned to each report, so that the calculated average treatment effect can depend more heavily on the findings of investigations of superior quality.[17,73] Alternatively, the studies could be stratified by quality score, so that an average treatment effect can be calculated separately for each stratum of quality. If the effects differ across strata, the average effect calculated from studies of superior quality can be considered to be the valid one.

Overviews in the health field have only rarely adjusted for the quality of the combined studies by using statistical techniques.[77] Experts have recommended that minimal quality standards be set in advance, in the form of criteria for inclusion, and that studies that do not meet them be excluded.[8,17,63] Others have proposed that only the "best" of the available studies be used.[78,79] Reports with a quality score below a certain threshold are often excluded in practice, but the scores and the threshold are often not stated explicitly in medical reports of overviews.

Quality scores have been criticized as being based on the report of a study, which is not necessarily an accurate measure of the truth about some elements of quality. The standards for reporting details of the methods used have become more stringent over the past decade,[80,81] and more recently published studies tend to attain higher quality scores for that reason. Liberati et al[82] used the method of Chalmers et al[64] to grade 63 RCTs of primary treatment of breast cancer, and they found an average quality score of 0.50 (95% CI = 0.46-0.54), on a scale from 0 to 1. Telephone calls to the principal investigator improved the quality scores by an average of

0.07, because information learned during the call clarified that some of the deficiencies lay in the reporting of a study, rather than in its performance. A more important criticism of quality scores is that they may exaggerate the quality of a reviewed study, because a study may suffer from bias even if evidence of that bias cannot be detected from the report of the study.

In the specific context of RCTs of platelet transfusion, study characteristics specific to platelet transfusion are at least as relevant as the generic aspects of study quality[63-68,80,81] discussed hitherto. Delaney et al[83] proposed a list of items for assessing the quality of reporting by RCTs of platelet transfusion that is based on both the CONSORT-Statement checklist[80,81] and a checklist specific for platelet transfusion.

The meta-analysis of RCTs of the hemostatic efficacy and capacity of pathogen-reduced platelets[23] included all studies meeting the aforementioned eligibility criteria, regardless of their quality. Three[32,33,35] of the five RCTs were double-blinded, and two[31,36] were open-label investigations. Only two of the studies[31,34] had optimally determined the occurrence of bleeding complications: the SPRINT RCT[33] and the RCT of Kerkhoffs et al.[31] These RCTs ascertained bleeding daily, by using trained assessors. Of those two studies, however, only the SPRINT RCT[33,34] had used blinded assessors. The euroSPRITE trial[32] and the Mirasol study,[36] as well as the expanded safety analysis of the SPRINT RCT,[34] supplemented the observations made by the investigators with hemorrhagic events recorded as part of the documentation of adverse events. In the case of the SPRINT RCT, adverse events were recorded by study-site personnel blinded to the treatment assignment[34] (as had been the case with the data collected for the initial analysis of that study[33]). Janetzko et al[35] relied solely upon the recording of adverse events, because bleeding was not an endpoint for that trial.

With regard to the study characteristics most relevant to the PR of platelets (Table 5-4), the recent independently funded RCT of Kerkhoffs et al[31] differed from the other studies,[32,33,35,36] both in the source of funding and in five other study descriptors. The latter differences were that Kerkhoffs et al[31] had

1. Transfused platelets to the treatment arm stored for a longer period (>3.5 days compared to ≤3.5 days).
2. Transfused a lower mean platelet dose per component given to the treatment arm (<3.5×10^{11} rather than ≥3.5×10^{11}).
3. Enrolled unselected hemato-oncology patients.
4. Recorded a lower frequency of bleeding complications (<30% compared with ≥50%).
5. Committed a higher proportion of protocol violations (>25% compared with ≤25%).

The higher frequency of protocol violations would reduce any difference between the two randomization arms; the four other attributes peculiar to the study of Kerkhoffs et al[31] would favor the detection of a higher frequency of bleeding complications in the treatment arm of that study than in the treatment arm of the other trials[32-36] (see discussion in the section "Unit of Observation in Meta-Analysis").

The mean length of storage of transfused platelets was higher by only 0.1 day (p>0.05) in the treatment arm of Kerkhoffs et al[31] than in that study's control arm; this difference is similar to the difference (0.1-0.2 day) between the randomization arms in the other RCTs.[32-36] Similarly, the mean number of platelets in concentrates transfused to the treatment arm of Kerkhoffs et al[31] was lower by only 0.2×10^{11} (p>0.05) than the number in the concentrates given to the control arm; this difference is similar to the difference (0 to 0.4×10^{11} platelets per concentrate) between the randomization arms in the other RCTs.[32-36]

For the purpose of guiding public policy decision-making, the design of the RCT of Kerkhoffs et al[31] was superior to that of all of the other RCTs,[32,33,35,36] because that study[31] enrolled unselected hemato-oncology patients and therefore reflected "real-world" conditions. Because that study[31] was hitherto the only one to enroll unselected hemato-oncology patients, the difference between its findings and those of the other studies[32,33,35,36] (Fig 5-1) could be due to that aspect of its design. It is also possible that observation bias (and, more specifically, diagnostic suspicion bias) could have accounted for the higher frequency of bleeding complications in the treatment than in the control arm of the study by Kerkhoffs et al.[31] Such might be the case if the unblinded assessors of that study were preferentially finding or recording bleeding complications in the recipients of the pathogen-reduced (as opposed to the non-pathogen reduced) platelets.

Rationale for Quantitative Research Synthesis

An overview compares the effect of a treatment in one study with the effect of that intervention in other investigations. A meta-analysis by the fixed-effects method[75,76] combines a series of 2 × 2 contingency table counts (Table 5-3), as though the tables were strata of patients enrolled in the same study (and stratified according to the level of a confounding factor in an epidemiologic investigation[75] or, in a multicenter RCT,[84,85] according to the admitting hospital; see Chapter 2 in the electronic supplement). The findings from these individual strata are integrated, according each stratum a weight commensurate with its sample size.[4-6] An assumption is made that there is a uniform or "fixed" treatment effect in all of the strata (or in all of the studies included in the meta-analysis). Studies are thought to have generated different estimates of this fixed effect solely because of random sampling variation. The results of a meta-analysis by the fixed-effects method thus are valid only if this is a reasonable assumption to make.[6]

However, that assumption cannot reasonably be made if the combined studies differ with respect to important design attributes (Table 5-4). If current medical knowledge suggests that the effect of an intervention should differ in various situations (Table 5-4), it is probably unreasonable to assume that the treatment has the same effect in all of the studies. A meta-analysis by the random-effects method[17,86] is advocated for these circumstances–that is, when studies differ from each other "in ways too complex to capture by a few simple study characteristics."[6 (p526)] The assumption here is that the true treatment effects vary from study to study, being randomly positioned about some central value. This value is the summary or average effect of the treatment across the combined studies.

In a fixed-effects analysis, only within-studies variation influences the uncertainty of the summary treatment effect across the combined studies, as calculated by the overview. "Within-studies" variation refers simply to random sampling variation from study to study–that is, the variation that results each and every time a study sample is drawn, at random, from the target population of all eligible patients. This sampling variation is inversely proportional to the sample size of each report. No "between-studies" variation is presumed to exist when a fixed-effects analysis is undertaken, because all included studies are assumed to measure the same (fixed) effect of the intervention. Therefore, the differences among the studies in the magnitude and direction of the reported treatment effect do not influence the uncertainty that surrounds the summary effect calculated and reported by the meta-analysis.

In contrast, in a random-effects analysis, both within-studies and between-studies variation influence the uncertainty surrounding this summary treatment effect. The uncertainty associated with the measured estimate of the effect increases if the sample size of the combined studies is small, because small sample sizes mean large within-studies variation. The uncertainty increases further if the combined studies differ in important design characteristics (Table 5-4), because such differences among the reports mean that the individual studies should be expected to measure different treatment effects. The more the combined studies differ in important design characteristics, the greater the expected differences in the estimates of the treatment effect(s) calculated by these studies–and, therefore, the greater the between-studies variation, and the greater the uncertainty that surrounds the summary treatment effect calculated by the meta-analysis.

The 95% CI of the summary treatment effect measures this uncertainty that surrounds the average treatment effect reported by the meta-analysts. The 95% CI calculated from a fixed-effects analysis is an estimate of the within-studies variation in the combined studies. In contrast, the 95% CI calculated from a random-effects analysis is an estimate of both the within- and the between-studies variation, thus being, by necessity, wider than the 95% CI calculated from a fixed-effects analysis. The difference between these two 95% CIs is proportional to the between-studies variation–that is, it is proportional to the magnitude of the differences, among the combined reports, in study design attributes and in reported results.

Because the summary effect of an intervention calculated by a random- (compared to a fixed-) effects analysis is surrounded by a wider 95% CI, it is more difficult to detect a statistically significant ($p<0.05$) average treatment effect with a random-effects analysis than with any fixed-effects method.[86] Moreover, small studies have more of an impact on the calculated average treatment effect when a random-effects analysis, as opposed to a fixed-effects analysis, is undertaken. When the literature eligible for analysis consists of one (or a few) large investigations and many small studies, a single large report may dominate the findings of an overview conducted by a fixed-effects method. This analysis would take only the within-studies variation into account, and would thus weigh studies with large sample sizes (and small within-studies variation) more favorably than small reports. Therefore, the conclusions of the overview might primarily reflect the results of these few large studies, as opposed to the composite evidence from all completed investigations. In contrast, the findings of a meta-analysis calculated by the use of the random-effects method would reflect the combination of within- and between-studies variation. The more the combined studies differ in important design attributes, the more important the between-studies variation becomes, as compared to the within-studies variation. As a result, the influence of a single large study diminishes more, and the stated conclusions of the overview accomplish the purpose of the meta-analysis more, which is to examine the effect of a treatment in many different situations.

If there are no important design differences between the combined studies, random- and fixed-effects analyses will produce similar results. In contrast, if there are substantive differences among the studies, the two methods of analysis will produce disparate results.[86] Fixed- and random-effects analyses are based on different conceptions of the proper role, scope, and meaning of meta-analysis. Despite the differences in assumptions delineated above, there are strong opinions about the appropriateness of both lines of analysis. Several statisticians have expressed a preference for fixed-effects methods.[15,87,88] Others unconditionally favor random-effects analyses.[17,89] Bailey[90] discussed the circumstances, assumptions, and research questions under which one or the other approach is the more appropriate.

In the meta-analysis of studies of the hemostatic efficacy and capacity of pathogen-reduced platelets,[23] measures of hemostatic efficacy (1- and 24-hour CCIs, as well as the total number of platelet transfusions and the interval between platelet transfusions) were integrated by a fixed-effects method.[91] A fixed-effects method was used because the meta-analysis was undertaken to produce an estimate of the magnitude of the average effect of PR across the studies, as opposed to aiming to establish whether an effect of PR on the hemostatic efficacy of pathogen-reduced platelets exists. All studies had been consistent with regard to their findings vis-à-vis hemostatic efficacy (Figs 5-2 through 5-4), showing that PR reduces the hemostatic efficacy of the treated components owing to the incurred platelet losses.[29,30] Moreover, the four quantitative outcomes concerning hemostatic efficacy had been determined by similar criteria in all the available studies.[31-33,35,36] For these reasons, a fixed-effects method was used for the synthesis, so that each available study[31-33,35,36] would contribute to the calculation of the average effect of PR in proportion to its sample size.[15,87,88]

In contrast, study findings on bleeding complications[31,32,34-36] were integrated by using a random-effects method.[92] A random-effects method was used because the available RCTs had employed different criteria for determining the occurrence of bleeding complications (Table 5-4) and because the purpose of this part of the analysis was to investigate whether PR of platelets indeed results in a greater risk of bleeding complications than does transfusion of untreated components. An association of PR with a higher risk of bleeding complications (Fig 5-1) had not been established before the undertaking of the meta-analysis[23] and, when the results of Kerkhoffs et al[31] were presented, they appeared to contradict prevailing opinion.[24-28] Because of the variation in study characteristics (Table 5-4) and the integration of RCTs that had used two different PR technologies (Intercept[31-35] and Mirasol[36]), it was assumed that PR would have a different effect on bleeding complications in each study, depending on the study's characteristics. This assumption required the undertaking of a random-effects analysis.[17,89]

Assessment of the Combinability of the Reports Included in the Meta-Analysis

Statistical Homogeneity of RCTs That Were Eligible for Analysis

Regardless of whether a fixed- or a random-effects method is used to integrate the findings of eligible studies, results of separate investigations can be combined by the techniques of meta-analysis only when the estimates of effect size are sufficiently close to one another.[1-7,88,93-95] This prerequisite is referred to as the "homogeneity of effects." The opposite situation–that is, the existence of sizable differences between investigations in the estimate of the effect of an intervention–is known as the "heterogeneity of effects." A discussion of the issue of homogeneity must precede the pooling of the results of the studies in any report of a meta-analysis. Study results cannot be combined in the presence of unexplained heterogeneity, and homogeneity of effects is a prerequisite for undertaking a quantitative research synthesis. Statistical reviewers of the US Food and Drug Administration have denigrated as mere computational exercises all overviews that combined heterogeneous reports.[93-95]

Homogeneity is assessed statistically by the Q test statistic, which examines whether the variation in the findings of the studies is sufficiently modest to be attributed to chance.[1-7] If $p<0.10$ for the Q test statistic, there is a <10% probability that the disagreements among the results of the available studies might have arisen by chance. In this situation, the hypothesis of homogeneity of effects is rejected, and the results of the studies cannot be combined. If a large number of studies is available for analysis, meta-analysts may consider that the hypothesis of homogeneity of effects is rejected if $p<0.05$ for the Q test statistic. However, the power of the Q test statistic to detect differences among studies depends on the number of the reports that are available for analysis. If the number of eligible studies is small, the power of the Q test statistic becomes unacceptably low, and some other arbitrary cutoff point (eg, $p<0.10$ or even $p<0.20$) should be selected by the meta-analysts for determining whether the noted disagreements among eligible studies are sufficiently modest to be attributed to chance.

The Q test statistic is a chi-square test with $n-1$ degrees of freedom (where n = the number of studies included in the overview). Because the Q test statistic depends on the number of studies–being less sensitive to heterogeneity when the number of studies available for meta-analysis is small–an alternative test (I^2) has been proposed to assess the extent of heterogeneity among studies.[96,97] The I^2 test does not inherently depend on the number of studies included in the analysis, and its results are expressed as a percentage (ie, the percentage of total variation across studies attributed to heterogeneity). For this reason, it has intuitive meaning to the reader, and it can be directly compared between meta-analyses. Low heterogeneity corresponds to I^2 values of <25%, whereas high heterogeneity is reflected in I^2 values of >75%.[96] However, Higgins et al[96] did not indicate any specific cutoff value (eg, >75%) past which it is inappropriate to integrate studies, owing to heterogeneity. Instead, they suggested that quantification of heterogeneity is only one component of a wider investigation of variability across studies and that the interpretation of a given degree of heterogeneity will differ according to whether the estimates of effect from the various studies show the same direction of effects.

Meta-analysts should not rely on statistical tests alone for assessing the combinability of the available studies. Graphic displays of study-specific data (such as those shown in Figs 5-1 through 5-4) allow both analysts and readers to examine whether the available study findings are sufficiently close to one another, and whether the condition of homogeneity of effects is satisfied. For example, Fig 5-1 shows that the OR of bleeding complications in patients receiving pathogen-reduced platelets versus controls—although it did not attain statistical significance in most cases—has always been >1 in all RCTs, with the sole exception of all bleeding complications in the small RCT of Janetzko et al.[35] Thus, Fig 5-1 shows the typical situation that led to the introduction of statistical overviews in medicine. Before the findings of Kerkhoffs et al[31] were presented, treatment effects reported from all studies had operated in the same direction, but they had not attained statistical significance in any study, perhaps owing to the small sample size and inadequate statistical power of each report. (Although the frequency of clinically significant bleeding complications as defined in the meta-analysis[23] had differed significantly in the expanded safety analysis of the SPRINT RCT,[34] a significant difference had not been reported by the investigators in either the initial[33] or the subsequent[34] analysis of that study, because of the manner in which the outcome variable had been defined; see below.) Similarly, Figs 5-2 through 5-4 show that the results of all available studies[31-33,35,36] have been consistent (ie, they have always operated in the same direction as well as attained statistical significance in the large studies) with regard to the 1- and 24-hour CCIs, the total number of platelet transfusions, and the interval between platelet transfusions.

Because the results of the studies have always operated in the same direction (Fig 5-1), when the magnitude of the variation in reported results was quantified by a Q test statistic, there was ≥50% probability that the variation in the results of the available studies in all three analyses included in Fig 5-1 could have arisen by chance ($p \geq 0.50$ for the Q test statistic). Such was the case, despite the fact that there was a severalfold difference between the OR of bleeding complications found by Kerkhoffs et al[31] and the ORs found by the earlier studies.[32,34-36] Across the studies included in the meta-analysis of the 1-hour CCI, the 24-hour CCI, the interval between platelet transfusions, and the total number of platelet transfusions (Figs 5-2 through 5-4), there was similar homogeneity of effects (respectively, $p>0.10$, $p>0.75$, $p>0.50$, and $p>0.25$ for the Q test statistic). Moreover, the results of the SPRINT RCT[33] that could not be included in the latter meta-analysis—because that study[33] had not reported the SD of the mean difference between the arms for these quantitative outcomes—were the mirror image of the findings of the meta-analysis of the three or four other studies.[31,32,35,36]

Selection of Estimates of Effect Reported by RCTs That Were Eligible for Analysis

The complexity of using bleeding as an endpoint[54,55] is underscored by the categorization of hemorrhagic events in the SPRINT trial by system-organ-class Medical Dictionary for Regulatory Activities (MedDRA, Version 3.3[98]) category[34] in addition to CTC Version 2.0 grade[34] and WHO grade,[33] and the reporting of information on bleeding complications in two different periods (the "transfusion" period and the "surveillance" period; Table 5-6). Because of the difficulties in using bleeding as an endpoint,[54,55] only the SPRINT trial[33] used WHO Grade 2 bleeding as its primary outcome; all four other studies[31,32,35,36] used the 1-hour CCI as their primary endpoint. This outcome is both accurate and reproducible, and it was consistently presented in all reports.[31-33,35,36]

To address the complexity of using bleeding as an outcome,[54,55] the meta-analysis[23] extracted from the reports of the five RCTs the bleeding information that could be considered most comparable,[31-36] and it did so over a period of observation (Table 5-6) that also could be regarded as the most comparable. The latter was the maximal period of observation during which information on hemorrhagic events had been made

Table 5-6. Period of Reporting Bleeding Complications in RCTs of the Hemostatic Capacity of Pathogen-Reduced Platelets

RCT	Period Under Observation*	Period during Which Bleeding Complications Were Reported†
euroSPRITE trial[32]	Up to 56 days, followed by a 28-day surveillance period‡ (Cycle 1)	Cycle 1
SPRINT trial[33,34]	Up to 28 days or until transfusion independence (defined as 7 days without platelet transfusions); a 7-day surveillance period followed	Period of platelet transfusion support[33] or both transfusion and surveillance periods[34§]
Janetzko et al[35]	Up to 28 days; hemostatic efficacy analyses pertained to the first eight platelet transfusions	Period during which patients were monitored for adverse events (entire study period)‖
Kerkhoffs et al[31]	Up to 42 days or up to five platelet transfusions	Same as period under observation
Mirasol Clinical Evaluation Study Group[36]	Up to 28 days or until transfusion independence; a 28-day surveillance period followed; hemostatic efficacy analyses pertained to the first eight platelet transfusions	Same as period under observation, but with bleeding assessments performed before and after "on-protocol" (as opposed to "off-protocol") transfusions

*If patients in a particular study were under observation for a longer period than in the other studies, they could manifest bleeding complications over a longer interval, and the RCT would potentially record bleeding complications in a higher proportion of patients.

†If the period during which bleeding complications were recorded had been less than the total study period, the RCT could have recorded a lower frequency of bleeding complications than did RCTs that recorded bleeding complications over the entire study period.

‡If additional platelet transfusion support was required, patients were asked to enroll for a second 56-day transfusion period and an additional 28-day adverse event surveillance period (Cycle 2).

§Bleeding complications were graded on the World Health Organization scale during the transfusion period[33] and on the Common Toxicity Criteria scale during both the transfusion and surveillance periods.[34]

‖Bleeding complications were not an endpoint of this study.

RCT = randomized controlled trial.

available. The RCTs of the Intercept technology had either presented information on bleeding complications by using the CTC scale[31,34] or categorized bleeding complications[32,35] as all or severe. The single RCT of the Mirasol technology[36] (which enrolled 110 of the 1080 experimental subjects) had presented information on bleeding complications only on the WHO scale.

Accordingly, the meta-analysis categorized bleeding complications as all or severe (with severe bleeding complications not categorized as such by the investigators corresponding to a grade 3 or greater on the CTC scale[31,34] or–if grading on the CTC scale was also unavailable–corresponding to a grade 3 or greater on the WHO scale[36]). This approach ensured the inclusion of information on all and on severe bleeding complications from all five RCTs.[31,32,34-36] For three[31,34,36] of the five RCTs, information was also available on clinically significant (ie, grade 2 or greater on either the CTC[31,34] or the WHO[36] scale) bleeding complications. Although this information was included in the analysis (middle section in Fig 5-1), it is less reliable than the information on all and on severe bleeding complications (top and bottom sections in Fig 5-1), owing to the difficulty (and resulting interobserver variation) in distinguishing between grade 1 and grade 2 bleeding.[54,55]

WHO grade 2 (as opposed to grade 2 or greater–ie, clinically significant; Fig 5-1) bleeding had been the primary outcome in the initial report of the SPRINT RCT.[33] During the transfusion period (Table 5-6), the proportion of patients having WHO grade 2 bleeding did not differ between the arms, although grade 2 bleeding occurred on a mean of 3.2 days in the PR arm as compared with 2.5 days in the control arm ($p<0.05$).[33] During both the transfusion and surveillance periods (Table 5-6), comparisons of bleeding complications separately for each CTC Version 2.0 grade yielded no significant difference.[34] The investigators reported significant differences only in individual minor hemorrhagic events, such as petechiae and fecal occult blood.[34]

Thus, the difference in the OR of bleeding complications between recipients of pathogen-reduced and non-pathogen-reduced platelets, as presented in the abstracts of the two reports of the SPRINT RCT[33,34] and in Fig 5-1, is due to the difference in the definition of bleeding complications between the two reports of the SPRINT RCT[33,34] and the meta-analysis.[23] Neither report of the SPRINT RCT[33,34] reported on all, clinically significant, and severe bleeding complications as defined in the meta-analysis[23] and as depicted in Fig 5-1. All and severe bleeding complications (as defined in the meta-analysis[23]) can be considered to represent hard endpoints that do not depend on interobserver variation. In contrast, owing to the difficulty in distinguishing between grade 1 and grade 2 bleeding complications,[54,55] WHO grade 2 bleeding (as used in the initial report of the SPRINT RCT[33]) represents a "soft" endpoint that is greatly influenced by interobserver variation.

More important, the clinically significant bleeding complications (grade 2 or greater on the CTC or WHO scale) depicted in Fig 5-1 represent a clinically far more meaningful endpoint than do the WHO grade 2 bleeding complications presented in the initial report of the SPRINT RCT[33] or the bleeding complications pertaining separately to each CTC grade, as presented in the expanded safety analysis of that same trial.[34] Both of the recent RCTs of platelet dose[56,57] reported on grade 2 or greater bleeding complications, including both symptomatic grade 2 bleeding necessitating some medical intervention–yet not being severe enough to require RBC transfusion–and bleeding requiring RBC transfusion (grade 3) as well as catastrophic (grade 4) bleeding. Such information (on grade 2 or greater bleeding complications) was available for the SPRINT RCT, although it was not based on daily assessments of bleeding complications by trained assessors[33]; it derived instead from "spontaneous" reports of hemorrhagic events by blinded study personnel.[34] Although daily assessments by trained assessors are the optimal method for grading bleeding as an endpoint, results of this approach from the SPRINT RCT have been reported only in the narrow context of the grade 2 bleeding complications.[33]

Any integration of the information on grade 2 bleeding complications from the SPRINT study[33] with the information on either severe or all bleeding complications from the other RCTs[31,32,35,36] would have been medically meaningless. Such integration would mix symptomatic bleeding complications severe enough to require some intervention (albeit not RBC transfusion) from the SPRINT RCT[33] with either bleeding complications requiring RBC transfusion and catastrophic bleeding complications from the other studies[31,32,35,36] or clinically unimportant (in addition to symptomatic, requiring RBC transfusion, and/or catastrophic) bleeding complications from the other RCTs.[31,32,35,36] The meta-analysis[23] avoided such a vacuous mathematical exercise by using the results from the expanded safety analysis of the SPRINT RCT,[34] which had presented information on all (grade 1 through 4), severe (grade 3 and 4), and clinically significant (grade 2 through 4) bleeding complications. Thus, all results on bleeding complications integrated by the meta-analysis[23] pertained to bleeding of similar severity. The downside of this approach was that the results on grade 2 bleeding from the SPRINT RCT,[33] which had been obtained by the optimal method for assessing bleeding complications–that is, through daily assessments of bleeding by trained and blinded assessors–were not used in the meta-analysis.[23]

Statistical Heterogeneity of RCTs That Were Eligible for Analysis

Unlike the situation with the RCTs of the hemostatic efficacy and capacity of pathogen-reduced platelets, when the studies available for meta-analysis are heterogeneous, any reported estimates of average treatment effects calculated across the studies should be regarded as fictional. Instead of pooling results, meta-analysts should present an analysis of the possible reasons for disagreements among the available investigations.[1-7,99-104] According to Ellenberg,[104] meta-analyses would be less controversial and more useful if they focused less on the overall results and more on the variation in the reported results. In Goodman's words, "regardless of the summary number, meta-analyses should shed light on why trial results differ."[7] The simplest method for explaining heterogeneity is a stratification of the eligible studies on the basis of design, quality, clinical profile of the enrolled patients, and/or other characteristics. Providing that the hypothesis of homogeneity of effects is not rejected within each stratum after such stratification of the available studies, the calculated stratum-specific average treatment effects may help explain the disagreements among the available reports (see Chapter 1 for a discussion of the situation of heterogeneity of effects). Regression techniques offer a more elegant method for explaining heterogeneity among studies, but their use requires that many studies have already become available.[99]

The Medical Interpretation of Overviews

In overviews addressing medical issues, research questions must be stated with "no less thorough a biologic discussion than would appear in a traditional review,"[7] and the findings must be discussed in the context of a review of pathophysiologic principles and results of basic laboratory research and individual trials.[105] Most important, the relevance of the findings to patient care must be explained to the reader. In addition, readers of overviews must be reminded that meta-analyses use historical material from studies published over a considerable period[105]; this historical nature of the material may influence the applicability of the findings of a meta-analysis to contemporary clinical care.

Medical Heterogeneity of the RCTs of the Hemostatic Efficacy and/or Capacity of Pathogen-Reduced Platelets

Although the RCTs of the hemostatic efficacy and capacity of pathogen-reduced platelets[31,32,34-36] were statistically homogeneous ($p \geq 0.50$ for the Q test statistic when bleeding complications were investigated), these same studies nonetheless were medically heterogeneous. They differed in the PR technology used (Intercept[31,32,34,35] or Mirasol[36]), the clinical profile of the enrolled patients (unselected,[31] moderately selected,[34] or selected[32,35,36] hemato-oncology patients with hypoproliferative thrombocytopenia), and the design aspects of the studies (ie, ascertainment of bleeding complications on a daily[31,34] or less frequent[32,35,36] schedule, and five study characteristics that differed between the RCT of Kerkhoffs et al[31] and the other studies).[32,34-36]

The difference between all and clinically significant bleeding complications across the four RCTs of the Intercept technology[31,32,34,35] did not attain significance (respectively, summary OR = 1.51; 95% CI = 0.99-2.31; and summary OR = 1.57; 95% CI = 0.97-2.54), although this difference did attain significance in the overall analysis of all five RCTs (Fig 5-1; respectively, summary OR = 1.58; 95% CI = 1.11-2.26; and summary OR = 1.54; 95% CI = 1.11-2.13). Although the results did not attain significance across the Intercept studies,[31,32,34,35] the findings of the integration of these four RCTs (Fig 5-5) were consistent with the results of the overall meta-analysis (Fig 5-1). It is possible that the results of the integration of these four RCTs, as opposed to all five RCTs, did not attain significance because the sample size was reduced from 1080 to 970 subjects.

The population of hemato-oncology patients enrolled in each study correlated with the reported results. As already discussed in the section on study quality and as shown in Table 5-6, at one end of the spectrum, three RCTs[32,35,36] had enrolled selected hemato-oncology patients, excluding patients with splenomegaly and DIC[32,35,36] and with infection/fever,[35,36] in addi-

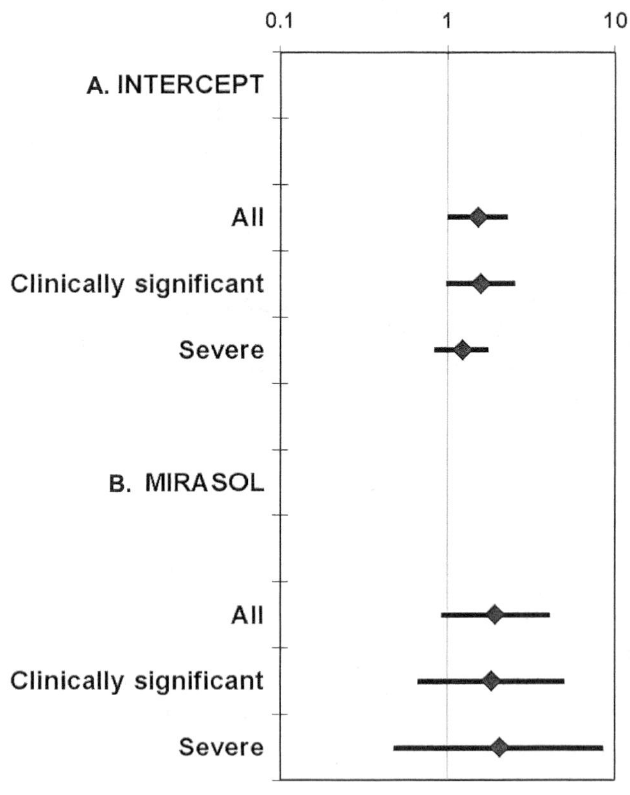

Figure 5-5. Odds ratios (ORs) of all bleeding complications, clinically significant bleeding complications, and severe bleeding complications in patients receiving pathogen-reduced or untreated platelets in the four randomized controlled trials (RCTs) of the Intercept tehnology[31,32,34,35] versus those in the single RCT of the Mirasol technology.[36] When the available RCTs[31,32,34-36] are stratified by employed PR technology, the trend toward an increase in bleeding complications in recipients of pathogen-reduced (rather than non-pathogen-reduced) platelets does not attain significance across the available studies. The studies of the Intercept technology were statistically homogeneous (p>0.10 for the *Q* test statistic) in all analyses.

tion to patients with other factors predisposing to platelet consumption. These studies[32,35,36] did not observe a difference between recipients of pathogen-reduced and non-pathogen-reduced platelets in all or clinically significant bleeding complications (Fig 5-6). In the middle of the road, the SPRINT RCT[34] did not list splenomegaly, DIC, or infection/fever among the exclusion criteria, and—in its expanded safety analysis[34]—it observed an increase in clinically significant bleeding complications in recipients of pathogen-reduced platelets. At the other end of the spectrum, Kerkhoffs et al[31] enrolled unselected hemato-oncology patients, using only the follow-

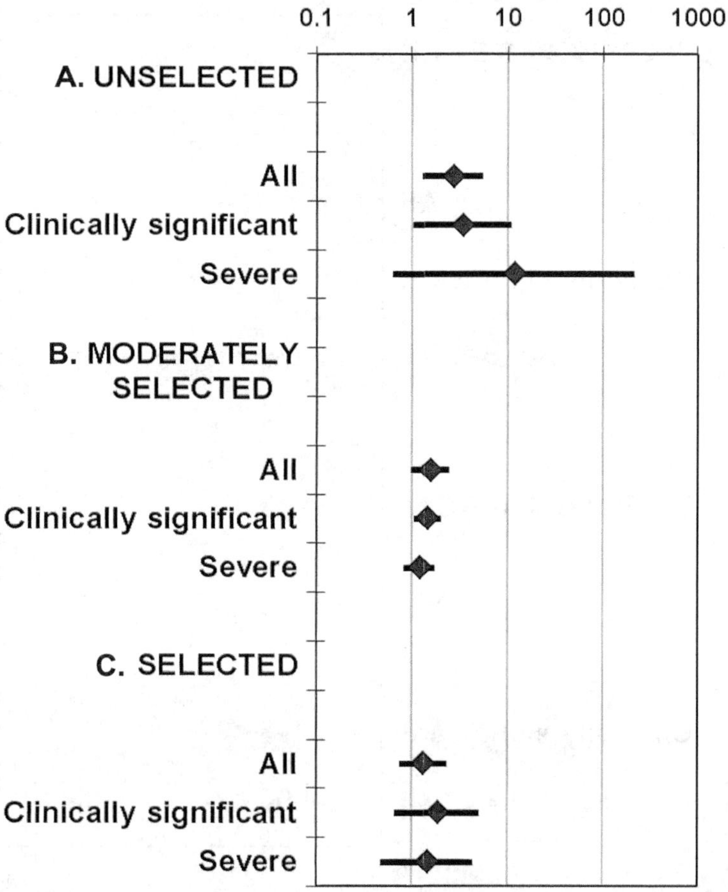

Figure 5-6. Correlation between the clinical profile of the enrolled hemato-oncology patients with hypoproliferative thrombocytopenia and the corresponding study findings in the five available randomized controlled trials (RCTs).[31,32,34-36] For each stratum, the figure shows the odds ratio (OR) of all bleeding complications, clinically significant bleeding complications, and severe bleeding complications in patients receiving pathogen-reduced platelets versus controls. Only Kerkhoffs et al[31] enrolled unselected hemato-oncology patients, and only the SPRINT RCT[34] enrolled moderately selected patients. Three studies[32,35,36] enrolled selected hemato-oncology patients. The difference attains statistical significance ($p<0.05$) only in the analysis of all and clinically significant bleeding complications in the RCT of Kerkhoffs et al[31] and in the analysis of clinically significant bleeding complications in the SPRINT RCT.[34] All integrated studies were statistically homogeneous ($p>0.10$ for the *Q* test statistic).

ing two exclusion criteria: 1) patients with HLA or platelet-specific alloantibodies and current refractoriness to platelet transfusions requiring support with apheresis components from matched donors and 2) pregnant or pediatric patients. Kerkhoffs et al[31] observed a greater incidence of both all and clinically significant bleeding complications in patients receiving pathogen-reduced than in those receiving non-pathogen-reduced platelets (Fig 5-7).

Although PR results in a predictable loss of platelets,[29,30] the euroSPRITE trial[32] and the RCT of Janetzko et al[35] reported no statistically significant reduction in the 1-hour CCI of

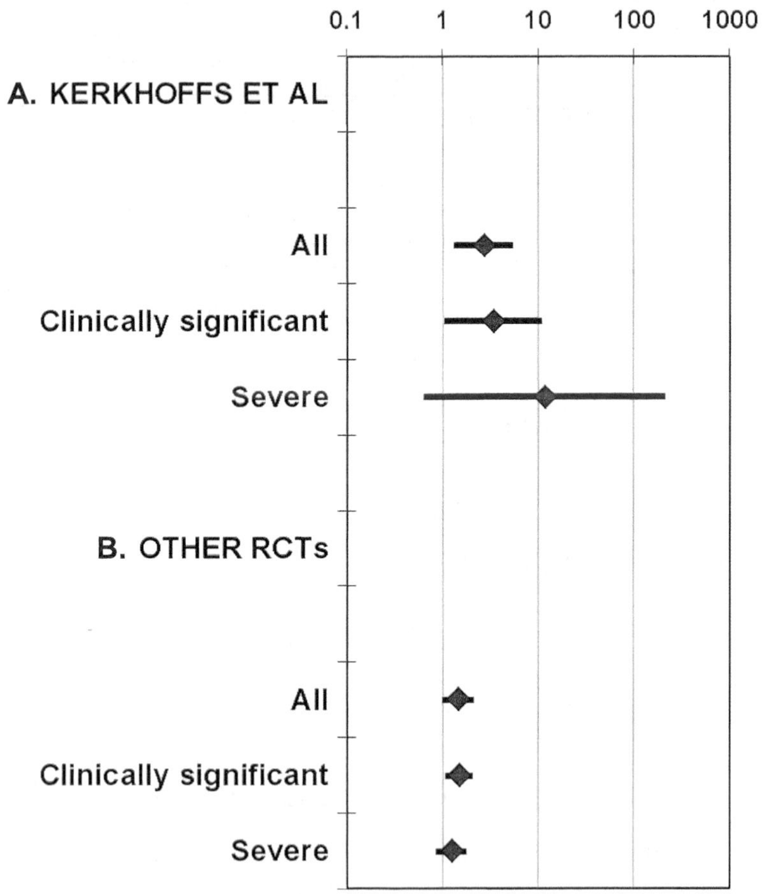

Figure 5-7. Odds ratios (ORs) of all bleeding complications, clinically significant bleeding complications, and severe bleeding complications in patients receiving pathogen-reduced or untreated platelets in the randomized controlled trial (RCT) of Kerkhoffs et al[31] versus those in the other studies.[32,34-36] Kerkhoffs et al[31] reported a statistically significant ($p<0.05$) difference for all and for clinically significant bleeding complications. The analysis shown for Kerkhoffs et al[31] is limited to a subgroup analysis of 179 of the 278 patients included in that study: patients receiving pathogen-reduced platelets were compared with patients receiving platelets suspended in a platelet additive solution (PAS-III). Across the four other studies,[32,34-36] the difference does not attain significance in the case of all bleeding complications (summary OR = 1.44; 95% CI = 0.98-2.12). Across the two RCTs that reported on clinically significant bleeding complications (the SPRINT trial[34] and the Mirasol RCT[36]), however, there is a significant difference in clinically significant bleeding (summary OR = 1.48; 95% CI = 1.06-2.07). All integrated studies were statistically homogeneous ($p>0.10$ for the *Q* test statistic).

patients receiving pathogen-reduced platelets as compared with the 1-hour CCI of patients receiving non-pathogen-reduced platelets (Fig 5-2). The euroSPRITE trial[32] increased the platelet dose given to the treatment arm (five to six buffy-coat WBD platelet concentrates, compared with four to five concentrates given to the control arm), and it transfused platelets with possibly impaired hemostatic capacity[38-43] (stored in PAS-II) to approximately half of the control patients (Table 5-4). Moreover, both the euroSPRITE trial[32] and Janetzko et al[35] transfused platelets prophylactically when the platelet count decreased to 20,000/µL (as opposed to 10,000/µL) (Table 5-4). These factors, along with the enrollment of selected hemato-oncology patients, could account for the lack of impairment in the hemostatic efficacy of the platelets given to the PR arm of these two RCTs.[32,35]

Totality of the Evidence on the Hemostatic Efficacy and/or Capacity of Pathogen-Reduced Platelets

The principal finding of the meta-analysis[23] of RCTs of the hemostatic efficacy and capacity of pathogen-reduced platelets was that the results of Kerkhoffs et al[31] were not inconsistent with the earlier literature. The five RCTs[31-36] integrated in that meta-analysis[23] were consistently homogeneous—that is, in all analyses, the variation in the findings of the studies could have arisen by chance. Concerning the studies of the Intercept technology,[31,32,34,35] the results of the studies represented a continuum, from the findings of the euroSPRITE trial[32] and Janetzko et al[35]—who observed no difference in the 1-hour CCI (Fig 5-2) or the bleeding complications (Fig 5-1)—to the middle-of-the-road results of the SPRINT RCT (Figs 5-1 and 5-2) and, further, to the recent findings of Kerkhoffs et al,[31] who observed larger differences between the randomization arms than had been reported by the SPRINT trial. The results of the single RCT of the Mirasol technology[36] were similar to the findings of the SPRINT study[33,34] (Figs 5-1 and 5-2).

Accordingly, because the five available RCTs[31-36] represent a continuum, the accumulated experience from all 1080 subjects included in the meta-analysis[23] should, in the future, always be considered in its entirety. Only when all 1080 subjects are considered together is the entire population of hemato-oncology patients represented. That population consists of selected,[32,35,36] moderately selected,[33] and unselected[31] patients (Table 5-4), which necessitates the consideration of all five available studies[31-36] together (Fig 5-5).

On the basis of the totality of the evidence hitherto adduced, the transfusion of pathogen-reduced platelets is associated with a 58% increase in the odds of all bleeding complications and a 54% increase in the odds of clinically significant bleeding complications than is the transfusion of non-pathogen-reduced platelets (Fig 5-1). This difference reflects the reduction in the hemostatic capacity of pathogen-reduced platelets that the transfusion-medicine community must explicitly tolerate to reap the benefits[24-28] of PR.

The meta-analysis showed a significant increase in all bleeding complications secondary to PR, but it also found that severe bleeding complications do not differ between subjects transfused with pathogen-reduced platelets and those transfused with untreated platelets. It is possible that the failure to detect a 25% (Fig 5-1) increase in the risk of severe bleeding complications may be due to the inadequacy of a sample of 1080 subjects for establishing such a small difference in risk. Alternatively, it is possible that PR is indeed not associated with an increased risk of severe bleeding complications. Two facts favor the latter possibility: 1) observational studies following the implementation of PR in some countries[61] did not record an increase in bleeding complications, and 2) the number of RBC transfusions administered to recipients of pathogen-reduced platelets was not greater than the number administered to recipients of non-pathogen-reduced platelets across the five available RCTs[31-33,35,36] (summary mean difference across four RCTs[31,32,35,36] was 0.31; 95% CI = –0.84-0.24; p>0.05). The summary mean difference calculated by the meta-analysis across these 4 studies is consistent with the difference reported by the SPRINT RCT[33] ($p = 0.13$).

Medical Implications of the Totality of the Evidence

The cellular losses with PR do not exceed one-third of the total platelets[29,30] and should not have produced the threefold increase in clinically significant bleeding (Fig 5-1) recorded in the trial of Kerkhoffs et al.[31] Because 1) the patients of Kerkhoffs et al [31] received prophylactic platelet transfusions when their platelet count fell to <10,000/µL, and 2) the Determination of the Optimal Prophylactic Platelet Dose to Prevent Bleeding in Thrombocytopenic Patients (PLADO) RCT showed that recipients of half the standard platelet dose have the same risk of bleeding as do recipients of the standard or double the standard platelet dose,[56] Kerkhoffs et al[31] would have been expected to find no increase in bleeding complications owing to the platelet losses induced by PR. If the expected platelet losses cannot account for the excess bleeding observed with PR, perhaps PR causes functional impairment of all the pathogen-reduced platelets in addition to causing loss of viability of a proportion of the treated platelets.[31] If that is the case, then—contrary to what we had previously assumed[24-28]—the platelet damage from PR cannot be overcome by merely increasing the platelet dose.[23,31] Introduction of PR in its current stage of development will result in an increase in mild and moderate—but perhaps not severe—bleeding complications, which we will have to explicitly tolerate to reap the benefits conferred by PR.[23]

It was known before the past 2 years that platelets have mRNA and mRNA splicing machinery and that they may translate mRNA into proteins affecting hemostasis and inflammation[106] (eg, platelets stored in the blood bank increase synthesis of integrin β3). It is now known, from data published in the past 2 years, that platelet microRNAs—small noncoding RNA species that play a key role in the posttranscriptional gene regulation for the majority of human genes[107,108]—are biologically and clinically relevant, both as potential regulators of platelet protein translation and expression and as biomarkers for platelet reactivity.[106]

Recently, Osman and Falker[109] identified 281 microRNA species in human platelets—a number corresponding to approximately 40% of all microRNAs listed in miRBase v14 (see http://www.mirbase.org), which is a relatively high number compared with the number of microRNA species found in nucleated cells. Nagalla et al[110] independently showed that platelet microRNA profiles are associated with, and may predict, platelet reactivity. They showed that platelets express 284 microRNAs, 74 of which were differentially expressed in 19 healthy subjects (such as blood donors) and spontaneously clustered into two groups according to platelet aggregation to epinephrine. A subset of these differentially expressed microRNAs predicted the platelet aggregation response. Moreover, platelet microRNAs were able to repress expression of platelet proteins. PR relies on the intercalation of chemicals into DNA and RNA, which is followed by exposure to ultraviolet light, to inhibit the DNA- and RNA-polymerase chain reaction and cell replication. In this way, PR prevents TAS and transfusion transmission of novel pathogens containing nucleic acids, but platelet microRNAs[106,109-112] may be as vulnerable to the effects of PR as are the nucleic acids of the pathogens themselves. (Double-stranded nucleic acids longer than 80 base pairs are the likely targets of Intercept; the precursor forms of microRNAs are double-stranded and close to 80 base pairs in length and thus potentially susceptible to inhibition by amotosalen in the presence of ultraviolet light.)

Platelet microRNAs inhibit protein synthesis by targeting mRNA for degradation or translational repression.[107,108] Because several different microRNAs may target one single mRNA, and because each microRNA may bind to several different mRNAs, a complex interaction network is created that is hard to unravel.[109] For this reason, a determination of whether inhibition of platelet microRNAs by PR systems can adversely affect platelet function (provided that continued synthesis of proteins by platelets stored in the blood bank affects platelet function) can be reached only by direct comparisons of the microRNA profiles (and ideally the proteome) of pathogen-reduced and non-pathogen-reduced platelets stored for 1 to 5 days after PR.[113] If the microRNA profiles (or proteome) differ between pathogen-reduced and non-pathogen-reduced platelets, an adverse effect of PR on platelet function (although not proven directly by such an experiment) can be indirectly inferred from the increase in bleeding complications in association with PR that was reported by Kerkhoffs et al[31] and by the meta-analysis of the five available RCTs (Fig 5-1).[23] A difference in microRNA profiles (or proteome) between pathogen-reduced and non-pathogen-reduced platelets would permit an inference that PR leads to functional impairment of all treated platelets because—despite the greater number of platelet transfusions given to recipients of pathogen-reduced platelets than to recipients of non-pathogen-reduced platelets to maintain a platelet count of $\geq 10{,}000/\mu L$[113] (Fig 5-4)—bleeding complications occurred more often in recipients of treated platelets than in those of untreated platelets.

The study of the riboflavin-UVA light (Mirasol) technology[36] accounted upfront for the platelet losses inflicted by PR by not transfusing the pathogen-reduced components in which the platelet content was below the minimum allowed by French standards (3.0×10^{11} platelets per transfused component). Despite this, the study of the Mirasol technology[36] failed to show noninferiority of the pathogen-reduced platelets. What the transfusion medicine community is willing to tolerate to reap the benefits of PR was a priori stated to be a 20% reduction in the 1-hour posttransfusion CCI. However, the mean difference in the 1-hour CCI between recipients of treated and untreated platelets was 5214, and the 95% CI of the mean difference (2887-7452) contained the a priori specified upper limit (2940) of the zone of noninferiority. Although a subsequent RCT administering a single experimental transfusion of platelets stored beyond the allowed storage period (and either pathogen-reduced with the Intercept technology or not) found noninferiority of the pathogen-reduced platelets, that study[60] had defined noninferiority as a "tolerable" 30% reduction in the 1-hour posttransfusion CCI.

Whether a 30%[60] or 20%[36] reduction in 1-hour CCI secondary to PR is "tolerable" is in the eye of the beholder. As AuBuchon said, "The proof of the pudding for a platelet component is its ability to prevent and treat hemorrhage,"[28] and, accordingly, the meta-analysis[23] (Fig 5-1) concentrated on the hemostatic capacity (rather than the efficacy) of pathogen-reduced (as compared with non-pathogen-reduced) platelets.

Because platelet losses alone cannot account for the finings of Kerkhoffs et al,[31] the research question continues to be whether pathogen-reduced platelets are capable of preventing bleeding, and investigations of the cost-effectiveness of PR (such as whether PR can permit extension of the allowed storage period of platelets[58,60]) are premature. Further research and development are needed vis-à-vis the PR of platelets. It is hoped that transfusion of pathogen-reduced platelets will eventually emerge as the optimal risk-reduction strategy for TAS and TTIs after the PR technologies have been licensed by the FDA. To choose between pathogen-reduced and non-pathogen-reduced platelets, the nature of the platelet damage caused by PR (cellular losses compared with functional impairment of the surviving platelets) and the increased risk of bleeding complications need to be, respectively, elucidated and more precisely quantified, so that they can be weighed against the competing risks of TAS and emerging TTIs (Chapter 2).

Observational studies after the implementation of PR in some countries[61] did not observe an increase in mild and moderate bleeding complications among the recipients of pathogen-reduced platelets, as would have been expected from the totality of the evidence on the hemostatic capacity of treated platelets hitherto adduced (Fig 5-1). However, these studies[61] also did not document the expected increase in the number of platelet transfusions owing to the platelet losses caused by PR. Most likely, platelet transfusions had been previously overused, so that the effective reduction in platelet dose caused by PR did not result in a visibly greater need for platelets.[28] It is also possible that the expected increase in mild and moderate (as opposed to severe) bleeding complications might have gone unnoticed outside the framework of an RCT.

The meta-analysis[23] was criticized[114] for having integrated RCTs that used two different PR technologies (Intercept[31,32,34,35] and Mirasol[36]) and for excluding the RCT of Lozano et al.[60] Insofar as different mechanisms of action are postulated for the Intercept and the Mirasol) technologies,[115] it can be argued[114] that the findings of the Intercept RCTs (Fig 5-5) should be considered alone—no matter whether eligibility is limited, for the aforementioned reasons, to the four studies[31,32,34,35] shown in Fig 5-5, or whether the RCT of Lozano et al[116] is included as well (see Fig 4-1). Whether it is appropriate to consider the RCTs of the Intercept technology[31,32,35,36] separately from the RCT(s) of the Mirasol technology[36] will perhaps depend on whether the results from experimental studies comparing the microRNA profiles (and ideally the proteome) of platelets stored for 1 to 5 days after PR with the Intercept versus the Mirasol technology show a difference in the microRNA profiles or proteome according to technology. (If Mirasol alters the proteome of stored platelets and Intercept does not, the argument of Corash[114] will be proven correct.) The argument that it is inappropriate to combine the results of both Intercept and Mirasol studies[114] could also be deemed reasonable, on the basis of what we already know about the differences in the mechanism of action between these two PR systems.[115]

Whether the conclusions vis-à-vis any increase in bleeding complications secondary to treatment with Intercept are based on the findings depicted in Fig 5-5 or in Fig 4-1, the available RCTs of the Intercept technology indicate a trend toward a greater risk of bleeding complications in association with PR. Therefore, before PR is adopted for routine use, further RCTs need to be conducted[117] to investigate whether this trend represents a true increase in the risk of bleeding or whether it should be ascribed to random variation.

Bias in Meta-Analytic Research

The value of meta-analysis in combining patient populations enrolled in separate studies for the purpose of documenting the existence of a treatment effect has been questioned.[118,119] This scrutiny of the value of overviews in the medical literature was in part provoked by three discordant reports[120-122] on the degree of agreement between overviews of small trials and subsequently published large RCTs.[123] Meta-analyses and large trials disagree 10% to 35% of the time—that is, more often than would be expected by chance.[120-122] Until the reasons for the disagreements are better understood, medical practitioners should not rely on meta-analyses for concluding that the existence of a treatment effect has been established. As discussed below, the findings of meta-analyses are susceptible to the effects of selection bias and observation bias, in a manner similar to the results of traditional observational original reports.

An observational study conducted at a single institution and investigating the effect of a treatment on a disease must enroll all patients who are sequentially admitted to that hospital with a specific diagnosis. If subjects are missed or excluded, selection bias may occur.[124(pp194-219)] Similarly, the validity of a meta-analysis depends on complete sampling of all studies performed on a particular topic. Validity can be preserved if a representative sample is obtained, but any incomplete sample is a potentially biased one.[125] Unfortunately, meta-analysts may not be able to locate all published studies, because computerized databases do not cover all periodicals, search algorithms often fail to identify relevant articles, and the indexing of studies is imperfect.[126-130] Even if the literature is optimally searched, studies published as government reports, book chapters, dissertations, conference proceedings, and such may not be captured, and unpublished studies will not be identified. Published trials differ systematically from unpublished ones, in that they are more likely both to have a larger sample and to have generated statistically significant results.[131] Systematic exclusion of small and negative studies from a meta-analysis that conditions eligibility on achievement of publication status is referred to as "publication bias."[131-141]

There is ample evidence of publication bias in the medical literature. Easterbrook et al[142] documented 3.8-fold better odds of publication (95% CI = 1.5-9.8) for observational studies reporting statistically significant findings than for studies with null results. Multivariate analysis showed that the better odds of publication could not be explained by the quality of study design. On the contrary, there was a trend toward a greater number of statistically significant results with poorer-quality studies.[142] Chalmers et al[143] corroborated the finding of Easterbrook et al[142] that achievement of publication status does not depend on the quality of study design. They also detected publication bias favoring studies with larger samples but no such bias for studies with statistically significant results.[143]

This author is not aware of any concrete examples of publication bias favoring investigations with null findings. However, Detsky et al[144] reported that studies of parenteral nutrition that were presented as abstracts had shown larger differences than did trials published in complete form. Begg and Berlin[132] speculated that, in past decades, publication bias might have favored the reporting of studies that had observed no association between asbestos and cancer.

Long-term solutions to the problem of publication bias must involve editors,[145] investigators,[146] and sponsors of research.[147,148] For example, editors could provide space for short reports of negative studies and could encourage peer review on the basis of methods, rather than results.[149] Investigators could report all trials in summary form,[143] providing that the summary is structured and contains specific methodologic details.[150] Interim solutions might involve attempts, on the part of meta-analysts, to locate unpublished data sets. For example, analysts could contact registries of clinical trials[139,151] or experts conducting original research on a particular hypothesis.[152] However, these attempts often are laborious and unsuccessful.[152] In addition, unpublished data sets must be assessed for quality—an often formidable task.[144]

A specific type of publication bias is the "Tower of Babel"[153] (ie, English-language[154]) bias. Although differences in quality between English and non-English reports are small,[154,155] authors are more likely to publish RCTs in English-language journals if the results are statistically significant.[154,155] Accordingly, if RCTs published in languages other than English are excluded, the findings of meta-analyses may be biased toward the reporting of statistically significant results. Grégoire et al[153] reported that 72% of the meta-analyses in their survey had restricted the literature search to studies published in English.

Selection bias can arise not only during retrieval of studies from the literature, but also during assessment of the eligibility of the retrieved reports. In evaluating the quality of investigations, analysts may be influenced by knowledge of the results of a study or by the journal of publication. They may even be inclined to modify eligibility criteria, so as to include in the overview reports from prestigious journals. According to Felson,[125] selection bias is the principal reason for discrepant results in meta-analyses. Different teams of analysts may base their conclusions on alternative sets of original reports, generating either statistically significant or null (ie, statistically insignificant) findings.

Information bias similar to that arising in clinical observational research[124(pp220-241)] can also occur in meta-analysis.[125] Data extracted from the same original report can vary among analysts.[156,157] However, information bias is investigator-initiated and thus is preventable by the use of a strict working protocol. Specific recommendations for its prevention have been offered.[125,156-158]

Conclusions

Meta-analyses are a supplement to RCTs, which remain the gold standard for evaluating the efficacy of therapeutic interventions, but which need to be supplemented by meta-analyses in order to broaden the applicability of their findings. Furthermore, meta-analyses can be an important research tool for the systematic evaluation of the quality of published studies and for the disciplined investigation of reasons for disagreements among reports. Overviews can identify errors and shortcomings in completed studies and may be able to explain why trial results differ. In the past, narrative reviews of the literature served these functions in a less formal manner. Because of their objective and quantitative nature, meta-analyses are much better suited for these purposes.

Meta-analyses also have been used to establish the existence of a treatment effect in situations where multiple small RCTs have been conducted but have not demonstrated a statistically significant effect, perhaps because of their small sample size. The value of meta-analysis in this area has been questioned.[118-120,132] However, the controversy over this specific use of meta-analysis should not detract from the value of overviews in assessing the quality of completed studies and the reasons for disagreements among reports. Future meta-analyses will likely find a more suitable role in addressing potential sources of heterogeneity, in lieu of trying to fit a summary estimate of the effect of an intervention among diverse studies.[123]

Guidelines for the conduct of meta-analyses have been developed[1-7,20,21] so that the two recurrent criticisms of the method (ie, the "garbage in–garbage out"[18] and "apples and oranges"[19] metaphors) can be avoided. Certainly, in mixing apples and oranges–and an occasional lemon–one does end up with an artificial product that probably has no biologic meaning whatsoever. However, the existing guidelines[1-7,20,21] require that the quality of eligible studies be assessed before the inclusion of the studies in an overview and also that the combinability of the subset of acceptable studies be shown before any quantitative research synthesis. If these two rules are followed, they should preclude any apple–orange–lemon combination. In fact, it might be impossible to publish any bad meta-analyses in the future if analysts managed to always resist the temptation to include poor-quality studies and/or to combine treatment effects in the presence of unexplained heterogeneity.

Critics of overviews should recognize that, had it not been for meta-analysis, many of the deficiencies in the quality of published research would not have been identified. In addition, investigators, editors, and readers might not have become aware of the extent of publication bias in medical research and of its implications for health policy formulation and the organization of patient care.[142] Meta-analyses are, and should be treated as, observational and retrospective original reports. Quantitative results from overviews (including p values and 95% CIs for summary treatment effects) should be considered as hypothesis-generating, rather than hypothesis-testing. A hypothesis formulated by a meta-analysis may or may not be corroborated when a "definitive" RCT is conducted. However, the limitations of the reported research and the reasons for disagreements among the studies–as identified by a meta-analysis–can guide the design and conduct of such a "definitive" RCT in the future. Meta-analysts can make a substantial contribution to the literature and may even overcome the aversion of clinicians for statistical reports, if they concentrate on the qualitative aspects of the analysis and "use statistics to clarify, not to obfuscate."[7]

Because meta-analysis is a partially technical method, many clinicians find themselves unable to appreciate its nuances and limitations in the same way that they can appreciate the nuances and limitations of a traditional original report. However, it is possible to critically read a report of a meta-analysis, by simply determining the extent to which the analysts have followed the sequence of required steps listed in Table 5-1. Readers of the medical literature need to be familiar with the definitions and assumptions of fixed- and random-effects analyses and with the meaning of the results of the Q or the I test statistic.[159] Indeed, it is necessary for readers of the medical literature to develop the skills necessary to comprehend and evaluate published reports of meta-analyses, because health policy guidelines–and perhaps also recommendations for patient management–are already based and are likely to be increasingly based in the future on input from statistical overviews.

References

1. Goodman SN. Meta-analysis in health services research. In: Armenian HK, Shapiro S, eds. Epidemiology and health services. New York: Oxford University Press, 1998:229-59.
2. Jenicek M. Meta-analysis in medicine: Where we are and where we want to go. J Clin Epidemiol 1989;42:35-44.
3. L'Abbé KA, Detsky AS, O'Rourke K. Meta-analysis in clinical research. Ann Intern Med 1987;107:224-33.
4. Glass GV, McGraw B, Smith ML. Meta-analysis in social research. Beverly Hills, CA: Sage Publications, 1981.
5. Light RJ, Pillemer DB. Summing up: The science of reviewing research. Cambridge, MA: Harvard University Press, 1984.
6. Cooper H, Hedges LV, eds. The handbook of research synthesis. New York: Russell Sage Foundation, 1994.
7. Goodman SN. Have you ever meta-analysis you didn't like? (editorial) Ann Intern Med 1991;114:244-6.
8. Glass GV. Primary, secondary, and meta-analysis of research. Educ Res 1976;5:3-8.
9. Fleiss JL, Tytum A, Ury HK. A simple approximation for calculating sample sizes for comparing independent proportions. Biometrics 1980;36:343-6.
10. Freiman JA, Chalmers RC, Smith H Jr, et al. The importance of beta, the type II error and sample size in the design and interpretation of the randomized controlled trial: Survey of 71 "negative" trials. N Engl J Med 1978;299:690-4.
11. Passamani E. Clinical trials: Are they ethical? N Engl J Med 1991;324:1589-91.
12. Hellman S, Hellman DS. Of mice but not men: Problems of the randomized clinical trial. N Engl J Med 1991;324:1585-9.
13. O'Rourke K, Detsky AS. Meta-analysis in medical research: Strong encouragement for higher quality in individual research efforts. J Clin Epidemiol 1989;42:1021-4.
14. Chalmers TC, Levin H, Sacks HS, et al. Meta-analysis of clinical trials as a scientific discipline. I. Control of bias and comparison with large co-operative trials. Stat Med 1987;6:315-25.
15. Peto R. Why do we need systematic overviews of randomized trials? Stat Med 1987;6:233-40.
16. Yusuf S. Obtaining medically meaningful answers from an overview of randomized clinical trials. Stat Med 1987;6:281-6.
17. Fleiss JL, Gross AJ. Meta-analysis in epidemiology, with special reference to studies of the association between exposure to environmental tobacco smoke and lung cancer: A critique. J Clin Epidemiol 1991;44:127-39.
18. Eysenck HJ. An exercise in megasilliness. Am Psychol 1978;35:517.
19. Wachter KW. Disturbed by meta-analysis? Science 1988;241:1407-8.
20. Moher D, Olkin I. Meta-analysis of randomized controlled trials: A concern for standards. JAMA 1995;274:1962-4.
21. Sacks HS, Berrier J, Reitman D, et al. Meta-analyses of randomized controlled trials. N Engl J Med 1987;316:450-5.
22. Proceedings of Methodologic Issues in Overviews of Randomized Clinical Trials Workshop. The National Heart, Lung, and Blood Institute and the National Cancer Institute. Bethesda, MD, May 15-16, 1986. Stat Med 1987;6:217-409.
23. Vamvakas EC. Meta-analysis of the randomized controlled trials of the hemostatic efficacy and capacity of pathogen-reduced platelets. Transfusion 2011;51:1048-71.
24. Allain JP, Bianco C, Blajchman MA, et al. Protecting the blood supply from emerging pathogens: The role of pathogen inactivation. Transfus Med Rev 2005;19:110-26.
25. McCullough J. Pathogen inactivation: A new paradigm for blood safety. Transfusion 2007;47:2180-4.
26. Klein HG, Anderson D, Bernardi MJ, et al. Pathogen inactivation: Making decisions about new technologies. Report of a consensus conference. Transfusion 2007;47:2338-47.
27. Vamvakas EC, Blajchman MA. Transfusion-related mortality: The on-going risks of allogeneic blood transfusion and the available strategies for their prevention. Blood 2009;113:3406-17.
28. AuBuchon JP. Current status of pathogen inactivation methods. ISBT Sci Series 2010;5:125-33.
29. Murphy S, Snyder E, Cable R, et al. Platelet dose consistency and its effect on the number of platelet transfusions for support of thrombocytopenia: An analysis of the SPRINT trial of platelets photochemically treated with amotosalen HCl and ultraviolet A light. Transfusion 2006;46:24-33.
30. Pineda A, McCullough J, Benjamin RJ, et al. Pathogen inactivation of platelets with a photochemical treatment with amotosalen HCl and

ultraviolet light: Process used in the SPRINT trial. Transfusion 2006;46:526-71.

31. Kerkhoffs JLH, van Putten WLJ, Novotny VMJ, et al. Clinical effectiveness of leukoreduced, pooled donor platelet concentrates, stored in plasma or additive solution with and without pathogen reduction. Br J Haematol 2010; 150:209-17.
32. van Rhenen D, Gulliksson H, Cazenave JP, et al. Transfusion of pooled buffy-coat platelet components prepared with a photochemical pathogen inactivation treatment: The euroSPRITE trial. Blood 2003;101:2426-33.
33. McCullough J, Vesole DH, Benjamin RJ, et al. Therapeutic efficacy and safety of platelets treated with a photochemical process for pathogen inactivation: The SPRINT trial. Blood 2004;104:1534-41.
34. Snyder E, McCullough J, Slichter SJ, et al. Clinical safety of platelets photochemically treated with amotosalen HCl and ultraviolet A light for pathogen inactivation: The SPRINT trial. Transfusion 2005;45:1864-75.
35. Janetzko K, Cazenave JP, Kluter H, et al. Therapeutic efficacy and safety of photochemically treated apheresis platelets processed with an optimized integrated set. Transfusion 2005;45: 1443-52.
36. The Mirasol Clinical Evaluation Study Group. A randomized controlled clinical trial evaluating the performance and safety of platelets treated with MIRASOL pathogen reduction technology. Transfusion 2010;50:2362-75.
37. Schrezenmeier H, Seifried E. Buffy-coat-derived pooled platelet concentrates and apheresis platelet concentrates: Which product type should be preferred? Vox Sang 2010;99:1-15.
38. van der Meer PF, Pietersz RNI, Reesink HW. Storage of platelets in additive solution up to 12 days with maintenance of good in vitro quality. Transfusion 2004;44:1204-11.
39. de Wildt-Eggen J, Gulliksson H. In-vivo and in-vitro comparison of platelets stored in either synthetic media or plasma. Vox Sang 2003;84: 256-64.
40. Wagner T, Vetter A, Dimonic N, et al. Ultrastructural changes and activation differences in platelet concentrates stored in plasma and additive solution. Transfusion 2002;42:719-27.
41. Bunescu A, Hild M, Lunbahl J, et al. Platelet storage in PAS-2 or autologous plasma: Impact on functional parameters. Transfus Med 2001;11:105-10.
42. Kerkhoffs JLH, Eikenboom JC, Schipperus MS, et al. A multicenter randomized study of the efficacy of transfusions with platelets stored in platelet additive solution II versus plasma. Blood 2006;108:3210-15.
43. van der Meer PF, Pietersz RNI, Tiekstra MJ, et al. WBC-reduced platelet concentrates from pooled buffy coats in additive solution: An evaluation of in vitro and in vivo measures. Transfusion 2001;41:917-22.
44. Turner VS, Mitchell SG, Hawker RJ. More on the comparison of Plasma-Lyte A and PAS 2 as platelet additive solutions. Transfusion 1996; 36:1033-4.
45. van Der Meer PF, Kerkhoffs JL, Carvers J, et al. In vitro comparison of platelet storage in plasma and in four platelet additive solutions, and the effect of pathogen reduction: A proposal for an in vitro rating system. Vox Sang 2010;98:517-24.
46. Dijkstra-Tiekstra MJ, Pietersz RN, Hendriks EC, et al. In vivo PLT increments after transfusions of WBC-reduced PLT concentrates stored for up to 7 days. Transfusion 2004;44:330-6.
47. Hogge DE, Thompson BW, Schiffer CA. Platelet storage for 7 days in second-generation blood bags. Transfusion 1986;26:131-5.
48. Slichter SJ, Davis K, Enright H, et al. Factors affecting post-transfusion platelet increments, platelet refractoriness, and platelet transfusion intervals in thrombocytopenic patients. Blood 2005;105:4106-14.
49. Klumpp TR, Herman JH, Innis S, et al. Factors associated with response to platelet transfusion following hematopoietic stem-cell transplantation. Bone Marrow Transplant 1996;17:1035-41.
50. Norol F, Kuentz M, Cordonnier C, et al. Influence of clinical status on the efficacy of stored platelet transfusion. Br J Hematol 1994;86: 125-9.
51. Bishop JF, Matthews JP, McGrath K, et al. Factors influencing 24-hour increments after platelet transfusion. Transfusion 1991;31:392-6.
52. Trotti A, Byhardt R, Stetz J, et al. Common toxicity criteria version 2.0. An improved reference for grading the acute effects of cancer treatment: Impact on radiotherapy. Int J Radiat Oncol Biol Phys 2000;47:13-47.
53. Miller AB, Hoogstraten B, Staquet M, et al. Reporting results of cancer treatment. Cancer 1981;47:207-14.
54. Webert KE, Cook RJ, Sigouin CS, et al. The risk of bleeding in thrombocytopenic patients with

acute myeloid leukemia. Haematologica 2006; 91:1530-7.
55. Heddle NM. Optimal timing and dosing of platelet transfusions. ISBT Sci Ser 2010;5:88-94.
56. Slichter SJ, Kaufman RM, Assmann SF, et al. Dose of prophylactic platelet transfusions and prevention of hemorrhage. N Engl J Med 2010; 362:600-13.
57. Heddle NK, Cook RJ, Tinmouth A, et al. A randomized controlled trial comparing standard- and low-dose strategies for transfusion of platelets (SToP) to patients with thrombocytopenia. Blood 2009;113:1564-73.
58. Simonsen AC, Johansson PI, Conlan MG, et al. Transfusion of 7-day-old amotosalen photochemically treated buffy-coat platelets to patients with thrombocytopenia: A pilot study. Transfusion 2006;46:424-33.
59. Slichter SJ, Raife TJ, Davis K, et al. Platelets photochemically treated with amotosalen HCl and ultraviolet A light correct prolonged bleeding times in patients with thrombocytopenia. Transfusion 2006;46:731-40.
60. Lozano M, Knutson N, Tardivel R, et al. A multicenter study of therapeutic efficacy and safety of platelet components prepared with pathogen inactivation (Intercept) stored for 6-7 days prior to transfusion. Vox Sang 2010;99(Suppl 1):13.
61. Osselaer JC, Messe N, Hervig T, et al. A prospective observational cohort safety study of 5106 platelet transfusions with components prepared with photochemical pathogen inactivation treatment. Transfusion 2008;48:1061-71.
62. AuBuchon JP, Herschel L, Roger J, et al. Efficacy of apheresis platelets treated with riboflavin and ultraviolet light for pathogen reduction. Transfusion 2005;45:1335-41.
63. Gerbarg ZB, Horowitz RI. Resolving conflicting clinical trials: Guidelines for meta-analysis. J Clin Epidemiol 1988;41:503-9.
64. Chalmers TC, Smith H Jr, Blackburn B, et al. A method for assessing the quality of a randomized controlled trial. Control Clin Trials 1981; 2:31-49.
65. Detsky AS, Naylor CD, O'Rourke K, et al. Incorporating variations in the quality of individual randomized trials into meta-analysis. J Clin Epidemiol 1992;45:255-65.
66. Zelen M. Guidelines for publishing papers on cancer clinical trials: Responsibilities of editors and authors. J Clin Oncol 1983;1:164-9.
67. Moher D, Jadad AR, Nichol G, et al. Assessing the quality of randomized controlled trials: An annotated bibliography of scales and checklists. Control Clin Trials 1995;16:62-73.
68. Moher D, Jadad AR, Tugwell P. Assessing the quality of reports of randomized trials. Int J Technol Assess Health Care 1996;12:195-208.
69. Lichtenstein MJ, Mulrow CD, Elwood PC. Guidelines for reading case-control studies. J Chron Dis 1987;40:893-903.
70. Feinstein AR. Clinical epidemiology: The architecture of clinical research. Philadelphia: Saunders, 1985:543-7.
71. Jadad AR, Moore RA, Carroll D, et al. Assessing the quality of reports of randomized trials: Is blinding necessary? Control Clin Trials 1996; 17:1-12.
72. Moher D, Jones BA, Cook DJ, et al. Does quality of reports of randomized trials affect estimates of intervention efficacy reported in meta-analyses? Lancet 1998;352:609-13.
73. Steinberg KK, Thacker SB, Smith SJ, et al. A meta-analysis of the effect of estrogen replacement therapy on the risk of breast cancer. JAMA 1991;265:1985-90.
74. Berlin JA, Colditz GA. A meta-analysis of physical activity in the prevention of coronary heart disease. Am J Epidemiol 1990;142:612-28.
75. Mantel N, Haenszel W. Statistical aspects of the analysis of data from retrospective studies of disease. J Natl Cancer Inst 1959;22:719-48.
76. Yusuf S, Peto R, Lewis J, et al. Beta blockade during and after myocardial infarction: An overview of the randomized trials. Prog Cardiovasc Dis 1985;27:335-71.
77. Klein S, Simes J, Blackburn GL. Total parenteral nutrition and cancer clinical trials. Cancer 1986;58:1378-86.
78. Slavin RE. Best-evidence synthesis: An alternative approach to traditional and meta-analytic reviews. Educ Res 1986;15(9):5-11.
79. Slavin RE. Best-evidence synthesis: Why less is more. Educ Res 1987;16(5):15-16.
80. Begg C, Cho M, Eastwood S, et al. Improving the quality of reporting of randomized controlled trials: The CONSORT statement. JAMA 1996;276:637-9.
81. Moher D, Schulz KF, Altman DG. The CONSORT statement: Revised recommendations for improving the quality of reports of parallel-group randomized trials. J Am Podiatr Med Assoc 2001;91:437-42.
82. Liberati A, Himel HN, Chalmers TC. A quality assessment of randomized controlled trials of primary treatment of breast cancer. J Clin Oncol 1986;4:942-51.

83. Delaney M, Meyer E, Cserti-Gazdewich C, et al. A systematic assessment of the quality of reporting for platelet transfusion studies. Transfusion 2010;50:2135-44.
84. Howard VJ, Grizzle J, Diener HC, et al. Comparison of multicenter study designs for investigation of carotid endarterectomy efficacy. Stroke 1992;23:583-93.
85. Fleiss JL. Multicenter clinical trials: Bradford Hill's contributions and some subsequent developments. Stat Med 1982;1:353-9.
86. Berlin JA, Laird NM, Sacks HS, Chalmers RC. A comparison of statistical methods for combining event rates from clinical trials. Stat Med 1989; 8:141-51.
87. Thompson SG, Pocock SJ. Can meta-analysis be trusted? Lancet 1991;338:1127-30.
88. Demets DL. Methods for combining randomized clinical trials: Strengths and limitations. Stat Med 1987;6:341-8.
89. Meier P. Commentary on "Why do we need systematic overviews of randomized trials?" Stat Med 1987;6:329-31.
90. Bailey KR. Inter-study differences: How should they influence the interpretation and analysis of results? Stat Med 1987;6:351-8.
91. Cochran WG. The combination of estimates from different experiments. Biometrics 1954; 10:101-29.
92. DerSimonian R, Laird N. Meta-analysis in clinical trials. Control Clin Trials 1986;7:177-88.
93. Huque MF. Experiences with meta-analysis in FDA submissions. Proc Biopharmaceutical Section Am Stat Assoc 1988;2:28-33.
94. Dubey S. Regulatory considerations on meta-analysis and multicenter trials. Proc Biopharmaceutical Section Am Stat Assoc 1988;2:18-27.
95. Stein RA. Meta-analysis from one FDA reviewer's perspective. Proc Biopharmaceutical Section Am Stat Assoc 1988;2:34-8.
96. Higgins JPT, Thompson SG, Deeks JJ, Altman DG. Measuring inconsistency in meta-analyses. Br Med J 2003;327:557-60.
97. Altman DG, Bland MJ. Interaction revisited: The difference between two estimates. Br Med J 2003;326:219.
98. MedDRA MSSO. MedDRA™ Introductory Guide. Version 3.3. Reston, VA: MedDRA MSSO, 2002.
99. Greenland S. Quantitative methods in the review of epidemiologic literature. Epidemiol Rev 1987;9:1-30.
100. Abramson JH. Meta-analysis: A review of pros and cons. Public Health Rev 1990/91;18:1-47.
101. Greenland S, Longnecker MP. Methods for trend estimation from summarized dose-response data, with applications to meta-analysis. Am J Epidemiol 1992;135:1301-9.
102. Greenland S, Salvan A. Bias in the one-step method for pooling study results. Stat Med 1990;9:247-52.
103. Cook TD, Cooper H, Cordray DS, et al. Meta-analysis for explanation: A casebook. New York: Russell Sage Foundation, 1992.
104. Ellenberg SS. Meta-analysis: The quantitative approach to research review. Semin Oncol 1988;15:472-81.
105. Borzak S, Ridker PM. Discordance between meta-analyses and large-scale randomized controlled trials: Examples from the management of acute myocardial infarction. Ann Intern Med 1995;123:873-7.
106. Edelstein LC, Bray PF. MicroRNAs in platelet production and activation. Blood 2011;117: 5289-96.
107. Friedman RC, Farh KK, Burge CB, et al. Most mammalian mRNAs are conserved targets of microRNAs. Genome Res 2009;19:92-105.
108. Fabian MR, Sonenberg N, Filipowicz W. Regulation of mRNA translation and stability by microRNAs. Annu Rev Biochem 2010;79:351-79.
109. Osman A, Falker K. Characterization of human platelet microRNA by quantitative PCR coupled with an annotation network for predicted target genes. Platelets 2011;22:433-41.
110. Nagalla S, Shaw C, Kong X, et al. Platelet microRNA-mRNA co-expression profiles correlate with platelet reactivity. Blood 2011;117: 5189-97.
111. Landry P, Plante I, Ouellet DL, et al. Existence of a microRNA pathway in anucleate platelets. Nat Struct Mol Biol 2009;16:961-6.
112. Ryan P, Atreya C. Blood cell microRNAs: What are they and what future do they hold? Transfus Med Rev 2011;25:247-51.
113. Hitzler W, Vamvakas EC. Platelet microRNA profiles and the effect of pathogen reduction on platelet function. Clin Lab 2011;57:451-4.
114. Corash L. The hemostatic efficacy of platelet components prepared with pathogen inactivation. Transfusion 2011;51:1355-6.
115. Kumar V, Lockerbie O, Keil SD, et al. Riboflavin and UV-light based pathogen reduction: Extent and consequence of DNA damage at the molecular level. Photochem Photobiol 2004; 80:15-21.

116. Lozano M, Knutson F, Tardivel R, et al. A multicenter study of the therapeutic efficacy and safety of platelet components treated with amotosalen and ultraviolet-A pathogen inactivation stored for 6 or 7 days prior to transfusion. Br J Haematol 2011;153:393-401.
117. Food and Drug Administration. Study designs (phases 3 and 4) for product development of human platelets using the Cerus INTERCEPT blood system for pathogen inactivation. Meeting of the Blood Products Advisory Committee. November 16, 2009. Rockville, MD: CBER Office of Community Outreach and Development, 2009:158-345. [Available at http://www.fda.gov/downloads/AdvisoryCommittees/CommitteesMeetingMaterials/BloodVaccinesOtherBiologics/BloodProductAdvisoryCommittee/ucm193385.pdf (accessed October 10, 2011).]
118. Bailar JC III. The promise and problems of meta-analysis. N Engl J Med 1997;337:559-61.
119. Meta-analysis under scrutiny (editorial). Lancet 1997;350:675.
120. Villar J, Carrolli G, Belizan JM. Predictive ability of meta-analyses of randomized controlled trials. Lancet 1995;345:772-6.
121. Cappelleri JC, Ioannidis JPA, Schmid CH, et al. Large trials versus meta-analyses of small trials: How do their results compare? JAMA 1996;276:1332-8.
122. LeLorier J, Grégoire B, Benhaddad A, et al. Discrepancies between meta-analyses and subsequent large randomized, controlled trials. N Engl J Med 1997;337:536-42.
123. Ioannidis JPA, Cappelleri JC, Lau J. Issues in comparisons between meta-analyses and large trials. JAMA 1998;279:1089-93.
124. Kleinbaum DG, Kupper LL, Morgenstern H. Epidemiologic research. New York: Van Nostrand Reinhold Co, 1982:194-219.
125. Felson DT. Bias in meta-analytic research. J Clin Epidemiol 1992;45:885-92.
126. Hewitt P, Chalmers TC. Using MEDLINE to peruse the literature. Control Clin Trials 1985;6:75-83.
127. Hewitt P, Chalmers TC. Perusing the literature: Methods of accessing MEDLINE and related data bases. Control Clin Trials 1985;6:168-77.
128. Poynard T, Conn HO. The retrieval of randomized clinical trials in liver disease from the medical literature: A comparison of MEDLARS and manual methods. Control Clin Trials 1985;6:271-9.
129. Dickersin K, Kewitt P, Mutch L, et al. Perusing the literature: Comparison of MEDLINE searching with a perinatal database. Control Clin Trials 1985;6:306-17.
130. Haynes RB, McKibbon KA, Walker CJ, et al. Computer searching of the medical literature: An evaluation of MEDLINE search systems. Ann Intern Med 1985;103:812-16.
131. Begg CB, Berlin JA. Publication bias and dissemination of clinical research. J Natl Cancer Inst 1989;81:107-14.
132. Begg CB, Berlin JA. Publication bias: A problem in interpreting medical data. J Royal Statist Soc Ser A 1988;151:419-63.
133. Simon R. Randomized clinical trials and research strategy. Cancer Treat Rep 1982;66:1083-7.
134. Zelen M. Strategy and alternate randomized designs in cancer clinical trials. Cancer Treat Rep 1982;66:1095-100.
135. Fleming TR. Historical controls, data banks and randomized clinical trials in clinical research: A review. Cancer Treat Rep 1982;66:1101-5.
136. Dickersin K, Chan S, Chalmers TC, et al. Publication bias and clinical trials. Control Clin Trials 1987;8:343-53.
137. Simes RJ. Confronting publication bias: A cohort design for meta-analysis. Stat Med 1987;6:11-29.
138. Pocock SJ, Hughes MD. Estimation in clinical trials and overviews. Stat Med 1990;9:657-71.
139. Simes RJ. Publication bias: The case for an international registry of trials. J Clin Oncol 1986;4:1529-41.
140. Koren G, Shear H, Graham K, et al. Bias against the null hypothesis: The reproductive hazards of cocaine. Lancet 1989;334:1440-2.
141. Dickersin K, Min YI, Meinert CL. Factors influencing publication of research results: Follow-up of applications submitted to two institutional review boards. JAMA 1992;267:374-8.
142. Easterbrook PJ, Berlin JA, Copalan R, et al. Publication bias in clinical research. Lancet 1991;337:867-72.
143. Chalmers I, Adams M, Dickersin K, et al. A cohort study of summary reports of controlled trials. JAMA 1990;263:1401-5.
144. Detsky AS, Baker JP, O'Rourke K, et al. A meta-analysis of perioperative parenteral nutrition. Ann Intern Med 1987;107:195-203.
145. Dickersin K. The existence of publication bias and risk factors for its occurrence. JAMA 1990;263:1385-9.

146. Chalmers I. Underreporting research is scientific misconduct. JAMA 1990;263:1405-8.
147. Davidson RA. Source of funding and outcome of clinical trials. J Gen Intern Med 1986;1:155-8.
148. Lauritsen K, Havelund T, Larsen LS, et al. Withholding unfavourable results in drug company sponsored clinical trials (letter). Lancet 1987; 329:1091.
149. Kochar MS. The peer review of manuscripts: In need for improvement. J Chron Dis 1986;39: 147-9.
150. Ad Hoc Working Group for Critical Appraisal of the Medical Literature. A proposal for more informative abstracts of clinical articles. Ann Intern Med 1987;106:626-7.
151. Easterbrook PJ. Reducing publication bias (letter). Br Med J 1987;295:1347.
152. Hetherington J, Dickersin K, Chalmers I, et al. Retrospective and prospective identification of unpublished controlled trials: Lessons from a survey of obstetricians and pediatricians. Pediatrics 1989;84:374-80.
153. Grégoire G, Derderian F, LeLorier J. Selecting the language of publication included in a meta-analysis: Is there a Tower of Babel bias? J Clin Epidemiol 1995;48:159-63.
154. Egger M, Zellweger-Zatner T, Schneider M, et al. Language bias in randomized controlled trials published in English and German. Lancet 1997;350:326-9.
155. Moher D, Fortin P, Jadad AR, et al. Completeness of reporting of trials published in languages other than English: Implications for conduct and reporting of systemic reviews. Lancet 1996;347:363-6.
156. Stock WA, Okun MA, Haring MJ, et al. Rigor in data synthesis: A case study of reliability in meta-analysis. Educ Res 1982;11:10-14, 20.
157. Smith ML, Glass GV. Meta-analysis of psychotherapy outcome studies. Am Psychol 1977;32: 752-60.
158. Littenberg B. Aminophylline treatment in severe, acute asthma: A meta-analysis. JAMA 1988;259:1678-84.
159. Moher D, Liberati A, Tetzlaff J, Altman DG, and the PRISMA Group. Preferred reporting items for systematic reviews and meta-analyses: The PRISMA statement. PLoS Medicine 2009;6: e1000097, pp.1-6. [Available at www.plosmedicine.org (accessed August 29, 2011).]

In: Vamvakas EC.
Decision Making in Transfusion Medicine
Bethesda, MD: AABB Press, 2011

6

Have Policy Makers Been Selectively Precautionary in Indefinitely Deferring Men Who Have Had Sex with Men (MSM) from Donating Blood?

BEFORE 1996-2000, EACH AUSTRALIAN state employed its own criterion for deferring men who had ever had sex with men (MSM) from donating blood. At that time, the MSM deferral thus varied by state from 5 years since the last male-to-male sexual contact to lifetime; approximately three-quarters of Australian male donors were under deferral policies similar to those in the United States, that is, they were permanently deferred from donating blood if they had ever had sex with another man or if they had had sex with another man even once since 1977 or even once since 1980; approximately one-quarter of Australian men were being deferred from donating blood for 5 years following their last male-to-male sexual contact. In 1996-2000, a 1-year deferral for MSM was gradually implemented in all Australian states and territories where first-time donors are not screened for infectious disease markers the first time that they present to donate blood but, as in the United States, blood is collected from them and used for transfusion if all results for infectious disease markers are negative at the time of that first blood donation. In comparing the HIV prevalence among donations made by Australian blood donors during the 5 years before and the 5 years after the reduction in the MSM deferral to 1 year, Seed et al[1] did not detect any increase in the prevalence of human immunodeficiency virus (HIV) infection in collected units of blood. The HIV prevalence was 1 per 167,732 collected units when the deferral varied between states from 5 years to lifetime; and it remained virtually the same (1 per 206,860 collected units; $p = 0.47$) after the deferral was reduced to 1 year. When only donations made by male donors were considered, the HIV prevalence was 1 per 131,647 collected units before, compared with 1 per 199,421 collected units after the reduction in the MSM deferral to 1 year ($p = 0.27$). Two of 15 male donors in the 5 years before, compared with 5 of 16 male donors in the 5 years after the reduction in the MSM deferral to 1 year (13.3% vs 31.3%; $p = 0.22$) indicated on postdonation interviews that male-to-male sex had been their risk factor. All these five donors (who made HIV-positive donations after the deferral had been reduced to 1 year) had engaged in male-to-male sex during the year preceding their blood donation and would have been deferred from donating had they disclosed their risk activity correctly.

Accordingly, in July 2010, Seed et al[1] concluded that it was not the length of the deferral (1 year versus 5 years or lifetime), but the extent of noncompliance with the applied deferral that determined the risk of collecting an HIV-positive unit. Furthermore, after reviewing the literature on the current extent of nondisclosure of MSM activity by prospective blood donors,[2] Seed et al[1] contended that the five noncompliant donors (who had disclosed male-to-male sex as their risk factor and from whom blood had been collected after the MSM deferral had been reduced to 1 year) represented only the "tip of the iceberg" concerning the noncompliance of prospective donors with the MSM deferral. They also concluded that the change in policy implemented by the Australian blood authorities in 1996-2000 had therefore not resulted in any increased risk of HIV infection for transfusion recipients.

Seed et al[1] acknowledged that their findings might not apply to other countries in which the deferral would be changing country-wide from indefinite to 1 or 5 years and/or where the sociodemographics of the donor population might differ from that of Australia. They also acknowledged that, since they had conducted an observational "before-and-after" study, other changes might have coincided with the change in the MSM deferral so as to obscure any effect of the reduction in the MSM deferral on the prevalence of HIV infection in collected units. Nonetheless, the results of Seed et al[1] (showing no increased risk of HIV infection for transfusion recipients when the MSM deferral changes from 5 years or lifetime to 1 year in a country with a western-type health-care system) are the *only empirical* data hitherto presented on whether reducing the MSM deferral might result in increased risk of HIV transmission to transfusion recipients.

A person infected with HIV has a greater probability of transmitting HIV infection than a man who has had sex with another man at least once since 1977 and whose sexual history is otherwise unknown. Yet, in the United States, a female donor who has had sex with a man infected with HIV is eligible to donate blood 12 months after that contact if she tests negative for circulating HIV antibody and nucleic acid. In contrast, men who have had sex with men even once since 1977 are indefinitely deferred from donating blood. Since it was introduced as a temporary measure before testing for HIV antibody was available, the lifetime deferral for MSM has not been harmonized with the 1-year deferral for similar- or greater-risk activities through heterosexual contacts, because of concern that reducing the MSM deferral could increase the risk of transfusion transmission of:

1. Known sexually and transfusion-transmitted viruses (predominantly HIV[3-6]) for which blood donors are tested.
2. Known sexually and *potentially* transfusion-transmitted viruses for which blood donors are not tested: human herpesvirus-8 (HHV-8)[7,8] is currently the only agent in this category.
3. Emerging transfusion-transmitted agents that may share the transmission routes and long asymptomatic phase of HIV, thereby accumulating in the blood-donor population and being transmitted to transfusion recipients before becoming recognized (Chapter 3).[9]

The concern that the risk of transfusion-acquired HIV infection would increase if MSM were allowed to donate 1 or 5 years after their last male-to-male sexual contact has dominated the public debate.[10-13] This is because: 1) when they are considered as a homogeneous group, MSM have a *far* greater prevalence and incidence of HIV infection than the general population[14-16]; 2) at least in some countries, the majority of blood donors who test positive for HIV infection acknowledge male-to-male sex as their risk factor when they are questioned closely on postdonation interviews[17]; and 3) in mathematical models that distinguished between MSM who have abstained from male-to-male sex for 12 months[3,4] or 5 years[6] and all MSM, the increase in risk from a reduction in the MSM deferral, *albeit minimal*, was not 0%. Because of the assumptions made in these models, the prerequisite articulated by policy makers[18] for reducing the lifetime MSM deferral—that there be *no* increase in risk because of the change in policy—cannot be satisfied[4] by such models.[3-6]

Even if public-policy decision making is to be based on mathematical models[3-6] rather than empirical data,[1] however, the relevant question might *not* be *whether* there will be an increase in risk but *how big* that increase in risk will be.

More specifically, the appropriate question might be whether the increase in risk from allowing blood donation by MSM who have abstained from male-to-male sex for 1 or 5 years is smaller than the currently tolerated transfusion risk, which exceeds the "as-low-as-reasonably-achievable" (ALARA) risk.[19] This is because the previously articulated position of United States policy makers[18] assumes that our approach to blood safety consistently renders the risk of an infectious unit's being released for transfusion as small as the ALARA risk. However, if a *minimal* risk greater than the ALARA risk were *de facto* tolerated in situations similarly under the control of policy makers, a *minimal* increase in risk from reducing the MSM deferral–*smaller* than the currently tolerated transfusion risk which exceeds the ALARA risk–could be regarded as "tolerable" as well.[20]

This chapter examines the currently tolerated allogeneic blood transfusion (ABT) risk, which exceeds the ALARA risk in the United States and compares it to the risk engendered by reducing the MSM deferral to 1 or 5 years. The obtained relative-risk estimates pertain solely to the United States where: 1) women who have had sex with a man infected with HIV are deferred from donating blood for 12 months after that exposure; and 2) units of blood donated by first-time donors are released for transfusion to patients, despite the fact that–compared with repeat donors–first-time donors have a several-fold higher risk of transmitting infections to transfusion recipients,[21-24] however minimal the absolute difference in risk between first-time and repeat donors may be. Several European countries, including the United Kingdom[25] and The Netherlands, do not follow one or both of the aforementioned policies. Therefore, a different comparison of the risk from reducing the MSM deferral compared with the currently tolerated ABT risk that exceeds the ALARA risk pertains to their jurisdictions.

Currently Tolerated ABT Risk in the United States That Exceeds the ALARA Risk

As shown in Table 2-1 of Chapter 2, compared with apheresis (single-donor) platelets, pooled whole-blood-derived platelets have a five-fold higher risk of transfusion-transmitted infections (TTIs) because, to procure a therapeutic platelet dose that could have been harvested from a single apheresis donor, one would pool donations from four to six whole-blood donors–each one of whom could be the source of a TTI.[26] In many countries, pooled platelets provide a justifiable balance between safety and availability: for logistical and/or financial reasons, it is infeasible to recruit enough apheresis donors to meet all platelet transfusion needs. (In this same manner, it is infeasible to recruit enough repeat donors[21-24] to meet all red cell transfusion needs in the United States where 28.5% of collections come from first-time donors.[27]) The feasibility of exclusive reliance on apheresis (single-donor) platelets is well-established in the Unites States where 87.1% of all therapeutic platelet doses were provided as single-donor components in 2008.[28]

Of 2.021 million apheresis (single-donor) dose-equivalents transfused in the United States in 2008, 0.260 million (12.9%) were transfused as whole-blood-derived platelet pools.[28] Rather than relying on 1.3 million whole-blood donors to procure 12.9% of the therapeutic platelet doses in 2008, these platelet doses could have been collected from 260,000 plateletpheresis donors–thereby avoiding 1.04 million exposures of platelet transfusion recipients to allogeneic donors.

The risk from continuing to transfuse 12.9% of platelet doses as pools[28] is the annual number of infectious platelet pools that would no longer be transfused in the United States if all therapeutic platelet doses were transfused as apheresis (single-donor) platelets. These *preventable* donor exposures from the continued use of pools result in a small number of HIV, hepatitis C virus (HCV), and hepatitis B virus (HBV) transmissions through platelet transfusion, and in at least

86.7 cases of platelet transfusion-associated sepsis (TAS) per year (Fig 2-17 in Chapter 2). With regard to HIV, the continued use of pools in the United States results in 0.48 *preventable* HIV transmission through platelet transfusion annually (or 1 HIV transmission every 2 years on average). The 1.04 million preventable donor exposures from the continued use of pools would further generate 104 transmissions during the year preceding the introduction of blood donor screening if the next major transfusion-transmitted pathogen to emerge in the United States were "HIV-like"; and 18.7 transmissions during the agent's first epidemic prior to the introduction of blood donor screening if the next agent to emerge were "West-Nile-virus-like" (see calculations in Table 2-1 of Chapter 2).

Scope of the Comparison

A relative risk (RR) comparing the risk of reducing the lifetime blood donation deferral for MSM and the tolerated ABT risk has been reported[29] based on risk estimates available through August 31, 2009 and the data on blood components transfused in the United States presented in the 2007 Nationwide Blood Collection and Utilization Survey Report.[27] That analysis[29] relied solely on projections of risk based on mathematical models,[3-5] because no empirical data on the prevalence of HIV infection in MSM donors who have abstained for 1 year *and* self-select to donate[1] were available at the time that the analysis[29] was conducted. This chapter updates the previously reported RR calculation[29] with risk estimates available through September 30, 2011 and the data on blood components transfused in the United States presented in the 2009 National Blood Collection and Utilization Survey Report.[28] The *only empirical* findings on the increase in risk if the MSM deferral is reduced to 1 year[1] and the only mathematical model specifically projecting the increase in risk if the MSM deferral is reduced to 5 years[6] were published after the completion of the previous analysis.[29]

Only the possibilities of reducing the MSM deferral to 1 or 5 years are considered here, because the circumstances of the predonation interview preclude the use of eligibility criteria that rely on a more detailed sexual history such a monogamy of both partners involved in an MSM relationship or exclusive practice of safe sex by prospective donors. Perhaps more important, the initiative to *altogether* remove the MSM deferral in Spain, replacing it with a question about whether a prospective donor has had more than one homosexual or heterosexual partner in the preceding year, was followed by a gradual (over 10 years) and clinically important increase in HIV-positive donations, including window-period donations and donations from repeat donors.[30] A similar increase was observed for incident and prevalent syphilis infections.[31] The increase in infectious donations was concentrated in the MSM group.[30,31] Monogamy practiced by only one of the two partners in a homosexual relationship, test-seeking behavior, and/or untruthful responses on the blood-donor questionnaire may have been responsible for the rise in infectious donations.

For donors reporting risk activities for HIV, HCV, or HBV, a 1-year deferral ensures that—given the screening of all blood donations by two separate assays for each TTI (Table 6-1)—no incident (window-period) infection undetectable by current assays can occur if donors have not engaged in more recent risk activity.[32] The same assurance applies to window-period infections with HBV and HCV.[33-37] Compared with current donors, however, newly eligible MSM donors who have abstained from male-to-male sex for 1 year and self-select to donate could have increased frequency of undiagnosed (prevalent) HIV and HBV—and perhaps also HCV—infection, which would increase the risk of collecting an infectious unit.[3-6]

The additional risk of collecting an HIV-infectious unit would depend on the prevalence of undiagnosed HIV infection in *actual* MSM donors—that is, MSM who have both abstained for 12 months and self-select to donate. The additional risk of releasing an infectious unit for transfusion would depend on: 1) the probability of false-negative results on blood-donor testing

Table 6-1. Infectious Window Period* of Three Transfusion-Transmitted Viruses

Virus	Combination of Tests Currently Used in the US to Detect Virus	Window Period (Days) (95% CI)
HIV	Antibody to HIV-1/2 HIV-1 nucleic acid	9.5† (8.2-10.8)
HCV	Antibody to HCV HCV nucleic acid	8.0† (6.8-9.2)
HBV	HBsAg HBc	38.3‡ (33-43.7)

*The window period is the interval between the onset of virus replication in peripheral blood and the time when viral markers become detectable by our current screening assays. During this interval, a donation is infectious, yet undetectable by current screening tests.
†For nucleic-acid testing employing minipools of 24; the window period is 9.1 days for HIV and 7.4 days for HCV if the nucleic-acid test employs minipools of 16.[34]
‡For PRISM HBsAg (Abbott Laboratories, Abbott Park, IL).[35] Although such testing is not required, part of the US blood supply is further tested for HBV nucleic acid, which results in a further reduction in the window period by 5 to 8 days.[35-37]
CI = confidence interval; HBc = antibody to hepatitis B virus core; HBsAg = hepatitis B virus surface antigen; HBV = hepatitis B virus; HCV = hepatitis C virus; HIV = human immunodeficiency virus; HIV-1/2 = HIV type 1 or 2.
Initially published by Vamvakas in Transfus Med Rev 2011;25:47-60.[29]

for HIV infection, because of suboptimal sensitivity of the screening assays and/or human errors in performing these tests; and 2) the probability of release from quarantine of an HIV-positive unit because of human error. The probability of release of a unit for transfusion before the completion of donor testing also exists; however, repeat donors (tested recently or well-known to a blood bank) are used in these rare situations.

A 5-year MSM deferral is considered, because—as possible pathogens potentially transmissible by transfusion continue to emerge[38-40] after the completion of the review by the AABB Transfusion-Transmitted Diseases Committee[9]—the possibility that the next major transfusion-transmitted agent could be an "HIV-like" sexually transmitted virus with a long incubation period cannot be excluded. Deferral of MSM to protect recipients from a sexually and transfusion-transmitted agent that has not yet emerged and for which MSM activity places the donor at greater-than-average risk of exposure could be an appropriate *precautionary* measure. As discussed in Chapter 1, the precautionary principle states that—when a purported risk represents a threat of "serious or irreversible damage"—complete evidence of risk does not have to exist in order to institute measures to protect individuals and society from that risk.[41,42] Thus, from the precautionary principle perspective vis-à-vis emerging pathogens,[43] acceptance of blood donations from MSM might be safe only after a 5-year abstinence from male-to-male sex has elapsed. During this period, any emerging pathogen (other than pathologic prions) would be recognized as transfusion-transmissible and measures to prevent transfusion transmission would be implemented. Such was the case with the three major transfusion-transmitted pathogens that emerged in the United States in the last 30 years (Fig 6-1).

Human immunodeficiency virus	
1978	Spread to North American MSM community to a significant, epidemic extent
1983	Recognition of transmission by transfusion and implementation of preventive measures (high-risk donor deferral)
1985	Introduction of donor screening through laboratory testing
Variant Creutzfeldt-Jakob disease	
1994	First clinical case
1999	Beginning of implementation of precautionary measures to protect the North American blood supply
West Nile virus	
1999	Initial North American cases
2002	First major epidemic in North America; recognition of transmission by transfusion
2003	Implementation of donor screening by a laboratory test

Figure 6-1. Current 5-year interval between the emergence of a novel agent and the introduction of measures to protect US blood transfusion recipients: all three major transfusion-transmitted pathogens that emerged in the last 30 years were followed, within 4 to 7 years, by the implementation of measures to protect the blood supply. The interval for HIV was 5 years until the introduction of deferrals for high-risk donors and 7 years until the introduction of laboratory screening of donors. Geographic donor deferrals for vCJD were introduced on a precautionary basis before vCJD was proven to be transmissible through ABT.
HIV = human immunodeficiency virus; vCJD = variant Creutzfeldt-Jakob disease; WNV = West Nile virus.

HHV-8 and MSM

MSM transmission of HHV-8 does occur,[44-48] and HHV-8 seroprevalence in MSM donors could be up to 10-fold higher[49,50] than the 3.5% prevalence recorded in current United States blood donors.[51] Because donors are not screened for HHV-8 infection, accepting donations from MSM who have abstained for 1 or 5 years would increase any risk of HHV-8 transfusion transmission if HHV-8 were indeed transmissible by transfusion. If that were the case—whether transfusion transmission of HHV-8 were patterned after that of the distantly related cytomegalovirus (CMV)[52,53] or the more closely-related Epstein-Barr virus (EBV)[54-56]—only a small per-unit transmission risk would be expected because, in HHV-8-infected individuals, the virus is probably latently maintained at undetectable levels in peripheral blood B lymphocytes and monocytes. Asymptomatic virus activation probably occurs episodically (as it does with all other herpesviruses[53]), and HHV-8 DNA can be detected in peripheral blood from donors experiencing virus activation or primary infection.[57] It is only donations made during such periods that could potentially transmit HHV-8 to recipients, placing—at least immunocompromised—recipients at risk of developing transfusion-associated Kaposi's sarcoma (KS).[58] Also, transmission can be effected only by fresh blood components in which the white blood cells (WBCs) harboring the virus have not been removed by WBC reduction and have not yet deteriorated during storage.[53]

Although 3.5% of current United States blood donors are HHV-8-seropositive,[51] development of KS has not been documented in a patient contracting HHV-8 through transfusion,[59] despite the fact that it has been documented in patients who contracted HHV-8 through renal transplantation.[60,61] No United

States blood donor has been found to carry HHV-8 DNA,[51,62] although HHV-8 viremia[63-65] has been reported in up to 22.5%[65] of donors from sub-Saharan Africa. In such high-prevalence areas, HHV-8 is probably transmitted through saliva, with its seroprevalence increasing with age among children.[66-69] Likely sources of infection include the mother[67-72] and older siblings.[68]

Relative Risk

The risk from reducing the MSM deferral is the number of additional infectious (whole-blood) units that would be released for transfusion annually in the United States if the MSM deferral was reduced to 1 or 5 years. The risk from continuing to provide 12.9% of therapeutic platelet doses as pooled platelets is the annual number of infectious platelet pools that would no longer be transfused in the United States if all platelet doses were provided as apheresis (single-donor) platelets. This latter risk derives from incident ("window-period") infections missed by current screening assays (Table 2-1 and Fig 2-17 in Chapter 2). The relative risk of HIV, HBV, or HCV infection is thus defined as follows:

$$\text{RR} = \frac{\text{Additional risk from reducing the MSM deferral to 1 or 5 years}}{\text{Current risk from the excess donor exposures that can be prevented if the use of pooled platelets is discontinued}}$$

Any increased risk of HIV, HBV, or HCV transmission owing to a higher frequency of prevalent infection in donors pertains exclusively to reducing the MSM deferral, although—compared to plateletpheresis and other (non-double-red-blood-cell) apheresis donors—whole-blood donors have a 5.8- to 25.0-fold higher ($p<0.05$) prevalence of these TTIs.[73] Because increased prevalence (Figs 8-2, 8-3, and 8-4 in Chapter 8) does not correlate with increased incidence (Table 8-1 in Chapter 8) of HIV, HBV, or HCV infection in blood donors, the higher prevalence of HIV, HBV, or HCV infection in whole-blood (compared with plateletpheresis) donors[73] is not taken into account in the analysis. Any increased risk of HHV-8 transmission similarly relates exclusively to reducing the MSM deferral,[44-48] whereas the excess risk of transfusion-associated sepsis (TAS)[74] relates only to the continued use of pooled platelets.[26] TAS is a principal cause of transfusion-related deaths today.[75,76] The risk attributed to the continued use of pooled platelets (Fig 2-17 in Chapter 2) was based on the assumptions that the historical risk of 1 per 3000 TAS cases for pooled[77,78] and 1 per 15,000[77] for apheresis (single-donor) platelets was reduced by 50% by various process improvements introduced before or around 2004,[74] and by a further 50% by culture testing for bacteria[79,80] (Fig 2-16 in Chapter 2). It was further assumed that all pooled platelets distributed in the United States in the future will be: 1) prepooled and cultured; and 2) manufactured by the United States platelet-rich plasma method rather than the European buffy-coat method.[26]

TTIs for Which Blood Donors Are Tested

1-Year Deferral

The prevalence of undiagnosed HIV infection in MSM who have abstained for 12 months *and* self-select to donate if the MSM deferral is reduced to 1 year can be inferred from the empirical results of Seed et al.[1] Blood donors are not a random subset of individuals eligible to donate blood, but a highly self-selected subgroup cognizant of risk factors for TTIs and much less likely to be infected with TTIs than the general population of individuals eligible to donate.[81,82] Over a 5-year period after the MSM deferral had been reduced to 1 year in Australia, there were 24 HIV-positive donations among 4,964,628 donations.[1] Sixteen of the 24 donors acknowledged deferrable risk behaviors on postdonation interviews. Five of these 16 donors who acknowledged deferrable risk behaviors—and thus five of the 24 donors who had made HIV-positive donations after the MSM deferral had been reduced to 1 year—admitted in the course of their postdonation interview that they had engaged in male-to-male sex during the 12 months preceding their blood donation. Thus, if these five donors had been compliant with the employed 1-year deferral following their last male-to-male sexual contact and had disclosed their *recent* MSM activity before donating, they would have been deferred. Had this been the case, over 5 years following the reduction in the MSM deferral to 1 year in Australia, the change in policy would have resulted in *no* HIV-positive donation entering the blood supply because of prevalent—and undiagnosed—HIV infection in MSM donors who had abstained for 12 months *and* had self-selected to donate.

Because of the limited compliance of prospective blood donors with any applied MSM deferral,[2] the donors who made blood donations in Australia before 1996-2000 (when the MSM deferral varied by state from 5 years to lifetime) had undoubtedly included donors with both recent (in the previous 12 months) and distant (in the previous 1 to 5 or >5 years) MSM activity. After the MSM deferral was reduced to 1 year in 1996-2000, the donors who made blood donations during the ensuing 5 years also doubtless included donors with both recent (in the previous 12 months) and distant (in the previous 1 to 5 or >5 years) MSM activity. Although it is impossible to know how many MSM donors with *distant* MSM activity (>1 year before their blood donation) donated over 5 years in Australia after the change in policy, one can safely infer from the presented results that acceptance of these donors resulted in 0 HIV-positive donations. Therefore, it can also be inferred that the prevalence of undiagnosed HIV infection in the MSM donors who had abstained for 12 months *and* self-selected to donate in the sample of Seed et al[1] was 0%.

Two questions remain unresolved by the results of Seed et al.[1] First is the question whether the sample of these investigators[1] (4,964,268 donations made across Australia in the 5 years following the change in policy) was large enough to include any MSM donors who had undiagnosed HIV infection even though they had abstained for 1 year *and* had self-selected to donate. There are no estimates of the size of the increase in the blood donor population when the MSM deferral is reduced from 5 years (or lifetime, depending on the state) to 1 year—as was the case in Australia in 1996-2000. Germain et al[4] assumed that the blood donor population would increase by approximately 1% if the MSM deferral in Quebec was reduced from lifetime to 1 year. This estimate does not apply to the Australian situation because MSM who had abstained from male-to-male sex for 5 years were already eligible to donate in some Australian states (representing approximately one-quarter of the population) before the change in policy. Nonetheless, the estimate used by Germain et al[4] for the change from lifetime to 1-year deferral would correspond to 49,643 donations made by MSM who had abstained for 1 year *and* had self-selected to donate in Australia after the change in policy.

If 0.6% of MSM donors who abstained for 12 months *and* self-select to donate have undiagnosed HIV infection—as was assumed by Germain et al[4] for Quebec—there should have been at least 1 HIV-positive donation by Australian MSM donors (who had abstained for 12 months *and* had self-selected to donate) if the sample of Seed et al[1] (4,964,268 donations made after the change in policy) had included at least 167 donations made by MSM donors who had abstained for 12 months *and* had self-selected to donate. The 95% confidence interval (CI) of this minimum number of MSM donors who would have had to have been included in the sample for 1 HIV-positive donation to be detected would be very broad, and it cannot be calculated from the available data. Nonetheless, considering that close to 50,000 MSM donors would have been included in the sample if the estimate of Germain et al[4] were applied to the Australian situation, it is likely safe to assume that the sample of Seed et al[1] would include the upper 95% confidence limit (CL) of the minimum number of MSM donors for detecting one HIV-positive donation under any plausible—or even conceivable—scenario. Thus, this chapter assumes that the empirical results of Seed et al[1] have shown that the prevalence of undiagnosed

HIV infection in MSM donors who have abstained for 1 year *and* self-select to donate *cannot* exceed the 0.6% prevalence assumed in the model of Germain et al.[4]

A second question that cannot be answered from the findings of Seed et al[1] is whether the reduction in the MSM deferral to 12 months might have increased the likelihood of *noncompliance* with the new deferral criterion which required abstinence from male-to-male sex for 12 months. Five of 4,964,628 donations after the change in policy, compared with 2 of 4,025,571 donations before the change in policy, were made by MSM who made blood donations because they were *noncompliant* with the applied deferral criterion either before or after the change in policy. Although the difference between the two periods is not statistically significant, the possibility that MSM activity might have been perceived by prospective blood donors as "less risky" following the change in policy—with prospective blood donors thus having a greater likelihood to make *noncompliant* donations in violation of the deferral criterion—cannot be ruled out based on the results of Seed et al.[1]

The availability of the *empirical* findings of Seed et al[1] permits a re-examination of the *projected* risks derived from the previously published mathematical models.[3-5] Based on various assumptions, mathematical models had previously produced estimates of the increase in the risk of transfusion-acquired HIV infection if MSM who had abstained for 1 year[3-5] were accepted as donors. Anderson et al[5] had also reported on the additional risk of HBV infection. Two models[4,5] had assigned probabilities to all three principal sources of risk: the prevalence of undiagnosed HIV infection in MSM donors who have abstained for 1 year *and* self-select to donate; the possibility of false-negative laboratory test results on donated blood because of window-period infections in donors who have engaged in *recent* MSM activity or human error in laboratory testing; and the possibility of erroneous release of HIV-positive units from quarantine. Soldan and Sinka[3] did not consider the risk from erroneous release of HIV-positive units from quarantine (Fig 6-2).

Anderson et al[5] modeled a 2% prevalence of undiagnosed HIV infection for actual United States MSM donors. They considered that MSM donors would be a random subset of all MSM who thought that they were not infected—*regardless of whether they had abstained for 1 year or would self-select to donate.* They derived an 8% estimate for the prevalence of HIV infection in United States MSM from national surveys of the household population[83] and of clients attending publicly funded HIV counseling and testing sites,[84] and they assumed that 75%[85] of these HIV-positive MSM would not donate because they would be aware of their infection.

Germain et al[4] considered that the prevalence of undiagnosed HIV infection in actual MSM donors would be 0.6%, because the prevalence in self-selected donors after 1 year's abstinence would be less than the 1.45% prevalence observed in the Omega cohort[86] of sexually active, young, Montreal gay men—ie, men who had not abstained for 12 months and had not self-selected to donate—specifically among those who thought that they were not infected (unpublished data from the Omega cohort). Soldan and Sinka[3] modeled that the prevalence of undiagnosed HIV infection among actual MSM donors would be 0.07% outside London and 0.84% in London (1st and 2nd columns under HIV prevalence in Fig 6-2). The number of undiagnosed HIV infections in MSM who had had sex in the previous 1 year was based on estimates obtained from individuals attending the Unlinked Anonymous Testing of Genitourinary Medicine Clinic.[87] The number of undiagnosed HIV infections in MSM who had abstained for 1 year was then obtained by subtracting this estimate from the estimated total number of undiagnosed HIV infections acquired through male-to-male sex in the United Kingdom.[88]

The assumptions made by the early models[3,4] about false-negative results of blood-donor screening assays (Fig 6-2) are no longer plausible following the introduction of the nucleic-acid screening assay for HIV-1 and the process and quality improvements implemented by blood establishments in the last 15 years to prevent human errors in laboratory testing. The contem-

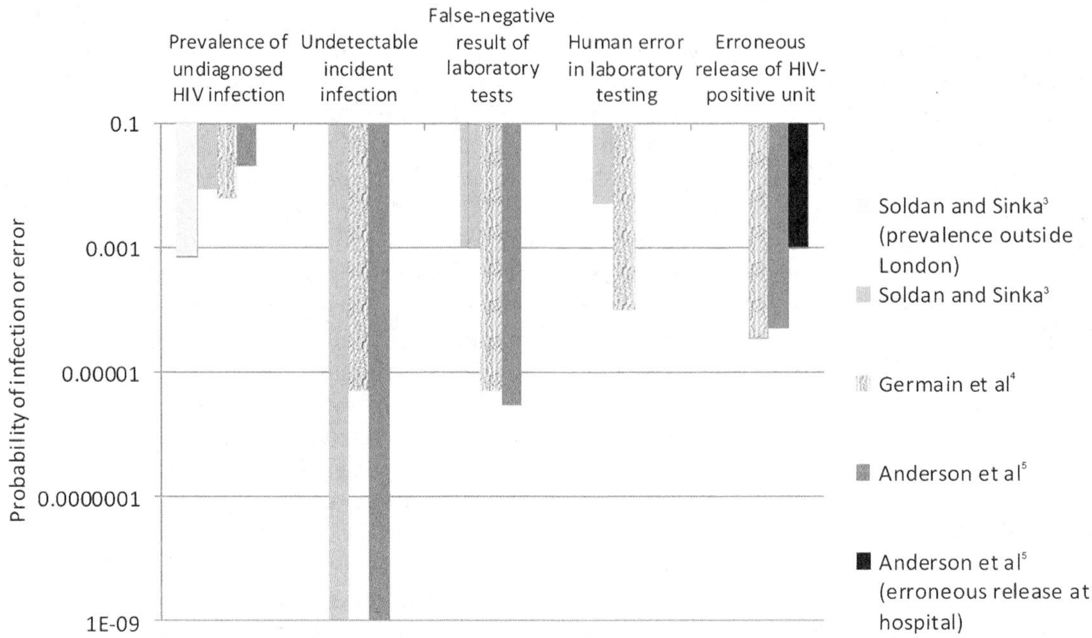

Figure 6-2. Comparison of the assumptions made in the published models[3-5] of the increase in the risk of transfusion-transmitted HIV infection if MSM who have abstained from male-to-male sex in the previous year are accepted as donors. Both Soldan and Sinka[3] and Anderson et al[5] assumed that the probability of an incident HIV infection's being undetectable by screening assays 1 year after contracting the infection is 0%; however these two columns terminate at 1 in 10^{-9} in the figure. Before the introduction of nucleic-acid testing, Soldan and Sinka[3] assumed a sensitivity of 99.9% for the antibody test. Germain et al[4] assumed a sensitivity of 99.99% for the antibody test, and of 95% for the (then recently implemented) nucleic-acid test, corresponding to a 1 per 200,000 probability of false-negative results occurring simultaneously on both tests because of suboptimal sensitivity of the assays. In addition to these false-negative results, both teams[3,4] modeled further false-negative results owing to human errors in test performance. Anderson et al[5] combined the false-negative results from these two sources into one estimate, derived from observing screening assay results on 17.8 million donations. The mean probability of an infectious unit's being missed by either the antibody or the nucleic-acid test was 1 per 1.72×10^3, and the probability of such a unit's being missed simultaneously by both tests is plotted in the figure. The human error component of this combined estimate was 1 per 10 million, compared to 1 per 200 in the early model of Soldan and Sinka[3] that had been based on pre-1994 New York State observations of laboratory error rates. Soldan and Sinka[3] did not include in their model the possibility of erroneous release of HIV-positive units from quarantine—a risk independent of the source of HIV infection in a donor.
Initially published by Vamvakas in Transfus Med Rev 2011;25:47-60.[29]

porary analysis of Anderson et al[5] revised these overly conservative assumptions made previously[3,4] (Fig 6-2). Similar quality improvements have been implemented by blood establishments in the last 15 years to prevent the release of HIV-positive units from quarantine owing to human error (Fig 6-3).

Based on the assumptions shown in Fig 6-2 about the contemporary performance of screening assays and probability of human errors, Anderson et al[5] calculated that, if the MSM deferral were reduced to 1 year, on average 1 additional HIV-infectious (whole-blood) unit would be released for transfusion in the United States every 5.55 years. However, only the two early analyses[3,4] had considered that the MSM who would actually donate would *not* be a random subset of MSM who thought that they were

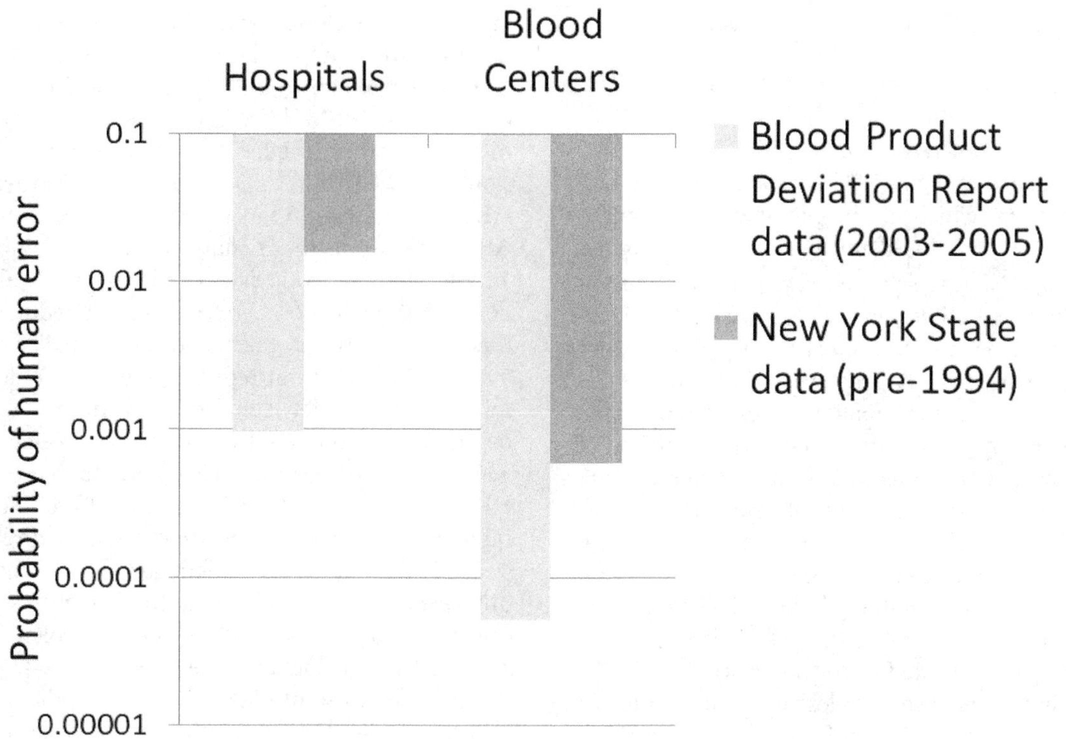

Figure 6-3. Comparison of 2003-2005 vs pre-1994 rates of erroneous release of TTI-reactive units from quarantine at hospitals and blood centers, as used by Anderson et al[5] to predict erroneous release of HIV-positive units. Based on nationwide mandatory reports of errors to the FDA[5] (filed as Biological Product Deviation Reports) or New York State,[89,90] respectively. Of 205,955 units (193,598 at blood centers and 12,357 at hospitals) quarantined in the United States over 2 years, nine HIV-, HBV-, HCV-, or human T-cell lymphotropic virus-reactive units were erroneously released from quarantine at blood centers and 11 at hospitals over 3 years.[5] The breakdown of these erroneous releases (in terms of the specific reactive screening test) was not reported. Initially published by Vamvakas in Transfus Med Rev 2011;25:47-60.[29]

not infected. Thus, had Anderson et al[5] employed the estimate of Germain et al[4] for the prevalence of undiagnosed HIV infection among MSM donors, the additional risk from reducing the MSM deferral to 1 year would have been 1 additional HIV-infectious (whole-blood) unit released for transfusion in the United States every 18.5 years. Because the *empirical* results of Seed et al[1] have shown that the prevalence of undiagnosed HIV infection in MSM donors who have abstained for 12 months *and* self-select to donate *cannot* exceed 0.6% (the prevalence assumed by Germain et al[4]), the increase in risk if the MSM deferral is reduced to 1 year is assumed here to be 1 additional HIV-infectious (whole-blood) unit released for transfusion in the United States every 18.5 years.

Uncertainty about such estimates does remain,[5] and it is highlighted by the 95% CI reported by Anderson et al[5]: although the most likely estimate of the increase in risk based on their model would be 1 additional HIV-infectious unit released in the United States every 5.55 years, the increase in risk in any 1 year could be as low as 0 and as high as one additional HIV-infectious unit. However, the risk of transfusion-transmitted HIV infection would decline four- to five-fold after the initial year of reducing the MSM deferral to 1 year.[5]

Relative Risk

The risk from reducing the MSM deferral to 1 year is 1 additional HIV-infectious whole-blood unit from which ≤1.5 manufactured components are transfused on average in the United States[27,28] and which are released for transfusion in the United States every 18.5 years. This HIV-infectious unit would infect ≤1.5 patients every 18.5 years or 1 patient every 12.3 years. The risk from the 1.04 million excess donor exposures resulting from the continued transfusion of pooled platelets (Table 2-1 in Chapter 2) is 1 HIV-infectious platelet pool transfused every 2.08 years (Fig 2-17 in Chapter 2). Thus, the risk from reducing the MSM deferral is 5.9 times smaller than the risk that—despite the fact that it exceeds the ALARA risk—is currently tolerated in the United States (Fig 6-4).

Male-to-male sex is a less frequent risk factor for HBV than for HIV infection,[17] whereas there are more HBV (than HIV) window-period infections in current donors (Fig 2-17 in Chapter 2). For these reasons, the additional HBV risk from reducing the MSM deferral to 1 year is 9.24 and 8.23 times, respectively, smaller than the risk from continuing to provide 12.9% of therapeutic platelet dose as pooled platelets (Fig 6-4).

Any association of HCV infection with MSM activity—if it exists at all—is much weaker[91] than the established relationship between MSM activity and HBV infection.[92,93] For this reason, Anderson et al[5] did not consider the possibility of an increase in the risk of transfusion-transmitted HCV infection if the MSM deferral were reduced to 1 year. Because the association of HCV infection with MSM activity is smaller than that of HBV infection,[91-93] and these authors[5] predicted 9.24 times more HIV- (than HBV-) infectious collections in the first year after reducing the MSM deferral to 1 year, there would be *at least* 9.24 times more HIV- (than HCV-) infectious collections made in the first year. Moreover, the risk of window-period HCV infection is approximately 10% higher than that of HIV infection.[31,32] Therefore, the risk of transfusion-transmitted HCV infection attributable to reducing the MSM deferral would be far less than the risk from the continued use of pooled platelets.

Figure 6-4 shows that the *average* risk from reducing the MSM deferral to 1 year is approximately six times smaller vis-à-vis HIV transmission, and well over 250 times smaller vis-à-vis HBV transmission, than the currently tolerated ABT risk from the continued transfusion of 12.9% of therapeutic platelet doses as platelet pools. Although the *average* risk from reducing the MSM deferral is calculated to be smaller on average, the risk from reducing the MSM deferral does not differ statistically from the risk owing to the continued use of pooled platelets. This is because the 95% CI for the increase in HIV risk secondary to reducing the MSM deferral to 1 year calculated by Anderson et al[5] (from 0 to 1 additional HIV-infectious whole-blood unit released for transfusion in the United States during any 1 year after the change in policy) is so broad that it includes the average risk from the continued use of platelet pools (1 additional HIV-infectious platelet pool transfused in the United States every 2.08 years). Even if the risk calculated by Anderson et al[5] were reduced by 3.3 times (to replace the estimate of the prevalence of undiagnosed HIV infection in MSM donors used by Anderson et al[5] with the estimate used by Germain et al[4]), the 95% CI for the increase in HIV risk would still include the average additional risk from the continued use of pooled platelets.

5-Year MSM Deferral

Anderson et al[5] further projected that, if the MSM deferral were reduced to 5 years, on average 1 HIV-infectious unit would be released for transfusion in the United States every 33.3 years. The associated 95% CI indicated that the increase in risk in any year could be as low as 0 and as high as 1 additional HIV-infectious unit. However, the authors themselves[5] considered this estimate an overestimate.

Previously, it had been reported that—of 25,000 male United States blood donors sent anonymous survey questionnaires after donating—those who disclosed MSM activity ≤5 years

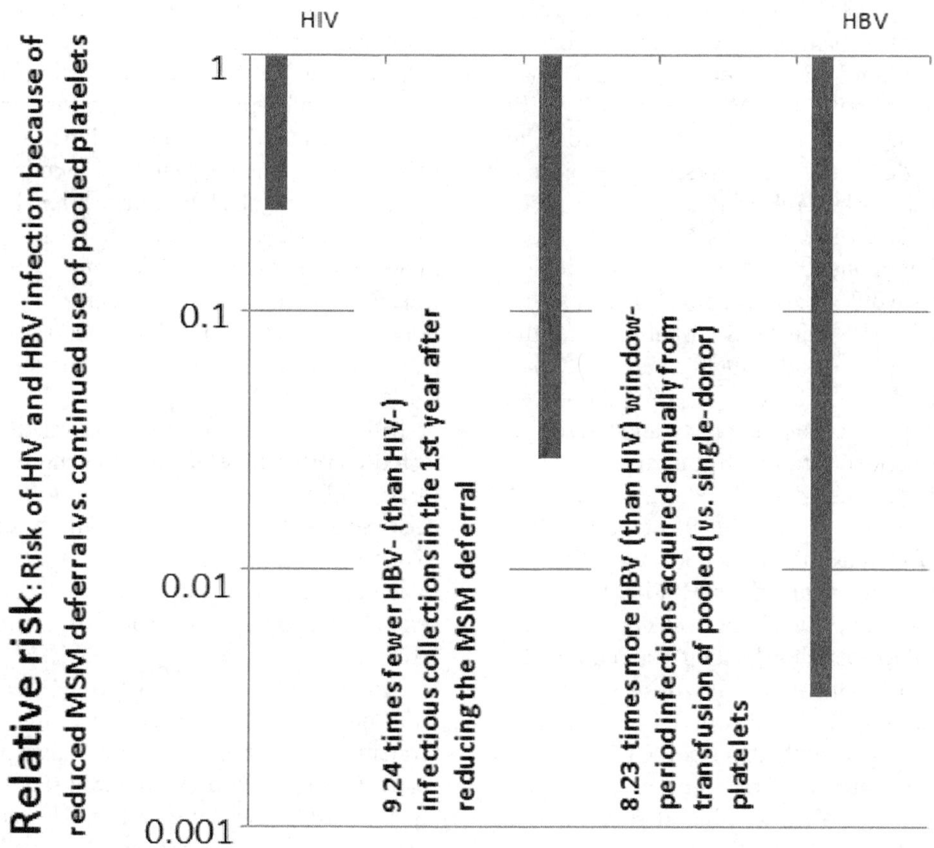

Figure 6-4. Risk of transfusion-transmitted HIV and HBV infection attributable to a reduced MSM deferral compared with the risk attributable to the continued transfusion of 12.9% of therapeutic platelet doses as pooled [rather than apheresis (single-donor)] platelets: ratio of the resulting number of transfusion-transmitted cases of infection per year. To calculate an estimate of the RR of HBV infection, the RR of HIV infection was reduced 9.24 times (because 9.24 times fewer HBV- than HIV-infectious collections would be made in the first year following a reduction of the MSM deferral to 1 year based on the model of Anderson et al[5]), and a further 8.23 times (because there are annually 8.23 times more HBV than HIV window-period infections attributable to the continued transfusion of pooled platelets—Fig 2-17 in Chapter 2).

before donating did not have a higher frequency of TTI markers than did donors who denied all MSM activity [odds ratio (OR) = 1.4; 95% CI, 0.7-2.6].[94] When the results were adjusted for HIV test-seeking behavior and donor status (first-time versus repeat), the adjusted OR was exactly 1.0 (95% CI, 0.5-2.2).

Recently, estimates were made available by Presanis et al[95,96] on the prevalence of undiagnosed HIV infection in UK MSM who had abstained from male-to-male sex for 5 years. Davison et al[6] used these figures[95,96] to estimate the projected increase in the risk of HIV transmission by ABT in the United Kingdom if the MSM deferral were reduced to 5 years. This was because, at the time their study was designed, a reduction in the MSM deferral to 5 years seemed to be a "plausible policy choice" for the United Kingdom.[6] Davison et al[6] projected that, if compliance with the MSM deferral policy remained the same following the reduction in the MSM deferral to 5 years, any projected change in the risk of releasing an HIV-infectious donation into the UK blood supply (from 1 per 4.41 million donations to 1 per 4.39 million donations) would be negligible. The risk of releasing an HIV-infectious donation into the UK blood supply could actually *decrease* if compliance with the HIV deferral policy improved as a result of the change in policy and/or educational efforts associated with the change in policy. However, the risk of releasing an HIV-infectious donation into the UK blood supply could also increase if the change in policy led MSM donors to regard their MSM activities as being "less risky" vis-à-vis transmitting HIV infection, thus perhaps leading them to make more noncompliant donations. In all cases (Fig 6-5), the 95% CIs for the projected risk estimates overlapped with the 95% CI associated with the current risk of releasing an HIV-infectious donation into the UK blood supply when donors with a history of MSM activity are indefinitely deferred from donating blood.

The last scenario depicted in Fig 6-5 is especially telling. If the MSM deferral is *altogether* removed, donors who have engaged in *recent* MSM activity (and could conceivably have a window-period HIV infection) would be eligible to donate. Therefore, an increase in risk would logically be expected from such a change in policy and it is reflected in the estimates generated by Davison et al[6]: 1 HIV-infectious donation per 3.48 million donations released into the UK blood supply if the MSM deferral were altogether removed compared with 1 HIV-infectious donation per 4.41 million donations currently released into the UK blood supply when a lifetime MSM deferral is applied. Although removing the MSM deferral altogether would thus increase the risk of an HIV-infectious donation being released for transfusion by 26.5%, the 95% CI of the risk of HIV transmission by ABT when the MSM deferral is altogether removed overlaps with the 95% CI of HIV transmission by ABT when a lifetime MSM deferral is employed. This situation demonstrates how difficult it is to document statistically significant ($p<0.05$) differences for events as rare as the release of an HIV-infectious donation into the blood supply. The projections shown in Fig 6-4—where the risk of HIV transmission by ABT if the MSM deferral is reduced to 1 year is six times smaller than the risk from the continued transfusion of 12.9% of therapeutic platelet doses as pools, but the difference is not statistically significant–should be understood in this spirit.

Davison et al[6] further compared the projected *increase* in risk from reducing the lifetime MSM deferral to 5 years to the projected *decrease* in risk from increasing, from 12 months to lifetime, the deferral for heterosexuals who have had sex with a partner who may have been sexually active in parts of the world where HIV/AIDS is "very common."[97] Because HIV/AIDS is "very common" in all sub-Saharan African countries, people who have had sex with a partner who may have been sexually active in one of many African countries arguably represents the "highest-risk" group among heterosexuals in the United Kingdom.[6] (In the United Kingdom, two-thirds of all new heterosexual diagnoses in 2010 were made in patient of African ethnicity, with the majority of those infected having acquired their infection abroad, mainly in sub-Saharan Africa.[6] These are predominantly prevalent infections and the frequency of sexual contact with people from sub-Saharan Africa in the United Kingdom is expected to be relatively high.[6] Exclusion of donors of African ethnic minorities is not an option, because these donors are needed to provide blood of compatible blood groups for patients from these minorities. However, people who have had sex in the United Kingdom with others who may have been sexually active in sub-Saharan Africa, and who are not of African ethnic minorities themselves, could be excluded without causing a shortage of critically needed blood groups.[6])

Acceptance of donations from this "high-risk" heterosexual group represents the currently tolerated ABT risk in the United Kingdom,[6] in the

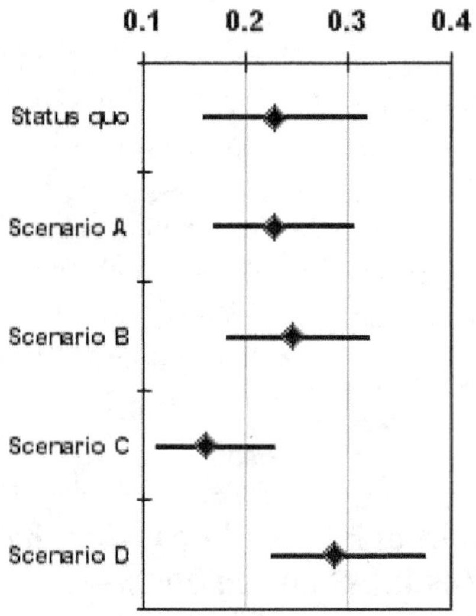

Figure 6-5. Projected estimates of the risk of releasing an HIV-infectious donation into the UK blood supply (per *million* donations) presented by Davison et al.[6] For both the status quo and four possible alternative scenarios, the figure depicts the point estimate of the risk and the associated plausible range. The plausible range is based on the upper and lower 95% CLs for the incidence and prevalence of HIV infection in UK blood donors, the upper and lower CLs for the prevalence of undiagnosed HIV infection among MSM, and the window period of HIV infection (9 vs 5.6 days) if minipool rather than single-unit testing is used to screen UK blood donors for HIV nucleic acid. The status quo pertains to the current lifetime MSM deferral, given the current compliance with the existing lifetime MSM deferral. Scenario A pertains to a reduction in the MSM deferral to 5 years, provided that the compliance with the new deferral criterion remains the same as with the existing deferral criterion. Scenario B pertains to a reduction in the MSM deferral to 5 years in the event that *noncompliance* with the new deferral criterion (compared with noncompliance with the existing lifetime deferral) is increased proportionately to the increase in HIV prevalence (in the newly eligible MSM donors plus the currently eligible donors vs the currently eligible donors alone). Scenario C pertains to a reduction in the MSM deferral to 5 years in the event that—thanks to the change in policy and educational efforts to better communicate to prospective blood donors what the policy is as well as why it has been formulated in this manner—*noncompliance* is decreased to zero and no MSM donors with *recent* MSM activity make blood donations in violation of the MSM deferral policy. Scenario D pertains to the use of *no* MSM deferral *at all.* The plausible range of the status quo overlaps with the plausible ranges of all alternative scenarios, including the scenario of *no* MSM deferral *at all.* The only difference that (only marginally) attains statistical significance ($p \leq 0.05$) in the figure is the difference between scenarios C and D—that is, the difference between a policy that achieves reduction of *noncompliance* with the MSM deferral policy to zero and a policy that altogether removes the MSM deferral criterion.

same manner that the continued transfusion of 12.9% of therapeutic platelet doses as pools represents the currently tolerated ABT risk in the US. Increasing the blood-donation deferral for this "high-risk" heterosexual group from 12 months to lifetime would decrease the risk of an HIV-infectious donation's being released into the UK blood supply by 7.2% (from 1 per 4.41 million to 1 per 4.75 million donations). In comparison, if there was no change in compliance with the applied MSM deferral, reducing the lifetime MSM deferral to 5 years would increase the current risk by only 0.4% (from 1 per 4.41 million to 1 per 4.39 million donations). The projected difference in risk between increasing the 12-month deferral for the "high-risk" heterosexual group to lifetime compared with reducing the lifetime MSM deferral to 5 years was not statistically significant, in the same manner that the projected difference in risk between reducing the lifetime MSM deferral to 1 year compared with continuing to transfuse 12.9% of therapeutic platelet doses as pools (Fig 6-4) is not statistically significant.

HHV-8 Transmission by ABT

Three studies[98-100] (the top three studies in Table 6-2) tested linked donor-recipient samples from repositories collected between the mid-1970s and mid-1980s–before the introduction of WBC reduction of cellular blood components,[98-100] and also before the deferral of donors reporting high-risk behaviors for HIV.[100] Considered together, these studies[98-100] indicate that blood from 151

Table 6-2. North-American Studies of Human Herpesvirus-8 (HHV-8) Transmission Through Transfusion Based on Testing of Linked Donor—Recipient Frozen Samples from Repositories[8]

Study	Repository	Period (Location) of Sample Collection	Number of Linked Donor—Recipient Pairs*	Number of Seroconverting Recipients†
Operskalski et al[98]	Transfusion Safety Study (TSS)	1984-1985 (Los Angeles, New York, San Francisco, Miami)	14 (11‡)	0
Engels et al[99]	Jamaican Transfusion Study	1987-1988 (Jamaica)	19 (12§)	0
Cannon et al[100]	Transfusion Transmitted Viruses Study (TTVS)	1974-1979 (Los Angeles, Houston, New York, St. Louis)	128	0
Dollard et al[101]	Frequency of Agents Communicable by Transfusion Study (FACTS)	1985-1991 (Baltimore, Houston)	NA‖	2

*Pairs of an HHV-8-seropositive donor and a recipient who tested HHV-8-seronegative before the transfusion of non-WBC-reduced cellular blood components.
†On subsequent testing for HHV-8 antibody, usually 6 months following the transfusion.
‡Three patients received plasma, washed red blood cells, or frozen red blood cells.
§One patient was HHV-8 seropositive before the transfusion; six patients received plasma or cryoprecipitate.
‖This repository consisted solely of recipient samples without linked donor samples.
Initially published by Vamvakas in Transfus Med Rev 2011;25:47-60.[29]

HHV-8-seropositive donors has been transfused to 151 HHV-8-seronegative patients with no documented case of HHV-8 transmission by transfusion.[8] The two seroconversions observed in the fourth North-American study[101] (Table 6-2) can be attributed to community or other nosocomial (ie, nontransfusion) sources (Fig 6-6). Thus, the *worst-case* scenario might be that the next (152nd) positive-donor/negative-recipient pair to be studied would coincide with HHV-8 transmission by transfusion. Such a risk (1/152 or 0.658% per HHV-8-seropositive donor)

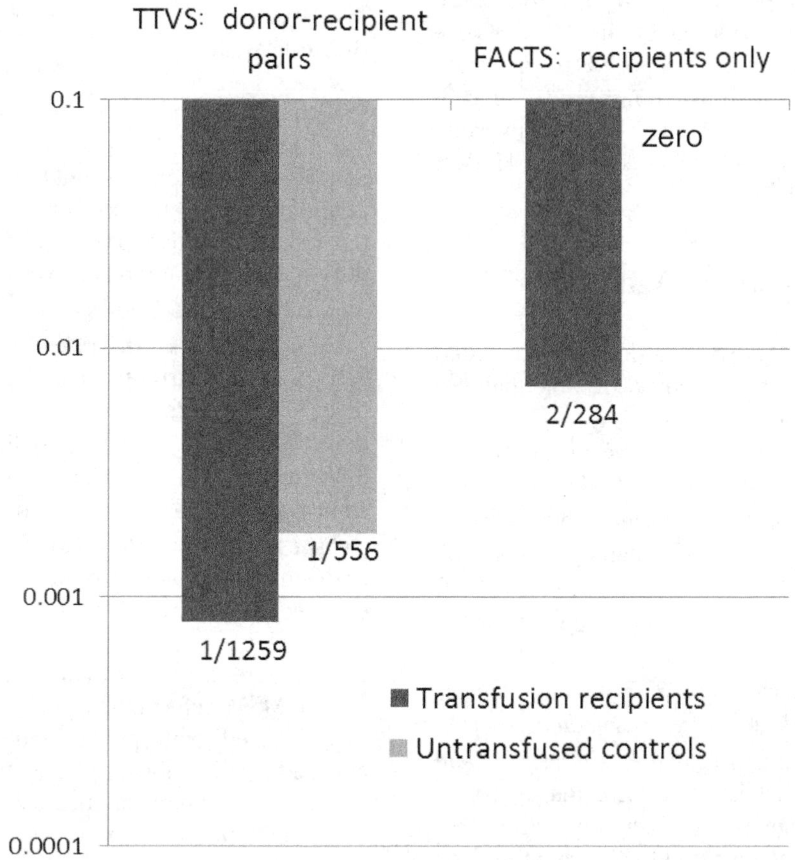

Figure 6-6. Possible attribution of the two seroconversions to HHV-8 observed among 284 perioperatively transfused patients (compared with 0 seroconversions among 75 untransfused controls) in the repository from the Frequency of Agents Communicable by Transfusion Study (FACTS)[101] to community or other nosocomial (ie, nontransfusion) sources, in the light of the results of testing of linked donor-recipient pairs from the repository of the Transfusion-Transmitted Viruses Study (TTVS).[100] In the latter study,[100] two seroconversions occurred over 6 months of follow-up in one recipient of HHV-8-seronegative blood and one untransfused control. Also, HHV-8 seroprevalence was 2.8% in blood donors, as compared with 7.1%, and 7.7%, respectively, in perioperatively transfused patients and untransfused surgical controls—indicating that it is likely for two postsurgical US patients (as observed in the FACTS[101]) to acquire HHV-8 infection over 6 months of follow-up from nontransfusion sources.

would be equivalent to a risk of 0.023% per current United States blood donor (since 3.5% of donors are HHV-8-seropositive[51]).

One cross-sectional study,[102] inferring the risk of HHV-8 transmission by transfusion through a mathematical model,[103] and one prospective cohort study[104] have been reported from Uganda (Fig 6-7). Over 24 weeks of follow-up, the latter study[104] observed a 2.8% per-unit absolute risk of HHV-8 seroconversion in exposed (compared with unexposed) patients (Fig 6-8). If this entire difference were attributed to the HHV-8-seropositive transfusion (as opposed to alternate infection sources such as the mother[67-72]—Fig 6-7 and Table 6-3), 12 of 24 seroconverting exposed patients would have contracted HHV-8 infection from the transfusion.

Emerging Agents

Recently, the AABB Transfusion-Transmitted Diseases Committee prioritized 68 potentially or actually transfusion-transmitted agents based on both the existing evidence of their transmissibility by transfusion and their potential for severe clinical outcomes.[9] Four priority categories were assigned to convey a particular agent's significance: white, yellow, orange, and red. The "red" agents were the variant Creutzfeldt-Jakob disease (vCJD) prions,[105] dengue-fever virus (DFV),[106] and *Babesia* species.[107-109] The "orange" agents were *Leishmania* species, *Plasmodium* species, *Trypanosoma cruzi*, Chickungunya virus,[110,111] and St. Louis encephalitis virus. With the exception of the last two agents, for which the concern was that they have the potential to replicate the West Nile virus experience of transfusion transmission,[112,113] all other "red" or "orange" agents have been shown to be transfusion-transmitted. None of these "red" or "orange" agents, however, is transmitted sexually like HIV or would be more likely to accumulate in MSM than in other donors.

Should the next pathogen be vector-, food-, or air-borne, pooled platelets will have a five times higher risk of transmitting the emerging agent (Table 2-1 in Chapter 2) than apheresis (single-donor) platelets collected from MSM. Should the next pathogen be transmitted sexually, MSM who have abstained for 5 years should carry the same risk as—if not a lower risk than—current donors (who would have continued to have heterosexual contacts during the period of the agent's silent accumulation in the population).

Discussion

Relative Risk

Whether the reason for indefinitely deferring MSM from blood donation has been: 1) the risk of HHV-8 infection (the only scientifically valid argument in the author's opinion, from the relative-risk perspective presented in this chapter, during the two-and-a-half years between the publication of the studies of Hladik et al[104] and Cannon et al[100]); 2) the risk of emerging pathogens (the only currently scientifically valid argument in the author's opinion when a 1-year deferral is considered); or 3) the risk of HIV infection (on which policy-makers[18] have concentrated, perhaps driven by public-health statistics[14-16] and models[114] of the prevalence of undiagnosed HIV infection in MSM *non-donors*); the risk from the continued provision of 12.9% of platelet doses as pooled platelets in the United States is greater than the risk from reducing the MSM deferral to 1 year.

Compared with pooled platelets, group O apheresis (single-donor) platelets given to group A patients may have an increased risk of hemolysis,[115] but this risk can be prevented by appropriate institutional policies.[116] Contrary to what has been postulated,[117] the higher risk of TTIs in association with pooled [compared with apheresis (single-donor)] platelets is most likely not offset by a higher risk of transfusion-related acute lung injury (TRALI)[118,119] from apheresis (single-donor) platelets.[26,120] A whole-blood-derived platelet concentrate contains four to six times less plasma from any *individual* donor (who may be a female donor alloimmunized to paternal WBC antigens during a previous pregnancy[117] and having circulating antibodies directed to the

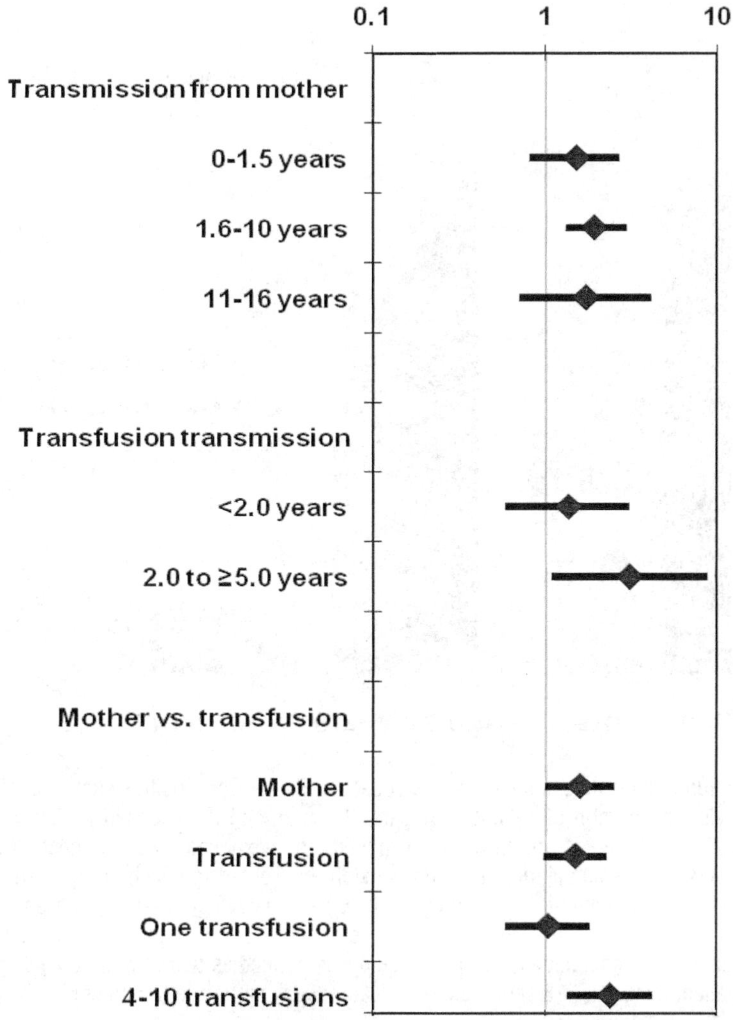

Figure 6-7. Probability of seroconversion to HHV-8 in association with either an HHV-8-seropositive mother or a blood transfusion in sub-Saharan Africa. Children were exposed to HHV-8 through: 1) their HHV-8-seropositive (compared to seronegative) mother in the cross-sectional study of Malope et al[131] (top panel in the figure); 2) one HHV-8-seropositive (compared to seronegative) transfusion in the prospective cohort study of Hladik et al[104] (middle panel); or 3) their HHV-8-seropositive (compared to seronegative) mother and/or *any* transfusion in the cross-sectional study of Mbulaiteye et al (lower panel).[102] Unlike older children, children ≤18 months[131] or <2 years[104] of age did not have a significantly higher risk of contracting HHV-8 from either one HHV-8-seropositive transfusion or their HHV-8-seropositive mother, perhaps owing to the persistence of some maternal antibodies.[102,104] When only one child was <1 year of age,[102] never-transfused (compared with transfused) children had about the same probability of HHV-8 seropositivity as children who had an HHV-8-seropositive (compared with seronegative) mother. Transfusion had a significant association with HHV-8 seropositivity only in children who had received ≥4 transfusions—a situation that is also a marker for poor health that predisposes a child to infection from community sources.

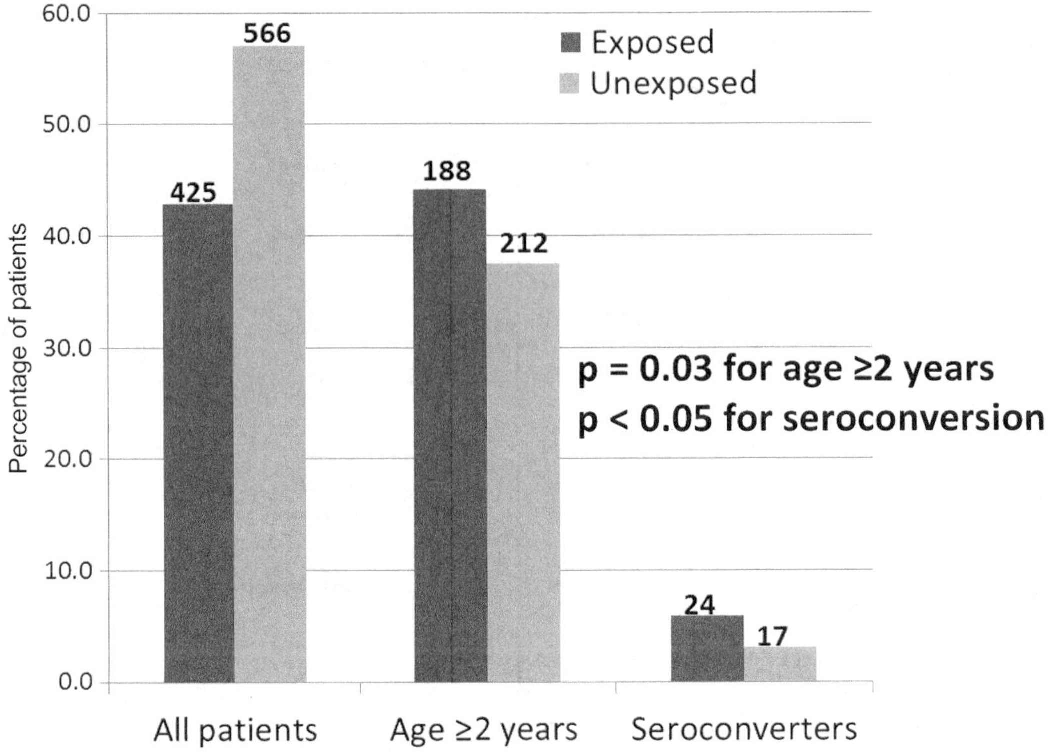

Figure 6-8. Proportion of patients exposed (vs unexposed) to HHV-8-seropositive blood transfusion in the study of Hladik et al[104]; also, proportion of patients ≥2 years of age among the exposed (vs unexposed) transfusion recipients included in the study, and proportion of exposed (vs unexposed) patients meeting the case definition of HHV-8 seroconversion. The actual number of transfusion recipients from each group is shown above the corresponding column. Exposed patients received one HHV-8-seropositive unit; additional transfusions to exposed patients were permitted provided that the donations were HHV-8 seronegative. Unexposed patients received solely HHV-8-seronegative transfusions. Seroconversion was defined as two or more consecutive follow-up visits on which the patient tested HHV-8 seropositive, at least 25 days after the transfusion.

transfusion recipient's WBC antigens[121]). However, a recipient of a platelet *pool* has a four to six times higher risk of receiving a 50-mL platelet concentrate from a female multiparous whole-blood donor with such WBC antibodies, and 50 mL of plasma are sufficient to cause TRALI.[122-125] The higher probability of exposure to 50 mL of plasma from such an alloimmunized donor probably carries as much TRALI risk on average as the receipt of ≤300 mL of plasma from a single donor who may be similarly alloimmunized.[26,120] The data[126-128] comparing the risk of TRALI from pooled compared with apheresis (single-donor) platelets (Table 4-2 in Chapter 4) demonstrated a similar risk from both components.[26]

Because mathematical models[3-5] project that acceptance of donations from MSM who have abstained from male-to-male sex for 1 year will increase the risk of TTIs, however *minimally*, one may wonder if a consistent approach to safety could be achieved by maintaining the current MSM deferral while reducing the use of pooled platelets. Even if transfusion of pooled platelets were banned, however, other examples—such as the delay[76] in implementing the

Table 6-3. Arguments for and Against Transmission of Human Herpesvirus-8 (HHV-8) Infection Through HHV-8-Seropositive Transfusion in the Study of Hladik et al[104]

Arguments for:	Arguments against:
1. Timing of seroconversion to HHV-8: Seroconversion peaked during weeks 3 through 10 after transfusion—a time consistent with the incubation period of other transfusion-transmitted herpesviruses[52] 2. Association of seroconversion with "fresh"(≤4-day-old) rather than "old" (>4-day-old) red blood cell units ($p<0.05$): Fresh units contain viable white blood cells that can harbor the virus	1. Lack of adjustment for the HHV-8 status of the mother in the analysis 2. Greater proportion of children aged ≥2 years among the exposed (compared with the unexposed: Fig 6-8) group: As a result (Fig 6-7), a greater proportion of exposed (compared with unexposed) children were likely to acquire HHV-8 infection from the mother, thereby leading to a higher overall incidence of seroconversion among the unexposed (compared with the exposed) children 3. Inconsistent results obtained with split components: Seroconversion did not occur in 12 patients who received half of split pediatric HHV-8-seropositive units, the other half of which was given to children who seroconverted*

*If these 12 seroconversions were excluded from the analysis—that is, considered to have acquired HHV-8 infection from other sources—the number of excess seroconversions attributed to HHV-8-seropositive transfusion by the authors[104] (n=12) would be reduced by exactly the same number, and patients exposed to HHV-8-seropositive transfusion would have the same probability of acquiring HHV-8 infection as would the unexposed patients.

AABB recommendations[129] for screening donors for WBC antibodies[130] to prevent TRALI from platelet transfusion–would show that the transfusion risk currently tolerated in the United States is higher than the ALARA risk.

HHV-8 Transmission through Transfusion

The interpretation of the results of Hladik et al[104] depends on the weight assigned to the arguments (Table 6-4) for and against attributing the observed difference in HHV-8 seroconversions between exposed and unexposed patients in that study (Fig 6-8) to the HHV-8-seropositive transfusion *per se.* The interpretation[59] of these results changes[8] as a better understanding of childhood HHV-8 infection in Africa is gained,[131,132] and as evidence on the absence of HHV-8 transmission by transfusion is adduced from settings where such alternate sources of infection are unlikely.[100] The alternative explanations listed in Table 6-4 do not rule out the possibility of a *small* risk of HHV-8 transmission by transfusion when the conditions for transmission by this route (high frequency of primary infection and episodic HHV-8 activation in blood donors, as well as transfusion of non-WBC-reduced fresh cellular blood components) are optimized. It is thus possible that HHV-8 might be *rarely* transmitted by transfusion similarly to EBV.[133,134] It is equally likely that the results of Hladik et al[104] reflect the risk of acquiring—over 24 weeks—HHV-8 infection from the alternate sources of infection available in a high-prevalence area.[8]

Concerning any purported HHV-8 risk, before the findings of Hladik et al[104] were reinterpreted in the manner presented in Table 6-3 and Fig 6-7, the balance of evidence—dominated by the study of Hladik et al[104]—favored the possibility of HHV-8 transmission by transfusion.[59] Yet, even if HHV-8 were transmitted by transfusion, acceptance of donations from MSM who have abstained for 1 year would increase the baseline risk of HHV-8 transmission through transfusion in the United States by less than 20%. This is because <2% of blood donors would be newly eligible MSM,[3,4,135] while 3.5% of current US donors are HHV-8 seropositive.[51] Even if the newly eligible MSM had 10 times the HHV-8 seroprevalence of current donors,[49-51] there would be >50 donations made by current donors for each donation made by a newly eligible MSM. Thus, a recipient would have a five times higher risk of contracting HHV-8 infection from current donors than from the newly eligible MSM. The absence of measures to prevent transmission of HHV-8 by transfusion reflects the tacit consensus among experts that HHV-8 is not transmitted by transfusion, or—if it is—that such transmission is extremely rare.[136]

Even if HHV-8 were rarely transmitted by transfusion in a manner akin to EBV, however, any risk of developing KS secondary to transfusion-acquired HHV-8 infection would be exceedingly small. The latter risk has not yet been clinically described, despite the fact that—in theory—up to 1 per 4343 current United States blood donors could have been transmitting infection for years. In contrast, the risk of TAS from the continued use of pooled platelets is a major transfusion risk,[26,75,76] and it far exceeds any purported HHV-8 risk from reducing the MSM deferral to 1 year.

Emerging Agents

In the absence of pathogen reduction of blood components, because emerging transfusion-transmitted (or potentially transfusion-transmitted) agents can be vector-borne,[106-113] food-borne,[105] or even air-borne[137]—rather than associated with identifiable high-risk groups (eg, MSM) that can be deferred from donating—limiting the number of donors to whom a patient is exposed is the most effective approach to protecting recipients from emerging agents.[76] Any speculation regarding the probability of emerging TTIs whose infectious agent would be concentrated within the MSM group is mere conjecture, and it is not supported by the TTIs (such as WNV infection and vCJD) that have emerged in the 3 decades since HIV. For this reason, pooled platelets pose a greater risk of transmitting the next major transfusion-transmitted pathogen than donations by MSM who have abstained for 5 years *and* self-select to donate.

Although men who have recently had sex with men (when considered as a homogeneous group) do have a higher prevalence of sexually transmitted infections (STIs) compared with many other sociodemographic groups, the most common STIs (including lymphogranuloma venereum, which currently represents an "emerging" STI in Europe and North America) are not transfusion transmissible. Outbreaks of syphilis among MSM have raised concerns about the possibility of MSM with early-stage syphilis infections making blood donations if the deferral were reduced, but *Treponema pallidum* does not survive in stored whole blood or blood components and the last case of transfusion-transmitted syphilis in the United States occurred in 1968.[138] With only one additional case in the developed world having been recorded since that time also in association with transfusion of fresh blood or components—in The Netherlands in 1977[139]—transfusion-transmitted syphilis had disappeared from the developed world before MSM were deferred from donating in 1983. The fact that syphilis testing of blood donors has not been eliminated[140] is a testament to the regulatory difficulties associated with the discontinuation of an existing blood-donor screening test when the test (much like the MSM deferral criterion) does not contribute to blood safety.

Although deferring MSM for 5 (rather than 1) year can be regarded as the safest option for addressing the possibility of emerging TTIs that have dual transmission modes (sexual as well as blood-borne), as well as a long incubation period akin to that of HIV infection, implementation of a 5-year deferral for MSM will be inconsistent with existing deferrals for similar-risk activities through heterosexual contacts. The latter were formulated based on the maximum window period of HIV, HBV, and HCV infection (Table 6-1); not to protect recipients from emerging agents. If the focus now moves to the prevention of emerging TTIs (and specifically TTIs with a dual mode of transmission: sexual as well as blood-borne), 5-year deferrals should be employed for all high-risk sexual contacts, whether homosexual or heterosexual. Recent empirical findings[141] (discussed in the next section) indicate that a 1-year MSM deferral (compared with any other deferral period) optimizes blood safety with regard to transfusion-transmitted HIV infection because it maximizes the probability of compliance with the applied MSM deferral. If transmission of HIV (rather than of emerging agents) is the primary concern, a 1- (rather than a 5-) year deferral may be the best option for ensuring overall blood safety.

Evidence Before July 2010

If the MSM deferral is reduced, there could be some *minimal* increase in the risk of TTIs. However, after the concern about HHV-8 transmission by ABT was alleviated in June 2009,[100] the risk from reducing the MSM deferral to 1 year is smaller than the transfusion risk which—despite exceeding the ALARA risk—is currently tolerated in the United States (Fig 2-17 in Chapter 2). Regarding HIV, if the assumptions made in the published models (Figs 6-2 and 6-3) were corroborated by empirical research, there could be some *minimal* increase in the risk of transfusion transmission if the MSM deferral were reduced. Not prohibiting transfusion of pooled platelets is currently causing a greater number of preventable TTIs (Fig 2-17 in Chapter 2), but reducing the MSM deferral is regarded as representing an *increase* in risk and this belief makes it hard for United States regulators to change the existing lifetime deferral. Implementing a policy that might increase risk is harder to accept than not implementing a policy that will reduce risk—even when the palpable risk to be prevented is greater than the postulated risk to be incurred. Furthermore, because the 95% CI for the increase in risk during the first year after the change in policy extended between 0 and 1 HIV-infectious whole-blood unit released for transfusion in the model of Anderson et al,[5] the possibility that 1 additional HIV-infectious unit could indeed be released for transfusion in the first year after the change in policy compounds the difficulty of implementing a reduction in the MSM deferral.

It is possible that reducing the MSM deferral might indeed increase risk because erroneous release from quarantine of TTI-reactive units predicts erroneous release of HIV-positive units[5] (Fig 6-3); and because those who have deferrable MSM risk and are currently donating will continue to donate as often as they do now after the MSM deferral is reduced.[5] Absent any empirical research findings on the effect that a change in policy might have had on compliance with the policy, Anderson et al[5] favored the speculation that reducing the MSM deferral to 1 year would have no effect on compliance with the policy. However, at the time of the publication of the model of Anderson et al,[5] it was equally plausible to speculate that the clarity of the *harmonized* criteria would enhance blood safety through improved comprehension of the questions and improved accuracy of the answers vis-à-vis recent risk activities on the part of both non-MSM and MSM donors.[142] After the model of Anderson et al was published, empirical findings from the United Kingdom[141] substantiated this latter thesis.[142]

Concerning the second assumption of Anderson et al,[5] erroneous release of HIV-positive units from quarantine is possible regardless of whether the donor acquired the infection through a homosexual or heterosexual contact; accordingly, investment in information-systems technologies for better inventory management at United States hospital blood banks is needed independently of whether donations by MSM are allowed. The 10-fold reduction in erroneous releases in 2003-2005 compared to a decade previously (Fig 6-3) underscores the preventable nature of these errors and the opportunity for major improvements through rigorous quality-assurance practices. Error rates at hospitals could be reduced to the level of blood centers, cutting the nationwide number of erroneous releases of TTI-reactive units in half. Errors could be further reduced by introducing electronic-barrier (or other) systems (Chapter 4).

When: 1) the risk attributed to erroneous releases (Fig 6-3) is removed from the MSM risk estimate; 2) the assumptions about suboptimal sensitivity of the screening tests and human errors in laboratory testing made in the older models[3,4] are harmonized with the assumptions made in the analysis of Anderson et al[5]; and 3) the estimate of Germain et al[4] is used for the prevalence of undiagnosed HIV infection in MSM donors who have abstained for 1 year *and* self-select to donate (Fig 6-2); the projected risk from reducing the MSM deferral to 1 year becomes 1 infectious donation per 56 million MSM donations.[29] This corresponds to 1 infectious donation released for transfusion in the United States every 280 years[29]—based on the assumption of 20 million donations per year and a 1% increase in donations owing to the reduction in the MSM deferral to 1 year.

Thus, in theory, and provided that reducing the deferral has no effect on compliance with the policy, any increase in risk attributable to a reduction in the MSM deferral to 1 year could be as high as 1 additional HIV-infectious unit released in the first year after the change in policy (the upper 95% CI of the estimate of Anderson et al[5]), or as low as 1 additional HIV-infectious unit released in the United States every 280 years.[29] Regardless of which of these estimates might represent the true increase in risk, before empirical research had documented that harmonized criteria most likely enhance blood safety (as well as maintain the credibility of blood agencies with donors through the application of donor selection criteria that are based on a clear rationale[141,142]), the increase in risk if the MSM deferral is reduced could never be shown to be zero[4] by mathematical models incorporating the three sources of risk and not considering the possibility of a decrease in risk thanks to improved donor compliance with the deferral. Even under these one-sided assumptions that were made in the models, either estimate of the increase in risk (1 additional HIV-positive unit released for transfusion in the United States in the first year after changing the policy or 1 additional HIV-positive unit released for transfusion in the United States every 280 years) was minimal and, if the policy debate had been framed in terms of *absolute* risk, the question would have been which of these two positions was the most *ethical* one: not to tolerate a minimal risk to protect transfusion recipients, or to tolerate a minimal risk to be fair to the MSM group. The answer to this policy dilemma represented a societal choice. Different countries made[143] (and will be making in the future) different policy decisions reflecting their respective societal values.

US policy makers have taken the position that, regarding the question of reducing the MSM deferral, a decision associated with any increase in risk—however *minimal*—is not acceptable.[18] This position may be less tenable, however, when the postulated increase in risk from reducing the MSM deferral is shown to be smaller than the currently tolerated transfusion risk that exceeds the ALARA risk (Fig 6-4). That is why, when the possibility of only an increase (as opposed to either an increase or a decrease) in risk is envisioned by theoretical models of the impact of a change in the MSM deferral, the policy debate ought to be framed in terms of the *relative* (in addition to *absolute*) risk. Furthermore, unlike what was done in the published models, removal of discrimination and fairness to the MSM group should be recognized as positive benefits to society; these benefits can compensate for any postulated increase in risk that might result from reducing the MSM deferral.[144-149] Such considerations do not apply to other indefinite deferrals (eg, the deferral for residence in Europe in 1980-1996), which are not associated with (nor do they reinforce) societal prejudice vis-à-vis the activity (MSM compared with travel to Europe) or the presumption of disease presence (HIV rather than vCJD).[150]

The Department of Health and Human Services Advisory Committee on Blood Safety and Availability voted 9 to 6 on June 11, 2010 against recommending any immediate change to the lifetime MSM deferral. The committee recognized, however, that the current policy is "suboptimal," because it permits "some potentially high-risk donations" (from heterosexual donors), "while preventing some potentially low-risk donations" (from MSM).[12] In an effort to improve blood safety while seeking to diminish the discriminatory aspects of the policy, the committee unanimously recommended a series of steps for moving toward taking individual behavior into account for donor selection rather than considering that all MSM (as well as all heterosexuals) have uniform behavioral characteristics.

Evidence Since July 2010

After the Blood Safety and Availability Committee made this recommendation in June 2010, the Department of Health and Human Services charged the Blood, Organ, and Tissue Safety Working Group to develop a plan based on the committee's recommendations. The Group recommended that three studies be conducted, to produce data needed for a re-evaluation of the current lifetime deferral for MSM and potentially lead to an interim change toward a shortened deferral since the last male-to-male sexual contact. These three studies are: 1) collection of baseline data on the risk of TTIs in relation to risk factors in blood donors; 2) root-cause analysis of erroneous releases from quarantine at blood collection centers; and 3) cognitive evaluation of the blood-donor history questionnaire. A study to better understand donation behavior by MSM is also under consideration.[151] These studies would generate valuable information for optimizing blood safety in the United States, although they would not provide a *direct* answer to the question whether the MSM deferral should be reduced to 1 or 5 years. The only study design that can produce findings as pertinent to US policy decision making as the study of Seed et al[1] would be a repetition in the United States of the same before-and-after design used in Australia.[1] This approach would require United States policy makers to change the MSM deferral based on the research findings reported from Australia[1] and the United Kingdom[141] and then compare HIV prevalence in collections made before with those made after the change in policy. The reason why only this research design can generate the answer needed for decision making is that only this design can study *actual* MSM donors who have abstained from male-to-male sex for 1 year and *self-select* to donate after the change in policy. No other research design can replicate this fundamental aspect of blood donation, that is, the self-selection of *actual* donors for making a blood donation based on altruism as well as perception of low self-risk for transmitting TTIs to transfusion recipients. Any pilot studies of MSM donors undertaken in the United States that do not employ such "real-world" conditions should strive to approximate the actual-donor self-selection process as closely as possible.

Recently Grenfell et al[141] published the *first* study reporting views on the MSM deferral criterion expressed by gay, bisexual, and other men who had had sex with men and who were identified through a *general population sample.* The design innovation of this study[141] lay in the use of a general population sample (as opposed to a "convenience" sample recruited from gay venues). In this way, the investigators captured the views and experiences of men who may not be publicly open about their sexual experiences with other men. Of 32,373 men from the general UK population, 1028 (3%) reported having had "any" sexual contact with a man and were routed to the blood donation module of the questionnaire. Almost half of the 1028 men reporting "any" sexual contact had had "penetrative" sex with another man, and 227 men had done so in the previous year; importantly, 23% of the latter 227 men described their sexual identity as heterosexual. Also, just under half of the 1028 men agreed to be re-contacted and 88 were selected for an in-depth interview. Of these 88 men, 30 participated in the interview (45 could not be contacted and 13 declined). Of the latter 30 men, 19 had complied with the UK lifetime MSM deferral and 11 had not.

Of the 474 respondents from the general male population who had had "penetrative" sex with other men, 50 (10.6%) had donated blood in the United Kingdom even though they were ineligible to donate. Ineligible donation was significantly less common among men who had had male penetrative sex in the past year compared with those who had done so longer previously (6.8% vs 15.1%; $p<0.01$); and among those who identified as gay compared with those who had not (5.2% vs 15.5%; $p<0.001$). "Noncompliers" described their reasons for having made ineligible donations in the course of the in-depth interviews. These reasons included self-categorization as low-risk, discounting the sexual experience that barred donation, need for discretion vis-à-vis sexual identity or practice, misconceptions related to procedures safeguarding blood, misunderstanding of the exclusion criterion, and resentment over the perceived inequity of the applied MSM deferral criterion. The current lifetime deferral was criticized by the participants who saw it as inequitable, discriminatory, and–above all–as lacking a clear rationale. Taking into account issues relating to feasibility, equity, and scientific coherence, the participants selected a 1-year deferral since the last male-to-male sexual contact as being the best policy option. A 5-year deferral was not considered acceptable. Lack of support for the 5-year option by the constituent group would not augur well for compliance with a 5-year deferral if a 5-year deferral were to be implemented in the United Kingdom.[141]

The UK study[141] further substantiated earlier Swedish conclusions. In Sweden, where rates and reasons for noncompliance among gay and bisexual men[142] are similar to those found by the UK investigators,[141] blood safety is predicted to be optimal under a 1-year MSM deferral (compared with any other deferral period). This is because a 1-year deferral maximizes compliance with the applied MSM deferral, and compliance with the deferral (as opposed to length of the deferral) is the critical factor determining blood safety.[1,6]

The UK study[141] was undertaken to inform a review of the UK blood donation policy with regard to men who have had sex with men. The authors concluded that replacing the lifetime MSM deferral with a 1-year deferral is seen as a fairer policy and it is thus likely to be welcomed by most gay, bisexual, and other men who have had sex with men; and that such increased endorsement by the constituency in question might improve compliance rates, particularly among men who are currently donating ineligibly owing to perceived discrimination.

Another finding of the study[141] was that some "noncompliers" dissociated past sexual experience with other men from the MSM deferral criterion because they identified as heterosexual and considered the MSM criterion to apply to gay men. The authors[141] urged health professionals to consider the possibility that men who do not identify themselves as gay, bisexual, or MSM may not absorb health information targeted to those groups.

Given these empirical findings,[141] and following a comprehensive evidence-based review by the Advisory Committee on the Safety of Blood, Tissues and Organs, the United Kingdom proceeded to reduce the MSM deferral to 1 year as of November, 2011.[152] Men who have had anal or oral sex with another man in the past 12 months, with or without a condom, will still not be eligible to donate blood, owing to the heightened risk of sexually active MSM–when considered as a homogeneous group–for sexually acquiring blood-borne viruses. In this way, the MSM criterion will be harmonized with the criteria used for other groups who are deferred from donating blood due to risks associated with sexual behaviors. The Advisory Committee (composed of experts in the field and joined by patient groups and key stakeholders) reviewed the risk of TTIs, donor attitudes toward complying (or not) with the donor selection criteria,[141] and the recent improvements in donor testing for TTIs. The UK National Blood and Transplant Service considered it essential that their donor selection criteria be based on evidence, so that the Service could maintain its credibility with donors.

The UK decision has thus been the first evidence-based decision vis-à-vis the MSM deferral policy. It relied on *empirical* findings from Australia[1] (showing that reducing the MSM deferral to 1 year does not result in increased collections of HIV-positive units) and from the United Kingdom[141] (showing that a 1-year deferral is likely to improve compliance with the MSM deferral policy and thus increase the safety of the blood supply). These empirical findings[1,141] apply directly to North America because Australia–like the United States and Canada–does not "prescreen" first-time donors for infectious disease markers before collecting blood from them; and because findings vis-à-vis compliance with the same lifetime deferral policy derived from UK gay and bisexual men, as well as other men who have had sex with men, can be reasonably extrapolated to the United States and Canada. These empirical findings[1,141] contradict the results of the earlier mathematical models[3-5] on which United States policy has hitherto relied. More specifically, these empirical findings[1,141] challenge both principal assumptions of Anderson et al[5]: unlike what was presumed by Anderson et al,[5] reducing the MSM deferral to 1 year does *not* result in increased collections of HIV-positive units[1]; furthermore, after a reduction of the deferral to 1 year, those with deferrable risk behaviors who used to donate ineligibly are *not* likely to continue donating as often as they did before the change in policy.[141] The empirical nature of these new findings[1,141] provides a new evidence base for policy change, as research into the question of MSM deferral has moved from theoretical models to empirical findings.

References

1. Seed CR, Kiely P, Law M, et al. No evidence of significantly increased risk of transfusion-transmitted human immunodeficiency virus infection in Australia subsequent to implementing a 12-month deferral for men who have had sex with men. Transfusion 2010;50:2722-30.
2. Polizzoto MN, Wood EM, Ingham H, Keller AJ. Reducing the risk of transfusion-transmissible viral infection through blood donor selection: The Australian experience 2000 through 2006. Transfusion 2008;48:55-63.
3. Soldan K, Sinka K. Evaluation of the de-selection of men who have had sex with men from blood donation in England. Vox Sang 2003; 84:265-73.
4. Germain M, Remis RS, Delage G. The risks and benefits of accepting men who have had sex with men as blood donors. Transfusion 2003; 43:25-33.
5. Anderson SA, Yang H, Gallagher LM, et al. Quantitative estimate of the risks and benefits of possible alternative blood donor deferral strategies for men who have had sex with men. Transfusion 2009;49:1102-14.
6. Davison KL, Brant LJ, Presanis AM, Soldan K. A re-evaluation of the risk of transfusion-transmitted HIV prevented by the exclusion of men who have sex with men from blood donation in England and Wales, 2005-2007. Vox Sang 2011;101:291-302.
7. Busch M, Glynn S. Use of the blood-donor and transfusion-recipient biospecimen repositories to address emerging blood-safety concerns and advance infectious disease research: The National Heart, Lung, and Blood Institute Biologic Specimen Repository. J Infect Dis 2009; 199:1564-6.
8. Vamvakas EC. Is human herpesvirus-8 transmitted by transfusion? Transfus Med Rev 2010; 24:1-14.
9. Stramer SL, Hollinger FB, Katz LM, et al. Emerging infectious disease agents and their potential threat to transfusion safety. Transfusion 2009;49(Suppl 2):1S-236S.
10. Wainberg MA, Shuldiner T, Dahl K, et al. Reconsidering the lifetime deferral of blood donation by men who have sex with men. CMAJ 2010;182:1321-4.
11. Neill US. Don't ask, don't tell...and don't donate (editorial). J Clin Invest 2010;120:1364.
12. US Department of Health and Human Services. Blood Safety and Availability Committee 39th Meeting Summary. June 10-11, 2010. Rockville, MD: DHHS, 2010. [Available at: http://hhs.gov/ash/bloodsafety/advisorycommittee/past meetings/pastmeetings.html#jun10 (accessed November 8, 2011).]
13. Brooks J. Should men who have ever had sex with men be allowed to give blood? No. Br Med J 2009;338:b318.
14. Centers for Disease Control and Prevention (CDC). Prevalence and awareness of HIV infection among men who have sex with men—21

cities, United States, 2008. MMWR Morbid Mortal Wkly Rep 2010;59:1201-7.
15. Health Protection Agency. Sexually transmitted infections and men who have sex with men in the UK: 2008 Report. London, UK: Health Protection Agency, 2008. [Available at: http://www.hpa.org.uk/webc/HPAwebFile/HDAweb_C/1227515298225 (accessed November 8, 2011).]
16. Murphy G, Charlett A, Jordon LF, et al. HIV incidence appears constant in men who have sex with men despite widespread use of effective antiretroviral therapy. AIDS 2004;18:265-72.
17. Van der Bij AK, Coutinho RA, van der Poel CL. Surveillance of risk profiles among new and repeat blood donors with transfusion-transmitted infections from 1995 through 2003 in the Netherlands. Transfusion 2006;46:1729-36.
18. Presented by the United States Food and Drug Administration at the United States Food and Drug Administration Workshop on Behavior-Based Donor Deferrals in the NAT Era. Lister Hill Auditorium National Institutes of Health, Bethesda, Maryland, March 8, 2006.
19. Leiss W, Tyshenko M, Krewski D. Men-having-sex-with-men donor-deferral risk assessment: An analysis using risk management principles. Transfus Med Rev 2008;22:35-57.
20. Vamvakas EC. Scientific background on the risk engendered by reducing the lifetime blood donation deferral period for men who have sex with men. Transfus Med Rev 2009;23:85-102.
21. Williams AE, Thomas RA, Schreiber GB, et al. Estimates of infectious disease risk factors in United States blood donors. JAMA 1997;277: 967-72.
22. Soldan K, Barbara JAJ, Ramsay ME, Hall AJ. Estimation of the risk of HBV, HCV and HIV infectious donations entering the blood supply in England, 1993-2001. Vox Sang 2002;84: 274-86.
23. Stramer SL, Glynn SA, Kleinman SH, et al. Detection of HIV-1 and HCV infections among antibody-negative blood donors by nucleic-acid amplification testing. N Engl J Med 2004;351: 760-8.
24. Wang B, Schreiber GB, Glynn SA, et al. Does prevalence of transfusion-transmitted viral infection reflect corresponsing incidence in United Stated blood donors? Tranfusion 2005;45: 1089-96.
25. James V, ed. Guidelines for the blood transfusion services in the UK. 7th ed. London, UK: The Stationery Office, 2005. [Available at: http://www.official-documents. gov.uk/documents/other/0117033715.asp (accessed November 8, 2011).]
26. Vamvakas EC. Relative safety of pooled versus single-donor (apheresis) platelets in the United States: A systematic review of disparate risks. Transfusion 2009;49:2743-58.
27. US Department of Health and Human Services. The 2007 Nationwide Blood Collection and Utilization Survey Report. Washington, DC: DHHS, 2008.
28. US Department of Health and Human Services. The 2009 National Blood Collection and Utilization Survey Report. Washington, DC: DHHS, 2011.
29. Vamvakas EC. Relative risk of reducing the lifetime blood donation deferral for men who have had sex with men versus currently tolerated transfusion risks. Transfus Med Rev 2011;25: 47-60.
30. Vesga MA. Requirements for donor selection in relation to human immunodeficiency virus in Spain. Presented at the 21st Congress of the Spanish Society of Blood Transfusion and Cellular Therapy. Valladolid, Spain, 11 June 2010. SETS 2010;22(2):64-6.
31. Jimenez Del Bianco A, Martin G, Lamamié De Clairac L, et al. Epidemiological profile and sexual conduct of ELISA/TPHA-positive donors. Presented at the 21st Congress of the Spanish Society of Blood Transfusion and Cellular Therapy. Valladolid, Spain, 11 June 2010. SETS 2010;22(2):171.
32. Coutlee F, Olivier C, Cassol S, et al. Absence of prolonged immunosilent infection with human immunodeficiency virus in individuals with high-risk behaviors. Am J Med 1994;96:42-8.
33. Dodd RY, Notari EP 4th, Stramer SL. Current prevalence and incidence of infectious disease markers and estimated window-period risk in the American Red Cross blood donor population. Transfusion 2002;42:975-9.
34. Busch MP, Glynn SA, Wright DJ, et al. Relative sensitivities of licensed nucleic-acid amplification tests for detection of viremia in early human immunodeficiency virus and hepatitis C virus infection. Transfusion 2005;45:1853-63.
35. Kleinman SH, Busch MP. Assessing the impact of HBV NAT on window-period reduction and residual risk. J Clin Virol 2006;36(Suppl):S523-S9.
36. Assal A, Barlet V, Deschaseaux M, et al. Sensitivity of two hepatitis B virus, hepatitis C virus

(HCV), and human immunodeficiency virus (HIV) nucleic-acid test systems relative to hepatitis B surface antigen, anti-HCV, anti-HIV, and p24/anti-HIV combination assays in seroconversion panels. Transfusion 2009;49:301-10.
37. Kleinman SH, Leslie N, Busch MP. Infectivity of human immunodeficiency virus-1, hepatitis C virus, and hepatitis B virus and risk of transmission by transfusion. Transfusion 2009;49: 2454-89.
38. Simmons P, Manning A, Kenneil R, et al. Parental transmission of the novel human parvovirus, PARV4. Emerg Infect Dis 2007;13:1386-8.
39. Sharp CP, Lail A, Donfield S, et al. High frequencies of exposure to the novel human parvovirus PARV4 in hemophiliacs and injection drug users, as detected by a serological assay for PARV4 antibodies. J Infect Dis 2009;200:1119-25.
40. Lombardi VC, Ruscetti FW, Das Gupta J, et al. Detection of an infectious retrovirus, XRMV, in blood cells of patients with chronic fatigue syndrome. Science 2009;326:585-9.
41. United Nations Conference on Environment and Development. Earth Summit. Rio Declaration on Environment and Development, Rio de Janeiro, Brazil. Publ. no. E.73II.A.14. New York: United Nations, 1992.
42. Foster KR, Vecchia P, Repacholi MH. Risk management. Science and the precautionary principle. Science 2000;288:979-81.
43. Wilson K, Wilson M, Hébert PC, Graham I. The application of the precautionary principle to the blood system: The Canadian blood system's vCJD deferral policy. Transfus Med Rev 2003;17:89-94.
44. Martin JN, Ganen DE, Osmond DH. Sexual transmission and the natural history of human herpesvirus 8 infection. N Engl J Med 1998; 338:948-54.
45. Smith NA, Sabin CA, Gopal R, et al. Serologic evidence of human herpesvirus 8 transmission by homosexual but not heterosexual men. J Infect Dis 1999;180:600-6.
46. Martin JN, Osmond DH. Determining specific sexual practices associated with human herpesvirus 8 transmission. Am J Epidemiol 2000; 151:225-9.
47. Grulich AE, Cunningham P, Munier ML, et al. Sexual behavior and human herpesvirus infection in homosexual men in Australia. Sex Health 2005;2:13-8.
48. Martro E, Esteve A, Schultz TF, et al. Risk factors for human herpesvirus 8 infection and AIDS-associated Kaposi's sarcoma among men who have sex with men in a European multicenter study.
49. Dukers NHTM, Rezza G. Human herpesvirus epidemiology: What we do and do not know. AIDS 2003;17:1717-30.
50. Martin JN. Diagnosis and epidemiology of human herpesvirus 8 infection. Semin Hematol 2003;40:133-42.
51. Pellett PE, Wright DJ, Engels EA, et al. Multicenter comparison of serologic assays and estimation of human herpesvirus-8 seroprevalence among United States blood donors. Transfusion 2003;43:1260-8.
52. Adler SP, McVoy MM. Cytomegalovirus infections in seropositive patients after transfusion: The effect of red-cell storage and volume. Transfusion 1989;29:667-71.
53. Vamvakas EC, Tegtmeier GE. Herpes viruses. In: Barbara JAJ, Regan FAM, Contreras MC, eds. Transfusion microbiology. Cambridge, UK: Cambridge University Press, 2008:35-58.
54. Pearson HA, Wood C, Andeman W, et al. Low risk of hepatitis B from blood transfusions in thalassemic patients in Connecticut. J Pediatr 1986;108:252-3.
55. Papaevangelou G, Economidou J, Roumeliotou A, et al. Epstein-Barr infection in polytransfused patients with homozygous beta-thalassemia. Vox Sang 1979;37:305-9.
56. Henle W, Henle G. Epstein-Barr virus and blood transfusions. In: Dodd RY, Barker LF, eds. Infection, immunity, and blood transfusion. New York: Alan R. Liss, 1985:201-9.
57. Blackbourn DJ, Ambroziak J, Lennette E, et al. Infectious human herpesvirus 8 in a healthy North-American blood donor. Lancet 1997; 349:609-11.
58. Cannon MJ, Laney AS, Pellett PE. Human herpesvirus 8: Current issues. Clin Infect Dis 2003: 37: 82-7.
59. Blajchman MA, Vamvakas EC. The continuing risk of transfusion-transmitted infections. N Engl J Med 2006;355:1303-5.
60. Luppi M, Barozzi P, Santagostino G, et al. Molecular evidence of organ-related transmission of Kaposi sarcoma-associated herpesvirus or human herpesvirus 8 in transplant patients. Blood 2000;96:3279-81.
61. Barozzi P, Luppi M, Facchetti F, et al. Post-transplant Kaposi's sarcoma lesions from renal transplant recipients barcoded either genetic or antigenic markers of the matched donors. Nat Med 2003;9:554-61.

62. Hudnall SD, Chen T, Rady P, et al. Human herpesvirus 8 seroprevalence and viral load in healthy adult blood donors. Transfusion 2003; 43:85-90.
63. Ferreira S, Sanabani S, Reis AD, et al. Human herpesvirus type 8 among Brazilian blood donors. Transfusion 2003;43:1764-5.
64. Enbom M, Urassa W, Massambu C, et al. Detection of human herpesvirus 8 DNA in serum from blood donors with HHV-8 antibodies indicates possible bloodborne virus transmission. J Med Virol 2002;68:264-7.
65. Belec L, Cancre N, Hallouin MC, et al. High prevalence in Central Africa of blood donors who are potentially infectious for human herpesvirus 8. Transfusion 1998;38:771-5.
66. Whitby D, Luppi M, Sabin C, et al. Detection of antibodies to human herpesvirus 8 in Italian children: Evidence of horizontal transmission. Br J Cancer 2000;82:702-4.
67. Mayama S, Cuevas LE, Sheldon J, et al. Prevalence and transmission of Kaposi's sarcoma associated herpesvirus (human herpesvirus 8) in Ugandan children and adolescents. Int J Cancer 1998;77:817-20.
68. Plancoulaine S, Abel L, van Beveren M, et al. Human herpesvirus 8 transmission from mother to child and between siblings in an endemic population. Lancet 2000;356:1062-5.
69. Martro E, Bultreys M, Stewart JA, et al. Comparison of human herpesvirus 8 and Epstein-Barr virus seropositivity among children in areas endemic and non-endemic for Kaposi's sarcoma. J Med Virol 2004;72:126-31.
70. Mbulaiteye SM, Pfeiffer RM, Whitby D, et al. Human herpesvirus 8 infection within families in rural Tanzania. J Infect Dis 2003;187:1780-5.
71. Plancoulaine S, Abel L, Trégouët D, et al. Respective roles of serological status and blood specific antihuman herpesvirus-8 antibody levels in human herpesvirus-8 intrafamilial transmission in a highly endemic area. Cancer Res 2004;64:8782-7.
72. Bourboulia D, Whitby D, Boshoff C, et al. Serologic evidence for mother-to-child transmission of Kaposi sarcoma-associated herpesvirus infection. JAMA 1999;280:31-2.
73. Zou S, Musavi F, Notari E, Stramer S, Dodd R. Prevalence, incidence, and residual risk of major blood-borne infections among apheresis collections to the American Red Cross Blood Services, 2004-2008. Transfusion 2010;50: 1487-94.
74. McDonald CP, Blajchman MA. Bacterial contamination in blood and blood components. In: Barbara JSJ, Regan FAM, Contreras MC, eds. Transfusion microbiology. Cambridge, UK: Cambridge University Press, 2008:87-115.
75. Food and Drug Administration. Fatalities reported to the FDA following blood collection and transfusion. Annual summary for fiscal year 2008. Rockville, MD: CBER Office of Communication, Outreach, and Development, 2008. [Available at: http://www.fda.gov/Biologics BloodVaccines/SafetyAvailability/ReportaProblem/TransfusionDonationFatalities/UCM 113649.htm (accessed November 8, 2011).]
76. Vamvakas EC, Blajchman MA. Transfusion-related mortality: The on-going risks of allogeneic blood transfusion and the available strategies for their prevention. Blood 2009;113: 3406-17.
77. Ness P, Braine N, King K, et al. Single-donor platelets reduce the risk of septic platelet transfusion reactions. Transfusion 2001;41:857-61.
78. Robillard P, Nawej KI, Jochem K. The Quebec hemovigilance system: Description and results from the first two years. Transfus Apher Sci 2004;31:111-22.
79. Murphy WG, Foley M, Doherty C, et al. Screening platelet concentrates for bacterial contamination: Low numbers of bacteria and slow growth in contaminated units mandate an alternate approach to product safety. Vox Sang 2008;95:13-19.
80. Benjamin RJ, Wagner SJ. The residual risk of sepsis: Modeling the effect of concentration on bacterial detection in two-bottle culture systems and an estimation of false-negative culture rates. Transfusion 2007;47:1381-9.
81. Seed C, Lee J, Buring M, Keller A. Do prospective blood donors understand HCV and HIV risk factors? The Austrialan experience (abstract). Transfusion 2002;42(Suppl):72S.
82. Musto JA, Seed CR, Law M, et al. Estimating the risk of blood donation associated with HIV risk behaviors. Transfus Med 2008;18:49-54.
83. McQuillan GM, Kruscon-Moran D, Kottiri B, et al. Prevalence of HIV in the United States household population. J Acquir Immune Defic Syndr 2006;41:651-6.
84. Valdiserri RO, Weber T, Frey R. Trends in HIV seropositivity in publicly-funded HIV counseling and testing program: Implications for prevention policy. Am J Prev Med 1998;14:31-42.

85. Health Protection Agency. HIV in the United Kingdom: 2008 Report. London, UK: Health Protection Agency, 2009.
86. Weber AE, Chan K, George C, et al. Risk factors associated with HIV infection among young gay and bisexual men in Canada. J Acquir Immune Defic Syndr 2001;28:81-8.
87. Unlinked Anonymous HIV Surveys Steering Group. Prevalence of HIV in the United Kingdom, data to end of 1998. London, UK: Department of Health, Public Health Laboratory Service, Institute of Child Health, Scottish Center for Infection and Environmental Health, 1999.
88. Petruckevitch A, Nicoll A, Johnson A, Bennett D. Direct estimates of prevalent HIV infection in adults in England and Wales for 1991 and 1993: An improved method. Genitour Med 1997;73:348-54.
89. Linden JV, Kaplan HS. Transfusion errors: Causes and effect. Transfus Med Rev 1994;34: 169-83.
90. Linden JV. Error contributes to the risk of transmissible disease. Transfusion 1994;34:1016.
91. Buffington J, Murray PJ, Schlanger K, et al. Low prevalence of hepatitis C virus antibody in men who have sex with men who do not inject drugs. Public Health Rep 2007;122(Suppl 2):63-7.
92. Mackellar DA, Valleroy LA, Secura GM, et al. Two decades after vaccine license: Hepatitis B immunization and infection among young men who have sex with men. Am J Pub Health 2001;91:965-71.
93. Alter MJ. Epidemiology of viral hepatitis and HIV co-infection. J Hepatol 2006;44:56-9.
94. Sanchez AM, Schreiber GB, Nass CC, et al. The impact of male-to-male sexual experience on risk-profiles of blood donors. Transfusion 2005; 45:404-13.
95. Presanis A, De Angelis D, Spiegelhalter D, et al. Conflicting evidence in a Bayesian synthesis of surveillance data to estimate human immunodeficiency virus prevalence. J R Stat Soc Ser A 2008;171:915-37.
96. Presanis AM, Gill ON, Chadborn TR, et al. Insights into the rise in HIV infections, 2001 to 2008: A Bayesian synthesis of prevalence evidence. AIDS 2010;24:2849-58.
97. Health Protection Agency. HIV in the United Kingdom: 2010 Report. London, UK: Health Protection Agency, 2010.
98. Operskalski EA, Busch MP, Mosley JW, Kedes DH. Blood donations and viruses. Lancet 1997; 349:1327.
99. Engels EA, Eastman H, Ablashi DV, et al. Risk of transfusion-associated transmission of human herpesvirus 8. J Natl Cancer Inst 1999;91: 1773-5.
100. Cannon MJ, Operskalski EA, Mosley JW, et al. Lack of evidence for human herpesvirus-8 transmission via blood transfusion in a historical United States cohort. J Infect Dis 2009;199: 1592-8.
101. Dollard SC, Nelson KE, Ness PM, et al. Possible transmission of human herpesvirus 8 by blood transfusion in a historical United States cohort. Transfusion 2005;45:500-3.
102. Mbulaiteye SM, Biggar RJ, Bakaki PM, et al. Human herpesvirus 8 infection and transfusion history in children with sickle-cell disease in Uganda. J Natl Cancer Inst 2003;95:1330-5.
103. Pfeiffer RM, Mbulaiteye S, Engels E. A model to estimate risk of infection with human herpesvirus 8 associated with transfusion from cross-sectional data. Biometrics 2004;60:249-56.
104. Hladik W, Dollard SC, Mermin J, et al. Transmission of human herpesvirus 8 by blood transfusion. N Engl J Med 2006;355:1331-8.
105. Zou S, Fang CT, Schoenberger LB. Transfusion transmission of prion diseases. Transfus Med Rev 2008;22:58-69.
106. Tambyah PA, Koay ESC, Poon MLM, et al. Dengue hemorrhagic fever transmitted by blood transfusion. N Engl J Med 2008;359:1526-7.
107. Gubernot DM, Lucey CT, Leek C, et al. Babesia infection through blood transfusions: Reports received by the United States Food and Drug Administration, 1997-2007. Clin Infect Dis 2009;48:25-30.
108. Tonnetti L, Eder AF, Dy B, et al. Transfusion-transmitted *Babesia microti* identified through hemovigilance. Transfusion 2009;49:2557-63.
109. Gubernot DM, Nakhasi HL, Mied PA, et al. Transfusion-transmitted babesiosis in the United States: Summary of a workshop. Transfusion 2009;49:2759-71.
110. Peterson LR, Stramer SL, Powers AM. Chikungunya virus: Possible impact on transfusion medicine. Transfus Med Rev 2010;24:15-21.
111. Brouard C, Bernillon P, Quatresous I, et al. Estimated risk of Chickungunya viremic blood donation during an epidemic on Reunion Island in the Indian Ocean, 2005 to 2007. Transfusion 2008;48:1333-41.

112. Pealer LN, Martin AA, Petersen LR, et al. Transmission of West Nile virus through blood transfusion in the United States in 2002. N Engl J Med 2003;349:1236-45.
113. Biggerstaff BJ, Petersen LR. Estimated risk of transmission of West Nile virus through blood transfusion in the US, 2002. Transfusion 2003; 43:1007-17.
114. Goubar A, Ades AE, De Angelis D, et al. Estimates of HIV prevalence and proportion diagnosed based on Bayesian multi-parameter synthesis of surveillance data. J R Stat Soc Ser A 2008;171:541-80.
115. Fung MK, Downes KA, Shulman IA. Transfusion of platelets containing ABO-incompatible plasma: A survey of 3,156 North-American laboratories. Arch Pathol Lab Med 2007;131:909-16.
116. Josephson CD, Mullis NC, van Demark C, Hillyer CD. Significant numbers of apheresis-derived group O platelet units have high-titer anti-A/A,B: Implications for transfusion policy. Transfusion 2004;44:805-8.
117. Popovsky MA, Chaplin HC Jr., Moore SB. Transfusion-related acute lung injury: A neglected, serious complication of chemotherapy. Transfusion 1992;32:589-92.
118. Toy P, Popovsky MA, Abraham E, et al. Transfusion-related acute lung injury: Definition and review. Crit Care Med 2005;33:721-6.
119. Kleinman S, Caulfield T, Chan P, et al. Toward an understanding of transfusion-related acute lung injury: Statement of a consensus panel. Transfusion 2004; 44:1774-89.
120. Kleinman S, Dumont LJ, Tomasulo P, et al. The impact of discontinuation of 7-day storage of apheresis platelets (PASSPORT) on recipient safety: An illustration of the need for proper risk assessments. Transfusion 2009;49:903-12.
121. Middleberg RA, van Stein D, Briët E, van der Bom JG. The role of donor antibodies in the pathogenesis of transfusion-related acute lung injury: A systematic review. Transfusion 2008; 48:2167-76.
122. Win N, Chapman CE, Bowles KM, et al. How much residual plasma may cause TRALI? Transfus Med 2008;18:276-80.
123. Ramanthan RK, Triulzi DJ, Logan TF. Transfusion-related acute lung injury following random-donor platelet transfusion: A report of two cases. Vox Sang 1997;73:43-5.
124. Lin Y, Kanani N, Naughton F, et al. Case report: Transfusion-related acute lung injury (TRALI)—A clear and present danger. Can J Anesth 2007;J4:1011-16.
125. Salman SS, Fernandez-Perez ER, Stubbs JR, Gajic O. The practice of platelet transfusion in the intensive care unit. J Intensive Care Med 2007;22:105-10.
126. Robillard P, Hyson C, McCombie N. TRALI, possible TRALI and respiratory complications of transfusion reported to the Canadian Transfusion-Transmitted Injuries Surveillance System (abstract). Transfusion 2007;47(Suppl):5A.
127. Gajic O, Rana R, Winters JL, et al. Transfusion-related acute lung injury in the critically ill: Prospective nested case-control study. Am J Respir Crit Care Med 2007;176:886-91.
128. Eder AF, Herron R, Strupp A, et al. Transfusion-related acute lung injury surveillance (2003-2005) and the potential impact of the selective use of plasma from male donors in the American Red Cross. Transfusion 2007;47:599-607.
129. Transfusion-related acute lung injury. AABB Association Bulletin #06-07 (November 3, 2006). Bethesda, MD: AABB, 2006. [Available at: http://www.aabb.org/resources/publications/bulletins/Pages/ab06-07.aspx (accessed November 8, 2011).]
130. Murphy MF, Navarette C, Massey E. Donor screening as a TRALI reduction strategy. Transfusion 2009;49:1779-82.
131. Malope BI, Pfeiffer RM, Mbisa G, et al. Transmission of Kaposi sarcoma-associated herpesvirus between mothers and children in a South African population. J Acquir Immune Defic Syndr 2007;44:351-5.
132. Minhas V, Crabtree KL, Chao A, et al. Early childhood infection by human herpesvirus 8 in Zambia and the role of human immunodeficiency virus type 1 co-infection in a highly endemic area. Am J Epidemiol 2008;168:311-20.
133. Alfieri C, Tanner J, Carpenter L, et al. EBV transmission from a blood donor to an organ-transplant recipient with recovery of the same virus strain from the recipient blood and oropharynx. Blood 1996;87:812-17.
134. Tattevin P, Cremieux AC, Descamps D, et al. Transfusion-related infectious mononucleosis. Scand J Infect Dis 2002;34:777-8.
135. Spencer B, Rios J, Cable R. Marginal recruitment impact of potential alterations to FDA deferral criteria for men who have sex with men. Transfusion 2006;46:869-70.
136. Dodd RY. Human herpes virus 8: What (not) to do? Transfusion 2005;45:463-5.

137. Food and Drug Administration. Guidance for Industry. Revised recommendations for the assessment of donor suitability and blood product safety in cases of suspected severe acute respiratory syndrome (SARS) or exposure to SARS. Rockville, MD: CBER Office of Community Outreach and Development, 2003. [Available at: http://www.fda.gov/BiologicsBloodVaccines/GuidanceRegulatoryInformation/Guidances/Blood/ucm075016.htm (accessed November 8, 2011).]
138. Chambers RW, Foley HT, Schmidt PJ. Transmission of syphilis by fresh blood components. Transfusion 1969;9:32-4.
139. Risseeuw-Appel IM, Kothe FC. Transfusion syphilis: A case report. Sex Transm Dis 1983; 10:200-1.
140. Katz LM. A test that won't die: The serologic test for syphilis. Transfusion 2009;49:617-19.
141. Grenfell P, Nutland W, McManus S, et al. Views and experiences of men who have sex with men on the ban on blood donation: A cross-sectional survey with qualitative interviews. Br Med J 2011;343:d5604.
142. National Board of Health and Welfare, Sweden. Summary of analyses on selection criteria for blood donors and requirements for methods of testing. Stockholm: Unit for Communicable Disease Prevention and Control, 2009.
143. Pillonel J, Semaille C. [Access to blood donation of men who have sex with men and impact on the risk of HIV transmission by transfusion: International overview.] Transfus Clin Biol 2011;18:151-7.
144. Galarneau C. Blood donation, deferral, and discrimination: FDA deferral policy for men who have sex with men. Am J Bioethics 2010;10:29-39.
145. Fisher C, Schonfeld T. A deeper exploration of discrimination in the FDA donor deferral policy. Am J Bioethics 2010;10:40-2.
146. Fox D. The expressive dimension of donor deferral. Am J Bioethics 2010;10:42-3.
147. Vernillo A. Blood is a precious resource—Does it really matter who donates it? Am J Bioethics 2010;10:44-5.
148. Klugman CM. Blood donation and its metaphors. Am J Bioethics 2010;10:46-7.
149. Galarneau C. A response to the commentaries on "Blood Donation, Deferral, and Discrimination." Am J Bioethics 2010;10:W4-W5.
150. Knowles LP. Ethical and societal considerations. Presented at the United States Department of Health and Human Services Blood Safety and Availability Committee 39th Meeting. Rockville, MD, June 11, 2010.
151. Secretary of Health and Human Services. Correspondence from Kathleen Sebelius to Representative Anthony D. Weiner. June 7, 2011.
152. UK Department of Health. Lifetime blood donation ban lifted for men who have had sex with men. [Available at: http://mediacentre.dh.gov.uk/2011/09/08/lifetime-blood-donation-ban-lifted-for-men-who-have-had-sex-with-men (posted September 8, 2011; accessed November 8, 2011).]

In: Vamvakas EC.
Decision Making in Transfusion Medicine
Bethesda, MD: AABB Press, 2011

7

Equipoise and the Continued Transfusion of "Old" Blood

Equipoise is a state of professional uncertainty about the therapeutic merits of two alternative treatments compared in a randomized controlled trial. Traditionally, it has been defined as pertaining to the interaction between a physician and a patient.

IN 1991, THE BLOOD PRODUCTS Advisory Committee (BPAC) of the Food and Drug Administration (FDA) reviewed all cases of transfusion-associated sepsis (TAS) secondary to contamination of Red Blood Cell (RBC) units with *Yersinia enterocolitica*.[1,2] At that time, all such cases reported from the United States had been due to transfusion of RBC units that had been stored at 4 C for >25 days. The five cases reviewed by Arduino et al[1] had all been associated with septic shock, and three of those five patients had died. Arduino et al[1] inoculated two RBC units with *Y. enterocolitica* and one RBC unit with *Enterobacter agglomerans* (to a concentration of approximately 1 CFU/mL) and stored the 3 units at 4 C for 60 days, sampling them periodically for bacteria and endotoxin. The logarithmic phase of bacterial growth was not reached until 14 to 21 days after inoculation, and it lasted for about 3 weeks. No endotoxin could be detected for 21 days after inoculation. After 21 days, however, the levels of endotoxin rose rapidly, reaching a peak at 6 weeks after inoculation.

Because of the length of storage necessary for the bacteria to attain a lethal concentration in RBC units,[1,2] the BPAC proposed a reduction in the allowed RBC storage period from 42 to 25 days. This recommendation was not endorsed by the FDA, however, because a questionnaire distributed at that time showed that 20% of RBC units in the inventory of more than 1500 US blood banks and transfusion services were >28 days old.[3,4] To make up for this loss of inventory and the expected increase in outdated units if the allowed RBC storage period was reduced from 42 to 25 days, it would have been necessary to recruit new donors to ensure 0.25 million additional donations per year. Recruitment of so many additional first-time donors would increase the risk of transfusion-transmitted infections (TTIs), because—compared with repeat donors—first-time donors are more likely to have chronic asymptomatic infection with transfusion transmitted viruses, (because their blood has not been repeatedly tested for TTIs). Moreover, units <25 days old can also cause TAS, and reducing the allowed RBC storage period to 25 days would lower the risk of TAS but would not eliminate it.[5,6] Finally, older units are less likely than newer units to transmit viruses such as human immunodeficiency virus (HIV) and human T-cell lymphotropic virus (HTLV).[7,8] Because of these three arguments, a case could be made[3,4] that there might not be a net reduction in transfusion-related risk if the allowed RBC storage period was reduced from 42 to 25 days.

The risk of RBC TAS secondary to *Y. enterocolitica* decreased since 1991, thanks to improved screening of prospective blood donors for asymptomatic donor bacteremia[9] and perhaps also thanks to the implementation of prestorage white blood cell (WBC) reduction for the majority of transfused RBC units.[10-12] Prestorage WBC reduction would, in theory, be expected to increase the risk of bacterial contamination of blood components by removing the phagocytic WBCs that eliminate low levels of bacteria from collected units of blood. However, in the case of *Y. enterocolitica*—the organism most extensively studied—prestorage WBC reduction through filtration is actually associated with a decrease in bacteria growth in experimentally inoculated units.[10-12] Whatever the reason for the reduction in risk may be, a cluster of deaths secondary to transfusion of RBCs contaminated with *Y. enterocolitica* (such as that reported in the late 1980s in the United States[1,2]) has not recurred. However, the possibility of such deaths remains when RBCs units >25 days old are transfused. In more recent years, the 2004-2005 United Kingdom Serious Hazards of Transfusion (SHOT) Report[13] and the French BACTHEM study[14] reported two cases of RBC TAS secondary to *Y. enterocolitica*, one of which was fatal.[15]

In summary, death from TAS following receipt of an "old" RBC unit contaminated with psychrophilic bacteria that grow in the cold is a proven,[1,2] but exceedingly rare,[16] risk of transfusion. Another rare and postulated risk of the transfusion of RBCs that have been stored for a long period is transfusion-related acute lung injury (TRALI) secondary to bioactive lipids that accumulate in the supernatant fluid of stored RBCs over time.[17-19] In vitro, the latter risk has been shown to persist even with WBC-reduced RBC units.[19] These known[1,2] or postulated,[17-19] but rare, risks of the transfusion of RBCs stored for long (>28- or >25- or even >14-day[1,5,6]) periods fall in the category of the currently tolerated allogeneic blood transfusion (ABT) risk that perhaps exceeds the as-low-as-reasonably-achievable (ALARA) risk (defined in Chapter 6). These risks could be reduced by decreasing the allowable period of RBC storage, but other risks would be engendered by the change in policy, including a reduction in inventory and a need to recruit additional first-time donors to make up for the expected increase in outdated units.[3,4]

In addition to these known[1,2] or postulated[17-19]—but rare—risks of old RBCs, observational studies[20-22] have also attributed to the transfusion of old (rather than fresh) RBCs such common (and nonspecific) adverse outcomes as a greater risk of mortality, organ failure, and/or in-hospital infection. Plausible biologic mechanisms that can account for such an association(s) include the following:

1. Proinflammatory,[23-26] procoagulant,[23] and/or immune[24] effects of old (rather than fresh) RBCs secondary to the development of microparticles[23,27] in old blood.
2. An increase in iron load from hemolyzed stored RBCs.
3. Activation of complement and neutrophils[26] and/or depletion of nitric oxide[26,28] or S-nitrosylated hemoglobin[29] in stored RBCs, which reduces the ability of the transfused RBCs to induce vasodilation (thereby resulting in inadequate blood flow and impaired oxygen delivery).[30]

If these associations of old (rather than fresh) RBCs with common adverse outcomes were shown to be causal, the allowed storage period of RBCs would have to be promptly reduced, and greater reliance would have to be placed on approaches to patient blood management,[31] because the patient's own freshly shed blood is the freshest blood possible.

Prompt policy intervention would be required because the effect of old (rather than fresh) RBCs on common adverse outcomes reported from some observational studies[32-36] far exceeds the risks due to the reduction in inventory and the need to recruit additional first-time donors, as well as the cost of producing more RBC units to make up for the expected increase in outdated units after the allowed RBC storage period is reduced. Thus, in the words of Ness, the question of whether old blood is less safe than fresh blood is the most critical issue facing transfusion medicine today.[37] He said, "Although we worry about other important issues such as emerging infectious risks..., there is nothing more important to our patients than making sure that the RBCs that we provide are collected and stored in ways that do not impair their transport of vital respiratory gases."[37] Several large randomized controlled trials (RCTs) comparing the frequency of common adverse outcomes (mortality, organ failure, and/or in-hospital infection) are currently enrolling patients in Canada and the United States.[38,39]

Is it appropriate to wait for the results of these ongoing RCTs[38,39]—which will take years to complete—before moving toward transfusing fresher blood and adopting further approaches to patient blood management? Isbister et al[31] argued that it is injudicious to wait. Instead of waiting for the definitive evidence that the ongoing RCTs[38,39] will produce, inference of cause should be made from passive observation (ie, from the results of the available observational studies), so that policy decisions can be made in the manner that they are made in risk-factor epidemiology when policymakers deal with deleterious exposures.[31] In other words, transfusion of old (in lieu of fresh) RBCs should be treated as a deleterious exposure, given the compelling biologic rationale for postulating an association between transfusion of old blood and common adverse outcomes,[23-30] as well as the findings of observational studies that have shown large increases in mortality and serious morbidity for patients receiving old (rather than fresh) RBCs.[32-36] Using this example of the "most critical issue facing transfusion medicine today,"[37] this chapter debates which of the following policy directions might be the more ethical: 1) proceeding with reduction in the allowed storage period of RBCs to mitigate known[1,2] or postulated[17-19] (but rare), in addition to common (but hitherto inferred solely from passive observation), risks of the transfusion of old (rather than fresh) RBCs; or 2) waiting for the completion of the RCTs currently under way in the United States[38] and Canada[39] and following up with a reduction in the allowed storage period of RBCs only if those RCTs generate evidence of a relationship between transfusion of old blood and the common adverse outcomes of mortality, organ failure, and/or in-hospital infection.

Equipoise as a Prerequisite for Undertaking RCTs

Two designs are being used in the RCTs currently under way in the United States[38] and Canada.[39] The design of the US study randomly assigns patients to receive "fresh" or "old" RBCs. The design of the Canadian study randomly assigns patients to receive "fresh" or "standard" RBCs. Standard RBCs are those issued for transfusion on the basis of current blood bank practices—that is, according to the rule that the oldest compatible unit in inventory is issued for transfusion first. However, patients are enrolled in the "standard" arm only on days during which the oldest compatible unit in inventory is older than a specified number of days. Thus, a patient not assigned to receive fresh RBCs receives the treatment that he or she would have received outside the trial. The patient is not denied access to fresher blood because of the trial, because he or she would not have received fresher blood had it not been for the trial. In contrast, when the alternative design is used,[38] a patient not assigned to receive fresh RBCs always receives

RBCs older than a specified number of days. Had it not been for the trial, this latter patient would not always have received RBCs older than the specified number of days; in fact, most likely he or she would have received RBCs ≤ 14 days old at most US hospitals.[40] The rationale for this latter allocation of patients is that subjects who have agreed to participate in the RCT receive one FDA-licensed RBC product rather than another FDA-licensed RBC product.

Equipoise for Clinical Decision-Making

If equipoise exists, physicians ethically can randomly assign patients to receive a new treatment (fresh RBCs) rather than a standard treatment (RBCs issued per current blood-bank inventory management practice). Equipoise is a state of professional uncertainty about the therapeutic merits of two alternative treatments compared in an RCT.[41] It has been traditionally defined as pertaining to the interaction between a physician and a patient. In numerous clinical situations, physicians—when presented with the alternative treatments available—make decisions about which alternative might most benefit their patients, no matter how much uncertainty there exists about the benefits (and risks) of the alternative treatments.

If a relevant "expert" community can be identified, and there is approximately a 50/50 split among the experts concerning their choice of fresh or standard RBCs, then there is definitely "no consensus within the expert clinical community about the comparative merits of the alternatives to be tested."[41] Lack of consensus does not require a 50/50 split, although the proportion of experts who need to favor the minority opinion for lack of consensus to be considered to exist has not been defined.[42] Nonetheless, if an expert community can be identified, and if data are developed to document sufficient lack of consensus among experts, it is ethical for physicians to enroll their patients into a trial that randomly assigns them to receive fresh or standard RBCs. The reason this is ethical is that, because equipoise has been documented to exist, no patient enrolled in such a trial knowingly receives "inferior" treatment. Therefore, physicians' ethical duties to their patients are discharged.

Evidence-based medicine considers RCTs to be the highest level of evidence (see Tables 1-1 through 1-4 in Chapter 1), and at least one hierarchy of the strength of evidence[43] explicitly lists expert opinion as representing the lowest level of evidence. Yet, the concept of equipoise[41] relies on canvassing expert opinion to document the existence of a state of professional uncertainty about the therapeutic merits of old RBCs compared with standard RBCs. The fallibility of expert opinion has been amply demonstrated vis-à-vis widely used treatments that have subsequently been proven to be ineffective or harmful. Such treatments include hormone-replacement therapy to promote cardiovascular health (later shown to be associated with multiple adverse outcomes[44,45]); high-dose chemotherapy with marrow transplantation for metastatic breast cancer (later shown to be no more effective, and considerably more toxic, than standard chemotherapy[46]); and antiarrhythmia drugs (later shown to be associated with greater mortality than placebo).[47] If experts consider an (ineffective or harmful) treatment to be beneficial, equipoise does not exist for the purpose of undertaking RCTs of hormone-replacement therapy or placebo, high-dose chemotherapy with marrow transplantation or standard chemotherapy for metastatic breast cancer, or antiarrhythmia drugs or placebo. By the same token, if experts consider as superior a treatment not proven to be superior, equipoise does not exist for the purpose of undertaking RCTs of fresh or standard RBCs.

There are examples of drugs that have received regulatory approval without results from RCTs.[48] Such drugs include cisplatin for testicular cancer[49] and bortezomib for multiple myeloma.[50] Recently, an article in *The New York Times*[51] prompted a discussion in *The New England Journal of Medicine*[42] about the ethics of conducting an RCT in a condition that is uniformly fatal (ie, metastatic melanoma) for the purpose of documenting the life-extending potential of a new treatment (PLX4032) when the standard treatment (dacarbazine) is only 15% effective. It was argued that virtually all physicians–when presented with impressive evidence about the potential of PLX4032 from a Phase I trial, and given the dismal prognosis and the lack of efficacy of the currently available standard treatment–would opt to use the alternative treatment rather than the marginally effective and toxic standard chemotherapy.[51] In such a case, equipoise does not exist, and PLX4032 should arguably receive regulatory approval without results from RCTs.[51] Additional, albeit less rigorous evaluation of the effectiveness of PLX4032 could perhaps be accomplished by requiring that all patients receiving the new drug be enrolled in a data registry, so that their outcomes can be compared with those of historical controls.

The New England Journal of Medicine editorialists concluded that PLX4032 is a genuinely difficult case and that reasonable people may differ over whether evaluation in RCTs is needed for establishing that the drug offers a survival benefit.[42] For clinicians and ethicists who espouse the concept of clinical equipoise, an RCT comparing PLX4032 with standard chemotherapy is indisputably unethical, because equipoise does not exist in this situation.

Equipoise for Policy Decision-Making

Clinicians make the best decisions for their individual patients in the here and now. In contrast, regulators approving a new treatment and health plans offering coverage for the new treatment adopt a population perspective. The FDA is charged with determining that new drugs are safe and effective for defined groups of patients before these drugs may receive regulatory approval. Public and private insurers then make decisions about coverage based on "medical necessity"–which generally rests on the availability of "convincing" evidence that a new treatment offers a net health benefit for a defined patient population.[42]

For such convincing evidence to be generated, both the benefits and the risks of a new treatment are rigorously studied. To inform regulatory and insurance decision-making, the evaluation of the new treatment continues past the point at which physicians would choose the new treatment over the standard treatment based on initial efficacy data.[42] Expert opinion often relies on early-phase trials that have not accumulated sufficient endpoints and that may even have been based on surrogate endpoints that do not reflect improved survival or enhanced quality of life.[52-54] In contrast, policy decisions should be based on rigorous knowledge from RCTs for two reasons: 1) the cost of new treatments is often big or prohibitive and 2) the new treatments can introduce new (and unanticipated) risks.[42]

The introduction to this chapter–even when limited to the known[1,2] and postulated,[17-19] but rare, risks of old (compared with fresh) RBCs–would probably convince a large majority of clinicians to consider fresh RBCs as superior to standard RBCs for their own individual patients. However, the endorsement of fresh (over standard) RBCs for regulatory and reimbursement purposes on the basis of the evidence hitherto adduced would introduce cost, RBC scarcity, and perhaps also other risk(s). As already discussed, endorsement of fresh RBCs was considered by the FDA BPAC in 1991, and the risks from a reduced supply and recruitment of additional first-time donors were thought to exceed the benefit of preventing RBC TAS that, in at least some cases, is fatal.[3,4] The risks associated with a reduced supply and recruitment of additional first-time donors probably continue to exceed the risk of RBC TAS and perhaps even the incremental risk of TRALI (as long as the mechanism attributing TRALI to bioactive lipids accumulating over time during storage[17-19] remains postulated rather than proven).

It could be argued, however, that–when the possibility of a nonspecific association of old (rather than fresh) RBCs with the common adverse outcomes of mortality, organ failure, and/or in-hospital infection is added–the criteria proposed by Miller and Joffee[42] for approving new treatments on the basis of nonrandomized evidence are met.[31] Table 7-1 shows these criteria[42] and the corresponding arguments for satisfying them in the case of fresh (compared with old) RBCs. Whether these criteria are indeed met–as they would appear to be, with the sole exception of a "well-understood" outcome–is examined in this chapter by means of a

Table 7-1. Application of the Criteria for Approving New Treatments Based on Nonrandomized Evidence[42] to a Reduction of the Allowed Red Blood Cell (RBC) Storage Period in the Absence of Results from Randomized Controlled Trials (RCTs)

Criteria of Miller and Joffee[42]	Arguments for Reducing the Allowed RBC Storage Period on the Basis of Results of Observational Studies Alone
The criteria for approving new treatments based on nonrandomized evidence pertain to treatments intended to treat life-threatening conditions	Transfusion of old (rather than fresh) RBCs is associated with greater mortality or life-threatening conditions (organ failure, in-hospital infection)[32-36]
There must be a compelling, mechanism-based rationale favoring the efficacy of the new treatment	The association of transfusion of old (rather than fresh) RBCs with an increase in the aforementioned common adverse outcomes can be accounted for by plausible biologic mechanisms[23-30] that could be deemed to be compelling
Given current theory, the outcome must be poor, well-understood, and with limited interpatient variability	In the studied settings of critical care and cardiac surgery, poor outcomes (eg, mortality, organ failure, and/or in-hospital infection) do occur in apparent association with transfusion of old (rather than fresh) RBCs; however, these outcomes have a multifactorial etiology[31] that is *poorly* understood
There must be one or more available concurrent or historical control groups with characteristics similar to those of the patients to be enrolled in a proposed RCT(s)	The available observational studies reporting common adverse outcomes in association with transfusion of old (rather than fresh) RBCs[32-36] used concurrent or historical control groups of patients undergoing cardiac surgery or admitted to the intensive care unit (ie, patients similar to those enrolled in the RCTs currently under way in the United States[38] and Canada[39])
The study or studies producing the nonrandomized evidence must have used clinical (or validated surrogate) endpoints	The available observational studies[32-36] used clinical endpoints: mortality, organ failure, or infection

review of the methods and meta-analysis of the observational studies reported through December 31, 2008,[55] and some more recent reports.[35,36,56-58]

Miller and Joffee[42] concluded that RCTs that violate equipoise are both ethical and necessary for the development of the evidence needed to support health policy decisions—which are made on behalf of populations of patients rather than individual patients. This chapter reaches the same conclusion vis-à-vis the RCTs of fresh (rather than standard) RBCs currently under way in the United States[38] and Canada.[39] Clinical equipoise may not exist with either the design allocating patients to receive fresh or standard RBCs or the design assigning patients to receive fresh or old RBCs. The reason is that a large majority of informed clinicians treating their own patients would likely opt for fresh (rather than standard or old) RBCs, owing to the wide dissemination of the results of some observational studies published in prominent journals.[33] Proposals that fresh RBCs are more likely to transmit viruses such as HIV and HTLV[7,8] or to result in microchimerism in patients transfused in the setting of trauma[59] would be unlikely to sway expert opinion, because of the extremely low incidence of HIV and HTLV infection in blood donors and because transfusion-associated microchimerism has not been convincingly linked to adverse clinical outcomes.

No patient is knowingly harmed when patients who are not given fresh RBCs are given standard treatment. The situation is different when patients randomly assigned to receive old RBCs always receive RBCs stored for longer than a specified number of days. The latter patients are perhaps knowingly exposed to the known[1,2] or postulated,[17-19] but rare, risks of old RBCs.

The ethical position of always allocating some experimental subjects to receive old RBCs could be deemed untenable if—in addition to the known[1,2] or postulated,[17-19] but rare, risks of old RBCs—one considered that sufficient evidence has already been adduced (Table 7-1) to infer a relationship between the transfusion of old or fresh RBCs and common adverse outcomes.[31] However, systematic reviews of the observational studies[20-22,55]—updated in this chapter—have concluded that the totality of the evidence hitherto adduced is not consistent with the findings of selected but widely publicized studies.[33] Despite the lack of clinical equipoise even when the risks of old RBCs are limited to the rare risks of TAS and TRALI, the RCTs currently under way[38,39] are indeed necessary for guiding public-policy decision making.[60] If interim analyses of the ongoing RCTs showed a large difference in favor of fresh (rather than old) RBCs, Data Safety Monitoring Boards (DSMBs) would recommend early interruption of the RCTs so that all patients could receive fresh RBCs. One must be prepared, however, for the possibility that the RCTs currently under way show no difference, as well as for the (physiologically unappealing) possibility that the direction of any difference may be the opposite of what is expected. Even if the ongoing RCTs show no benefit from fresh (rather than old) RBCs, we will still have learned a tremendous amount about the reality of oxygen delivery in patients,[37] and that new knowledge will guide future research.

Preliminary Results from RCTs

Table 7-2 shows the design and conclusions of RCTs that have reported on the mortality of patients allocated to receive old or fresh RCBs.[58,61,62] These RCTs have been pilot studies intended to investigate the feasibility of conducting large RCTs of the relationship between transfusion of old or fresh RBCs and common adverse outcomes. All three studies[58,61,62] showed no difference in mortality between recipients of old RBCs and recipients of fresh RBCs (Fig 7-1). It is important that none of the three studies[58,61,62] showed a trend toward increased mortality in association with receipt of old (rather than fresh) RBCs. In all three studies, the mortality of the recipients of fresh RBCs was higher than that of the recipients of old RBCs, although the difference did not attain significance in any of the studies. Results on organ failure or in-hospital infection have not been reported from such pilot RCTs.

Mou et al[63] randomly assigned infants with congenital heart disease to undergo circuit priming with fresh whole blood (stored for 45.8 to 50.7 hours) or RBCs stored for 117.0 to 162.7 hours and reconstituted with Fresh Frozen Plasma (FFP). Both arms of this RCT received RBCs <7 days old. The study included 200 infants with a median age of 2.7 months and a median weight of 4.3 kg, many of whom underwent the equivalent of a complete exchange transfusion with one whole-blood unit used for priming. On the basis of an intention-to-treat analysis, recipients of fresh whole blood had a greater length of stay in the intensive care unit (ICU) and more generalized edema ($p<0.05$) than did recipients of older (yet <7-day-old) RBCs reconstituted with FFP. Transfusion

Table 7-2. Pilot Randomized Controlled Trials (RCTs) Investigating the Feasibility of Conducting an RCT of Patients Allocated to Receive Fresh or Old RBCs

RCT	Comparison Arms	Sample Size	Conclusions	Other Findings or Comments
Schulman et al[61]	Trauma patients receiving ≥2 units of <11-day-old or >20-day-old WBC-reduced RBCs	17	Conduct of an RCT is not feasible in a single-center US setting	Recipients of fresh RBCs received 9.3 units and had four deaths; recipients of old RBCs received 10.6 units and had two deaths
Hébert et al[62]	Cardiac-surgery *or* ICU patients receiving <8-day-old or standard-issue RBCs (but randomly assigned only when >15-day-old RBCs were available in the blood bank) after implementation of universal WBC reduction	57	Conduct of an RCT is feasible in a multicenter Canadian setting, because: 1) the median storage time was 4 or 19 days, in recipients of <8- or >15-day-old RBCs, respectively; and 2) 59% and 91%, of the subjects allocated to receive <8- or >15-day-old RBCs, respectively, received the appropriate component >90% of the time	Compared with the recipients of old RBCs, recipients of *fresh* RBCs had *more* in-hospital deaths (Fig 7-1; p = 0.45), as well as more in-hospital deaths together with life-threatening complications (27% vs 12%, respectively; p = 0.31), but they were 5 years older on average as well as sicker [co-morbid illness(es) present in 85% vs 65%, respectively] and they received a higher transfusion dose (5.5 vs 3.3 units, respectively)
Heddle et al[58]	Unselected patients (ie, all transfused hospitalized patients) receiving the freshest or the oldest RBC unit available in inventory on the day of their transfusion; patients needing fresh blood or receiving massive transfusion or uncrossmatched RBCs were excluded	910	Conduct of a *pragmatic* RCT, addressing the question of adverse effects of transfusing fresh or old blood in an *unselected* hospital population, is feasible in a Canadian setting. The mean ± SD age of RBCs differed by 12.0 days between recipients of the freshest (11.3 ± 6.4 days) and the oldest (23.3 ± 7.3 days) RBCs	Mortality was 10.1% and 11.3% in recipients of the oldest and the freshest RBCs, respectively (p>0.05)

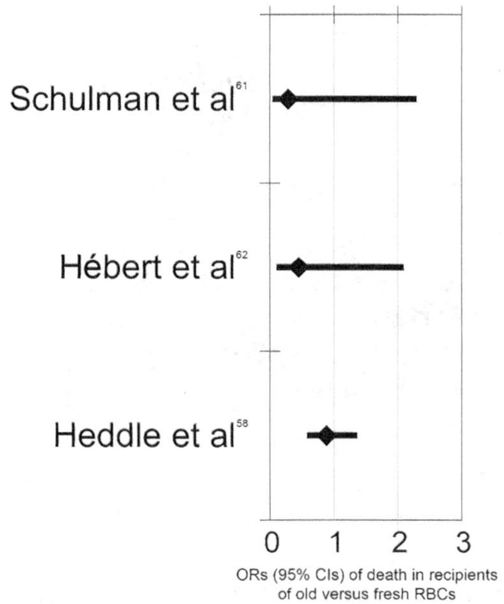

Figure 7-1. Randomized controlled trials (RCTs) investigating the association of Red Blood Cell (RBC) storage with in-hospital mortality.[58,61,62] For each RCT, the figure shows the odds ratio (OR) of occurrence of the adverse outcome (death) in recipients of old vs fresh RBCs and the associated 95% confidence interval (CI). If the 95% CI includes the null value of 1, the difference is not statistically significant. If the difference is statistically significant, an OR >1 indicates that old RBCs are associated with a worse outcome than are fresh RBCs, and an OR <1 indicates that old RBCs are associated with a better outcome than are fresh RBCs. Both of the smaller studies[61,62] reported only "as-treated" analyses, which included the transfusion recipients from among the subjects randomly assigned to receive old or fresh RBCs. All randomly assigned subjects in the study of Heddle et al[58] were transfused.

requirements, postoperative bleeding, and indicators of myocardial injury or systemic inflammation did not differ between the study arms.

Three more RCTs[40,64,65] have reported on a comparison between older and fresher RBCs. One RCT[40] did not report on any clinical or physiologic endpoints; one[64] reported on physiologic endpoints but not on clinical outcomes; and one[65] was conducted in healthy volunteers. Two of these RCTs[64,65] did not detect any clinical or physiologic difference between the recipients of old RBCs and the recipients of fresh RBCs.

Observational Studies

A meta-analysis of the observational studies of the association between transfusion of old or fresh RBCs and common adverse outcomes (mortality, organ failure, or infection) reported through December 31, 2008,[55] limited eligibility to studies that had presented results adjusted for the effects of confounding factors (provided that the adequacy of the adjustment for the effects of confounders could be assessed from the report of each study). Eligible studies had defined RBC storage as the mean ± SD duration of storage of all transfused RBCs, the age of the oldest transfused RBC unit, and/or the transfusion of RBCs, all of which (or the oldest unit of which) had been stored for more than, compared with less than, a specified number of days. Studies were integrated in a meta-analysis if they had defined RBC storage in the same manner, had reported on the same adverse outcome in the same clinical setting, and had included either children only or adults only.[55]

Adjustment for the effects of confounders could have been accomplished through matching or multivariate analysis. The meta-analysis assessed the adequacy of the adjustment for confounding factors based on the balance in prognostic factors between comparison groups (for matched analyses) or based on the variables included in the final statistical model (for multivariate analyses). (For more information, see Chapter 2 in the electronic supplement.) Provided that there was ≥5% probability that the variation in the findings of the studies could have arisen by chance ($p>0.05$ for the *Q* test statistic), adjusted findings of observational studies that had reported odds ratios (ORs) of adverse outcomes occurring in recipients of old or fresh RBCs were integrated by the fixed-effects method of Prentice and Thomas.[66] A

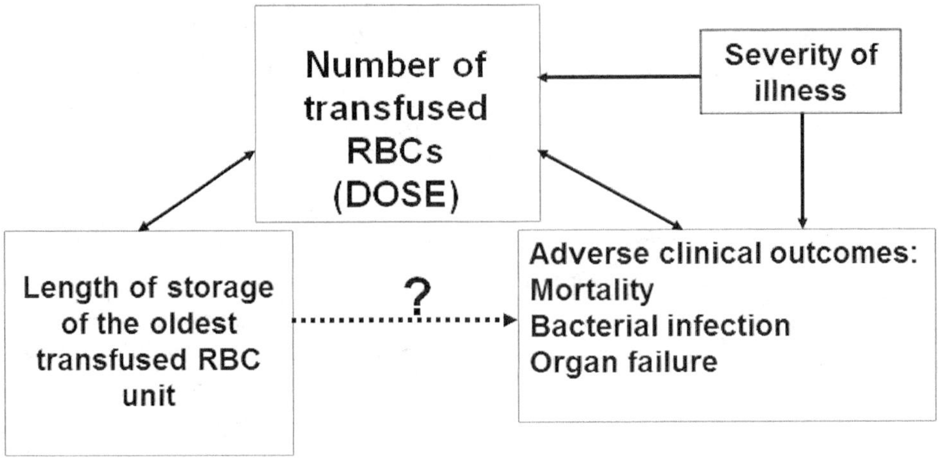

Figure 7-2. Confounding of the association between the oldest Red Blood Cell (RBC) unit transfused to each patient and common adverse outcomes by the number of transfused RBC units in observational studies. Each time a request for transfusion is received by the hospital blood bank, the blood bank issues for transfusion the oldest compatible unit in inventory. The purposes of this standard inventory-management practice are to minimize wastage of RBC units and thus avoid RBC shortages, delay of RBC transfusions, and/or postponement of surgeries. Although the impact of this standard practice on patient outcomes is unknown, the result of the practice is that the transfusion of fresh RBCs is the exception rather than the rule: each time a patient is transfused, he or she is a candidate for receiving the oldest RBC unit available at that time. Thus, the more often a patient is transfused, the more likely he or she is to receive an RBC unit at a time when the oldest available unit is "old." (At the same time, the more often a patient is transfused, the more likely he or she is to receive an RBC unit at a time when the oldest available unit is "fresh.") Because of these situation(s) engendered by the inventory-management practices of US and Canadian blood banks, recipients of more RBC units are more likely to have received some of the oldest, as well as some of the freshest, RBC units. In contrast, there is no a priori reason for the mean age of all transfused RBCs to be associated with the number of transfused RBC units. In addition to correlating with the length of storage of the oldest transfused unit, the number of transfused RBC units is the best predictor of common adverse outcomes[67-69]—mortality, organ failure, or in-hospital infection—because need for transfusion reflects the presence of co-morbidities and the severity of the underlying illness. (Stated another way, patients with higher acuity receive more RBC transfusions—a situation that was recently referred to in the literature as "confounding by indication.") The age of the oldest unit is thus bound to be associated with adverse outcomes because it is associated with the number of transfused RBC units (which is itself associated with adverse outcomes). To investigate the possibility of an independent association between the age of the oldest unit and adverse outcomes, investigators must adjust for the effect of the number of transfused RBC units. This adjustment is accomplished by matching patients according to the number of transfused RBC units that they have received in the matched analyses or by testing the age of the oldest unit for entry into a multivariate regression model in which the number of transfused RBC units is already physically present (see Chapter 2 in the electronic supplement).

fixed-effects method was used for the synthesis to maximize the probability of detecting a difference in outcome between recipients of old RBCs and recipients of fresh RBCs.

Observational studies suffer from the inability to separate any effect of the oldest transfused RBC unit from the effect of the number of transfused RBCs (Fig 7-2). In most observational studies, the number of transfused RBCs is the best predictor of adverse outcomes,[67-69] including the three outcomes considered in the meta-analysis.[55] The need for RBC transfusion reflects presence of co-morbidities, more-severe illness, and a poorer baseline prognosis, at least in addition to any postulated adverse effect(s) of the RBC transfusion per se.[67-69] Moreover, as illustrated by the data of van de Watering et al,[70] in observational studies studying the effect of the oldest transfused unit (as opposed to the effect of the mean length of storage of all transfused RBCs), there is a predictable association between the number of transfused RBCs and the length of storage of the oldest unit. That is to say, as patients receive a total transfusion dose of 1, 2, 3...10, or >10 RBC units, the oldest transfused RBC unit gets, progressively and without fail, older and older, because, each time a request for transfusion is received by the blood bank, the blood bank issues for transfusion the oldest compatible unit in inventory. Therefore, the more often a patient is transfused, the more likely he or she is to be issued blood at a time that the oldest compatible unit is "old" (Fig 7-2).

To establish a valid association between the length of storage of the oldest transfused unit and adverse outcomes in observational studies, it is therefore necessary to adjust any reported relationship for the number of transfused RBCs. Any effect on outcome mediated jointly by the number of transfused RBCs and the oldest RBC unit must be attributed to the number of transfused RBCs. Therefore, investigators should choose between not adjusting for the effect of the most important confounder and reducing the power of their study to detect an adverse effect of old RBCs. Hitherto, investigators have erred overwhelmingly in the direction of not adjusting for the number of transfused RBCs.[22,55] Only Offner et al[71] considered this question explicitly, and they justified their decision not to introduce the number of transfused RBCs into their statistical model by invoking the high degree of correlation between the age of the oldest transfused RBC unit and the number of transfused RBCs. Owing to the high correlation between these two candidate independent variables, their joint presence in a multivariate regression model predicting the occurrence of a common adverse outcome (eg, mortality, organ failure, or in-hospital infection) would violate the assumptions of logistic regression. More recently, Gauvin et al[36] showed the same close correlation between the number of transfused RBCs and the length of storage of the oldest transfused RBC unit as previously shown by van de Watering et al.[70] Gauvin et al stated that—owing to this high degree of correlation between the two candidate independent variables for entry into their regression model—their statistical analysis could not "deconstruct the interaction between length of storage and the effect due to the number of units of RBCs administered in [their] study."[36]

The second limitation of observational studies pertains to the definition of the transfusion of "old" or "fresh" RBCs. Because most patients receive >1 RBC unit, included patients receive RBCs stored for various lengths of time. As shown in Fig 7-2, the mean duration of storage of all transfused RBCs could be a measure of the effect of RBC storage that is not intrinsically confounded by the number of transfused RBCs and that thus is amenable to statistical adjustment for the effects of confounding factors via multivariate regression analyses. However, only a minority of observational studies investigated the effect of the mean duration of storage of all transfused RBCs. Most studies examined instead the effect of the oldest transfused RBC unit, under the assumption that a single "old" unit can adversely affect mortality, organ failure, or nosocomial infection—regardless of the age of the remainder of the units that a patient has received during his or her hospitalization. By focusing exclusively on the oldest unit, investigators could include the entire population of transfused patients available to them. Patients whose oldest transfused unit was older than a specified number of days were categorized as recipients of "old" RBCs, and patients whose oldest transfused unit was fresher than a specified number of days were categorized as recipients of "fresh" RBCs. A minority of studies restricted eligibility of patients to those who had exclusively received units stored for more (compared with less) than a specified number of days. In this case, if the cutoff was set at 14 days, all patients categorized as recipients of "fresh" blood had exclusively received RBCs stored for ≤14 days, and all patients categorized as recipients of "old" blood had exclusively received RBCs stored for >14 days. Patients who had received a mixture of RBCs (ie, some stored for ≤14 days and some stored for >14 days) were excluded from the analysis—an approach that resulted in a substantial reduction in sample size.

Finally, when the outcome studied by the observational studies was organ failure or nosocomial infection, rather than mortality, investigators could not be certain that the outcome followed (rather than preceded) the transfusion of the oldest unit on the effect of which they based the premise of their entire analysis. Data on the length of storage of all transfused RBCs usually were collected without regard to the timing of the receipt of the oldest unit vis-a-vis the timing of the development of nosocomial infection or organ failure.[36]

Twenty-two observational studies[32-34,70-88] were included in the meta-analysis[55] and involved a variety of patient groups. Six were conducted in ICU patients,[72-77] eight in trauma patients,[34,71,78-83] six in cardiac surgery,[32,33,70,84-86] and two in colorectal surgery.[87,88] Further studies have been conducted in the ICU[35,36] and cardiac surgery[56,57] settings; they reported adverse effects exclusively attributable to the transfusion of old WBC-reduced RBC units.[35,36]

Mortality

Eight studies[33,34,70,73,76,81,82,86] reported unadjusted results for in-hospital, ICU,[76] or 30-day[70] mortality. The investigators defined old RBCs as those more than 14,[33,82] 18,[70] 19,[81] 20,[73] 21,[76] 28,[34] or 30[86] days old. Only four[33,70,81,82] of the eight studies compared groups of patients who had exclusively received RBCs older or fresher than a specified number of days.

Solely for the purpose of illustration, Figs 7-3 and 7-4 show the reported unadjusted findings on the association between transfusion of old or fresh RBCs and mortality. Of the eight studies, only two[33,34] had reported an unadjusted association between transfusion of old or fresh RBCs and increased mortality. The medical heterogeneity of the eight studies in terms of the definitions of "old" and "fresh" RBCs and the clinical setting was reflected in statistical heterogeneity. The hypothesis of homogeneity was rejected across all eight studies ($p<0.05$ for the Q test statistic), and the results could not be integrated in a meta-analysis. Figure 7-3 stratifies the studies based on the manner that they defined old (rather than fresh) RBCs, and it also separately considers the studies that exclusively transfused RBCs older or fresher than a specified number of days. Figure 7-4 stratifies the studies by clinical setting.

The impact of not adjusting the effect of RBC storage for the effect of transfusion can be illustrated with the data of Koch et al.[33] They considered that recipients of RBCs stored for >14 or ≤14 days had received the same RBC transfusion dose (median of 2 units, interquartile range of 2-4 units), and they did not control for the number of transfused RBCs. However, recipients of old RBCs had received, on average, 0.38 unit,[89] or 0.25 unit according to the reply of Koch et al to four letters to the editor[90]—more RBCs on average than recipients of fresh RBCs. As Fig 1(A) in the report of Koch et al[33] illustrated, the higher transfusion dose among the recipients of old blood was concentrated among the patients who had received >9 RBC units. Thus, there were more multitransfused patients (with a worse baseline prognosis; Fig 7-2) among the recipients of old RBCs than among recipients of fresh RBCs, and the investigators did not adjust statistically for this cardinal difference between their comparison groups.

Seven studies[32-34,80,83] had reported adjusted results for the effect of old (rather than fresh) RBCs at the time of the meta-analysis,[55] and additional adjusted results[35,36,56,57] have been reported since then. After the adequacy of the adjustment for the effects of confounding factors was questioned,[91] one cardiac surgery study was retracted.[92] Adjusted results from trauma studies[34-36,82,83] have consistently supported an association between transfusion of old (rather than fresh) RBCs and increased mortality. However, in only one of these studies (the smallest study[34]) was the effect of RBC storage adjusted for the number of transfused RBCs. There are now four cardiac surgery studies[56,57,70,86] that

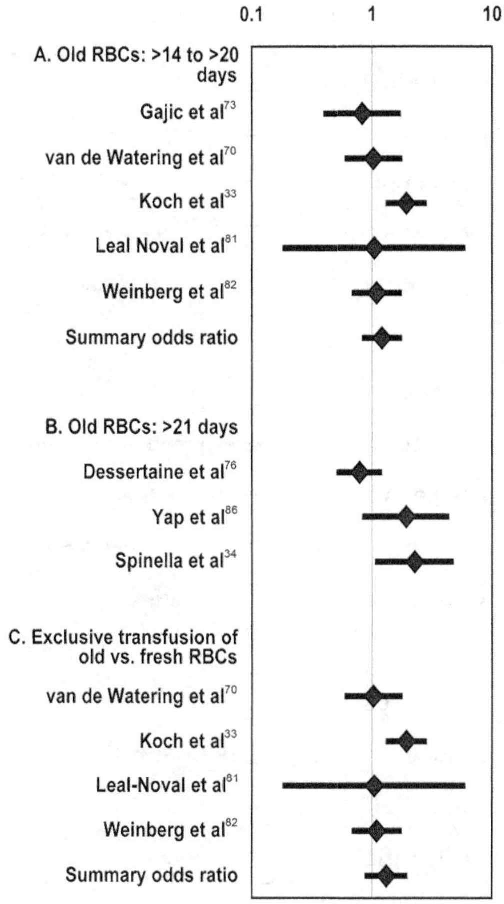

Figure 7-3. Observational studies reporting unadjusted findings on in-hospital, intensive care unit,[76] or 30-day[70] mortality, stratified according to the employed definitions of old and fresh Red Blood Cells (RBCs), and a subgroup of the observational studies reporting unadjusted results on mortality in which the comparison groups had exclusively received RBCs older or fresher than a specified number of days. For each study, the figure shows the odds ratio (OR) of mortality in recipients of old or fresh RBCs and the associated 95% confidence interval (CI). When the 95% CI of the OR does not include the null value of 1, the effect of old or fresh RBCs on morality is statistically significant ($p<0.05$). Provided that the effect is significant, an OR >1 indicates that old (rather than fresh) RBCs are associated with greater mortality. Studies defining old RBCs as those >14 to >20 days old (or even older)[33,70,73,81,82] were statistically homogeneous ($p > 0.10$ for the Q test statistic), and they did not support an adverse effect of old (rather than fresh) RBCs (summary OR = 1.21; 95% CI = 0.86-1.70; $p>0.05$). Studies defining old RBCs as those >3 weeks old[34,76,86] were statistically heterogeneous ($p = 0.025$ for the Q test statistic); integration of their results under conditions of heterogeneity would not support an adverse effect of old (rather than fresh) RBCs (summary OR = 1.38; 95% CI = 0.62-3.04; $p>0.05$). The four studies[33,70,81,82] in which the comparison groups had exclusively received RBCs older or fresher than a specified number of days were statistically homogeneous ($p>0.10$ for the Q test statistic), and they did not support an adverse effect of old RBCs (summary OR = 1.31; 95% CI = 0.91-1.89; $p>0.05$). Because these results are unadjusted results from observational studies, they are presented solely for the purpose of illustration.

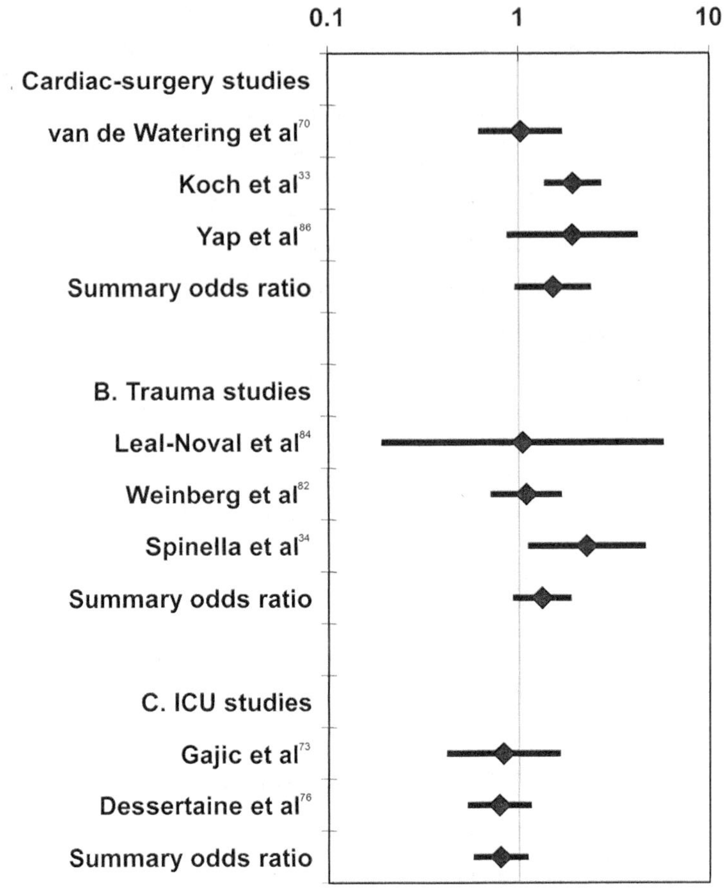

Figure 7-4. Observational studies reporting unadjusted findings on in-hospital, intensive care unit (ICU),[76] or 30-day[70] mortality in cardiac surgery,[33,70,86] trauma,[34,81,82] or ICU[75,76] patients. Studies conducted at each of the three clinical settings were statistically homogeneous (p>0.10 for cardiac surgery, p>0.25 for trauma, and p>0.99 for ICU patients), and findings are integrated across studies from the same clinical setting. In no setting was an unadjusted increase in mortality detected in association with old vs fresh Red Blood Cells (RBCs): OR = 1.32 [95% confidence interval (CI) = 0.95-2.42] for cardiac surgery; OR = 1.32 (95% CI = 0.93-1.89) for trauma; and OR = 0.80 (95% CI = 0.57-1.12) for ICU patients. Because these results are unadjusted results from observational studies, they are presented solely for the purpose of illustration.

have adequately adjusted for the effects of confounding factors, including adjustment for the number of transfused RBCs.[93] These studies are homogeneous, and no effect of transfusion of old (rather than fresh) RBCs is detected across the studies (Fig 7-5).[93] Figure 7-6 depicts the results of a different approach to the analysis: RBC storage is defined here as mean storage of all transfused RBCs (Section A) or length of storage of the oldest transfused RBC unit (Section B).

Figure 7-7 shows the results of the important study of Edgren et al.[56] These investigators included all patients receiving RBCs in Denmark and Sweden between 1995 and 2002, thereby including 404,959 transfusion episodes.

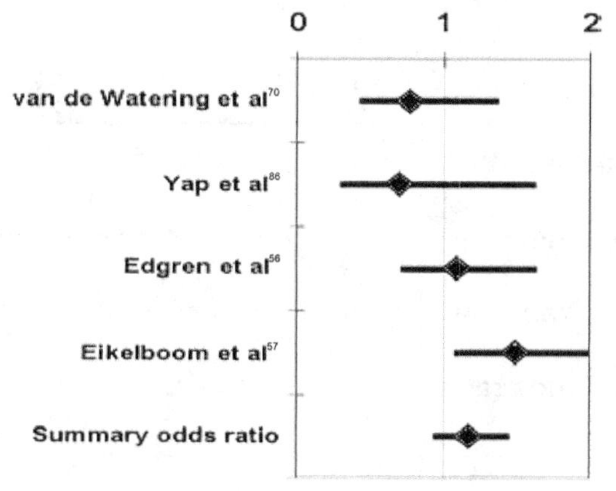

Figure 7-5. Observational studies reporting adjusted findings on in-hospital,[57,86] 7-day,[56] or 30-day[70] mortality of patients receiving Red Blood Cells (RBCs) stored for more or less than a specified number of days. For each study,[56,57,70,86] the figure shows the odds ratio (OR) of mortality in recipients of old vs fresh RBCs. The figure also shows the summary OR across the studies, calculated by the fixed-effects method of Prentice and Thomas.[66] When the 95% confidence interval (CI) of an OR does not include the null value of 1, the effect of RBC storage is significant ($p<0.05$). Old blood was >18 days old in the study of van de Watering et al[70] and >30 days old in the study of Yap et al.[86] In the analysis of all patients receiving RBCs in Denmark and Sweden between 1995 and 2002,[56] old blood (30-42 days old) was compared to RBCs stored for 10 to 20 days, because fresher units are usually issued for special indications. Results were reported on all patients, patients undergoing coronary artery bypass graft (CABG) surgery, and patients undergoing extracorporeal circulation. Eikelboom et al[57] found a significant association of in-hospital mortality of patients with cardiovascular disease who received old (≥23-day-old) rather than fresh (<14-day-old) blood (the oldest quartile compared with the freshest quartile of the RBC units transfused to this patient population). When CABG patients, patients undergoing extracorporeal circulation, or all patients from the study of Edgren et al were included,[56] the four studies[56,57,70,86] were homogeneous ($p \geq 0.10$ for the *Q* test statistic), and there was no increase in mortality across the studies [summary OR = 1.16 (95% CI = 0.92-1.46); summary OR = 1.14 (95% CI = 0.91-1.42); and summary OR = 1.06 (95% CI = 0.98-1.14)].[93]

Because WBC reduction was introduced during this period, Edgren et al[56] reported separately on the outcome of the recipients of WBC-reduced units. The investigators also reported separately on the effect of transfusion of 1 to 2, 3 to 4, or ≥5 RBC units. They found no effect of old RBCs on short-term (7-day) mortality (Section A). This short-term mortality from the study of Edgren et al[56] is comparable to the in-hospital mortality reported by the other observational studies reviewed here, and it was integrated in the meta-analysis shown in Fig 7-5.

Edgren et al[56] also presented results on long-term (2-year) mortality (Section B, Fig 7-7). In that case, there was a significant ($p<0.05$) effect of RBC storage that was evident only in recipients of 1 to 2 (as opposed to more) RBC units. This excess 2-year mortality seemed more compatible with a higher baseline risk among the recipients of the oldest units than with a deleterious effect of the oldest units themselves. The authors acknowledged that they were "unable to adjust directly for disease severity," and they stated their interpretation of the findings vis-à-vis long-term mortality as follows: "[A]ny excess mortality truly caused by the transfusion of 30- to 42-day-old RBCs, if it exists at all, was inflated by undocumented confounding by indication."[56]

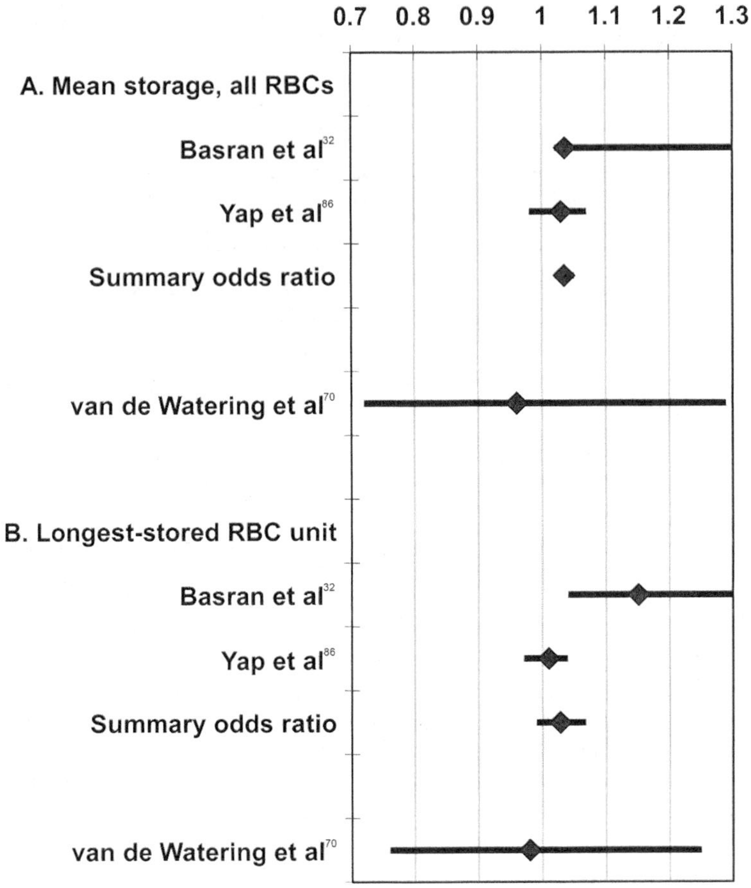

Figure 7-6. Observational studies reporting adjusted results of the effect of the mean duration of storage of all transfused Red Blood Cells (RBCs) (Section A) and of the duration of storage of the oldest transfused RBC unit on the mortality of patients undergoing cardiac surgery.[32,70,86] In the analysis of the mean storage of all transfused RBCs (Section A), the largest study[70]—which had produced negative results—could not be integrated with the other two reports[32,86] because it had presented the adjusted effect per additional week (rather than per additional day) of storage. Integration of the later-retracted study[32] with the third study[86] produced a significant ($p < 0.05$) adverse effect of RBC storage on mortality [summary OR = 1.035; 95% confidence interval (CI) = 1.020-1.051; $p<0.05$]. In the analysis of the oldest transfused RBC unit (Section B)—in which the largest study[70] again could not be integrated, for the same reason—no effect of RBC storage on mortality was detected across the studies (summary OR = 1.028; 95% CI = 0.99-1.068; $p>0.05$). When RBC storage is defined as the mean duration of storage of all transfused RBCs (Section A) or as the duration of storage of the oldest transfused unit (Section B), the reported adjusted ORs express the increase or decrease in mortality per additional day (or, in the study of van de Watering et al,[70] per additional week) in the mean duration of storage of all transfused RBCs or in the duration of storage of the oldest unit.

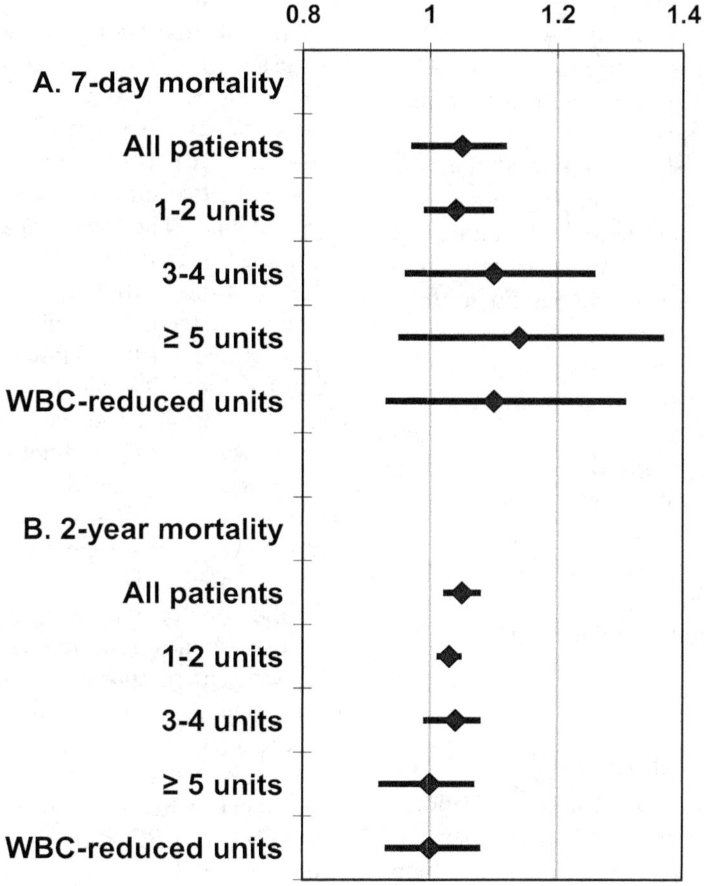

Figure 7-7. Odds ratios (ORs) and their 95% confidence intervals (CIs) for the effect of Red Blood Cell (RBC) storage on short-term (7-day) and long-term (2-year) mortality of all transfusion recipients, recipients stratified by number of transfused RBC units, and recipients of white blood cell (WBC)-reduced units. The figure is based on the analysis of all patients receiving RBC transfusions in Denmark and Sweden between 1995 and 2002, as reported by Edgren et al.[56]

With >400,000 transfusion episodes and 100,000 deaths, the database of Edgren et al[56] allowed for a finer categorization of RBC storage time, permitted elaborate statistical modeling to adjust for confounding factors (including the number of transfused RBCs), and offered unprecedented statistical precision as well as maximum generalizability of the findings. The investigators established four mutually exclusive transfusion categories (recipients of RBCs <9, 10-19, 20-29, and 30-42 days old), excluding patients who had received units with mixed storage times. Because fresh RBC units are usually issued for special indications, patients who had exclusively received RBCs stored for 10 to 19 days were considered to represent the appropriate "reference" group in the study of Edgren et al[56]; patients who had exclusively received RBCs stored for 30 to 42 days were designated as recipients of "old" RBCs. However, all patient groups (ie, recipients of RBCs <9, 20-29, and 30-42 days old, as well as the recipients of mixed-age units) were compared with the "reference" group of patients. In no case did an association between an RBC storage category and short-term mortality attain significance.

Finally, one ICU study[80] reported that the effect of a composite variable defined as the mean storage of all transfused RBCs multiplied by the number of transfused units was not significant. Two medically heterogeneous studies (one in cardiac surgery[86] and one in the pediatric ICU[77]) reported the unadjusted mean ± SD duration of storage of all RBCs transfused to survivors or nonsurvivors, and it observed no difference between the groups. One study enrolling 31 ICU patients[72] reported that the median storage of RBCs transfused to nonsurvivors was significantly ($p<0.05$) longer than that of RBCs administered to survivors, but a multivariate analysis was not included in the report.

Organ Failure

Seven studies presented adjusted[32,33,73,75,78,86] or unadjusted[83] results for the effect of RBC storage on single- or multi-organ failure or a similar outcome. Gajic et al observed no association between storage and acute lung injury (ALI) in a matched[75] and a univariate[73] analysis; the latter study was not followed by a multivariate analysis because no univariate association was recorded. In the matched analysis,[75] the median (interquartile range) duration of storage of transfused RBCs was 22.9 (17-31) days in subjects with ALI and 22.9 (15-30) days in controls (n = 35 matched pairs of ICU patients). In addition, among 181 ICU patients,[73] those who developed ALI had received RBCs stored for a mean (range) of 17.7 (13-22) days, as compared with 18.5 (15-23) days for subjects who did not develop ALI. In that study, there also was no association between transfusion of RBCs stored for >20 days and ALI (OR = 0.83; 95% CI = 0.42-1.66). A multivariate analysis of trauma patients[83] also failed to detect an association between transfusion of RBCs stored for >14 days and acute respiratory distress syndrome (ARDS) (OR = 1.03; 95% CI = 0.89-1.19).

Two cardiac surgery studies[32,86] reported adjusted associations between RBC storage and renal failure. The studies were homogeneous in the duration of storage of the oldest transfused RBC unit ($p>0.05$ for the Q test statistic), and—across the two studies—the age of the oldest unit was not associated with renal failure (summary OR = 0.993; 95% CI = 0.963-1.024). The two studies were extremely heterogeneous in the mean storage of all transfused RBCs ($p<0.00001$ for the Q test statistic), as the 95% CIs for the ORs calculated from within each study[32,86] did not even overlap. For this reason, these two studies could not be combined in the analysis of mean storage. A relationship between transfusion of RBCs stored for >14 days and renal failure was reported in trauma patients from a multivariate analysis that did not adjust for the number of transfused RBC units.[83]

Two studies reported adjusted associations between a composite outcome[33] or multiple-organ failure (MOF)[78] and RBC storage. In cardiac surgery,[33] the odds of occurrence of the composite outcome were greater (p = 0.03) in recipients of RBCs stored for >14 days than in recipients of RBCs stored for <14 days, but this analysis did not adjust for the effect of the number of transfused RBC units or of multiple comparisons. In trauma,[78] 23 subjects who developed MOF received older RBCs than did 40 (matched-for-transfusion-dose) controls who did not develop MOF (mean ± SD RBC age: 30.5 ± 7.68 and 24.0 ± 3.16 days, respectively).

In a study in a pediatric ICU, Gauvin et al[36] recently reported an association between duration of storage of the oldest (WBC-reduced) RBC unit and development of new or progressive multiple-organ dysfunction score (MODS). These authors reported multiple analyses, defining transfusion of old RBCs as receipt of ≥1 unit stored for ≥7 days, ≥1 unit stored for ≥14 days, or ≥1 unit stored for ≥21 days. They also reported on a subgroup analysis of critically ill children transfused with 1 RBC unit. In that patient subgroup, the effect of the duration of storage of the single transfused RBC unit was not confounded by the number of transfused RBC units. There was no difference in new or progressive MODS when ≥7- or ≥14-day-old RBCs were compared with fresher (<7 or <14-day-old, respectively) RBCs. However, when old RBCs included only ≥21-day-old RBCs and were compared to units stored for <21 days, the OR of developing new or progressive MODS was significantly increased (OR = 3.27; 95% CI = 1.38-7.74; $p<0.05$). There was also a significant association between transfusion of RBCs >14 days old and FFP transfusion—probably reflecting the fact that sicker children (who were at greater risk of needing FFP transfusion) were also more likely to receive an older RBC unit.[36] This finding led the authors to conclude that—without conducting an RCT—"[I]t is not possible to discern the impact of older blood from the possible impact of FFP transfusion on outcome."[36] ABO blood group [owing to the higher Factor VIII levels in non-group O (compared with group O) individuals—an attribute that may predispose to thrombosis] is another possible confounder not controlled but commented upon in the discussion by Gauvin et al.[36]

Concerning the question of multiple comparisons in the analysis of Koch et al,[33] it is noted that most published observational studies had considered several adverse outcomes and had presented adjusted results for only some of them. Thus, Koch et al[33] reported on six outcomes in their abstract (ie, in-hospital mortality, 1-year mortality, intubation for >72 hours, renal failure, sepsis, and a composite of complications), only one of which (a composite of complications) had been adjusted for the effects of confounding factors[94] (albeit not for the number of transfused RBCs[20,22,55,89]). Even if the lack of adjustment for this latter (and most important) confounder were to be ignored, the reported adjusted finding ($p = 0.03$) would no longer be significant if it were adjusted further for the effect of multiple comparisons.[94,95] The same concern about multiple comparisons[95] would apply to the results of the meta-analysis,[55] had the findings of the overview been positive. When synthesis of results from multivariate analyses was feasible, however, the results of the meta-analysis[55] were either negative or impossible to evaluate because of the effects of uncontrolled confounders.

Nosocomial Infection

Figure 7-8 shows the unadjusted results of observational studies reporting on the association between RBC storage and postoperative pneumonia in cardiac surgery.[84-86] Although there was an association between the oldest[85,86] (or oldest and second-oldest[84]) transfused RBC unit and postoperative pneumonia before adjustment for the effects of confounding factors, no association was detected when the adjusted results from the same observational studies[84-86] were integrated (Fig 7-9). Four studies[83-86] have presented adjusted results on the effect of RBC storage on pneumonia, but one of them, a trauma study,[83] did not adjust for the number of transfused RBCs. Weinberg et al[83] reported an association between transfusion of RBCs stored for >14 days and pneumonia (OR = 1.10; 95% CI = 1.04-1.17; $p<0.05$).

A study of 61 trauma patients[71] found an association ($p<0.05$) between the transfusion of RBCs older than 14 or 21 days and major infection, after adjustment for patient age and Injury Severity Score, but not for the number of transfused RBCs. In contrast, a study of 448 ICU patients that evaluated the effect of both the length of storage and the number of transfused RBCs concluded that only the number of transfusions was associated with major infection.[74] One[87] of two[87,88] colorectal surgery studies reported an association between transfusion of RBCs stored for >21 days and postoperative infection (excluding urinary tract infection), on the basis of a multivariate analysis that did not adjust for the number of transfused RBCs.

RCTs Currently Under Way in the United States and Canada

Several RCTs comparing recipients of fresh RBCs with recipients of standard or old RBCs are currently ongoing (see http://www.clinicaltrials.gov and http://www.controlled-trial. com).[96]

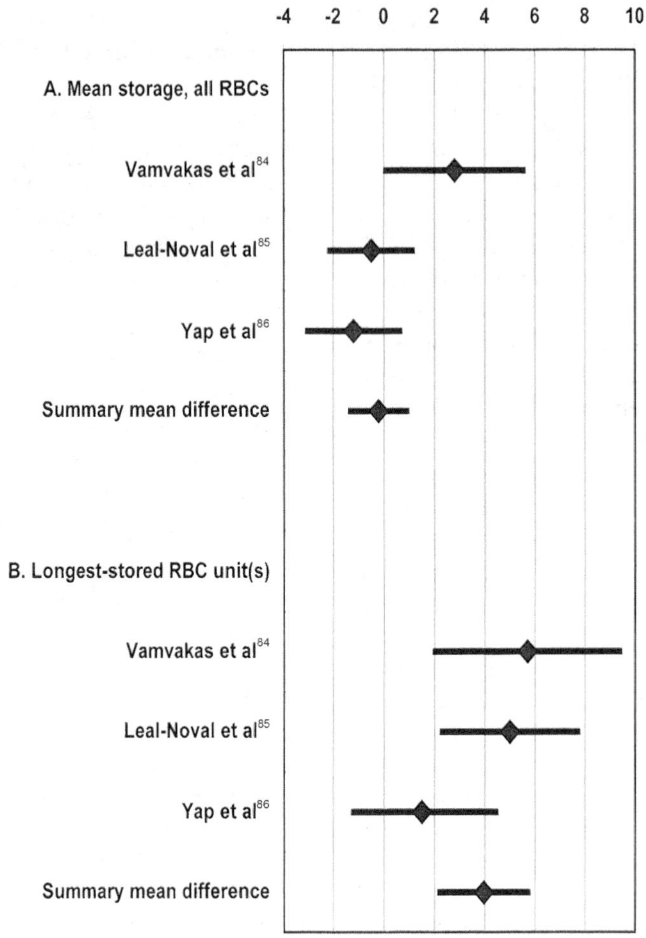

Figure 7-8. Observational cardiac-surgery studies reporting unadjusted findings on the association between the mean duration of storage of all transfused Red Blood Cells (RBCs)[84-86] (Section A) or the duration of storage of the oldest[85,86] (or oldest and second-oldest[84]) transfused RBC unit(s) (Section B) and postoperative pneumonia. For each study, the upper section shows the difference between the mean duration of storage of all RBCs administered to patients who developed pneumonia and the mean duration of storage of all RBCs transfused to patients who did not develop pneumonia. The lower section shows the difference in the duration of storage of the oldest (or oldest and second-oldest) unit(s) received by subjects who did or did not develop pneumonia. Each mean difference is surrounded by its 95% confidence interval (CI). If the CI does not include the null value of 0, the effect of RBC storage is statistically significant ($p<0.05$). Each section also shows the summary mean difference across the studies.[84-86] The studies were statistically homogeneous ($p>0.05$ and $p>0.25$ for the mean storage and the age of the oldest unit, respectively). Across the three studies, the duration of storage of the oldest (or oldest and second-oldest) unit(s) was associated with postoperative pneumonia (summary mean difference: 3.95; 95% CI = 2.20-5.71; lower section), but the mean storage of all transfused RBCs did not show such a significant association with the development of pneumonia (summary mean difference: –0.21; 95% CI = –1.32 to 0.90; upper section). Because these are unadjusted results from observational studies, they are presented solely for the purpose of illustration.

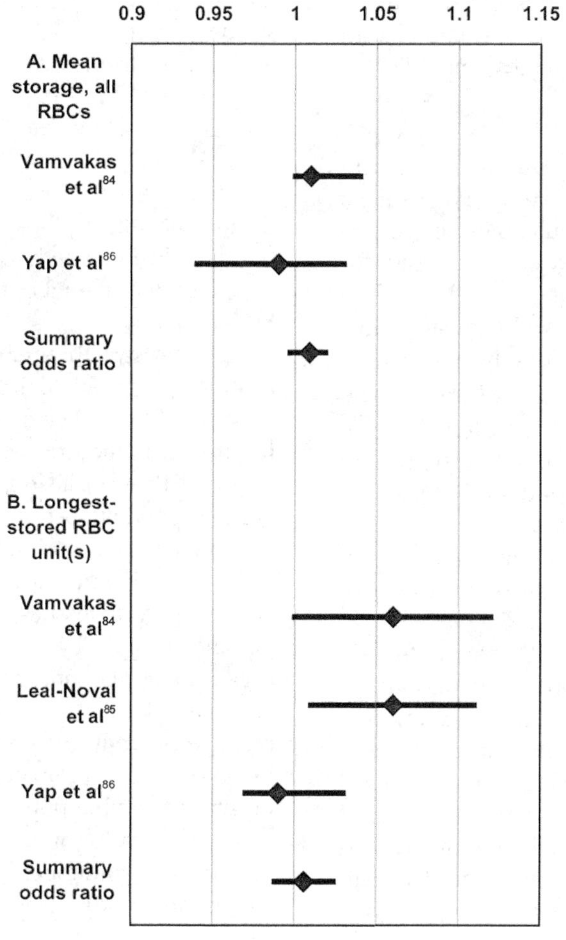

Figure 7-9. Observational cardiac surgery studies reporting adjusted results for the association between the mean storage of all transfused Red Blood Cells (RBCs)[84,86] (Section A) or the duration of storage of the oldest[85,86] (or oldest and second-oldest[84]) transfused RBC unit(s) (Section B) and postoperative pneumonia. For each study, the figure shows the odds ratio (OR) of postoperative pneumonia and the associated 95% confidence interval (CI). If the 95% CI does not include the null value of 1, the association between RBC storage and the development of pneumonia is statistically significant ($p<0.05$). The studies were homogeneous in the mean storage of all transfused RBCs ($p>0.50$ for the Q test statistic), and, across the two studies,[84,86] mean storage was not associated with pneumonia (summary OR = 1.009; 95% CI = 0.999-1.019). The studies were heterogeneous in the duration of storage of the oldest[85,86] (or oldest and second-oldest[84]) transfused RBC unit(s) ($p<0.005$ for the Q test statistic). Yet, integration of their findings under conditions of heterogeneity would not support an adverse effect of the oldest transfused RBC unit on pneumonia (summary OR = 1.006; 95% CI = 0.988-1.024). When RBC storage is defined as the mean storage of all transfused RBCs (Section A) or as the duration of storage of the oldest transfused unit (Section B), the reported adjusted ORs express the increase (or decrease) in the risk of postoperative pneumonia per additional day of the mean duration of storage of all transfused RBCs or the duration of storage of the oldest unit.[55]

Enrollment of patients into the Age of Red Blood Cell in Premature Infants (ARIPI) RCT[97] has been completed. This study was intended to recruit 450 premature neonates and allocate them to receive fresh RBCs stored for <7 days or RBCs issued per standard blood-bank policy.[97] The Red Cell Storage Duration and Outcomes in Cardiac Surgery study is a single-center RCT comparing outcomes in 2800 patients allocated to receive RBCs stored for <14 or >20 days (see websites above). The Red Cell Storage Duration Study will compare 1434 cardiac surgery patients randomly assigned to receive RBCs stored for <10 or >21 days.[98] The Age of Blood Evaluation (ABLE) RCT[39] is randomly assigning patients admitted to the ICU to receive RBCs stored for ≤7 days or RBCs issued per standard blood-bank policy.

Before the early 1980s, it was standard policy to transfuse low-birthweight premature neonates with the freshest blood available in inventory and to aim for RBCs stored for <7 days. There were (and still are) three reasons for such a policy when it comes to premature neonates: 1) the increase (over time) in the level of potassium in the supernatant fluid of stored RBCs; 2) the decrease (over time) in the level of 2,3-diphosphoglycerate (2,3-DPG) in stored RBCs; and 3) the possible risks associated with the use of additives (such as mannitol) and the relatively large amounts of glucose (dextrose) and phosphate present in the RBC preservative solutions used for storing RBCs for up to 42 days [additive solution (AS)-1, -3, or -5 compared with the citrate-phosphate-dextrose (CPD) medium previously used for storing RBCs for 21 days for transfusion to neonates]. Although these concerns are legitimate for large-volume (≥25 mL/kg) transfusions given rapidly, they do not apply to small-volume (10-20 mL/kg) transfusions infused slowly over 2 to 4 hours.[99-101]

In the 1980s, when the risks of transfusion-transmitted viral diseases became paramount, the policy for transfusion of low-birthweight neonates changed from transfusing the freshest RBCs available (to prevent the aforementioned adverse metabolic effects of transfusion of stored RBCs) to transfusing RBCs from "dedicated donors." The latter (current) policy calls for allocating a fresh RBC donor unit to a particular neonate through its expiration at 42 days, so that aliquots of 10-20 mL/kg can be repeatedly drawn from this same unit each time that the designated newborn needs to be transfused. In this way, a neonate's exposure to allogeneic blood donors is minimized because—despite the fact that multiple RBC transfusions are needed during the infant's hospitalization—all of his or her transfusion needs can possibly be met by exposing the neonate to only one allogeneic blood donor.

Low-birthweight premature neonates thus are routinely exposed to transfusions of old RBCs because of the policy of "dedicated donors." Furthermore, premature neonates are very likely to require RBC transfusion, and they are also a vulnerable population most likely to suffer serious morbidities and mortality. If the RBC storage lesion[102-105] can be expected to compromise oxygen delivery to tissues, thereby perhaps resulting, nonspecifically, in increases in mortality, organ failure, and/or infection,[32-36] these adverse effects of old RBCs should be most readily apparent in the susceptible population of low-birthweight premature neonates. Moreover, in this susceptible population, a composite measure of severe morbidities (eg, necrotizing enterocolitis, retinopathy of prematurity, bronchopulmonary dysplasia, intraventricular hemorrhage, and mortality) is expected to occur in up to 65% of the enrolled patients. Therefore, a 15% reduction in the occurrence of this composite measure—thanks to the transfusion of fresh (rather than old) RBCs—can be established (with 80% power) by including only 450 neonates (225 in each arm).[97]

Thus, the ARIPI RCT[97] was the first study randomly assigning recipients to transfusion of old or fresh RBCs to be initiated in Canada. It is intended to determine which of the following strategies is associated with the best clinical outcomes in low-birthweight premature neonates: transfusing these susceptible newborns with RBCs <7 days old (to prevent the purported adverse effects of RBC storage[32-36]) or transfusing them per standard blood-bank policy (to minimize allogeneic donor exposures). The ARIPI RCT[97] was conducted at six neonatal

ICUs across Canada. Low-birthweight (<1250 g) premature neonates needing at least one RBC transfusion were randomly assigned to the study if they were not expected to need exchange transfusion. For the control arm, donor units divided into 4 (quad-pack) or ≤8 (pedi-pack) aliquots were stored for up to 42 days after collection (or up to 28 days after gamma-irradiation), and they were used to meet all of a neonate's transfusion needs.

The ARIPI RCT[97] is unique among the RCTs currently under way in Canada or the United States, in that clinical equipoise for conducting this trial truly did exist among neonatologists. Regardless of opinions about the purported nonspecific adverse effects of old blood,[32-36] opinions varied among neonatologists about the optimal transfusion policy.[106] Some neonatologists favored the traditional blood-bank policy of transfusing neonates with the freshest blood available (aiming for blood <7 days old to prevent the aforementioned adverse metabolic effects of stored RBCs in patients whose premature liver and kidneys have difficulty handling the potassium, dextrose, and preservatives infused with old RBCs stored in additive solutions). Other neonatologists favored the "dedicated-donor" policy introduced in the 1980s to mitigate the risk of TTIs. Now that there has been a ≥3-log reduction in the risk of viral TTIs since the 1980s,[107] the benefits of avoiding the metabolic effects of transfusion of stored RBCs may outweigh the benefits of minimizing donor exposures.

The reason that equipoise exists in the ARIPI RCT[97] is precisely the reason that the results of this trial cannot inform RBC transfusion policy for adult transfusion recipients. Neither a dedicated-donor policy for minimizing allogeneic-donor exposures nor a policy for transfusing fresh RBCs to prevent the metabolic effects of stored RBCs is relevant to adult patients. If the ARIPI RCT establishes poor clinical outcomes in association with the transfusion of old RBCs, those adverse effects of old blood may simply reflect the metabolic effects of stored RBCs on the premature liver and kidneys of vulnerable newborns. Accordingly, such adverse effects cannot be generalized to adult patients.

As of January 2011, the ABLE RCT[39] had enrolled 492 patients from 23 Canadian ICUs. The investigators planned to enroll 2510 patients in order to detect a 5% absolute risk reduction (from 25% to 20%) in the mortality of ICU patients. Patients admitted to the ICU and having an anticipated requirement for mechanical ventilation exceeding 48 hours continue to be enrolled into this study when the first request for an RBC transfusion is received. Assuming that enrollment continues at the rate of 40 to 50 patients per month, recruitment of 2510 patients will be completed in 3 to 4 years. Additional sites from Canada, France, and the United Kingdom are being asked to participate in the ABLE RCT. The primary outcome measure is 90-day mortality, but additional data are collected on organ failure and nosocomial infection.

The DSMB of the ABLE RCT requested that an interim analysis be conducted each time 500 new patients are enrolled. In this way, there will be four interim analyses and one final analysis of the data. The DSMB will interrupt the study if a difference is detected at the $p = 0.00001$ significance level at the time of the first interim analysis; at the $p = 0.0008$ significance level at the time of the second interim analysis; at the $p = 0.007$ significance level at the time of the third interim analysis; at the $p = 0.022$ significance level at the time of the fourth interim analysis; and at the $p = 0.0423$ significance level at the time of the final analysis.[39]

If a difference is detected by the ABLE RCT, the findings will apply only to critically ill patients. To inform policy for all RBC transfusion recipients, a pragmatic RCT (along the lines of the pilot completed by Heddle et al[58]; Table 7-2) will need to be conducted to study the same question in an unselected hospital population including all transfused patients. Because the mortality of all transfused patients is 10.6%[58] (compared with 25% for patients transfused in the ICU[39]), this latter trial will need to enroll 25,000 patients to detect a 15% reduction in mortality in association with transfusion of fresh (rather than old) RBCs.[58] With such a large sample, indications for RBC transfusion can be assumed to be equally distributed between the two trial arms, thanks to the play of chance.

Patients randomly assigned to the "fresh" arm of the ABLE RCT receive RBCs stored 2 to 7 days; subjects randomly assigned to the "old" arm of the trial receive the oldest compatible unit available in inventory (which can be as old as 42 days but which, in theory, also could be only 2 days old). Randomly assigning patients to always receive RBCs stored for more than a specified number of days (eg, >14 or >21 days) was deemed to be unethical by the ABLE investigators, transfusion-medicine physicians, critical-care physicians, and research ethics boards (which would not consider ethical the transfusion of RBCs that had been intentionally held for 2 to 3 weeks to become "old").[39]

Discussion

Subjects randomly assigned to always receive old RBCs in RCTs allocating patients to receive fresh or old RBCs are knowingly exposed to the proven or probable–but rare–risks of TAS[1,2] and TRALI.[16-19] The ethical justification for knowingly exposing half of the experimental subjects to these risks is that, if the purportedly far more frequent adverse effects of old RBCs vis-à-vis the common outcomes of mortality, organ failure, and in-hospital infection are indisputably documented, appropriate measures will follow for their abrogation. Therefore, the benefit to society from documenting the existence of the purported common adverse effects of old RBCs[32-36] is deemed to be sufficiently worthy to allow for exposing >2000 subjects enrolled in the ongoing RCTs to the known[1,2] and probable[16-19] risks of transfusion of old RBCs.

The ethical justification for allocating patients to receive fresh or old (rather than fresh or standard) RBCs is that a design maximizing the difference between the treatments given to the two trial arms also maximizes the power of the study to detect a difference between the two treatments. If an RCT randomly assigns patients to receive RBCs stored for ≤10 or >21 days,[38] that RCT is more likely to detect a small difference between the arms than is an RCT randomly assigning patients to receive RBCs stored for ≤7 days or standard RBCs. If the latter RCT is completed without establishing a difference between the study arms, no benefit is accrued to society, because the evidence needed for policy decision-making has not been produced.

Three recent systematic reviews[20-22] of the available clinical studies concluded that the existence of the purported common adverse effects of old RBCs *cannot* be adequately inferred from the available data. Two of these systematic reviews[20,22] did not include a meta-analysis, whereas the authors of the third review[21] deemed that the available studies are too heterogeneous to allow for meta-analysis. These three systematic reviews refuted the earlier conclusion[108] that had supported an association between transfusion of old (rather than fresh) RBCs and common adverse outcomes–and on the basis of which the Canadian and US RCTs of the effect of RBC storage were initiated. A meta-analysis[55] subsequently showed that integration of adjusted findings from observational studies reporting on the same outcome in the same setting and defining transfusion of old or fresh RBCs in the same manner (ie, of observational studies that can be legitimately combined) produced summary results that were negative in six of eight analyses. The two situations in which positive findings were produced–namely, 1) the analysis of the effect of the mean storage of all transfused RBCs on mortality (Fig 7-6), and 2) the synthesis of trauma studies[34,82,83] that had presented adjusted results on mortality–did not integrate studies that had adjusted for the effect of the most important confounder (ie, the number of transfused RBCs[109]). Accordingly, it would be injudicious for policy-makers to endorse such a radical change in policy (mandating transfusion of fresh rather than old or standard RBCs) without waiting for definitive evidence to be produced from randomized studies.[60]

Given the paucity of evidence on any association between transfusion of old RBCs and common adverse outcomes,[20-22,55] the ongoing RCTs will likely generate null findings and, when their results are reported, the transfusion medicine community will probably have to grapple, once more, with the issue of whether to transfuse

RBCs older than 28 (or even 21) days when fresher units are available. The question of whether RBC storage should be limited to 28 (or fewer) days to prevent the known[1,2] or probable[16-19]—but rare—risks of transfusion of old RBCs will remain unanswered if the ongoing RCTs find no association between old RBCs and the common adverse clinical outcomes that they were designed to target. As evidence is presented that the RBC inventories of transfusion services in the United States are fresher[40] than previously thought, if conversion to a "fresh" RBC inventory is appropriate, it may be indicated for reasons[1,2,16-19] other than those investigated by the RCTs currently under way in the United States and Canada.[32-36]

As discussed in Chapters 2 and 4 of this book, 12 years after the publication of the Transfusion Requirements in Critical Care (TRICC) RCT,[110] the findings of that seminal RCT concerning an association of a liberal or restrictive RBC transfusion strategy with adverse outcomes remain unconfirmed by another RCT of adult transfusion recipients. In the TRICC RCT, the receipt of 3 more RBC units on average by ICU patients randomly assigned to receive RBC transfusion per liberal criteria than by those transfused per restrictive criteria was associated with an increase in several secondary outcomes: in-hospital mortality, myocardial infarction, pulmonary edema, and MODS, as well as any studied complication. The mechanism of this effect of RBC transfusion has not been elucidated. Because the TRICC RCT transfused RBCs according to standard inventory policy, it is possible that patients transfused by the liberal RBC transfusion strategy—that is, receiving 3 more RBC units on average than those transfused by the restricted RBC criteria—also received more old RBC units on average (Fig 7-2). If that was the case, it is possible that the purported adverse effects of old (rather than fresh) RBCs could be the basis of the association between RBC transfusion and the adverse outcomes observed in the TRICC study. Fergusson et al[97] also offered the hypothesis that prolonged RBC storage might exacerbate the effect of transfusing non-WBC-reduced RBCs, because there may be an interaction between the duration of RBC storage and the effect of soluble mediators released from deteriorating WBCs during storage (Fig 2-15 in Chapter 2). In an earlier before-vs-after observational study,[111] Fergusson et al had observed a trend toward a more frequent occurrence of the composite of complications used in the ARIPI study[97] before rather than after the implementation of universal WBC reduction in Canada.

Such possibilities concerning the origin of the previously reported associations between liberal or restrictive RBC transfusion strategies[110] or non-WBC-reduced or WBC-reduced ABT[111] are currently being investigated in critically ill patients[39] and subjects undergoing cardiac surgery.[38] Negative results of the ongoing RCTs may reassure clinicians and blood bankers about the safety and efficacy of transfusing both fresh and standard (or old) RBCs. Positive results may have major implications with regard to RBC inventory management and may also prompt research to gain better understanding of the RBC storage lesion in the hope of minimizing its clinical consequences through the development of better storage methods.

References

1. Arduino MJ, Bland LA, Tipple MA, et al. Growth and endotoxin production of *Yersinia enterocolitica* and *Enterobacter agglomerans* in packed erythrocytes. J Clin Microbiol 1989;27: 1483-5.
2. Centers for Disease Control and Prevention. Update: *Yersinia enterocolitica* bacteremia and endotoxin shock associated with red blood cell transfusion—United States, 1991. MMWR Morb Mortal Wkly Rep 1991;40:176-8.
3. Council of Community Blood Centers. FDA committee endorses education and research to combat rare bacterial reaction: Rejects operational changes for now. CCBC Newsletter 1991; May 10:1-4.
4. AABB. FDA Blood Products Advisory Committee supports educational efforts on *Yersinia enterocolitica*. Blood Bank Week 1991;20:1-3.
5. Jensenius M, Hoel T, Heier HE. *Yersinia enterocolitica* septicemia after blood transfusion. Tidsskr Nor Laegeforen 1995;115:940-2.

6. Jacobs J, Jamaer D, Vandeven J, et al. *Yersinia enterocolitica* in donor blood: A case report and review. J Clin Microbiol 1989;27:1119-21.
7. Donegan E, Lenes BA, Tomasulo PA, et al. Transmission of HIV-1 by component type and duration of shelf storage before transfusion. Transfusion 1991;30:851-2.
8. Donegan E, Lee H, Operskalski EA, et al. Transfusion transmission of retroviruses: Human T-lymphotropic virus types I and II compared with human immunodeficiency virus type 1. Transfusion 1994;34:478-83.
9. Centers for Disease Control and Prevention. Red blood cell transfusions contaminated with *Yersinia enterocolitica*—United States, 1991-1996, and initiation of a national study to detect bacteria-associated transfusion reactions. MMWR Morb Mortal Wkly Rep 1997;46:553-5.
10. Hogman CF, Gong J, Hambraeus A, et al. The role of white cells in the transmission of *Yersinia enterocolitica* in blood products. Transfusion 1992;32:654-7.
11. Kim DM, Brecher ME, Bland LA, et al. Prestorage removal of *Yersinia enterocolitica* from red cells with white cell-reduction filters. Transfusion 1992;32:658-62.
12. Buchholz DH, AuBuchon JP, Snyder EL, et al. Removal of *Yersinia enterocolitica* from AS-1 red cells. Transfusion 1992;32:667-72.
13. Serious Hazards of Transfusion (SHOT). SHOT Report for 2004-2005. Manchester, UK: SHOT Office, 2005. [Available at http://www.shotuk.org/shot-reports/report-and-summary-2005/ (accessed November 2, 2011).]
14. Perez P, Salmi LR, Follea G, et al. Determinants of transfusion-associated bacterial contamination: Results of the French BACTHEM case-control study. Transfusion 2001;41:862-71.
15. Brecher ME, Hay SN. Bacterial contamination of blood components. Clin Microbiol Rev 2005;18:195-204.
16. Kuehnert MJ, Roth VR, Haley NR, et al. Transfusion-transmitted bacterial infection in the United States, 1998 through 2000. Transfusion 2001;41:1493-9.
17. Silliman CC, Clay KL, Thurman GW, et al. Partial characterization of lipids that develop during the routine storage of blood and prime the neutrophil NADPH oxidase. J Lab Clin Med 1994;124:684-94.
18. Kelher MR, Masuno T, Moore EE, et al. Plasma from stored packed red blood cells and MHC class I antibodies causes acute lung injury in a 2-event in vivo rat model. Blood 2009;113:2079-87.
19. Silliman CC, Moore EE, Kehler MR, et al. Identification of lipids that accumulate during the routine storage of prestorage-leukoreduced red blood cells and cause acute lung injury. Transfusion 2011;51:2549-54.
20. Zimrin AB, Hess JR. Current issues relating to the transfusion of stored red blood cells. Vox Sang 2009;96:93-103.
21. Lelubre C, Piagnerelli M, Vincent JL. Association between storage of transfused red blood cells and morbidity and mortality in adult patients: Myth or reality? Transfusion 2009;49:1348-94.
22. van de Watering L. Red cell storage and prognosis. Vox Sang 2011;100:36-45.
23. Jy W, Ricci M, Shariatmandar S, et al. Microparticles in stored red blood cells as potential mediators of transfusion complications. Transfusion 2011;51:886-93.
24. Spinella PC, Sparrow RL, Hess JR, Norris PJ. Properties of stored red blood cells: Understanding immune and vascular reactivity. Transfusion 2011;51:894-900.
25. Hod EA, Spitalnik SL. Harmful effects of transfusion of older stored red blood cells: Iron and inflammation. Transfusion 2011;51:881-5.
26. Weinberg JA, Barnum SR, Patel RP. Red blood cell age and potentiation of transfusion-related pathology in trauma patients. Transfusion 2011;51:867-73.
27. Grimshaw K, Sahler J, Spinella SL, et al. New frontiers in transfusion biology: Identification and significance of mediators of morbidity and mortality in stored red blood cells. Transfusion 2011;51:874-80.
28. Kim-Shapiro DB, Lee J, Gladwin MT. Storage lesion: Role of red blood cell breakdown. Transfusion 2011;51:844-51.
29. Reynolds JD, Hess DT, Stamler JS. The transfusion problem: Role of aberrant S-nitrosylation. Transfusion 2011;51:852-8.
30. Roback JD, Neuman R, Quyyumi A, Sutliff R. Insufficient nitric oxide bioavailability: A hypothesis to explain adverse effects of red blood cell transfusion. Transfusion 2011;51:859-96.
31. Isbister JP, Shander RA, Spahn DR. Adverse blood transfusion outcomes: Establishing causation. Transfus Med Rev 2011;25:89-101.
32. Basran S, Frumento RJ, Cohen A, et al. The association between duration of storage of transfused red blood cells and morbidity and

mortality after reoperative cardiac surgery. Anesth Analg 2006;103:15-20 [Retracted].
33. Koch CG, Li L, Sessler DI, et al. Duration of red-cell storage and complications after cardiac surgery. N Engl J Med 2008;358:1229-39.
34. Spinella PC, Carroll CL, Staff I, et al. Duration of red blood cell storage is associated with increased incidence of deep-vein thrombosis and in-hospital mortality in patients with traumatic injuries. Crit Care 2009;13:R151.
35. Karam O, Tucci M, Bateman ST, et al. Association between length of storage of red blood cell units and outcome of critically-ill children: A prospective observational study. Crit Care 2010;14:R57.
36. Gauvin F, Spinella PC, Lacroix J, et al. Association between length of storage of transfused red blood cells and multiple-organ dysfunction syndrome in pediatric intensive-care patients. Transfusion 2010;50:1902-13.
37. Ness PM. Does transfusion of stored red blood cells cause clinically important adverse effects? A critical question in search of an answer and a plan. Transfusion 2011;51:666-7.
38. Stein ME, Stowell C. Does red blood cell storage affect clinical outcome? When in doubt, do the experiment. Transfusion 2009;49:1286-90.
39. Lacroix J. Hebert P, Fergusson D, et al. The Age of Blood Evaluation (ABLE) randomized controlled trial: Study design. Transfus Med Rev 2011;25:197-205.
40. Bennet-Guerrero E, Stafford-Smith M, Waweru P, et al. A prospective, double-blind randomized feasibility clinical trial of controlling the storage age of red blood cells for transfusion in cardiac surgical patients. Transfusion 2009;49:1375-83.
41. Freedman B. Equipoise and the ethics of clinical research. N Engl J Med 1987;317:141-5.
42. Miller FG, Joffee S. Equipoise and the dilemma of randomized clinical trials. N Engl J Med 2011;364:476-80.
43. Sackett DL. Rules of evidence and clinical recommendation on the use of antithrombotic agents. Chest 1989;95(Suppl 2):2S-4S.
44. Rossouw JE, Anderson GL, Prentice RL, et al. Risks and benefits of estrogen plus progestin in healthy postmenopausal women: Principal results from the Women's Health Initiative randomized controlled trial. JAMA 2002;288:321-33.
45. Manson JE, Hsia J, Johnson KC, et al. Estrogen plus progestin and the risk of coronary heart disease. N Engl J Med 2003;349:523-34.
46. Stadtmauer EA, O'Neill A, Goldstein LJ, et al. Conventional-dose chemotherapy compared with high-dose chemotherapy plus autologous hematopoietic stem-cell transplantation for metastatic breast cancer. N Engl J Med 2000;342:1069-76.
47. Echt DS, Liebson PR, Mitchell LB, et al. Mortality and morbidity in patients receiving encainide, flecainide, or placebo—the Cardiac Arrhythmia Suppression Trial. N Engl J Med 1991;324:781-8.
48. Tsimberidou AM, Braiteth F, Stewart DJ, Kurzrock R. Ultimate fate of oncology drugs approved by the US Food and Drug Administration without a randomized trial. J Clin Oncol 2009;27:6243-50.
49. Einhorn LH, Donohue J. Cis-diamminedichloroplatinum, vinblastin, and bleomycin combination chemotherapy in disseminated testicular cancer. Ann Intern Med 1977;87:293-8.
50. Richardson PG, Barlogic B, Berenson J, et al. A phase 2 study of bortezomib in relapsed, refractory myeloma. N Engl J Med 2003;348:2609-17.
51. Harmon A. New drugs stir debate on rules of clinical trials. New York Times 2010;Sept 18:A1.
52. Buyse M, Thirion P, Carlson RW, et al. Relation between tumor response to first-line chemotherapy and survival in advanced colorectal cancer: A meta-analysis. Lancet 2000;356:373-8.
53. Shanafelt TD, Loprinzi C, Marks R, et al. Are chemotherapy response rates related to treatment-induced survival prolongations in patients with advanced cancer? J Clin Oncol 2004;22:1966-74.
54. Tang PA, Bentzen SM, Chen EX, Siu LL. Surrogate endpoints for median overall survival in metastatic colorectal cancer: Literature-based analysis from 39 randomized controlled trials of first-line chemotherapy. J Clin Oncol 2007;25:4562-8.
55. Vamvakas EC. Meta-analysis of clinical studies of the purported deleterious effects of "old" (versus "fresh") red blood cells: Are we at equipoise? Transfusion 2010;50:600-10.
56. Edgren G, Kamper-Jorgensen M, Eloranta S, et al. Duration of red-blood-dell storage and survival of transfused patients. Transfusion 2010;50:1185-95.
57. Eikelboom J, Cook RJ, Liu Y, Heddle NM. Duration of red-cell storage before transfusion and in-hospital mortality. Am Heart J 2010;159:737-43.

58. Heddle NM, Eikelboom JW, Cook RJ, et al. Can we do a 25,000-patient pragmatic study to address the age of blood and mortality controversy? A pilot to determine feasibility. Transfusion 2011;51(Suppl):193A.
59. Lee TH, Paglieroni T, Ohto H, et al. Survival of donor leukocyte subpopulations in immunocompetent transfusion recipients: Frequent long-term microchimerism in severe trauma patients. Blood 1999;93:3127-39.
60. Glynn SA. The red blood cell storage lesion: A method to the madness. Transfusion 2010;50:1164-9.
61. Schulman CI, Nathe K, Brown M, Cohn SM. Impact of age of transfused blood in the trauma patient. J Trauma 2002;52:1224-5.
62. Hébert PC, Chin-Yee I, Fergusson D, et al. A pilot trial evaluating the clinical effects of prolonged storage of red cells. Anesth Analg 2005;100:1433-8.
63. Mou SS, Giroir BP, Molitor-Kirsch EA, et al. Fresh blood versus reconstituted blood for pump priming in heart surgery in infants. N Engl J Med 2004;351:1635-44.
64. Walsh TS, McArdle F, McLellan SA, et al. Does the storage time of transfused red blood cells influence regional or global indexes of tissue oxygenation in anemic critically ill patients? Crit Care Med 2004;32:364-71.
65. Weiskopf RB, Feiner J, Hopf H, et al. Fresh blood and aged stored blood are equally efficacious in immediately reversing anemia-induced brain oxygenation deficits in humans. Anesthesiology 2006;104:911-20.
66. Prentice RL, Thomas DB. On the epidemiology of oral contraceptives and disease. Adv Cancer Res 1986;49:285-401.
67. Koch CG, Li L, Duncan AI, et al. Transfusion in coronary-artery bypass grafting is associated with reduced long-term survival. Ann Thorac Surg 2006;81:1650-7.
68. Koch CG, Li L, Duncan AI, et al. Morbidity and mortality risk associated with red-blood-cell and blood-component transfusion in isolated coronary-artery bypass grafting. Crit Care Med 2006;34:1608-16.
69. Marik PE, Corwin HL. Efficacy of red-blood-cell transfusion in the critically ill: A systematic review of the literature. Crit Care Med 2008;36:2667-74.
70. van de Watering L, Lorinser J, Versteegh M, et al. Effects of storage time of red-blood-cell transfusions on the prognosis of coronary-artery bypass-graft patients. Transfusion 2006;46:1712-8.
71. Offner PJ, Moore EE, Biffl WL, et al. Increased rate of infection associated with transfusion of old blood after severe injury. Arch Surg 2002;137:711-6.
72. Purdy FR, Tweeddale MG, Merrick PM. Association of mortality with age of blood transfused in septic ICU patients. Can J Anaesth 1997;44:1256-61.
73. Gajic O, Rana R, Mendez JL, et al. Acute lung injury after blood transfusion in mechanically ventilated patients. Transfusion 2004;44:1468-74.
74. Taylor RW, O'Brien J, Trottier SJ, et al. Red blood cell transfusions and nosocomial infections in critically ill patients. Crit Care Med 2006;34:2302-8.
75. Gajic O, Rana R, Winters JL, et al. Transfusion-related acute lung injury in the critically ill: Prospective nested case-control study. Am J Respir Crit Care Med 2007;176:886-91.
76. Dessertaine G, Hammer L, Chenais F, et al. Does red-blood-cell storage time still influence ICU survival? Transfus Clin Biol 2008;15:154-9.
77. Kneyber CJ, Gazendam RP, Markhorst DG, Plotz FB. Length of storage of red blood cells does not affect outcome in critically ill children. Intensive Care Med 2009;35:179-80.
78. Zallen G, Offner PJ, Moore EE, et al. Age of transfused blood is an independent risk factor for post-injury multiple-organ failure. Am J Surg 1999;178:570-2.
79. Keller ME, Jean R, LaMorte WW, et al. Effects of age of transfused blood on length of stay in trauma patients: A preliminary report. J Trauma 2002;53:1023-5.
80. Murrell Z, Haukoos JS, Putnam B, Klein SR. The effect of older blood on mortality, need for ICU care, and the length of ICU stay after major trauma. Ann Surg 2005;71:781-5.
81. Leal-Noval SR, Munoz-Gomez M, Allerano-Orden V, et al. Impact of age of transfused blood on cerebral oxygenation in male patients with severe traumatic brain injury. Crit Care Med 2008;36:1290-6.
82. Weinberg JA, McGwin G Jr, Griffin RL, et al. Age of transfused blood: An independent predictor of mortality despite universal leukoreduction. J Trauma 2008;65:279-82.
83. Weinberg JA, McGwin G Jr, Marques MB, et al. Transfusion in the less severely injured: Does age of tranfused blood affect outcomes? J Trauma 2008;65:794-8.

84. Vamvakas EC, Carven JH. Transfusion and postoperative pneumonia in coronary artery bypass graft surgery: Effect of the length of storage of transfused red cells. Transfusion 1999;39:701-10.
85. Leal-Noval SR, Jara-Lopez I, Garcia-Garmendia JL, et al. Influence of erythrocyte concentrate storage time on post-surgical morbidity in cardiac-surgery patients. Anesthesiology 2003;98:815-22.
86. Yap CH, Lau L, Krishnaswamy M, et al. Age of transfused red cells and early outcomes after cardiac surgery. Ann Thorac Surg 2008;86:554-9.
87. Mynster T, Nielsen HJ. The impact of storage time of transfused blood on postoperative infectious complications in rectal cancer surgery. Danish RANX05 Colorectal Cancer Study Group. Scand J Gastroenterol 2000;35:212-17.
88. Edna TH, Bjerkeset T. Association between transfusion of stored blood and infective bacterial complications after resection for colorectal cancer. Eur J Surg 1998;164:449-56.
89. Hall SW. Red-cell storage and complications of cardiac surgery (letter). N Engl J Med 2008;358:2841.
90. Koch CG, Li L, Blackstone EH. Red-cell storage and complications of cardiac surgery (reply to letters). N Engl J Med 2008;358:2841-2.
91. Rothmann M, Braun MM, Ng T-H. On the hazard ratios and corresponding confidence intervals that appear in Basran et al (2006). Anesth Analg 2007;104:1597.
92. Shafer SL. Occam's razor (letter). Anesth Analg 2007;104:1597-8.
93. Vamvakas EC. Purported deleterious effects of old versus fresh red blood cells: An updated meta-analysis. Transfusion 2011;51:1122-3.
94. Benjamin RJ, Dodd RY. Red-cell storage and complications of cardiac surgery (letter). N Engl J Med 2008;358:2840-1.
95. Kanter M. Accuracy of statistical methods in *Transfusion*: A review of articles from July/August 1992 through June 1993. Transfusion 1994;34:697-701.
96. Steiner ME, Stowell C. Does red blood cell storage affect clinical outcome? When in doubt, do the experiment. Transfusion 2009;49:1286-90.
97. Fergusson D, Hutton B, Hogan DL, et al. The age of red blood cells in premature infants (ARIPI) randomized controlled trial: Study design. Transfus Med Rev 2009;23:55-61.
98. Steiner ME, Assmann SF, Levy JH, et al. Addressing the question of the effect of RBC storage on clinical outcomes: The Red Cell Storage Duration Study (RECESS). Transfus Apher Sci 2010;43:107-16.
99. Luban NLC, Strauss RG, Hume HA. Commentary on the safety of red blood cells preserved in extended storage media for neonatal transfusions. Transfusion 1991;31:229-35.
100. Strauss RG, Burmeister LF, Johnson K, et al. Randomized trial assessing feasibility and safety of biological parents as red-blood-cell donors for their preterm infants. Transfusion 2000;40:450-6.
101. Strauss RG, Burmeister LF, Johnson K, et al. Feasibility and safety of AS-3 red blood cells for neonatal transfusions. J Pediatr 2000;136:21509.
102. Wolfe LC. The membrane and the lesions of storage in preserved red cells. Transfusion 1985;25:185-203.
103. Card RT. Red cell membrane changes during storage. Transfus Med Rev 1988;2:40-7.
104. Chin-Yee I, Arya N, D'Almeida M. The red cell storage lesion and its implication for transfusion. Transfus Sci 1997;18:447-58.
105. Bennett-Guerrero EB, Veldman TH, Doctor A, et al. Evolution of adverse storage in stored RBCs. Proc Natl Acad Sci U S A 2007;104:17063-8.
106. Levy GJ. National survey of neonatal transfusion practice: I. Red blood cell theory. Pediatrics 1993;91:532-9.
107. Kleinman S, Chan P, Robillard P. Risks associated with transfusion of cellular blood components in Canada. Transfus Med Rev 2003;17:120-62.
108. Timmouth A, Fergusson D, Yee IC, Hébert PC. Clinical consequences of red-cell storage in the critically ill. Transfusion 2006;46:2014-27.
109. Middelburg RA, van de Watering LMG, van der Bom JG. Blood transfusions: Good or bad? Confounding by indication, an underestimated problem in clinical transfusion research. Transfusion 2010;50:1881-3.
110. Hébert PC, Wells G, Blajchman MA, et al. A multicenter randomized controlled trial of transfusion requirements in critical care. N Engl J Med 1999;340:409-17.
111. Fergusson D, Hébert PC, Lee SK et al. Clinical outcomes following institution of universal leukoreduction of blood transfusions for premature infants. JAMA 2003;289:1950-6.

In: Vamvakas EC.
Decision Making in Transfusion Medicine
Bethesda, MD: AABB Press, 2011

8

Paradigm Shifts in Transfusion Medicine

IN A RECENT ARTICLE, FARRUGIA[1] identified the following six characteristics of the current "transfusion paradigm": 1) centralized blood systems, 2) blood component therapy, 3) manufacturing culture, 4) focus on the product, 5) primacy of inventory, and 6) detachment from the clinical environment. The cursory overview of transfusion medicine that standard textbooks of medical education embedded in the minds of transfusion-medicine professionals educated after the early 1980s included the principles of blood component therapy on which this paradigm is based before those professionals entered the field and acquired the knowledge that would allow them to assess the validity of the paradigm's assumptions. Thus, these tenets became the "common sense" of transfusion medicine for all professionals who—like this author—are now in their forties or early fifties. These professionals hardly ever encountered any questioning or re-evaluation of the assumptions of the common sense of transfusion medicine, and they are not old enough to remember the debates from the 1970s about whether, as Grindon posited, "one-third to one-half of all transfusions in the operating room" can be given in the form of Red Blood Cells (RBCs) rather than whole blood.[2] The mention of such debates in current specialized textbooks of transfusion medicine is typically relegated to the "history" of blood transfusion.

Yet, the established common sense of transfusion medicine—or, rather, of blood component therapy—might defy ordinary common sense. Based as it is on the rationale that whole blood can be reconstituted by mixing RBCs and Fresh Frozen Plasma (FFP)—as well as platelets, when needed—from different allogeneic donors, the established common sense of transfusion medicine calls for exposing patients who need multiple transfusions of various blood components to as many allogeneic donors as the number of individual blood components that the patients receive. Moreover, the established common sense of transfusion medicine calls for transfusing to patients the oldest compatible RBC or platelet unit available in inventory, so as to preserve inventory and avoid wastage of units and blood component shortages. Regardless of whether "old" RBCs are associated with the purported common adverse effects of old blood discussed in Chapter 7, old RBCs are indisputably an inferior-quality product from the vantage points of laboratory parameters and their expected ability to deliver oxygen to tissues. This is because the extended-storage conditions of RBCs were approved on the basis of the laboratory standard that 75% of the transfused stored RBCs should still be circulating 24 hours after the allogeneic blood transfusion (ABT), regardless of the fact that—as discussed in Chapter 7—RBCs stored for >25 days are associated with a higher risk of transfusion-associated sepsis (TAS), while RBCs stored for prolonged periods may be associated with a higher risk of transfusion-related acute lung injury (TRALI).

In a similar vein, as discussed in Chapter 2, platelets stored for >3 days are indisputably associated with a higher risk of TAS than are fresh platelets. [In fact, Germany and Japan have limited the storage period of platelets (which is 5 days in the United States) to 4 and 3 days, respectively, to reduce the risk of TAS.[3]] Furthermore, the longer platelets are stored, the lower the resulting posttransfusion 1-hour corrected count increment (CCI) becomes, especially when platelet additive solutions (PASs) rather than plasma are used to support platelet metabolism during storage.[4] Ordinary common sense—in contrast to the established common sense of transfusion—would favor exposure to as few allogeneic donors as possible if the ABT needs of multitransfused patients (for example, those with acute blood loss) could be met by transfusing actual whole blood (rather than whole blood "reconstituted" from RBCs and FFP collected from different allogeneic donors). The same ordinary common sense also would favor the avoidance of products of inferior quality, such as old RBCs or old platelets.

Nonetheless, the established common sense of transfusion has been aimed at avoiding blood shortages and, by so doing, saved many lives in the 20th and early 21st centuries. The risk due to the nonavailability of the blood components needed for a bleeding patient *far* exceeds the infectious and noninfectious risks of unnecessarily exposing a bleeding patient to multiple allogeneic donors, as well as the greater risk of TAS or any other risk(s) associated with the transfusion of components that represent the oldest compatible units in inventory. Equally important, many transfusion recipients need transfusion of only one blood component: RBCs (for anemia), platelets (for thrombocytopenia), or FFP (for deficiency of coagulation factors). In such patients (who do not need reconstituted whole blood through receipt of a combination of RBC and FFP components and sometimes platelets as well), each donor's gift of whole blood is arguably maximized by having a single whole-blood unit serve the needs of as many as three recipients.[5] Furthermore, when this approach is followed, recovered plasma from whole-blood collections supplements the source plasma collected through plasmapheresis for fractionation, ensuring that all Factor VIII needs of patients with hemophilia are met.

In the absence of considerations of cost, insofar as each whole-blood donation is split into three components solely for the purpose of meeting supply needs for Factor VIII and platelets, which cannot be harvested through demonstrated efforts to recruit plasmapheresis and plateletpheresis donors, the established common sense of transfusion indisputably serves the needs of patients today in the same manner that it served the needs of transfusion recipients when it was initially introduced in the late 1970s. If, however, each whole-blood donation is split into three components for reasons other than supply needs, transfusion medicine professionals could question whether continued reliance on the aforementioned six tenets that define the current transfusion paradigm[1] best serves the interests of their patients.

It is possible to identify economic (rather than supply) reasons for the continued use of the two "by-products" of RBC collection, that is, recovered plasma and whole-blood-derived (WBD) platelets. Use of these by-products as source material for Factor VIII concentrates or for creating a therapeutic platelet dose from a pool to which four to six allogeneic whole-blood donors have contributed, certainly helps to subsidize the cost of manufacturing all the various blood components needed by the entire population of a country or region, and thus helps to meet all of the supply needs of that population at a reasonable total cost for all transfused blood components and without incurring the risk of blood shortages. In this way, all of a country's patient needs for blood components are met at a total expenditure that the country's health-care system can afford. If no additional resources are made available by that country's health-care system for the provision of blood components, any change to the manner in which RBCs, FFP, and/or platelets are procured for multitransfused recipients in need of various blood components must be feasible without an increase in the total cost of components. Alternatively, if the change requires an increase in the total cost of components, the benefit derived from avoiding the exposure of multitransfused patients to as many allogeneic donors as the number of components that each patient receives should be deemed worth paying for by the patients, the clinicians, and also the policy makers who work within the fiscal constraints imposed by each country's health-care system.[6]

Every patient has the right to know the risks and benefits of any recommended treatment, as well as those of any possible alternative treatments.[7] Thus, when transfusion of platelet pools is not mandated by supply needs or by the economic constraints imposed by a particular country's health-care system, the choice between pooled WBD and apheresis (single-donor) platelets should be made by each individual patient in the context of informed consent. Patients appear to be poorly informed about transfusion choices, however, and clinicians and institutions are not *systematically* attempting to improve the information provided to prospective transfusion recipients. A study in Western Australia in 1998 found that 96% of patients would avoid ABT if possible, although only 4% were aware that alternatives to ABT were available; similar findings have been obtained from Europe[8] and North America.[9]

There is certainly discord between the public's perception of ABT as being an inherently "unsafe" intervention (a perception that calls for the avoidance of ABT whenever possible) and the transfusion medicine professionals' conviction that "blood is safer than ever" (on which the premise of the current transfusion paradigm rests). It is as much because of this conviction as because of the constraints imposed by supply needs and economic considerations that the current transfusion paradigm in the United States or countries with a similar health-care system continues to split each unit of whole blood into three components and then "reconstitute" whole blood by mixing RBCs, platelets, and FFP—thereby exposing each multitransfused ABT recipient to many more allogeneic donors than would be necessary if "patient blood management" (PBM) along with multicomponent apheresis (Table 8-1) were used to meet all of a multitransfused patient's transfusion needs. Although, as described in this chapter, patient blood management combined with multicomponent apheresis could certainly reduce both the infectious and noninfectious risks associated with each allogeneic-donor exposure, what remains to be determined is whether the reduction in risk that would result from the transition from a "component-centric" to a "patient-centric" transfusion medicine paradigm (Table 8-1) is sufficiently large to justify such a radical and disruptive move away from the existing component-centric infrastructure of a blood supply system that has become entrenched as the common sense of transfusion.

Expanding on the information presented in Chapters 2, 3, 4, and 7, this chapter presents three currently debated paradigm shifts in transfusion medicine and the overall contrast between a component-centric and a patient-centric approach to meeting patient transfusion needs (Table 8-1). The three paradigm shifts discussed here are PBM, multicomponent apheresis, and pathogen reduction (PR). PBM minimizes allogeneic-donor exposures and transfusion complications through the enforcement of restrictive transfusion thresholds, preoperative correction of anemia, and perioperative minimization of blood loss through various methods [including pharmacologic alternatives to transfusion, preoperative acute normovolemic hemodilution (ANH), and perioperative recovery of the patient's own blood]. Multicomponent apheresis collects RBCs along with platelets and/or plasma during the same donor apheresis procedure and may eventually minimize allogeneic-donor exposures (and the resulting transfusion complications) by reserving and transfusing to the same transfusion recipient all of the components collected during a single apheresis procedure. Although PBM and multicomponent apheresis share the same patient-centric approach to meeting patient transfusion needs (Table 8-1), they are discussed in this chapter as individual paradigm shifts because of the changes in infrastructure and philosophy that they impose, respectively, on the transfusion and

Table 8-1. Transfusion-Medicine Paradigms

Component-Centric	Patient-Centric
Blood component therapy:	Patient blood management:
• Each whole-blood donation is split into RBCs, platelets, and plasma to meet the transfusion needs of three different patients for combating anemia, thrombocytopenia, and coagulopathy, respectively	• Each patient's total transfusion needs are met through an individualized combination of approaches, including preoperative correction of anemia and methods to minimize blood loss, perioperative blood recovery, and transfusion of blood components collected from as few allogeneic donors as possible
• Each blood component is a drug that will equally benefit every recipient and has the same indications for every recipient with the same disease classification	• Each blood component is an allogeneic donor exposure (potentially associated with infectious and/or immunologic complications) to which each individual patient may need to be subjected to a larger (or—alternatively—smaller) extent compared with other patients with the same disease classification
• Stored RBCs and plasma units from different allogeneic donors (as well as platelets when appropriate) are used in acute blood loss	• According to some experts, fresh whole blood could (or even should) be used instead of a combination of stored blood components from different donors in acute blood loss
• Multitransfused patients needing RBCs, plasma, and/or platelets are transfused with blood components collected from different donors	• Multicomponent apheresis is used to collect any combination of RBCs, plasma, and/or platelets through one apheresis procedure; all components collected from the same donation are reserved for transfusion to the same multitransfused patient
Focus on the blood component:	Focus on the individual patient:
• Each blood component meets or exceeds specified standards for that component (ie, minimum hemoglobin content, proportion of RBCs surviving at 24 hours, minimum platelet content, or minimum content of coagulation factors)	• The combination of approaches used for patient blood management meets or exceeds therapeutic targets (set for each individual patient) with exposure to as few allogeneic donors as possible
• Centralized blood systems excel at a manufacturing culture that requires adherence to current good manufacturing practice regulations for the production of blood components from allogeneic whole blood	• Each patient's transfusion needs are met individually, in a clinical environment in which a medical culture is paramount
• Centralized decision making at the point of component manufacture aims at the production of components that meet uniform standards	• Decentralized decision making close to the patient permits each patient's transfusion needs to be met by an individualized combination of approaches

Table 8-1. Transfusion-Medicine Paradigms (Continued)

Component-Centric	Patient-Centric
Primacy of inventory: • The objective of a country's (or a region's) centralized blood supply system is to avoid blood shortages and to always meet *all* transfusion needs of *all* patients • The longest-stored compatible blood component available in inventory is routinely issued for transfusion to avoid outdates of units and any shortages of blood components that could result from such outdates	Primacy of individual needs: • An *individual* patient's transfusion needs for RBCs, platelets, and plasma are met in an *optimal* manner that is decided individually for each patient • According to some experts, fresh RBC units would be preferred to stored RBC units to improve clinical outcomes

collection sides of the current blood procurement system.

PR inactivates transfusion-transmitted pathogens to eliminate the most common transfusion-associated infection (TAS secondary to platelet transfusion; Chapter 2) and to protect the blood supply from the next major transfusion-transmitted pathogen to emerge in the future (Chapter 3). PR builds upon the existing component-centric infrastructure to minimize the infectious (and some noninfectious) risks of ABT so as to make each transfused component safer for the recipient. It is a component-centric approach that does not seek to reduce the number of allogeneic-donor exposures or in any way to implement the tenets of a patient-centric (Table 8-1) transfusion medicine paradigm. Instead, it improves the safety of the existing blood supply system and reinforces the established common sense of transfusion. If PR is not associated with any new risks, introducing PR (at a very considerable cost) would improve transfusion safety without changing the blood supply system's infrastructure and philosophy. All manufactured blood components would be produced according to uniform standards, but they would be safer than they are today. Each patient's transfusion needs would be met in the same manner as now, although the aggregate risk from the transfusion of RBCs, plasma, and platelets (for a multitransfused patient needing transfusion of all these various blood components) would be lower than it is today.

In contrast to PR, both PBM and multicomponent apheresis change the blood system's infrastructure and philosophy by concentrating on how to optimally meet the transfusion needs of each individual patient. Implementation of PBM and multicomponent apheresis (reserving for transfusion to the same recipient all of the components collected during a single apheresis procedure) may result in increased total costs for blood components, although the costs of a complete paradigm change have not yet been predicted, quantified, or compared to the cost of introducing PR. The three debated paradigm shifts thus appear to compete with one another and—worse yet—to involve competing commercial interests as the recipients of any additional monies that may be expended on meeting the US total needs for blood components. [Depending on what paradigm shift(s) prevail(s), the recipients of any such additional monies may include manufacturers of cell separators used for multicomponent apheresis and manufacturers of other technologies used in PBM approaches, manufacturers of PR systems for individual blood components, or both.] The debate on the appropriateness of the PBM paradigm shift[10-15] has hitherto concentrated on the setting of RBC transfusion. The arguments advanced for the setting of RBC transfusion are reviewed in this chapter, but briefly, because they have been presented extensively in the literature.[10-15] Multicomponent apheresis is discussed next, because an understanding of this fundamental concept is needed before PBM in platelet transfusion is covered. After looping back to PBM, this time in the setting of platelet transfusion, the final paradigm of pathogen reduction is explored in the context of platelet components. In fact, platelet transfusion is used to contrast the different philosophies underlying each paradigm shift and to illustrate how these shifts could, at least in the absence of cost considerations, complement one another for the benefit of patients.

Patient Blood Management in RBC Transfusion

PBM is a patient-specific, multidisciplinary, multimodal approach to optimizing the care of patients who might need ABT, including the appropriate conservation and management of a patient's own blood as a vital resource.[11-13] PBM is applied to both surgical and medical patients and aims at achieving better patient outcomes by identifying patients who are at risk of ABT and then formulating a management plan to reduce or eliminate the need for ABT. In the specific context of RBC transfusion, PBM strives to reduce the impact of three major contributors to a negative clinical outcome: anemia, blood loss, and ABT.[16-18] Thus, preoperative anemia is identified, evaluated, and treated before admission, as it represents (in the PBM context) an explicit contraindication to elective hospital admission. The expected iatrogenic, interventional, surgical, and disease-related blood loss is estimated for each individual patient, and the patient-specific postoperative hemoglobin is calculated by using algorithms.[19] The patient-specific physiologic reserve is also assessed and—if the expected postoperative hemoglobin indicates a need for ABT—three preventive countermeasures are taken, which are referred to as the "three pillars" of PBM.[13]

These three pillars are 1) optimizing the patient's endogenous red cell mass, 2) minimizing bleeding and blood loss, and 3) harnessing and optimizing the patient-specific physiologic tolerance of anemia through the adoption of restrictive transfusion thresholds and other means.[13] Through a combination of methods used preoperatively, intraoperatively, and postoperatively for each pillar, PBM preempts and significantly reduces the need to resort to ABT. PBM encourages physicians to transfuse blood components only when a documented medical need exists and when proven benefit of the receipt of ABT—established by clinical studies rather than postulated on the basis of any current understanding of pathophysiology—is expected for the individual patient. PBM also encourages physicians to avoid blood use altogether in selected surgical situations and for specific patients.[10,14,15]

PBM must be distinguished from the isolated adoption and use of evidence-based, restrictive transfusion guidelines for RBC, platelet, and plasma transfusion as discussed in Chapter 4. Such published guidelines aim at administering "appropriate" transfusions—that is, at defining transfusion indications for and thresholds at which transfusions cannot be withheld without causing harm to the recipient. The Transfusion Requirements in Critical Care (TRICC)[20] randomized controlled trial (RCT) and, more recently, the Transfusion Requirements After Cardiac Surgery (TRACS) RCT[21] showed that the clinical outcome in patients receiving RBC transfusion on the basis of a restrictive transfusion threshold was not inferior to that in subjects transfused on the basis of a liberal transfusion threshold. No data from RCTs are available for patients who received transfusion(s), on the basis of their own physicians' judgment, at a threshold between the restrictive and liberal thresholds used in these published RCTs[20,21] (see Fig 4-5 in Chapter 4). No data are available from subjects randomly assigned not to receive RBC transfusion for a hemoglobin level falling below the thresholds used in these studies.[20,21] Yet a threshold of 7 g/dL is now generally accepted as appropriate for normovolemic, hemodynamically stable patients admitted to the intensive care unit (ICU).[22,23]

PBM incorporates the adoption and enforcement of such evidence-based, restrictive transfusion guidelines for all blood components as one of its necessary components, but it is not limited to the enforcement of such guidelines. Stated another way, the adoption of evidence-based, restrictive transfusion guidelines does not equate to the implementation of a PBM program. PBM is much broader (and requires much more labor and commitment from many different hospital departments) than is the adoption of restrictive transfusion guidelines alone.

Table 8-2 summarizes the components of a hospital blood management program; detailed guidelines for surgeons and anesthesiologists are available in the literature.[24] For example, the 2011 update to the blood-conservation clinical practice guidelines of the Society of Thoracic Surgeons and the Society of Cardiovascular Anesthesiologists[24] made revisions to the previous guidelines in eight main areas:

1. Management of antiplatelet therapy given to patients before a surgical procedure.
2. Use of drugs that augment red cell volume or limit blood loss.
3. Use of blood derivatives including Factor XIII, recombinant Factor VIII, antithrombin, and Factor IX concentrates, in addition to use of FFP, apheresis (single-donor) platelets, and white blood cell (WBC)-reduced RBCs.
4. Changes to the management of blood recovery.
5. Use of minimally invasive procedures to limit perioperative bleeding and ABT.
6. Recommendations for blood conservation related to extracorporeal membrane oxygenation and cardiopulmonary perfusion.

Table 8-2. Summary of the Elements of a Patient Blood Management Hospital Program

- Having the hospital's Transfusion Committee or another entity assess all the methods for meeting patient transfusion needs and determine what methods or combination of methods will be offered at the hospital so that admitted patients have sufficient access to alternatives to allogeneic blood transfusion (ABT).
- Having the hospital's medical staff adopt and enforce restrictive transfusion thresholds for the administration of all blood components (Chapter 4).
- Using pharmacologic alternatives to correct anemia* and coagulopathy before admission (if admission is elective).
- Scheduling preoperative autologous blood donations (in selected cases or when this is the patient's own choice) optimally around the anticipated surgery date to permit collection of an appropriate number of units as well as allow the patient time to recover.
- Minimizing blood losses through laboratory sampling during the entire hospitalization.
- Providing the patient with current, accurate, understandable, and complete information on why ABT is necessary, what is the proven benefit from ABT, what are the risks of receiving (or refusing) ABT, and what alternatives to ABT are available; obtaining informed consent for ABT after such a discussion of all the available options/alternatives.
- Using drugs (eg, antifibrinolytics) to minimize perioperative blood loss; optimal and blood-sparing surgical techniques; anesthetic blood conservation strategies; meticulous surgical hemostasis; and vigilant monitoring for prevention and management of postoperative bleeding.
- Optimizing the patient's intraoperative cardiac output, ventilation, and oxygenation.
- Using perioperative blood recovery and acute normovolemic hemodilution where indicated.

*Through the use of such drugs as folate, iron, and erythropoiesis-stimulating agents (ESAs).

7. Use of topical hemostatic agents to augment good surgical technique.
8. Insights into the value of team interventions in PBM.

Although the specific management recommendations presented in such updated guidelines[24] (eg, the revisions made in the main areas 1 through 7 mentioned above) are beyond the scope of this chapter, a listing of the eight main areas in which revisions were made is provided here to highlight the multidisciplinary and multimodal character of PBM. An important premise of PBM is that a multidisciplinary team made up of a broad base of stakeholders ensures better utilization of blood resources than does a single decision maker who makes transfusion decisions about ABT and blood conservation in bleeding patients. Many decisions about transfusion are not made by surgeons. Recognizing the multitude of practitioners who participate in the transfusion decisions is an important step in managing valuable blood resources. Moreover, massive bleeding is life-threatening and should prompt the involvement of expert team members to improve outcomes.[24]

Proponents of PBM have identified five drivers shifting the paradigm from component-centric transfusion practice to PBM.[13] These drivers are 1) the continuous effort to protect the allogeneic blood supply from known, new, or re-emerging pathogens, while facing uncertainty about their potentially long silent-carrier states; 2) a lack of evidence of ABT's benefit for many transfusion recipients[25,26]; 3) the aging population that generates an increasing demand for blood products[27] while the donor base is shrinking[28]; 4) the growing awareness that transfusion is a complex service involving many different cost centers within a hospital and representing a multiple of the cost of the administered blood component per se[29,30]; and 5) the emerging evidence that ABT is an independent risk factor for adverse outcomes.[31-34]

Of these five drivers,[13] the first and second have been discussed in Chapters 3 and 4, respectively. The third and fourth drivers (that is, concern over the future adequacy of the blood supply[28] and the debate over whether PBM can result in lower total transfusion costs than does ABT, beyond the reduction in costs achieved by simply enforcing restrictive transfusion thresholds for allogeneic blood-component transfusion), are beyond the scope of this book. The focus of this chapter is on the difference in philosophy between the two paradigms: the component-centric paradigm (that aims to meet all of the transfusion needs of the entire population of a country or region and that is supported by a supply shortfall of up to 47% that is expected over the next 20 years in such countries as Germany[28]) and the patient-centric paradigm (that aims to meet individual patient needs in a manner that is most beneficial for the particular patient). The fifth driver (ie, the thesis that ABT is an independent risk factor for adverse outcomes,[35] whereas PBM can prevent the purported deleterious immunomodulatory effects of ABT[36] and/or the purported adverse effects of old RBCs; Chapter 7) is considered in detail in Chapter 2 of the electronic supplement, has been discussed in Chapter 1, and also is briefly commented upon here.

Regardless of whether the purported benefits of PBM as compared with those of ABT (with regard to the prevention of the deleterious immunomodulatory ABT effects[36] and the common adverse effects of old blood on morbidity and mortality) are established (or not) by future research, the minimization (or elimination) of exposures to allogeneic donors indisputably reduces both the infectious and immunologic risks of ABT, as discussed in Chapters 2 and 4. Thus, the potential for implementing PBM raises important ethical questions.[7] 1) What is the obligation of a hospital (or the hospital's medical staff) to offer the hospital's patients access to PBM methods, including perhaps bloodless surgery for selected patients (such as Jehovah's Witnesses)? 2) Are physicians permitted to provide only one type of blood service (ABT or a combination of PBM methods or one or another PBM method), despite the patient's stated wishes or even contrary to hospital policy? 3) Can physicians' blood-ordering practices be permitted to vary widely for the same diagnosis within the same institution?

Sazama[7] discussed the ethics of blood management, based on the four fundamental principles of biomedical ethics[37]: autonomy,[38,39] beneficence, nonmaleficence (ie, doing no harm), and justice (Table 8-3). In summary, a hospital should offer its patients access to PBM methods when such methods become feasible; a patient should be presented with all the options and alternatives available to him or her with regard to ABT; and physicians' blood-ordering

Table 8-3. Application of Ethical Principles to Allogeneic Blood Transfusion (ABT) and Patient Blood Management (PBM)

Autonomy: A competent adult has the right to determine what will (or will not) be done with his or her own person, including the right to make decisions based on his or her values, which may differ from societal norms

- The patient's right to choose or refuse any proposed medical treatment is based on a truthful and complete discussion of all material factors by the care team
- This care team veracity and the patient's right-to-know all information pertinent to exercising his or her choice are fundamental to the informed consent process
- The care team provides patients at risk for ABT with answers to the following questions: Why is ABT necessary? What is the proven benefit from ABT? What are the risks of receiving (or refusing) the ABT? What alternatives to ABT are available?

Beneficence: A physician must *do no* harm ("*primum non nocere*"); he or she can do or promote only good things for his or her patients

- When discussing ABT/PBM options and alternatives, a patient should expect that all recommendations offered by his or her physician are permissibly based on beneficence
- A patient without a documented medical indication for ABT should never be transfused
- When a documented medical indication for ABT is present, only the needed blood component (RBCs, platelets, *or* plasma) should be transfused
- Both the number of samples obtained for laboratory testing and the volume of blood per draw should be carefully monitored and minimized to prevent iatrogenic anemia

Nonmaleficence: A physician must *avoid* doing harm by taking no unnecessary risks with patients; that is, by taking no actions for which the benefits may be minimal or that can cause serious injury in the short term while the long-term effects are simply not known

- A physician should avoid the risks of "unnecessary" ABT (and avoid ordering practices that—for the same disease classification—vary widely from those of his or her peers within the same institution)
- A physician should avoid any risks possibly or potentially introduced by some PBM practices (eg, administration of erythropoiesis-stimulating agents) whose benefit-to-risk ratio compared to ABT has not been established in an evidence-based manner

Justice: All people should be treated justly, fairly, and equally for the same health condition; medical decisions are made based on diagnosis, prognosis, and available treatments, and not on some other impermissible basis such as age, ethnicity, skin color, race, or sexual orientation

- A hospital should offer its patients access to PBM methods (or at least those PBM methods considered by its medical staff to have an adequately established benefit-to-risk ratio compared to ABT)
- All patients with a given diagnosis and prognosis are given equal access to the PBM methods offered at a particular hospital

practices should not be permitted to vary widely for the same diagnosis within the same institution. Otherwise, the ethical principles of justice, autonomy, and beneficence and nonmaleficence, respectively, are violated. An approach to ABT and PBM based on the principles listed in Table 8-3 should prevent the legal, economic, and political harm (and public loss of confidence in blood services) that could result from the emergence of the next major transfusion-transmitted pathogen.

The feasibility and the capabilities of PBM programs have been amply demonstrated in the treatment of Jehovah's Witnesses, a religious denomination whose adherents now number more that 6 million worldwide. Many of the group's doctrines derive from literal interpretations of the Bible, several specific verses of which (Leviticus 17:19,12; Genesis 9:3-5; and Acts 15:29) prohibit the ingestion of blood. In response to the Jehovah's Witnesses' refusal of ABT, "bloodless surgery" programs implemented specifically to treat Jehovah's Witnesses were designed to be transfusion-free: ABT was strictly disallowed, despite actual risk of patient mortality. The risk of not giving transfusion(s) to Jehovah's Witnesses who are undergoing surgery is apparent from studies showing an inverse correlation between hemoglobin levels and mortality and reporting historical mortality as high as 33.3% in nontransfused Jehovah's Witnesses with a hemoglobin of <6 g/dL.[40] Nonetheless, between 1997 and 2005, the bloodless surgery program of the USC (University of Southern California) University Hospital performed >200 major surgical procedures on Jehovah's Witnesses, with a >99% success rate.[41-48] These impressive results[41-48] show the feasibility (Table 8-4) of performing major surgical procedures in a transfusion-free setting when a comprehensive PBM program is implemented.

Is it Time for a Paradigm Shift Toward PBM Rather than Allogeneic RBC Transfusion?

The combination of PBM approaches listed in Table 8-2 can minimize allogeneic-donor exposures or avoid ABT altogether. Complete avoidance of ABT has been achieved through these approaches in Jehovah's Witnesses, for whom bloodless surgery is necessary. For patients who

Table 8-4. Acute Normovolemic Hemodilution for Liver Resection in a *Transfusion-Free* Setting*†

	ANH (Non-ABT) Group	ABT Group
Number of patients	65	179
Proportion of patients receiving intraoperative ABT	0%	44%
Mean number of RBC units transfused (range)	0	3.3 (1-15)
Mean age (range)	47 (18-75)	55 (16-82)
Mean preoperative hematocrit (range)	37.5 (28.6-50)	39 (22-48.4)
Mean postoperative hematocrit (range)	31 (22.6-40.2)	31.3 (7.9-41.2)

*Based on data reported by Tokin et al.[48]
†ANH preserves the integrity of both RBCs and coagulation factors, thereby ensuring availability of a significant amount of fresh, autologous whole blood.
ANH = acute normovolemic hemodilution; ABT = allogeneic blood transfusion; RBC = Red Blood Cell.

do not refuse to receive ABT for religious or other reasons, the elimination of unnecessary transfusions and the minimization of allogeneic-donor exposures (through a combination of some of the PBM methods listed in Table 8-2) can reduce the risk of any ABT complication—whether infectious, noninfectious, or poorly understood (Chapter 2). If the patient is not exposed to infectious agents or antigens and antibodies found in the blood of an allogeneic donor(s), both infectious and immunologic transfusion complications (including some of the leading causes of ABT-related deaths: TRALI, mistransfusion owing to clerical error, and TAS) are prevented. Transfusion-associated circulatory overload (TACO) is also prevented by the attention afforded each individual patient for optimizing his or her cardiac output, ventilation, and oxygenation.

This reasoning makes the benefit of implementing PBM (as a concept or in principle) indisputable for the individual patient. Restrictive transfusion guidelines should be adopted by all hospital medical staffs to allow ABT only when the benefit resulting from ABT (in terms of ensuing oxygen consumption and function by tissues or—alternatively—in terms of hemorrhage prevention) is clinically proven by RCTs rather than presumed to exist according to the current understanding of pathophysiology. By reducing allogeneic-donor exposures, evidence-based, restrictive transfusion guidelines (Chapter 4) reduce all ABT risks without introducing any new risks. In addition to adopting such restrictive guidelines for the transfusion of all blood components, hospitals could make available to their patients access to some combination of the PBM approaches listed in Table 8-2. The choice of the approaches to offer would be based on an evaluation of the efficacy and safety of each listed component of PBM.

PBM—considered in principle or as a concept—thus benefits every transfusion recipient, but each individual component of PBM may (or may not) be beneficial for an individual patient, because of limited efficacy in reducing donor exposures in the setting of the procedure that the patient is scheduled to undergo or because of introduced risks. Thus, British guidelines no longer support preoperative autologous blood donation as an alternative to RBC transfusion.[49] Erythroid-stimulating agents (ESAs) and perioperative autologous blood recovery are widely used in many countries, but the extent to which these modalities prevent or reduce the use of ABT in settings where evidence-based, restrictive transfusion guidelines have already been implemented is disputed.[50] A meta-analysis of the earlier studies found that, although perioperative blood recovery produced a significant reduction in the likelihood of exposure to allogeneic RBCs, the mean reduction in the number of allogeneic-donor exposures achieved per patient was only 0.67 [95% confidence interval (CI), 0.45-0.89]. Moreover, the administration of ESAs creates new risks of deep vein thrombosis[51] and related adverse events, especially in patients with cancer[52] and renal[53] (albeit not heart[54]) disease.

To overcome such arguments concerning the limited efficacy of, or new risks associated with, individual components of PBM, advocates for PBM have usually emphasized the much greater benefit that would result from implementing all components of PBM (including components reported to introduce new risks, such as ESAs) if PBM prevented the increase in the common adverse outcomes of morbidity and mortality[35] that purportedly results from ABT and/or the transfusion of stored (rather than fresh) RBCs. In this context, advocates for PBM have argued that one should infer cause from passive observation (as is done in risk-factor epidemiology) and should accept that the associations reported from observational studies between ABT (and/or transfusion of old rather than fresh RBCs) and common adverse morbidity or mortality outcomes represent causal relationships.[35] Their proposal for a causal pathway linking ABT and the transfusion of old (rather than fresh) RBCs to increased mortality and morbidity[35] is that ABT is one of multiple contributing factors leading to an adverse outcome for the occurrence of which there are no necessary and/or sufficient conditions, but only a complex multifactorial etiology. On the basis of this rationale, Isbister et al[35] argued that a change in the transfusion medicine paradigm from component-centric to patient-centric (Table 8-1) is urgently needed, and, therefore, the implementation of this change should not wait for the publication of the results of RCTs that aim to establish causal relationships between ABT (or the transfusion of old rather than fresh RBCs) and the common adverse outcomes of major morbidity and mortality.

Isbister et al[35] highlighted the fact that observational studies have associated ABT with a greater risk of mortality [as well as with major morbidity that includes postoperative infection, acute respiratory distress syndrome (ARDS), and multiorgan failure and that results in the prolongation of ICU and hospital stays]. Probably, however, as discussed in detail in Chapter 2 of the electronic supplement, such a nonspecific association of ABT with virtually any adverse outcome(s) studied indicates that ABT is an excellent surrogate factor for illness severity. In the absence of randomization—as is the case in the observational studies on which Isbister et al[35] and other proponents of PBM have relied—selection bias in the allocation of subjects to treatment and control arms is unavoidable; any adjustment for differences in the levels of confounding factors occurring in patients who did or did not receive a new therapy is incomplete. Observational studies use statistical techniques to adjust for such baseline differences, and they control only for the effects of known and measurable confounders. The effects of unknown and/or poorly quantified confounding factors cannot be controlled statistically, and these variables always compromise, to some extent, the findings of observational studies. The need for a transfusion often reflects severity of illness—a factor that cannot be adequately quantified and controlled by statistical techniques. Either the need for transfusion (ie, a more-severe illness) or the receipt of transfusion can then be responsible for the various adverse outcomes seen in association with ABT in the observational studies hitherto quoted by PBM proponents.

Isbister et al[35] correctly pointed out, however, that neither the safety nor the efficacy of blood components is as established as it is assumed to be; each quality-adjusted life-year saved through the implementation of further measures for improving the safety of the blood components manufactured by our current component-centric paradigm costs far more than it does in any other sector of health care. Moreover, patients do not want to be exposed to ABT, and many of them do—or can do—just as well without it. Yet, inappropriate transfusion practices (contrary to guidelines) persist,[55] and there remains wide variation in transfusion practices across countries, hospitals, and individual clinicians.[56] The First Austrian Benchmark Study of elective orthopedic and coronary artery bypass graft (CABG) surgery[56] showed that the level of anemia before surgery, the volume of perioperative blood loss, and the employed transfusion thresholds predicted 97.4% of all RBC transfusions; the number of RBC units transfused to anemic patients in this study was fourfold the number given to nonanemic patients. In a follow-up study, after different hospitals adopted various levels of individual components of PBM (Table 8-2), many participating hospitals had significant reductions in the number of administered RBC transfusions (by as much as >50%).[57] In addition, other observational studies have reported on the success of PBM approaches in reducing the use of RBC transfusions and on an apparent improvement in patient clinical outcomes associated with the reduction in RBC transfusions.[58-61]

Yet, PBM approaches for avoiding or minimizing the use of ABT have not been widely adopted by either clinicians or blood bankers, who continue to use ABT as the "default" or "safe" option.[35] Although more research is needed into the safety and efficacy of various transfusion alternatives, such as ESAs, these alternatives (together with ABT) should be considered for future studies to be conducted on a "level playing field": that is, equal and due consideration should be given to the benefits and risks associated with each of these options that are open to a patient.[35]

Use of Fresh (as Opposed to Old) RBCs

All of the aforementioned arguments[35] underscore the benefits of moving toward a patient-centric transfusion medicine paradigm in the context of RBC transfusion. In this author's opinion, however, such a move is justified without engaging in a debate over whether to consider as established the purported association between the transfusion of old (rather than fresh) RBCs and an increase in the common adverse outcomes of morbidity and mortality.[62]

As discussed in Chapter 7, the alternative possibility that adverse effects of ABT may be associated with transfusion of fresh (rather than old) RBCs cannot be ruled out on the basis of preliminary findings from RCTs (see Table 7-2 and Fig 7-1 in Chapter 7), whereas the associations between the transfusion of old RBCs and common adverse outcomes reported by some of the published observational studies can be attributed to flaws in the design of those studies.[63] As shown in Fig 7-2 of Chapter 7, the reason that one cannot rely on the results of the observational studies that have reported an association between the age of the oldest unit and common adverse outcomes is that the age of the oldest unit is bound to be associated with adverse outcomes, because it is associated with the number of transfused RBCs. Each time a request for transfusion is received, as dictated by the tenets of the current component-based paradigm whose purpose is to preserve inventory for preventing blood shortages (Table 8-1), the blood bank issues for transfusion the oldest compatible unit in inventory. Thus, the more often a patient receives a transfusion, the more likely he or she is to receive blood at a time when the oldest compatible RBC unit available in the inventory is "old." At the same time, as discussed in detail in Chapter 2 of the electronic supplement, such need for more blood is always associated with adverse outcomes, because the sicker a patient is, the more blood he or she needs. Hardly any of the observational studies that reported an association between transfusion of old (rather than fresh) RBCs and common adverse outcomes had adjusted the reported association for the number of transfused RBCs (Chapter 7).

The substitution of fresh RBCs for old RBCs is therefore not appropriate unless it is supported in the future by the results of the RCTs that are currently under way. It is possible that these RCTs will not show a difference in the frequency of common adverse outcomes between recipients of old RBCs and recipients of fresh RBCs, or even that any recorded difference may be the opposite of the one expected by PBM advocates. Thus, if—rather than undertaking the ongoing RCTs (Chapter 7)—we had invoked the precautionary principle (Chapter 1) to reduce the allowed storage period of RBCs to <2 or 3 weeks on the basis of the findings of the available observational studies, we might be implementing a "safety" measure that could have deleterious effects on transfusion recipients, despite our good intentions.[62] Nonetheless, even if no greater benefit from fresh (as compared with old) RBCs is shown by the ongoing RCTs, moving toward a patient-centric transfusion medicine paradigm (Table 8-1) through the implementation of many other components of PBM (Table 8-2) would still be appropriate for the purpose of reducing ABT-related deaths from TRALI, other noninfectious causes, and emerging transfusion-transmitted infections (TTIs).[62]

Use of Fresh Whole Blood in Acute Blood Loss

The use of fresh whole blood or, alternatively, RBCs and FFP collected in the course of the same multicomponent donor apheresis procedure, instead of "whole blood" reconstituted from the RBC and FFP units collected from two different allogeneic donors, is another proposed element of the patient-centric paradigm (Table 8-1) that remains to be established by future research. In the era of blood component therapy, according to the ethical premise that a transfusion recipient should receive only the blood component that he or she needs (Table 8-3), and according to the doctrine of "less is more,"[64] FFP and RBCs have usually been administered in the setting of acute blood loss (eg, when trauma victims are resuscitated), by using an FFP-to-RBCs ratio of 1:3-4. During the recent wars in Iraq and Afghanistan, however, fresh whole blood was once more used to resuscitate military casualties. The use of FFP and RBCs at a 1:1 ratio (or even FFP, platelets, and RBCs at a 1:1:1 ratio) for the purpose of reconstituting whole blood was reported to be associated with lower mortality of such military casualties; that report led to a debate about whether a 1:1 (or even 1:1:1) ratio should be used in the trauma resuscitation protocols used in civilian settings. If an increased (1:1 rather than 1:3-4) plasma-to-RBCs ratio in the setting of trauma were indeed associated with lower mortality and morbidity of the trauma victims, the continued use of RBCs and FFP collected from two different allogeneic donors for such recipients (in lieu of fresh whole blood collected from one whole-blood donor or of stored RBCs and FFP collected from one donor in the course of the same multicomponent apheresis procedure) would defy ordinary common sense.

Evidence supporting a 1:1 ratio has, however, not yet been produced by RCTs. Figure 4-9 in Chapter 4 shows lower mortality after massive transfusion to trauma patients when a higher (closer to 1:1) rather than lower (closer to 1:4) plasma-to-RBCs ratio is used for the administered blood components. The unadjusted odds ratio (OR) of mortality is shown for each of the eight studies in the upper section of the figure,[65-72] but for the two studies in the lower section (Snyder et al[73] and Scalea et al[74]), the figure shows an adjusted OR calculated from a multivariate analysis. As presented in the figure, individual studies show a continuum from a 95% reduction ($p<0.05$) to a 50% increase ($p>0.05$) in mortality when a higher (compared with a lower) plasma-to-RBCs ratio is used.

The studies differed with respect to the clinical setting (military[68] or civilian), the specific plasma-to-RBCs ratio (or ratios) investigated, whether the studies considered only plasma ratio(s) or both plasma and platelet ratios, the time at which they recorded mortality (ie, 24 hours, in-hospital, 30-day, or other), and the patient population that they studied (ie, type of trauma, presence and severity of coagulopathy, and presence of physiologic aberrations or comorbidities). Of the studies that reported statistically significant ($p<0.05$) results—and for which the unadjusted OR is depicted in the figure—several[65-72] also reported multivariate analyses based on variously built statistical models. In all of those studies, the findings of the multivariate analyses supported the result of the univariate comparison, which indicated a benefit just as pronounced as (if not more pronounced than) that from early aggressive administration of plasma. Accordingly, the results of the unadjusted comparisons are depicted in the figure for these studies[65-72] as more comparable to one another, because the results shown in Fig 4-9 of Chapter 4 are intended solely for the purpose of illustration. In contrast, to be consistent with the conclusions of Snyder et al[73] and Scalea et al,[74] adjusted ORs are depicted for their studies.

Most studies reported several (both adjusted and unadjusted) ORs. According to the discussions accompanying the papers in the *Journal of Trauma, Injury, Infection, and Critical Care,* even more ORs (not reported) were often calculated by the authors, to examine the effects of additional plasma-to-RBCs ratios, times of recording mortality, and so on. The ORs shown in Fig 4-9 in Chapter 4 pertain to the subgroup analyses of the massively transfused patients (ie, the recipients of ≥10 RBCs over 24 hours) in the event that both massively transfused and non-massively transfused patients had been included in a study. When more than two comparison groups were employed (to investigate a continuum of more than two plasma-to-RBCs ratios), the results depicted in Fig 4-9 of Chapter 4 reflect the analysis most closely approximating a comparison of a high to low plasma-to-RBC ratios (ie, a ratio close to 1:1 rather than close to 1:4). For example, for the study of Dente et al,[66] a ratio of between 1:1 and 1:2 is compared with a ratio of >1:3, which excludes the patients who received plasma and RBCs at a ratio of between 1:2 and 1:3. In contrast, for the study of Maegele et al,[72] the patients whose transfusions had a ratio of >1.1 are compared to patients whose transfusions had ratios of approximately 1:1, as well as to subjects treated with even more aggressive administration of plasma.

Snyder et al[73] reported an analysis considering a fixed effect of the plasma-to-RBCs ratio on mortality [relative risk (RR) = 0.37; 95% CI, 0.22-0.64; $p<0.05$—an approximation of the unadjusted OR reported by the eight studies[65-72] in the upper section of the figure], only to contrast it with the adjusted OR calculated from their analysis and shown in Fig 4-9 of Chapter

4. The latter approach incorporated a time-varying covariate in an effort to adjust for the effect of survivor bias. Scalea et al[74] refrained altogether from presenting unadjusted ORs. The conclusion of Snyder et al[73] was, "[T]he nonsurvivors in our study population did not die because they got [FFP and RBCs at] a lower … ratio; they got [FFP and RBCs at] a lower ratio because they died." Trauma patients who survive long enough will receive additional plasma therapy; however, trauma patients who do not survive are assigned to lower plasma-to-RBC ratio groups in observational studies[65-74] and analyzed as treatment failures. Such an approach incorporates the effect of survivor bias into the results of the analysis, which generates a spurious survival benefit from the receipt of FFP and RBCs at higher plasma-to-RBCs ratios.[75]

Military casualties often have multiple penetrating wounds and massive orthopedic blast injuries—a situation not readily transferable to the civilian setting.[75] The "triage" that often occurs with military casualties does not occur as frequently with civilian trauma victims. In the treatment of the military casualties,[68] furthermore, there was an intermingling of fresh whole blood along with the use of recombinant Factor VIIa.[75] In addition, during the 2003-2005 period of the war in Iraq, a number of logistical changes occurred in the military trauma system, and changes also occurred in the medical management of these trauma patients. Finally, as Hannon said, "[T]rauma patients are a tremendously heterogeneous group (as opposed to, say, hip replacement patients), making comparisons across patient groups challenging at best."[75]

For all these reasons, caution is warranted in extrapolating from the management of military casualties to the civilian trauma setting. Kashuk et al[69] demonstrated a U-shaped curve, with an initial decline in mortality as the plasma-to-RBCs ratio increased toward 1:3; as the ratio climbed further toward 1:1, however, mortality increased. It is possible that any beneficial effect from the early administration of plasma has already peaked when a ratio of 1:3 is reached.[69] After this point, the deleterious effects of plasma transfusion (eg, TRALI and perhaps also multiple-organ failure) may predominate. If that were the case,[69] the early administration of plasma would have a very narrow therapeutic window, which would make the determination of a precise plasma-to-RBCs ratio that optimizes survival in trauma victims critically important.[75]

Demonstration of a benefit from a higher (compared with a lower) plasma-to-RBCs ratio—to justify the use of fresh whole blood as listed by some experts as an element of the patient-centric transfusion-medicine paradigm (Table 8-1)—is not necessary to the adoption of the overall philosophy and many other elements of the patient-centric paradigm. As in the case of fresh compared with old RBCs, in which a transition to the patient-centric paradigm would be beneficial for patients even if old (rather than fresh) RBCs were not shown to cause any increase in common adverse mortality and morbidity outcomes, the benefit from the reduction in allogeneic-donor exposures conferred by the patient-centric paradigm would remain even if a role for fresh whole blood (intended to replace the "whole blood" currently reconstituted from RBCs and FFP collected from two different donors) were not documented by future research. Every proposed element of the patient-centric paradigm (Table 8-1) must be individually evaluated and shown to benefit patients as compared with ABT. Although it is understandable that, as O'Keeffe et al[76] said, "[H]eroic new measures are aggressively sought after" when mortality rates in massively transfused trauma patients range from one-third to one-half of all victims, it is important that such new measures not be too easily embraced without proof of their benefits according to the tenets of evidence-based medicine.

Hospitals need to use the best available evidence to develop patient-centric massive-transfusion protocols and also to continually evaluate the effectiveness and appropriateness of these protocols. Independent of the plasma-to-RBCs ratio used, development of a protocol per se may convey some benefit by increasing communication among team members and by allowing quicker access to blood products.[77] Point-of-care testing of coagulation should be employed to change the treatment approach with regard to the administration of blood components in acute blood loss from empirical to goal-directed therapy at the earliest possible time.[78-81] A most promising development has been the reporting of a recent RCT[82] that showed the safe and effective use of the antifibrinolytic drug tranexamic acid in trauma patients to reduce transfusion requirements and to improve survival.

Multicomponent Apheresis

Multicomponent apheresis can collect any combination of RBCs, platelets, and/or plasma from a single donor during the same donation, and—combined with logistical and information systems improvements on both the blood center and hospital sides—it could eventually ensure that all components collected during the same apheresis donation are transfused to the same recipient.[83,84] Common protocols used in multicomponent apheresis permit the collection of 1) two (or three) units of single-donor platelets; 2) one unit of single-donor platelets and two units (or one double unit) of FFP; 3) three units (or one triple unit) of FFP; 4) one RBC unit and two FFP units; and 5) two RBC units. If a multitransfused patient (eg, a patient with acute blood loss) requires transfusion of both RBCs and FFP (and sometimes transfusion of platelets as well), the reduction in the number of allogeneic donor exposures that multicomponent apheresis allows is apparent.

In addition, multicomponent apheresis renders obsolete the debate presented in the previous section, as to whether blood services should revert to producing and distributing fresh whole blood, as opposed to reconstituting whole blood from RBCs and FFP collected from two different allogeneic donors. If the debated reasons for providing fresh whole blood in acute blood loss are vindicated by future research, multicomponent apheresis could do even better than could the provision of a unit of fresh whole blood, because the former can provide, for example, one RBC unit and two FFP units collected from the same donor for even more aggressive plasma resuscitation when needed. Overall, allogeneic donor exposures for multitransfused patients could be reduced by ≥50% when multicomponent apheresis is used, which will result in a ≥50% decrease in the risk of both TRALI[83] and all TTIs.

The technology to collect two or more doses of platelets in the course of the same plateletpheresis donation has been available since the early 1990s.[84] The definition of the minimum platelet dose as 3.0×10^{11} per transfused component was based on the capability of the technology more than on the data showing the minimum effective dose for patients needing platelet transfusion. As apheresis technology improved greatly over the years, in terms of both donor safety and efficiency of collection, blood services started subdividing ("splitting") plateletpheresis collections into two or three platelet components, and they routinely aimed to collect a "double" platelet unit in the course of the same donor apheresis procedure, so as to meet the platelet transfusion needs of two different patients. This practice was driven primarily by health-care economics—to such an extent that the potential it afforded for greater transfusion safety (if all collected platelet doses were reserved for a transfusion recipient who needed multiple, and closely spaced, platelet transfusions for maintaining a platelet count of ≥10,000/µL) went unmentioned for years.

The technology to collect two RBC units in the course of the same apheresis donation has been available since 1997.[84] The absolute red cell volume drawn during one collection is based on a Food and Drug Administration (FDA)-approved nomogram that takes into account the donor's gender, hematocrit, weight, and height. Compared with whole-blood donors, donors who qualify for double RBC collection are more often male than female, whereas male donors (especially first-time male donors) more often have prevalent human immunodeficiency virus (HIV), hepatitis C virus (HCV), or hepatitis B virus (HBV) infection than do female donors (Fig 8-1). Thus, some concern about the use of double-RBC apheresis collections was generated when an unexpectedly greater prevalence of known TTIs was observed in the early 21st century (as compared with the prevalance in previous years) among all apheresis donations.[85]

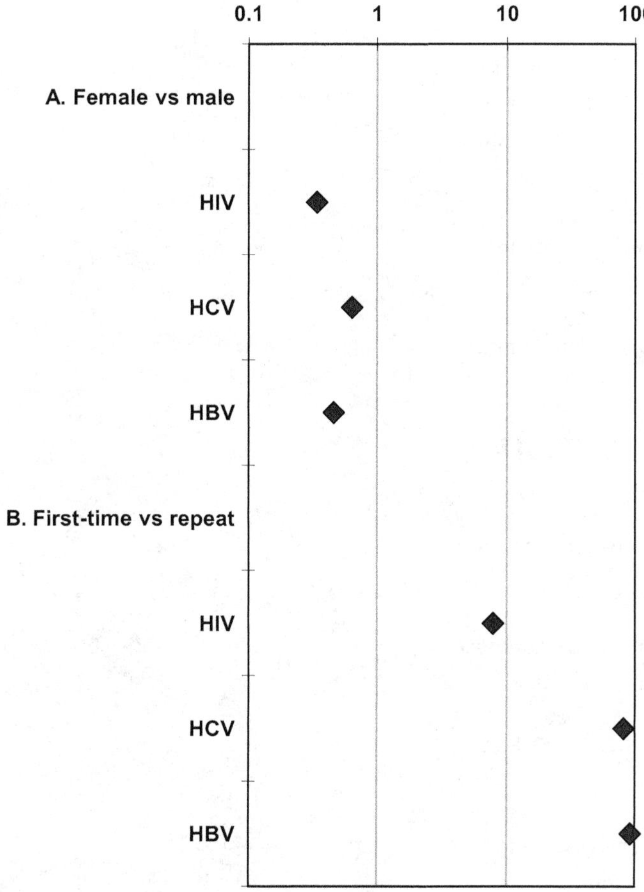

Figure 8-1. Risk factors for increased prevalence of known transfusion-transmitted infections (TTIs) in blood donors: male (vs female) gender and first-time (vs repeat) donor status. The figure shows the odds ratio (OR) of human immunodeficiency virus (HIV), hepatitis C virus (HCV), and hepatitis B virus (HBV) infection in female vs male donors and first-time vs repeat donors in all (whole-blood as well as apheresis) donations made to the American Red Cross between 2004 and 2008.[85] ORs [and 95% confidence intervals (CIs) surrounding the ORs] as reported by Zou et al[85] are shown; owing to the large sample size, the 95% CIs are narrow. Female donors had a lower ($p<0.05$) prevalence of HIV, HCV, and HBV infection than did male donors, and first-time donors had a higher ($p<0.05$) prevalence of HIV, HCV, and HBV infection than did repeat donors; for all comparisons shown in the figure, the 95% CI of the depicted OR does not include the null value of 1. The prevalence of HIV infection was almost 10 times as high in first-time donors than in repeat donors; the prevalence of HCV and HBV infection was almost 100 times as high in first-time donors than in repeat donors. The prevalence of HIV, HCV, and HBV infection was lower in female donors than in male donors by approximately two-thirds, one-third, and one-half, respectively.

This unexpected upward trend was investigated,[85] showing that the prevalence of HCV and HBV infection in double-RBC apheresis collections was significantly ($p<0.05$) lower than that in whole-blood collections, whereas the prevalence of HIV infection did not differ between double-RBC apheresis and whole-blood collections (Fig 8-2). As had long been the case, the prevalence of TTIs in non-double-RBC (predominantly plateletpheresis) collections was sig-

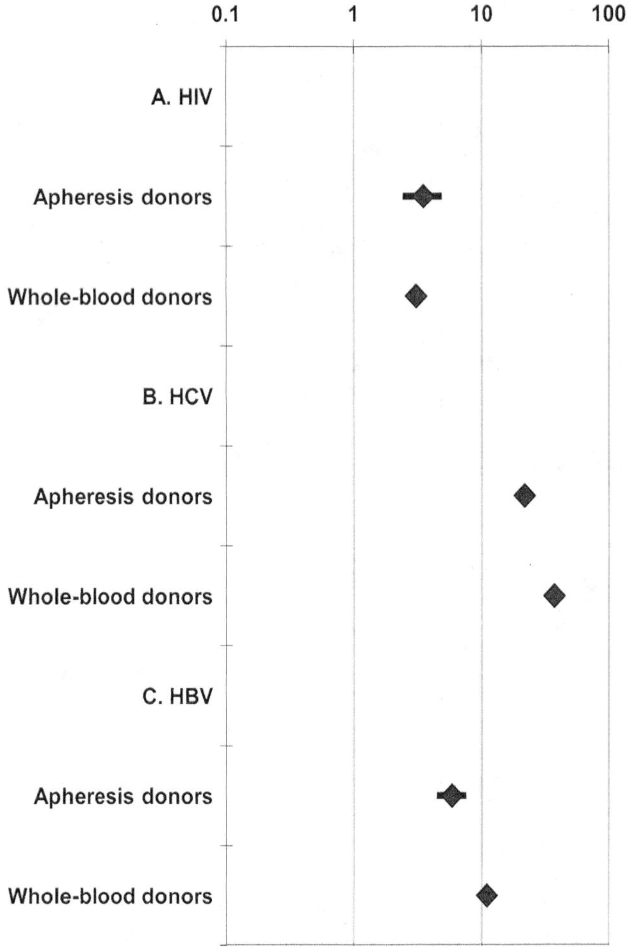

Figure 8-2. Prevalence of transfusion-transmitted infections (TTIs) in double-RBC apheresis and whole-blood donations made to the American Red Cross between 2004 and 2008.[85] For human immunodeficiency virus (HIV), hepatitis C virus (HCV), and hepatitis B virus (HBV), the prevalence of infection per 100,000 collections is given, surrounded by its 95% CI. The prevalence of HBV infection is based on the results of hepatitis B surface antigen testing. Compared with whole-blood donors, double-RBC apheresis donors had a significantly ($p<0.05$) lower prevalence of HCV and HBV infection (OR = 0.81; 95% CI, 0.71-0.93; and OR = 0.59; 95% CI, 0.45-0.77, respectively). However, in the case of HIV infection, the 95% CIs for double-RBC apheresis and whole-blood donors overlapped, which indicated no difference between the prevalence of infection in these two donor categories. Multivariate Poisson regression analysis with adjustment for the effects of donor gender, age, and first-time (rather than repeat) status corroborated the fact that double-RBC apheresis donors indeed had a lower prevalence of HCV and HBV infection than did whole-blood donors. Although double-RBC donors had a prevalence of TTIs lower than (or equal to) that calculated for whole-blood donors, the prevalence of HCV, HBV, and HIV infections was significantly ($p<0.05$) higher in double-RBC apheresis donors (above) than in non-double-RBC apheresis (predominantly plateletpheresis) donors (Fig 8-3). Depending on the year, first-time male double-RBC apheresis donors accounted for 25% to 100% of all recorded prevalent infections among apheresis donors, despite the fact that donations from first-time male donors represented only 1% to 5% of the total apheresis collections between 2004 and 2008.

nificantly ($p<0.05$) lower than that in whole-blood collections[85] (Fig 8-3). When the TTI marker results for double-RBC and non-double-RBC apheresis collections were combined, apheresis collections had a significantly ($p<0.05$) lower prevalence of HIV, HCV, and HBV infection than did whole-blood collections (Fig 8-4).

Despite these differences in the prevalence of known TTIs between double-RBC apheresis, non-double-RBC apheresis, and whole-blood collections, no difference was observed between these three donor categories in the incidence of newly acquired TTIs that could represent a potential risk of transmission to transfusion recipients[85] (Table 8-5). Thus, based on the evidence hitherto presented, the per-donor residual risk of transmission of HIV, HCV, and HBV infection is the same for all three donor categories; in calculations of the risk of transmission of TTIs, each allogeneic-donor exposure—regardless of whether it originates in a whole-blood, non-double-RBC apheresis, or double-RBC apheresis collection—should be counted as representing one unit of risk, as has been done in this book (eg, see Table 2-1 and Fig 2-17 in Chapter 2).

Reduction in ABT Risks Thanks to Multicomponent Apheresis

The principal argument for replacing the whole-blood-collection infrastructure of the 20th century with a new, multicomponent-apheresis-collection infrastructure in the 21st century is the improvement in patient safety that multicomponent apheresis can afford. The argument for adopting multicomponent apheresis collections to reduce the risk of TRALI is especially instructive.

Van Stein et al reported the best available passive-surveillance study of TRALI for the period of January 1, 2005, to July 1, 2007 (ie, the 30-month period before the introduction of male-only FFP in The Netherlands).[86] TRALI usually occurs in multitransfused patients who receive various combinations of different blood components (ie, RBCs, FFP, and/or platelets—5.3 units on average in the study of van Stein et al[86]). Contrary to what was done in most other TRALI hemovigilance studies, van Stein et al[86] performed a TRALI work-up on all implicated blood components: 129 RBC, 66 platelet (in platelet pools), and 64 FFP units. [That is, unlike what has usually been reported in the literature, these investigators[86] (Fig 2-7 in Chapter 2) did not selectively work up the "plasma-rich" components (FFP and single-donor platelets) or the components donated by female donors.] In addition to including all implicated components, van Stein et al[86] tested for actual WBC incompatibility between donor and recipient, not merely for the presence of WBC antibodies in the donor. Of 49 patients with a TRALI diagnosis based on the Canadian consensus criteria,[86] 36 (73.5%) were associated with an implicated donor who had WBC antibodies and, in 21 (43%), actual serologic WBC incompatibility existed between the recipient and at least one donor. The latter 21 cases were designated as "alloimmune" TRALI and were associated with 31 donors producing serologic WBC incompatibility with the recipient: 14 (45%) FFP, 14 (45%) RBC, and 3 (10%) platelet donors.

More important, perhaps, of 10 recorded TRALI deaths over these 2.5 years in The Netherlands,[86] two could have been prevented by FFP—and one by apheresis (single-donor) platelets—collected solely from male donors or female donors without a history of pregnancy or shown not to have WBC antibodies. Seven deaths, however, were ascribed to the transfusion of "buffy-coat" RBCs containing <20 mL of donor plasma; these deaths (Fig 2-10 in Chapter 2) could not have been prevented by the measures hitherto implemented in Europe and North America for TRALI prevention. As shown by further studies from The Netherlands,[87,88] these earlier measures (principally, the avoidance of "plasma-rich" components containing, or potentially containing, WBC antibodies; Chapter 4) prevent only one-third of the TRALI cases when TRALI diagnoses are based on strict adherence to the Canadian consensus criteria (adherence that removes the diagnostic suspicion bias favoring diagnoses of TRALI when a donor work-up identifies WBC antibodies or

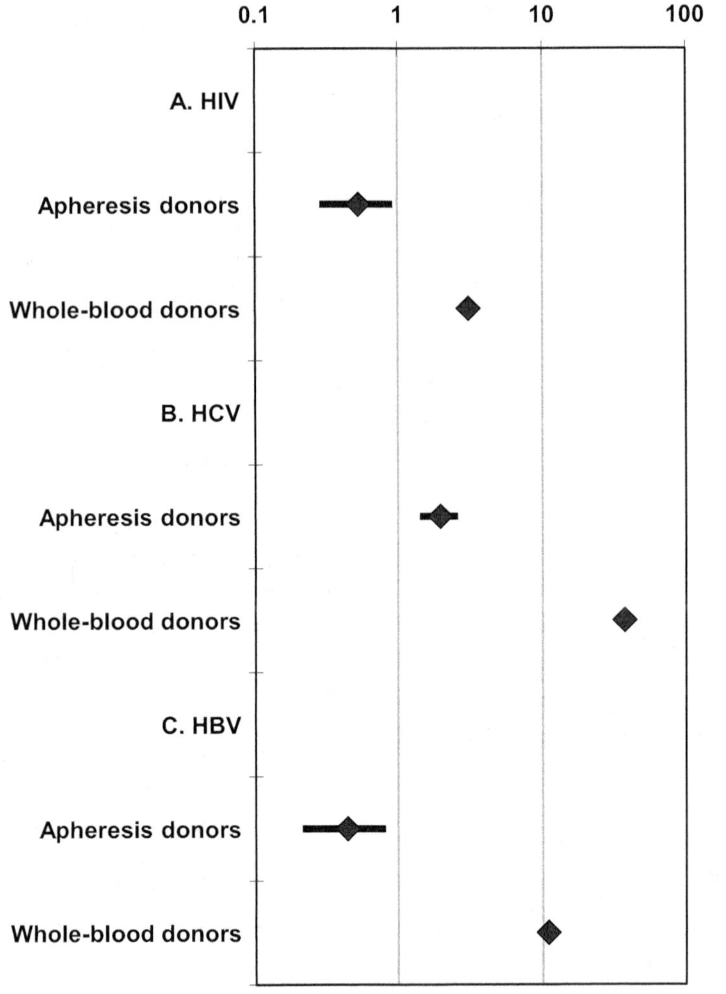

Figure 8-3. Prevalence of transfusion-transmitted infections (TTIs) in non-double-RBC apheresis (predominantly plateletpheresis) and whole-blood donations made to the American Red Cross between 2004 and 2008.[85] For human immunodeficiency virus (HIV), hepatitis C virus (HCV), and hepatitis B virus (HBV), the prevalence of infection per 100,000 collections is given, surrounded by its 95% CI. The prevalence of HBV infection is based on the results of hepatitis B surface antigen testing. There was a statistically significant ($p<0.05$) difference between non-double-RBC apheresis and whole-blood collections in the prevalence of all three infections: OR = 0.39 (95% CI, 0.22-0.69) for HIV; OR = 0.29 (95% CI, 0.22-0.37) for HCV; and OR = 0.37 (95% CI, 0.20-0.69) for HBV. Multivariate Poisson regression analysis with adjustment for the effects of donor gender, age, and first-time (rather than repeat) status corroborated the fact that non-double-RBC apheresis collections had a lower prevalence of HIV, HCV, and HBV infections than did whole-blood collections. Published initially by Vamvakas in Clin Lab 2010;56:263-79.[92]

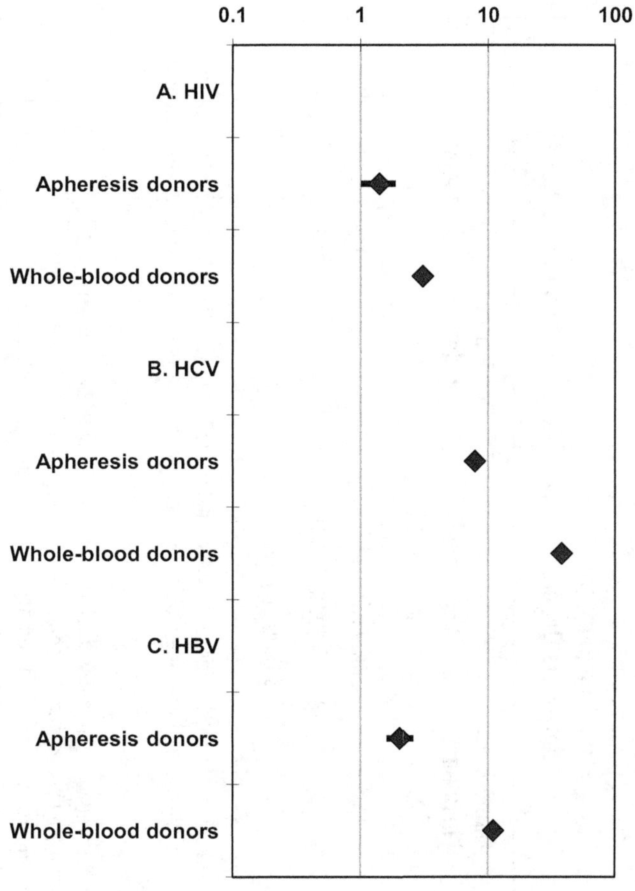

Figure 8-4. Prevalence of transfusion-transmitted infections (TTIs) in all [Red Blood Cell (RBC), platelet, and plasma] apheresis and whole-blood donations made to the American Red Cross between 2004 and 2008.[85] For human immunodeficiency virus (HIV), hepatitis C virus (HCV), and hepatitis B virus (HBV), the prevalence of infection per 100,000 collections is given, surrounded by its 95% CI. The prevalence of HBV infection is based on the results of hepatitis B surface antigen testing. Compared with whole-blood donors, apheresis donors have a significantly ($p<0.05$) lower prevalence of HIV, HCV, and HBV infections.

when the patient has received "plasma-rich" components).

Additive solutions have been used to replace more than two-thirds of donor plasma in units of platelets in an effort to reduce the risk of TRALI as well as other immunologic risks of transfusion (eg, anaphylactic or anaphylactoid reactions to plasma proteins). Because TRALI occurs with transfusion of <20 mL of donor plasma,[86,89] however, such attempts to minimize the residual volume of plasma in manufactured RBCs and platelets can (perhaps) reduce, but (certainly) cannot eliminate, the risk of TRALI from ABT. [As discussed in a subsequent section on allergic transfusion reactions (ATRs), to eliminate ATRs, 95% of the donor plasma from platelet components should be removed through washing.] For this reason, rather than removal—during compo-

Table 8-5. Incidence of HIV, HCV, and HBV Infection in Repeat Donors Making Double-RBC Apheresis, Non-Double-RBC Apheresis, and Whole-Blood Donations to the American Red Cross, 2007-2008*

	Double-RBC Apheresis Donors		Non-Double-RBC Apheresis Donors		Whole-Blood Donors	
TTI	Number of Incident Cases	Incidence† (95% CI)	Number of Incident Cases	Incidence† (95% CI)	Number of Incident Cases	Incidence† (95% CI)
HIV	9	3.80 (1.97-7.28)‡	6	3.86 (1.73-8.58)‡	77	1.99 (1.59-2.48)‡
HCV	4	1.69 (0.63-4.49)§	2	1.29 (0.32-5.13)§	121	3.12 (2.70-3.84)§
HBV	6	6.02 (2.71-13.41)‖	2	3.06 (0.76-12.23)‖	39	2.39 (1.75-3.28)‖

*Based on data reported by Zou et al.[85] The number of incident cases of each TTI for each donor category is included in the table to highlight the fact that—in the case of non-double-RBC (and also) double-RBC apheresis donors—the incidence calculations were based on a very small number of incident cases, which generated very wide 95% CIs.

†Per 100,000 person-years.

‡Apheresis donors had a somewhat higher HIV incidence compared with whole-blood donors, although the 95% CIs overlapped.

§Apheresis donors had a somewhat lower HCV incidence compared with whole-blood donors, although the 95% CIs overlapped.

‖Apheresis donors had a somewhat higher HBV incidence compared with whole-blood donors, although the 95% CIs overlapped.

RBC = Red Blood Cell; TTI = transfusion-transmitted infections; CI = confidence interval; HIV = human immunodeficiency virus; HCV = hepatitis C virus; HBV = hepatitis B virus.

nent manufacture—of all the plasma from donor units to prevent TRALI and other immunologic risks of ABT, the goal should be the removal of the immunologic exposures to the donors themselves.[83,90]

Multicomponent apheresis permits a reduction in the number of immunologic exposures to donors and therefore also in the corresponding immunologic ABT risks of TRALI, mistransfusion owing to clerical error, and anaphylactic or anaphylactoid reactions. The reduction in risk equals the reduction in the number of allogeneic-donor exposures: as the number of donors to whom a multitransfused recipient is exposed is reduced by ≥50%, the reduction in these immunologic risks of ABT also amounts to ≥50%. Therefore, for multitransfused recipients, the ≥50% reduction in the number of allogeneic-donor exposures that could eventually be made feasible by the replacement of the existing whole-blood collection and processing infrastructure with a new multicomponent-apheresis collection and processing infrastructure could reduce all infectious and all immunologic risks of ABT by ≥50%.[90-92]

Proponents of multicomponent apheresis[84] have advanced further arguments for such a paradigm change from whole-blood collections to multicomponent apheresis collections. Conceivably, multicomponent apheresis could help to mitigate blood shortages in the future (as the US population continues to age, increasing the demand for blood components, while the donor population is shrinking), as well as help to reduce the total costs for blood procurement and administration in an environment of limited reimbursement for blood services.[84] However, similar arguments (based equally on the widening "demographic gap" between donors and recipients) have also been made by the proponents of the status quo who adhere to the tenets of the current component-centric transfusion medicine paradigm: namely, a focus on the component (rather than the patient) and the primacy of inventory.[28] According to that view, to anticipate and prevent the inexorable supply shortages predicted for the future, efforts should concentrate on the recruitment of whole-blood donors,[28] as well as on the maximization of each donor's gift through the continued production, from each unit of whole-blood, of three blood components that will benefit three different patients.[5]

Possible Complications of Multicomponent Apheresis

Important to this position[5,28] is the argument that—because all of the platelet transfusion needs of patients who are not alloimmunized to human leukocyte antigens can be met by pooling already available WBD platelets—any donor reactions to plateletpheresis collections represent an additional and thus hard-to-justify risk.[5] However, multicomponent apheresis can meet all transfusion needs of US patients by subjecting to the rare risks of donation a number of donors that will not exceed the number of donors who donate today for producing the same number of components from whole-blood collections (Chapter 4).[90] This is the case because any country with a North American/Western European health-care system requires several times more RBC doses than platelet or plasma doses to meet the needs of all of its transfusion recipients.[90]

Equally important, and in contrast to the indications of the historical literature[5] on donor reactions [which preceded the advent of modern apheresis technology and reported increased frequency of donor reactions following apheresis (rather than whole-blood) collections], multicomponent apheresis collections are not associated with a greater incidence of donor reactions than are whole-blood collections (Fig 4-2 and Fig 4-3 in Chapter 4). Although severe donor reactions to apheresis collections that require hospitalization continue to be reported,[93] when all 793,293 allogeneic whole-blood and apheresis donations made to Blood Systems in 2007 were considered together, platelet/plasmapheresis collections as well as "double RBC" collections were associated with a lower ($p<0.05$) frequency of moderate and severe donor reactions compared with whole-blood donations, in a multivariate regression model that adjusted for all the usual predictors of adverse reactions to donation.[94]

In addition to such adverse reactions to donation, concerns have been expressed about the possibility of a sustained decrease in platelet count following repeat plateletpheresis donations,[95,96] as well as a decrease in bone mineral density in the lumbar spine and femoral neck owing to accumulating citrate toxicity in repeat apheresis donors.[97] Lazarus and colleagues[96] reported a mean decrease of 40,000/µL platelets in frequent plateletpheresis donors over 4 years, compared with these donors' baseline. Eighty-four of 939 (9%) frequent plateletpheresis donors were eventually deferred from donating because of a low platelet count, but most of them returned to donate successfully after being temporarily deferred. The investigators concluded that, although regular plateletpheresis donors develop sustained decreases in platelet count, clinically significant thrombocytopenia is unusual when rigorous ongoing review of platelet counts and prudent donor deferral policies are established and followed.[96] Previously, Stohlawetz and colleagues[95] had observed no difference in peripheral blood platelet counts between first-time and frequent plateletpheresis donors although, compared with first-time donors, repeat donors had significantly lower levels of reticulated platelets on Day 3 after apheresis, with their baseline values reached again on Day 4. These authors suggested that the levels of reticulated platelets could be used to monitor the thrombopoietic capacity of long-term platelet donors.[95]

Whether regular apheresis (in which citrate is routinely used for anticoagulation) affects bone and mineral metabolism remains unknown. A recent observational study found significantly ($p<0.05$) lower bone mineral density in the lumbar spine of regular plateletpheresis donors compared with matched controls; bone mineral density was also lower in the femur and femoral neck (albeit not significantly so).[97] Amrein and colleagues[97] concluded that, if their finding is confirmed, strategies to prevent such long-term effects of regular apheresis donations on bone and mineral metabolism will need to be formulated. Thus, in anticipation of moving toward an all-apheresis blood supply that relies on multicomponent-apheresis (rather than whole-blood) donations, such possibilities of long-term effects of regular apheresis donations need to be elucidated as soon as possible by further research. RCTs need to be employed whenever feasible, both to determine whether regular apheresis donations have cumulative adverse effects on the donors and to test the efficacy of possible strategies for ameliorating any such adverse effects.

Patient Blood Management in Platelet Transfusion

The current component-centric approach to platelet transfusion administers transfusions of either apheresis (single-donor) or pooled WBD allogeneic platelets to patients needing platelet transfusion. A single plateletpheresis donor, or, alternatively, four to six whole-blood donors, are needed for harvesting each platelet dose, so that the transfusion of one therapeutic platelet dose entails exposure to one or four to six allogeneic donors, respectively. Each successive platelet dose (often administered daily to patients needing chronic platelet transfusion support and having suboptimal posttransfusion platelet count increments) necessitates further exposures to one or four to six allogeneic donors, depending on whether apheresis or pooled WBD platelets are used; such a patient requiring a total of 10 platelet transfusions is thus exposed to 10, or 40 to 60, allogeneic donors, respectively. Moreover, the additional needs of these multitransfused patients for RBCs and plasma are met by exposing the recipient to a further (incremental) number of allogeneic donors that equals the number of RBC and plasma units received. When systems of PR of platelets become licensed by the FDA, both apheresis (single-donor) and pooled WBD platelets would presumably be subjected to PR, which would prevent the transfusion transmission of all pathogens containing nucleic acids (including viruses, protozoa, and bacteria, except for rare spore-forming bacteria and viruses circulating at virus loads exceeding the capacity of platelet PR systems for inactivation of viruses).

To the extent that plasma and apheresis (single-donor) platelets are collected from male donors or female donors who have no history of pregnancy or who are shown not to have WBC antibodies, cases of "alloimmune" TRALI[86] associated specifically with the transfusion of such "plasma-rich" components are prevented. The risk of TRALI associated with RBCs or pooled WBD platelets is not affected by these measures, however, either because the latter components contain some (<20 mL) plasma from unscreened female donors, or because TRALI can be caused by pathogenetic mechanisms other than WBC incompatibility between donor and recipient (Chapters 2 and 4). Also, to the extent that pooled WBD platelets continue to be used in the United States, each platelet dose transfused as a pool to which four to six allogeneic donors have contributed may expose the recipient to a risk of transmission of the next "HIV-like" transfusion-transmitted pathogen to emerge that would be four to six times as high as the risk afforded by the transfusion of a (therapeutically equivalent) platelet dose harvested from a single donor through plateletpheresis (Table 2-1 and Fig 2-17 in Chapter 2). An HIV-like pathogen would have the same long phase of asymptomatic pathogenemia as does HIV, although it would not have to be a virus or be transmitted sexually, as is HIV; variant Creutzfeldt-Jakob disease (vCJD; Chapter 3) is the agent best approximating the next major HIV-like transfusion-transmitted pathogen to emerge.

A completely patient-centric approach (Table 8-1) to platelet transfusion would combine two steps: 1) transfusing apheresis (single-donor) platelets collected from male or screened female donors to reduce the risk of TAS (Fig 2-5 in Chapter 2), TTIs (Fig 2-17 in Chapter 2), and TRALI; and 2) reserving the platelets and plasma (and/or RBCs) harvested from the same multicomponent apheresis collection for transfusion to the same recipient, to further reduce the risk of TTIs and TRALI. Moreover, when systems for PR of platelets become licensed by the FDA, apheresis (single-donor) as opposed to both apheresis and pooled WBD platelets—and, more specifically, apheresis (single-donor) platelets collected from male or screened female donors—would be subjected to PR, to prevent the transmission of all pathogens containing nucleic acids (except for rare, spore-forming bacteria and viruses circulating at excessively high virus loads).

Table 8-6 contrasts the component-centric and patient-centric philosophies on the best approach for optimally meeting patients' platelet transfusion needs. The fundamental premise of the component-centric paradigm is that "blood is safer than ever"—that is, 1) the residual risk of known TTIs is exceedingly small (Fig 2-17 in Chapter 2); 2) no HIV-like emerging transfusion-transmitted pathogen is currently on the horizon; and 3) thanks to the surveillance systems implemented since the emergence of HIV, any novel pathogen with a long asymptomatic phase will likely be detected much sooner than HIV was detected (ie, when the new pathogen's prevalence in the donor population is much lower than that attained by HIV in the year preceding the introduction of testing). Correspondingly, the fundamental premise of the patient-centric paradigm is that, although blood may be safer than ever, the determination of the magnitude of "acceptable" risk should be made by the prospective transfusion recipient, rather than by the officials of the blood system. Accordingly, the patient should be presented with the alternatives open to him or her with regard to platelet transfusion and with the risks associated with each alternative, and he or she should be allowed to choose between the platelet (and other) components administered. Table 2-1 in Chapter 2 provides calculations that could help guide this communication of risk to prospective platelet transfusion recipients. These calculations are based on the premise that (thanks to the surveillance systems implemented since the emergence of HIV) the next major HIV-like transfusion-transmitted pathogen will be confronted when it has reached a prevalence one-tenth that reached by HIV in the US blood donor population in the year preceding the introduction of HIV testing.

Nevertheless, rather than deferring the decision making entirely to the patient, policy decisions about optimal platelet transfusion could be made by clinicians and regulators on the basis of

Table 8-6. Component-Centric vs Patient-Centric Philosophies for Meeting Patient Needs for Platelet Transfusion

Component-Centric	Patient-Centric
• Either relies primarily (or exclusively) on transfusion of pooled WBD platelets (for all patients except patients needing HLA-matched platelet support), or permits the continued transfusion of pooled WBD platelets for reasons other than supply needs or the limited resources of a country's health-care system*	• Either prohibits the transfusion of pooled WBD platelets altogether, or limits the transfusion of pooled WBD platelets to the minimum imposed on policy-makers by supply needs or the limited resources of a country's health-care system*
• Suspends pooled WBD platelets in 100 mL of plasma from a male donor contributing to the pool, to *reduce* the risk of "alloimmune" TRALI†	• Limits transfused platelets to apheresis (single-donor) platelets collected from male donors or screened female donors, to *eliminate* the risk of "alloimmune" TRALI
• Administers RBCs and plasma from different allogeneic whole-blood donors to multitransfused platelet transfusion recipients needing transfusion of RBCs and plasma in addition to platelets	• Reserves the platelets and plasma (and/or RBCs) harvested from the same multicomponent apheresis collection for transfusion to the same recipient
• Will presumably pathogen-reduce pooled WBD (or both pooled WBD and single-donor) platelets when systems for PR of platelets are licensed by the FDA, for reasons not limited to supply needs or the limited resources of a country's health-care system	• Will pathogen-reduce *only* apheresis (single-donor) platelets (along with any minimum of pooled WBD platelets imposed on policy-makers by supply needs or the limited resources of a country's health-care system) when systems for PR of platelets are licensed by the FDA

*Preventing the recruitment of an adequate number of plateletpheresis donors or the acquisition of donor apheresis technology.

†The remaining <20 mL of plasma from each unscreened female donor contributing to the platelet pool are sufficient to cause TRALI.[86,89]

WBD = whole-blood derived; TRALI = transfusion-related acute lung injury; RBC = Red Blood Cell; PR = pathogen reduction; FDA = Food and Drug Administration.

the following considerations: 1) the incremental risk of TTIs and TAS associated with pooled WBD [rather than apheresis (single-donor)] platelets (Fig 2-17 in Chapter 2); 2) any risk of bleeding (Fig 4-1 in Chapter 4 and Fig 5-1 in Chapter 5), and possibly also acute respiratory distress syndrome (ARDS; see next section), associated with PR; 3) the question of whether PR can protect from all pathogens; and 4) the question of whether other benefits–noninfectious, that is immunologic, benefits, such as TRALI prevention–accrue from the reduction in donor exposures that results from the transfusion of apheresis (single-donor) rather than pooled WBD platelets (Chapter 4). Based on these four considerations, Table 8-7 contrasts the three possible risk-reduction strategies for platelet transfusion currently debated in the United States.

All four of these considerations have already been discussed in this book. The first consideration is the fact that the incremental risk of TTIs

Table 8-7. Three Risk-Reduction Strategies for Mitigating the Risks of TAS and Emerging TTIs Secondary to Platelet Transfusion*

- Transfusion of *non*-pathogen-reduced apheresis *(single-donor)* platelets if both the following conditions exist:
  - The available PR systems result in unacceptable risks of bleeding complications and/or ARDS.
  - There is no platelet PR system capable of inactivating all transfusion-transmitted pathogens.
- Transfusion of pathogen-reduced *pooled* WBD platelets if both the following conditions exist:
  - PR can be achieved with a tolerable increase in bleeding complications and/or ARDS, and it is capable of inactivating *all* emerging pathogens.
  - The reduction in the number of allogeneic-donor exposures does *not* result in other (eg, immunologic, such as TRALI prevention) benefits.
- Transfusion of pathogen-reduced apheresis *(single-donor)* platelets if either one of the following two conditions exist:
  - The reduction in the number of allogeneic-donor exposures results in other (eg, immunologic, such as TRALI prevention) benefits.
  - There is no PR system capable of inactivating all emerging pathogens, although PR can be achieved with a tolerable increase in bleeding complications and/or ARDS.

*Once systems for PR of platelets become licensed by the FDA. See Fig 2-5, Fig 2-17, and Table 2-1 in Chapter 2. TAS = transfusion-associated sepsis; TTI = transfusion-transmitted infection; PR = pathogen reduction; ARDS = acute respiratory distress syndrome; WBD = whole-blood derived; TRALI = transfusion-related acute lung injury.

from the pooled WBD platelets still transfused in the United States amounts to 104 and 18.7 annual transmissions, respectively, of the next HIV-like or West Nile virus (WNV)-like transfusion-transmitted pathogen (associated with chronic or acute pathogenemia, respectively) to emerge (Table 2-1 and Fig 2-17 in Chapter 2). In addition, as discussed in Chapters 4 and 5, the question of whether PR can be achieved with a tolerable increase in bleeding complications remains to be determined. Furthermore, of the two TTIs shown to be transmissible through transfusion in the 21st century and for which transfusion safety measures were implemented in the last decade, one (WNV) infection would have been prevented and one (vCJD) would not have been prevented by the implementation of PR for platelets prior to the corresponding agent's emergence. Finally, as discussed here and in Chapter 4, the reduction in the number of donor exposures afforded by the transfusion of apheresis (single-donor) rather than pooled WBD platelets, especially when combined with further reduction in the number of donor exposures through transfusion to the same recipient of the plasma and/or RBCs collected (together with the single-donor platelets) from the same male or screened female donor in the course of the same multicomponent apheresis donation, results in other (noninfectious: ie, immunologic) benefits for the patient, such as TRALI prevention.

All of these considerations combined might preclude the use of pooled WBD platelets in any (current or future) risk-reduction strategy for platelet transfusion.[91,92] If (or when) PR of platelets is adopted, PR could be applied only on apheresis platelets (not on platelet pools). Multicomponent apheresis is already available and its use will certainly benefit patients. What remains to be demonstrated now is that a paradigm change from a blood procurement system relying on whole-blood donations to a blood procurement system based on multicomponent-apheresis collections could be accomplished without adversely affecting the supply of all the blood components needed by all US transfusion recipients; and that any increase in cost required for achieving such a paradigm change would be deemed worth paying for by US patients, clinicians, and policy makers. If this research is completed and supports a change in paradigm, what would be needed next would be to change the existing paradigm of platelet transfusion from component-centric to patient-centric through the adoption of multicomponent apheresis as the standard of care.

Whether (or when) to adopt PR for apheresis (single-donor) platelets also represents a question requiring further research. The immediate benefit from PR would be the prevention of virtually all cases of platelet TAS [except for cases secondary to some rare spore-forming bacteria—a risk for which there is now an alternative solution that can be immediately implemented for apheresis (single-donor) platelets: implementation of a second bacteria detection test at the time of issue of the platelet component[98]; Chapters 2 and 4]. Equally important, if the next HIV-like major transfusion-transmitted pathogen to emerge has microbiologic properties akin to those of HIV (rather than the vCJD prions), PR would prevent that pathogen's transmission through platelet transfusion. The possible drawback of PR, however, is the greater risk of mild and moderate bleeding complications (and perhaps also ARDS), which is discussed in the next section.

Allergic Reactions to Platelets

As shown in the second column of Table 8-6, a possible future combination of the component-centric approach of PR (when systems for PR of platelets become licensed by the FDA) with the patient-centric approach of multicomponent apheresis would be to conduct PR of apheresis (single-donor) rather than pooled WBD platelets. Such a combination of the two paradigms in the future illustrates how transfusion-medicine paradigm shifts that initially appear to compete with one another for resources or in philosophy could eventually complement each other for the patient's benefit. One more element needs to be added to those of the patient-centric approach to platelet transfusion listed in the second column of Table 8-6. This last element pertains to the concentration (or washing, if necessary) of apheresis (single-donor) platelets for transfusion to patients who are prone to allergic transfusion reactions.[99]

ATRs are the most common transfusion complication. Although they are not usually serious, when cumulative, they can amount to significant morbidity for the multitransfused hospitalized patients who are the sickest of all patients. To prevent ATRs, diphenhydramine is administered before more than half of the transfusions given in the United States, despite the fact that pretransfusion medication with 25 mg of diphenhydramine was found not to prevent ATRs in two RCTs.[100,101] In a selected population of multitransfused hemato-oncology patients especially prone to ATRs, Tobian et al[102] found that concentrating apheresis platelets (to remove 73% of the donor plasma, leaving ≥100 mL of plasma in the component to resuspend the platelets) reduces the risk of ATRs by more than two-thirds (from 5.5% to 1.7%), while washing apheresis platelets (to remove 95% of the donor plasma) reduces the risk of ATRs by more than a further two-thirds, to 0.5%.

Recipient factors (as opposed to product or donor factors) are primarily responsible for ATRs. Over a period of 10 years in the Johns Hopkins oncology service, a minority (30%) of platelet transfusion recipients accounted for a majority (62.1%) of ATRs.[103] A total of 630 ATRs occurred when apheresis platelets split from the same plateletpheresis collection were transfused to two or more recipients. However, ATRs were observed in two or more different recipients of the same collection only six (0.95%) of 630 times—that is, as frequently as would have been expected from the overall incidence of ATRs (1.7%) in all clinical services of the Johns Hopkins hospital.[103]

Because recipient factors are primarily responsible for ATRs,[103] prevention efforts should focus on the patient rather than on the transfused component.[99] It is for the minority of patients who have already manifested severe ATRs that Tobian et al[102] recommended the removal of donor plasma from the platelet components for the prevention of ATRs. Concentrated apheresis platelets should be used first, and washed apheresis platelets (and RBCs) should be used for patients who fail to respond to concentrated apheresis platelets (as was the case for one-third of the patients of Tobian et al[102]). Washing platelets does reduce the risk of ATRs; however, it also decreases the number of platelets transfused to the patient (because 15% of platelets are lost during washing), and it may also reduce the survival of the washed platelets. Accordingly, patients who are chronically transfused with washed platelets should be monitored via daily platelet counts, so that—if necessary—they can receive a greater number of platelet transfusions to maintain adequate platelet counts.[102]

The approach recommended by Tobian et al[102] to prevent ATRs is patient-centric, because it selects the patents to whom concentrated or washed apheresis platelets are to be administered, and it monitors the recipients of washed platelets with daily platelet counts to ensure a compensatory increase in platelet transfusions when needed. Only a minority of patients are prone to ATRs, and therefore only a minority of patients would receive concentrated apheresis platelets if this approach is adopted. In this way, the majority of platelet transfusion recipients would benefit from any hemostatic contribution made by the two-thirds of donor plasma left in the unit (rather than removed at the stage of component manufacture for the purpose of reducing the risk of ATRs in recipients). Because platelet transfusion recipients who are not prone to ATRs would necessarily incur the allogeneic-donor exposure associated with the donor of the apheresis platelet concentrate that they are receiving, there is no reason for them not to receive the other two-thirds of the plasma from that donor (which some blood systems remove at the stage of component manufacture). Removing two-thirds of the plasma from a plateletpheresis unit would not prevent the transmission of either TRALI[86, 87] or vCJD (Fig 3-2 in Chapter 3). Untoward effects of ABO-incompatible plasma in ABO-incompatible apheresis platelets can be avoided by other means.[104]

Nonetheless, a component-centric approach to preventing ATRs treats the component rather than the recipient.[99] PASs have been used outside the United States for replacing approximately the same volume of donor plasma as that removed from the concentrated apheresis platelets of Tobian et al.[102] PASs have indeed been shown to reduce the risk of adverse reactions to platelets,[4,105] although only recently was a PAS (namely, PAS-III) developed that resulted in posttransfusion platelet CCIs equivalent to those—and prevention of bleeding as effective as that—achieved by platelets stored in plasma.[106] Previously available PASs (such as PAS-II) had resulted in lower posttransfusion platelet CCIs than did platelets stored in plasma,[4] yet several international blood operators had moved to the production of platelets stored in PAS-II. At any rate, approximately one-third of the patients prone to ATRs would not respond to platelets suspended in PAS (just as they did not respond to concentrated platelets in the study of Tobian et al[102]), and they would need to be identified and treated with washed platelets. Thus, settings in which a component-centric approach is used should implement at least some of the patient-centric steps recommended by Tobian et al[102]; these steps are the daily monitoring of platelet counts for recipients of washed platelets and an increase in the number of platelet transfusions when needed.

Pathogen Reduction of Platelet Components

Available systems for PR of platelets were discussed in Chapter 4. When PR systems are used, platelets are suspended in a plasma-reduced medium because plasma inhibits the inactivation of platelets. This is achieved either by conducting plasma reduction of a platelet component destined for PR or by using a PAS to replace approximately two-thirds of the plasma contained in the starting platelet component. Thus, pathogen-reduced platelets are usually suspended in a mixture of approximately 35% plasma and 65% PAS, and a major initial stimulus for the development of PASs was the desire to introduce (or to have the ability to introduce) PR of platelets. PASs consist of sodium chloride, acetate, and phosphate. The PR process damages platelets, although the conditions employed in the platelet PR systems licensed in Europe have been optimized to permit maximal inactivation of microorganisms along with minimal damage to platelets. Despite such optimization, however, there is a cellular loss of a proportion of the treated platelets, which results in 1) a reduction of the effective platelet dose administered to the recipient and thus in reduced 1- and 24-hour posttransfusion platelet CCIs (Table 5-2 in Chapter 5), 2) a need for a greater number of prophylactic platelet transfusions to maintain a platelet count of 10,000/µL (Fig 5-2 in Chapter 5), as well as 3) a shorter interval between platelet transfusions (Fig 5-3 in Chapter 5) during a period of hypoproliferative thrombocytopenia.

If the PR-induced platelet damage is limited to cellular losses of platelets, the increase in platelet transfusions for maintaining a platelet count of >10,000/µL should prevent any bleeding complications secondary to PR. Stated another way, if the PR-induced damage is limited to cellular losses of platelets, the corresponding increase in platelet transfusions should fully compensate for the platelet losses caused by PR. On the other hand, if the recipients of pathogen-reduced (compared with non-pathogen-reduced) platelets have increased bleeding complications despite the receipt of an increased number of platelet transfusions, PR may be causing functional impairment of all the treated platelets in addition to causing the loss of a proportion of the treated platelets. Two meta-analyses of the RCTs of the bleeding complications of pathogen-reduced (compared with non-pathogen-reduced) platelets[107,108] were undertaken to investigate this possibility of an increase in bleeding complications secondary to PR, despite the administration of a greater number of platelet transfusions.

The initial meta-analysis[107] (see Fig 5-1 in Chapter 5) included the RCT of the Mirasol (CaridianBCT, Lakewood, CO) system,[109] excluded the RCT of Lozano et al,[110] and integrated the results for 179 of the 278 patients of Kerkhoffs et al[106] (see Table 5-1 in Chapter 5), as well as data on bleeding complications from the SPRINT RCT as reported in the expanded safety analysis of that study.[111] The subsequent meta-analysis[108] (Fig 4-1 in Chapter 4), undertaken in response to criticisms[112] of the design of the initial meta-analysis,[107] excluded the Mirasol trial,[109] included the RCT of Lozano et al,[110] and integrated the results of all 278 patients of Kerkhoffs et al.[106] The primary analysis of the updated report[108] integrated the data on bleeding complications from the SPRINT RCT as presented in the expanded safety analysis of that study[111] (Fig 4-1 in Chapter 4); a sensitivity analysis in the updated report[108] further integrated the results of the SPRINT trial as presented in the initial report of that study.[113] When results on bleeding complications for the SPRINT trial were extracted from the expanded safety analysis[111]—but not the initial report[113]—of that RCT, the meta-analysis[107,108] showed an association between PR and clinically significant bleeding complications.

If this association is supported by future RCTs of the bleeding complications of PR, it would indicate that PR causes not only the loss of a proportion of the treated platelets but also the functional impairment of all the treated platelets.[106,107] A plausible hypothesis for such an increase in bleeding complications in association with PR (secondary to functional impairment of all the treated platelets) was recently advanced. MicroRNAs are small noncoding RNA species that play a role in posttranscriptional gene regulation for the majority of human genes.[114,115] Results made available in the past 2 years indicate that platelets contain microRNAs[116-118] that may regulate platelet protein translation and synthesis,[119-121] thereby affecting hemostasis.[122-124] Osman and Falker[125] identified 281 microRNA species in human platelets—a number corresponding to approximately 40% of all microRNAs listed in miRBase v14 (http://www.mirbase.org)—which is a relatively high number when compared with the number of microRNA species found in nucleated cells. Such platelet microRNAs might be as vulnerable to the effects of PR as are the nucleic acids of the pathogens themselves, and PR could alter the proteome of platelets stored after PR by inhibiting protein synthesis during storage.[126] If this were the case, and if proteins synthesized during storage affected platelet function, PR could indeed cause functional impairment of all of the treated platelets, thereby accounting for any observed increases in bleeding complications in association with PR.

An argument for why this may not be so, at least for the amotosalen/ultraviolet-A-light PR system (Intercept, Cerus Corp, Concord, CA), is that amotosalen forms adducts in double-stranded regions of DNA or RNA every 80 base-pairs on average, with larger nucleic-acid molecules (≥80 base-pairs) being more likely to be modified by amotosalen than are smaller molecules.[127] Bruchmuller et al showed that platelet nucleic-acid sequences of 100 base-pairs were not inhibited by amotosalen, and that consistent inhibition did not occur until nucleic-acid sequences of approximately 800 base-pairs were used as targets.[127] MicroRNAs (including their double-stranded precursors) are smaller than 80 base-pairs and thus not likely to be modified by amotosalen. Furthermore, the adhesion and aggregation of amotosalen-treated platelets to damaged endothelium were preserved,[128] whereas thrombotic events have not been reported from surveillance studies[129,130] conducted in areas routinely using the Intercept system. Nonetheless, no direct comparisons of the microRNA profiles and/or the proteome of pathogen-reduced with non-pathogen-reduced platelets over 1 to 5 days of platelet storage following treatment with Intercept have been conducted to investigate the potential for such a detrimental effect of Intercept treatment on platelet function.[126] Thus, the theoretical prediction that treatment with Intercept should not inhibit platelet microRNAs remains to be proven by laboratory experiments.

In summary, the totality of the evidence indicates that clinical equipoise[131] still exists vis-à-vis the undertaking of RCTs of platelets treated with PR. The concerns about emerging TTIs and platelet TAS that the PR would alleviate are balanced by the concern about increased bleeding complications in association with PR. Even if individual clinicians are sufficiently convinced about the benefit-to-risk ratio of PR to prescribe treated platelets for their own patients, policy makers—as discussed in Chapter 7—must demand more definitive evidence[132] (than the evidence hitherto adduced in the case of platelet PR; Fig 4-1 in Chapter 4 and Fig 5-1 in Chapter 5) about the lack of toxicity of a new treatment before they can approve such an expensive technology for routine clinical use. In this spirit, a new RCT of the Mirasol system is currently being conducted in The Netherlands, with US and Canadian participation.

Although the possible bleeding complications of PR have been discussed in detail in this book—because they have served as an example of the application of meta-analysis in transfusion medicine (Chapter 5)—they may not be the primary concern of US regulators with regard to the candidate systems for PR of platelets. A more serious concern to be addressed in ongoing and future RCTs is the possibility of a greater risk of ARDS in association with PR.[133] The SPRINT RCT[111] reported serious adverse events in 27% (86/318) of the recipients of pathogen-reduced platelets and in 25% (81/327) of the recipients of non-pathogen-reduced platelets ($p = 0.53$). Although the differences between the study arms in nearly all individual categories of adverse events were not significant, there were significant ($p<0.05$) differences in the risk of pleuritic pain, pneumonitis (not otherwise specified), and ARDS—all of which had occurred more frequently in recipients of pathogen-reduced platelets than in recipients of non-pathogen-reduced platelets. ARDS had occurred in 1.6% of recipients of pathogen-reduced platelets and in 0% of controls ($p = 0.03$); pneumonitis had occurred in 2.2% of recipients of pathogen-reduced platelets and in 0% of controls ($p<0.01$).

Additional investigation showed that there had been inconsistent use of the terms pneumonitis and ARDS among study sites in the reporting of adverse events.[111] A reanalysis of retrospectively collected pulmonary data on 148 patients (78 recipients of pathogen-reduced platelets and 70 recipients of non-pathogen-reduced platelets, all of whom had experienced potentially serious pulmonary adverse events) was conducted by expert physicians blinded to the treatment assignment.[111] The reanalysis found no significant difference in pleuritic pain, pneumonitis, or ARDS between these two selected patient sugroups.[111] Such a reanalysis, however, cannot entirely rule out the possibility of a greater risk of adverse pulmonary events secondary to the receipt of pathogen-reduced platelets compared with those secondary to the receipt of non-pathogen-reduced platelets, as recorded by the initial analysis of the data collected in the trial.

Conclusions

At any point in time, scientific thinking is reflected in a set of accepted and shared beliefs, which is called a "paradigm."[134] Scientific thinking thus goes through long periods of a stable, unquestioned status quo punctuated by paradigm shifts. During such paradigm shifts, the existing, dominant paradigm is brought under increasing pressure (as a result of anomalies that violate its assumptions) until it is replaced by another paradigm. According to Kuhn, who introduced the concepts of paradigm and paradigm shifts,[134] a change in paradigm amounts to no less than a scientific revolution. His examples included the progression of cosmologic theory through the Ptolemaic, Copernican, Newtonian, and Einsteinian models. No scientist works independently of theory, and all experimental work is therefore performed and interpreted within the disciplinary matrix of the prevalent paradigm. Once adopted as a paradigm, no theory is recognized as being testable by any quantitative tests that it has not already passed.[135] During the ensuing long period of status quo, adherents of the dominant paradigm elaborate upon, revise, and refine the current paradigm through experiment and measurement.

As Farrugia eloquently wrote,[1] since the late 1970s or early 1980s, transfusion medicine has been in a state of stasis: the currently dominant component-centric paradigm is deeply entrenched, and the tenets of blood component therapy, a focus on the quality of the blood component, and the primacy of inventory that make up this paradigm (first column in Table 8-1) are no longer regarded as "testable." As platelet TAS could now be confronted by means of implementing a second bacteria detection test at time of issue,[98] in the context of platelet transfusion both PR and the reduction in the number of donor exposures through the combined use of apheresis (single-donor) platelets and multicomponent apheresis represent either alternate or complementary solutions to the problem of emerging TTIs. When solutions to the problem of emerging TTIs are sought within the confines of the dominant paradigm, however, emerging TTIs can be regarded as a sufficiently significant problem for development of PR systems for treating each individual platelet component, although they may not necessarily be regarded as a sufficiently significant problem for discontinuing the production of pooled WBD platelets so as to reduce the number of allogeneic-donor exposures associated with the receipt of each platelet dose from four to six exposures to one exposure.

It might appear that PR applied to each platelet component at the stage of component manufacture is congruent with a focus on the quality of the blood component mandated by the current paradigm. Reducing the number of donor exposures associated with each platelet dose is important to the quality of the transfusion received by an individual patient, although not to the quality of the component manufactured by the current blood system. A reduction in donor exposures does not enhance the quality of a component as defined by good manufacturing practice regulations, and it may also affect adversely the total supply of blood components by diverting efforts from the recruitment of whole-blood donors (each of whom will benefit three patients, thereby maximizing both the "donor's gift" and the blood inventory) to the recruitment of plateletpheresis donors (who will provide a "redundant" product that is already available if we were to pool the WBD platelets that we already have). Although platelet PR systems are being developed to confront emerging TTIs, TTIs are nonetheless rare and blood is safer than ever. Given the exceedingly small magnitude of the risk of contracting a TTI from a platelet transfusion, four to six units of risk may be just as tolerable as is one unit of risk. Not the *individual* patient transfused today, but *all* patients transfused in the future might be better served once the quality of *all* distributed platelet components is improved by developing and implementing PR for both apheresis (single-donor) and pooled WBD platelets.

Yet, Farrugia[1] has argued that an alternative paradigm (based on the corresponding tenets of PBM, a focus on the individual patient, and the primacy of individual needs; second column of Table 8-1) is emerging. He predicted that the large "quality-control industry that has arisen around the current paradigm, the commercial agencies vested in supplying the myriad consumables needed for component manufacture, and the bureaucracies that fund the established centralized blood systems may resist the emergence of the new paradigm in which decision-making and the power to shape transfusion practice will be regained by clinicians."[1] The next few years will likely see whether the revolution in transfusion medicine indicated by this new patient-centric paradigm will occur, benefiting patients and discomforting many in what is often called the "blood industry."[1] The component-centric transfusion-medicine paradigm has delivered much good and saved many lives. Now, at least in the absence of considerations of cost, it could be said that transfusion-medicine professionals could deliver even safer transfusions than those using the "safer-than-ever" blood components still distributed by blood systems in the beginning of the 21st century. We now have the capability to do better than we were doing in the beginning years of this century—much as we were doing better in those years than we had been doing in the early 1980s. Stated another way, in the absence of considerations of cost, the recognition of our current (2011) capabilities could spearhead progression toward a better transfusion paradigm that, as Farrugia said, "should address the problems of the present while retaining the good of the past."[1]

Because the new paradigm of PBM and multicomponent apheresis [or PBM/multicomponent apheresis along with PR of apheresis (single-donor) platelets when PR systems for platelets are licensed by the US FDA] will be *both* safer *and* more costly than the components supplied by the current transfusion paradigm, we must do the research necessary for showing that the proposed paradigm change(s) are worth the added cost. This research would consist of estimating, based on the best available evidence, the cost incurred by each paradigm change(s) per year-of-life-saved. It would also involve operational research into the logistics of the change(s), to demonstrate that the proposed change(s) will not adversely affect the availability of all blood components needed for all US transfusion recipients; as well as further research into the efficacy and safety of the proposed change(s) along the lines discussed in this chapter. Namely, research to elucidate whether "fresh" RBCs (as well as RBCs transfused together with plasma at a 1:1 ratio in massive transfusion) are associated with better clinical outcomes than "old" RBCs or RBCs given at a ratio of (plasma to RBCs) 1 to 3-4; investigation of whether regular apheresis donations are associated with long-term adverse effects in donors, and—if so—evaluation of strategies to prevent such adverse effects; and research into whether the available PR systems for platelets are associated with impairment of the function of treated platelets and possibly also with development of ARDS in recipients.

Provided that this future research into the logistics, efficacy, and safety of the proposed change(s) supports a change(s) in paradigm, the judgment of whether the corresponding change(s) in paradigm is worth the added cost is not only an economic consideration, but primarily an ethical and moral one. Opinions about whether something is "worth" a certain amount of money are subject to variations in the perspective and the values of the person making the judgment of worth. What is an acceptable cost in one setting may be unacceptable in another setting. Moreover, what is an acceptable cost at one time may be unacceptable at another time.

Table 8-8 compares the cost-effectiveness ratios calculated for preoperative autologous blood donation[136] and nucleic-acid technology

Table 8-8. Estimated Cost Per Year of Life Saved Thanks to Various Interventions*

Intervention	Cost per Year of Life Saved
Mandatory seat belt use	$98
Mammography every 3 years for women 60 to 65 years of age	$2,700
Smoke detectors in airplane lavatories	$30,000
Prophylactic zidovudine following needlestick injury in health-care workers	$41,000
Flashing lights at railroad-highway crossings	$42,000
PAD for patients scheduled to undergo hip replacement surgery†	$235,000
Intensive care for seriously ill patients with multiple trauma	$460,000
PAD for patients scheduled to undergo CABG†	$494,000
Banning asbestos in roofing felt	$550,000
South Coast of California ozone control program	$610,000
Radionuclide emission control at Department of Energy facilities	$730,000
PAD for patients scheduled to undergo abdominal hysterectomy†	$1,358,000
Nucleic-acid technology (NAT) testing for HIV-1	$2,000,000
PAD for patients scheduled to undergo TURP†	$23,643,000

*Based on data reported by Tengs et al.[138]
†The cost-effectiveness ratios from the study of Etchason et al[136] (published in 1995) are used for PAD, because all other ratios shown are based on studies published before 1995. For the cost-effectiveness of NAT testing for HIV-1, the cost-effectiveness estimate of AuBuchon et al,[137] published in 1997, is used.
PAD = preoperative autologous blood donation; CABG = coronary artery bypass graft; HIV = human immunodeficiency virus; TURP = transurethral prostatectomy.

(NAT) testing for HIV[137] to the ratios calculated for other safety, environmental, and medical interventions.[138] All of the interventions listed in Table 8-8 (except, most likely, for preoperative autologous blood donation for patients scheduled to undergo transurethral prostatectomy) are "accepted" by society. Thus, there are large variations in the amount of money expended per year-of-life-saved for these "accepted" interventions. In fact, society makes decisions to allocate resources in ways that do not reflect the cost-effectiveness of the adopted measures.[6] Yet, at this time, we do not know where in the range of the cost-effectiveness ratios listed in Table 8-8 (from $98 to $2,000,000 per year-of-life-saved) the alternate paradigms discussed in this chapter might lie. These paradigms may even fall outside the range shown in Table 8-8—either because they are truly unaffordable or (as the proponents of multicomponent apheresis have argued[84]) because they offer a potential for cost-savings rather than for an increase in costs.

Both PR of platelets and multicomponent apheresis/PBM should thus be evaluated under the assumption of a "paradigm change"—with their costs estimated as they would pertain to a situation in which each of these alternate paradigms had become the dominant paradigm or the standard of care. It is critical that all these candidate paradigm changes undergo objective cost-effectiveness analyses free of any conflict of interest.[139] In conducting these analyses, we must remember that blood is transfused to patients who are invariably already ill, as well as elderly in most cases; and that the methods of cost-effectiveness analyses "discriminate" against the groups of patients whose life expectancy is shortest.[140] In preventing deaths from TRALI and TAS, the alternate transfusion-medicine paradigms may not save society many life-years, because transfusion recipients are old and sick. In preventing deaths from the next major HIV-like transfusion-transmitted agent to emerge, the alternate transfusion-medicine paradigms may benefit only those recipients who contract the infection through transfusion and survive long enough to develop (and ultimately die of) the associated disease. In either case, the number of life-years saved will be small, making the costs incurred owing to the change in paradigm appear too large in relation to the benefit accrued for society.

As with other transfusion safety measures before them,[136,141-146] the alternate transfusion-medicine paradigms reviewed in this chapter may thus look "ineffective" compared with other candidate health or safety measures, especially when compared with interventions outside the field of transfusion medicine. Yet, it is also possible that society may opt for improved blood safety and may implement the reviewed paradigm changes despite unfavorable cost-effectiveness ratios, as it has done before.[6] As the US FDA has articulated,[147] acceptance of risk is a political decision; acceptance of cost is also a political decision; and the role of transfusion-medicine professionals is to ensure that the best evidence is adduced for the making of policy decisions and also that such decisions are transparent. Once all the necessary evidence for each policy decision concerning a paradigm change becomes available, policy-makers will debate the merits of the evidence about whether a change in paradigm is appropriate, taking into account ethical, moral, and economic considerations.

References

1. Farrugia A. Falsification of paradigm shift? Toward a revision of the common sense of transfusion. Transfusion 2011;51:216-24.
2. Grindon AJ. The use of packed red cells (commentary). JAMA 1976;235:389.
3. Schmidt M. Comparison of different methods of bacterial detection in blood components. ISBT Sci Ser 2009;4:80-6.
4. Kerkhoffs JLH, Eikenboom JC, Schipperus MS, et al. A multicenter randomized study of the efficacy of transfusions with platelets stored in platelet additive solution II versus plasma. Blood 2006;108:3210-15.
5. Schrezenmeier H, Seifreid E. Buffy-coat-derived pooled platelet concentrates and apheresis platelet concentrates: Which product type should be preferred? Vox Sang 2010;99:1-15.
6. AuBuchon JP, Birkmeyer JD, Busch MP. Safety of the blood supply in the United States: Opportunities and controversies. Ann Intern Med 1997;127:904-9.
7. Sazama K. The ethics of blood management. Vox Sang 2007;92:95-102.
8. Eurobarometer: Europeans and blood. Prepared for the European Commission on Employment, Industrial Relations, and Social Affairs. Paris, France: Institut National de la Recherche Agronomique, 1995.
9. Lowe KC, Ferguson E. Benefit and risk perceptions in transfusion medicine: Blood and blood substitutes. J Intern Med 2003;253:498-507.
10. Isbister JP. The paradigm shift in blood transfusion. Med J Aust 1988;148:306-8.
11. Spahn DR, Moch H, Hofmann A, et al. Patient blood management: The pragmatic solution for the problems with blood transfusions. Anesthesiology 2008;109:951-3.
12. Thomson A, Farmer S, Hofmann A, et al. Patient blood management: A new paradigm for transfusion medicine? ISBT Sci Ser 2009;4: 423-35.
13. Hofmann A, Farmer S, Shander A. Five drivers shifting the paradigm from product-focused transfusion practice to patient blood management. Oncologist 2011;16(Suppl 3):3-11.
14. Shander A. Surgery without blood. Crit Care Med 2003;31(Suppl 12):S708-14.

15. Frenzel T, van Aken H, Westphal M. Our own blood is still the best thing to have in our veins. Curr Opin Anaesthesiol 2008;21:657-63.
16. Vincent JL, Baron JF, Reinhart K, et al. Anemia and blood transfusion in critically-ill patients. JAMA 2002;288:1499-507.
17. Taylor RW, O'Brien J, Trottier SJ, et al. Red blood cell transfusions and nosocomial infections in critically ill patients. Crit Care Med 2006;34:2302-8.
18. Vincent JL, Sakr Y, Sprung C, et al. Are blood transfusions associated with greater mortality rates? Results of the Sepsis Occurrence in Acutely Ill Patients Study. Anesthesiology 2008;108:31-9.
19. Mercuriali F, Ingilleri G. Proposal of an algorithm to help the choice of the best transfusion strategy. Curr Med Res Opin 1996;13:465-8.
20. Hébert PC, Wells G, Blajchman MA, et al, and the Transfusion Requirements in Critical Care Investigators Canadian Critical Care Trials Group. A multicenter, randomized, controlled clinical trial of transfusion requirements in critical care. N Engl J Med 1999;340:409-17.
21. Hajjar LA, Vincent JL, Galas FR, et al. Transfusion requirements after cardiac surgery: The TRACS randomized controlled trial. JAMA 2010;304:1559-67.
22. Napolitano LM, Kurek S, Luchette FA, et al. Clinical practice guidelines: Red blood cell transfusion in adult trauma and critical care. Crit Care Med 2009;37:3124-57.
23. Rossaint R, Bouillon B, Cerny V, et al. Management of bleeding following major trauma: An updated European guideline. Crit Care 2010; 14:R52.
24. Ferraris VA, Brown JR, Despotis GJ, et al, for the Society of Thoracic Surgeons Blood Conservation Guideline Task Force. 2011 update to the Society of Thoracic Surgeons and the Society of Cardiovascular Anesthesiologists Blood Conservation Clinical Practice Guidelines. Ann Thorac Surg 2011;91:944-82.
25. Wilkinson KL, Brunskill SJ, Dorée C, et al. The clinical effects of red blood cell transfusions: An overview of the randomized controlled trials evidence base. Transfus Med Rev 2011;35:145-55.
26. Curry N, Stanworth S, Hopewell S, et al. Trauma-induced coagulopathy—a review of the systematic reviews: Is there sufficient evidence to guide clinical transfusion practice? Transfus Med Rev 2011;25:217-31.
27. Ali A, Auvinen MK, Rautonen J. The aging population poses a global challenge for blood services. Transfusion 2010;50:584-8.
28. Greinacher A, Fendrich K, Brzenska R, et al. Implications of demographics on future blood supply: A population-based cross-sectional study. Transfusion 2011;51:702-9.
29. Shander A, Hofmann A, Ozawa S, et al. Activity-based costs of blood transfusions in surgical patients at four hospitals. Transfusion 2010;50: 753-65.
30. Shander A, Hofmann A, Gombotz H, et al. Estimating the cost of blood: Past, present, and future directions. Best Pract Res Clin Anaesthesiol 2007;21:271-89.
31. Malone DL, Dunne J, Tracy JK, et al. Blood transfusion, independent of shock severity, is associated with worse outcome in trauma. J Trauma 2003;54:898-905.
32. Marik PE, Corwin HL. Efficacy of red blood cell transfusion in the critically ill: A systematic review of the literature. Crit Care Med 2008; 36:2667-74.
33. Khorana AA, Francis CW, Blumberg N, et al. Blood transfusions, thrombosis, and mortality in hospitalized patients with cancer. Arch Intern Med 2008;168:2377-81.
34. Castillo JJ, Dalia S, Pascual SK. Association between red blood cell transfusions and development of non-Hodgkin lymphoma: A meta-analysis of observational studies. Blood 2010; 116:2897-907.
35. Isbister JP, Shander A, Spalin DR, et al. Adverse blood transfusion outcomes: Establishing causation. Transfus Med Rev 2011;25:89-101.
36. Vamvakas EC, Blajchman MA. Transfusion-related immunomodulation: An update. Blood Rev 2007;21:327-48.
37. Beauchamp TL, Childress JF. Principles of biomedical ethics. Oxford, UK: Oxford University Press, 1974.
38. Sazama K. Practical issues in informed consent for transfusion. Am J Clin Pathol 1997;107 (Suppl):S72-4.
39. Chan T, Eckert K, Venesoen P, et al. Consenting to blood: What do patients remember? Transfus Med 2005;15:461-6.
40. Carson JL, Duff A, Roses RM, et al. Effect of anemia and cardiovascular disease on surgical mortality and morbidity. Lancet 1996;348: 1055-60.
41. Jabbour N, Gagandeep S, Mateo R, et al. Live donor liver transplantation without blood products: Strategies developed for Jehovah's Wit-

nesses offer broad application. Ann Surg 2004; 240:350-7.

42. Jabbour N, Gagandeep S, Bramstedt KA, et al. To do or not to do: Living donor hepatectomy in Jehovah's Witnesses: Single institution experience of the first 13 resections. Am J Transplant 2005;5:1141-5.
43. Jabbour N, Gagandeep S, Thomas D, et al. Transfusion-free techniques in pediatric live donor liver transplantation. J Pediatr Gastroenterol Nutr 2005;40:521-3.
44. Jabbour N, Gagandeep S, Mateo R, et al. Transfusion-free surgery: Single institution experience of 27 consecutive liver transplants in Jehovah's Witnesses. J Am Coll Surg 2005;201:412-17.
45. Jabbour N, Gagandeep S, Mateo R, et al. Live donor liver transplantation in children—Guidelines for transfusion-free techniques. Hepatobiliary Pancreat Dis Int 2004;6(Suppl 1):67S.
46. Jabbour N, Gagandeep S, Peilin AC, et al. Recombinant human coagulation factor VIIa in Jehovah's Witness patients undergoing liver transplantation. Ann Surg 2005;71:175-9.
47. Strum E, Jabbour N, Gagandeep S, Selby R. Transplantation in Jehovah's Witness population: Bloodless surgery allows options. Semin Anesth Perioper Med Pain 2004;23:66-70.
48. Tokin C, Almeda J, Jain S, et al. Blood-management programs: A clinical and administrative model with program implementation strategies. Permanente J 2009;13:18-28.
49. Boulton FE, James V. Guidelines for policies on alternatives to allogeneic blood transfusion. 1. Predeposit autologous blood donation and transfusion. Transfus Med 2007;17:354-65.
50. Carless PA, Moxey A, O'Donnell D, et al. Autologous transfusion techniques: A systematic review of their efficacy. Transfus Med 2004;14: 123-44.
51. Stowell CP, Jones SC, Enny C, et al. An open-label randomized, parallel-group study of perioperative epoetin alfa versus standard of care for blood conservation in major elective spinal surgery: Safety analysis. Spine 2009;34:2479-85.
52. Hershman DL, Buono DL, Malin J, et al. Patterns of use and risks associated with erythropoiesis-stimulating agents among Medicare patients with cancer. J Natl Cancer Inst 2009; 101:1633-41.
53. Lipp G, Franchini M, Favaloro EJ. Thrombotic complications of erythropoiesis-stimulating agents. Semin Thromb Hemost 2010;36:537-49.
54. van der Meer P, Groenveld HF, Januzzi JL Jr, et al. Erythropoietin treatment in patients with chronic heart failure: A meta-analysis. Heart 2009;95:1309-14.
55. Jackson GN, Snowden CA, Indrikovs AJ. Prospective audit program to determine blood component transfusion appropriateness at a large university hospital: A 5-year experience. Transfus Med Rev 2008;22:154-61.
56. Gombotz H, Rehak P, Shander A, et al. Blood use in elective surgery: The Austrian benchmark study. Transfusion 2007;47:1468-80.
57. Gombotz H, Rehak P, Shander A. Blood use in elective surgery: The 2nd Austrian Benchmark Study. Vienna, Austria: Austrian Federal Department of Health, 2011.
58. Freedman J, Luke K, Monga N, et al. A provincial program of blood conservation: The Ontario Transfusion Coordinators (ONTraC). Transfus Apher Sci 2005;33:343-9.
59. Helm RE, Rosengart TK, Gomez M, et al. Comprehensive multimodality blood conservation: 100 consecutive CABG operations without transfusion. Ann Thorac Surg 1998;65:125-36.
60. Green JA. Blood conservation in cardiac surgery: The Virginia Commonwealth University (VCU) experience. J Cardiothorac Vasc Anesth 2004;8(Suppl 4):S18-S23.
61. Moskowitz DM, McCullough JN, Shander A, et al. The impact of blood conservation on outcomes in cardiac surgery: Is it safe and effective? Ann Thorac Surg 2010;90:451-8.
62. Vamvakas EC. Establishing causation in transfusion medicine and related tribulations. Transfus Med Rev 2011;25:81-8.
63. van de Watering L, for the Biomedical Excellence for Safer Transfusion (BEST) Collaborative. Pitfalls in the current published observational literature on the effects of red blood cell storage. Transfusion 2011;51:1847-54.
64. Corwin HL, Carson JL. Blood transfusion—When is more really less? N Engl J Med 1999; 356:1667-9.
65. Duchesne JC, Hunt JP, Wahl G, et al. Review of current blood transfusion strategies in a mature level I trauma center: Were we wrong for the last 60 years? J Trauma 2008;65:272-6.
66. Dente CJ, Shaz BH, Nicholas JM, et al. Improvements in early mortality and coagulopathy are sustained better in patients with blunt trauma after institution of a massive transfusion protocol in a civilian level I trauma center. J Trauma 2009;66:1616-24.

67. Teixeira PGR, Inaba K, Shulman I, et al. Impact of plasma transfusion in massively transfused trauma patients. J Trauma 2009;66:693-7.
68. Borgman MA, Spinella PC, Perkins JG, et al. The ratio of blood products transfused affects mortality in patients receiving massive transfusions at a combat support hospital. J Trauma 2007; 63:805-13.
69. Kashuk J, Moore E, Johnson J, et al. Post-injury life threatening coagulopathy: Is 1:1 fresh frozen plasma: Packed red blood cells the answer? J Trauma 2008;65:261-71.
70. Cotton B, Au B, Nunez T, et al. Predefined massive transfusion protocols are associated with a reduction in organ failure and post-injury complications. J Trauma 2009;66:41-8.
71. Holcomb JB, Wade C, Michalek J, et al. Increased plasma and platelet to RBC ratios improves outcome in 466 massively transfused civilian trauma patients. Ann Surg 2008;248: 447-58.
72. Maegele M, Lefering R, Paffrath T, et al. Red-blood-cell to plasma ratios transfused during massive transfusion are associated with mortality in severe multiple injury: A retrospective analysis from the Trauma Registry of the Deutsche Gesellschaft fur Unfallchirurgie. Vox Sang 2008;95:112-19.
73. Snyder CW, Weinberg JA, McGwin G Jr, et al. The relationship of blood product ratio to mortality: Survival benefit or survival bias? J Trauma 2009;66:358-62.
74. Scalea TM, Bochicchio KM, Lumpkins K, et al. Early aggressive use of fresh frozen plasma does not improve outcome in critically-injured trauma patients. Ann Surg 2008;248:578-84.
75. Hannon T. Trauma blood management: Avoiding the collateral damage of trauma resuscitation protocols. Hematology 2010:463-4.
76. O'Keeffe T, Refaai M, Tchorz K, et al. A massive transfusion protocol to decrease blood component use and costs. Arch Surg 2008;143:686-91.
77. Riskin DJ, Tsai TC, Riskin L, et al. Massive transfusion protocols: The role of aggressive resuscitation versus product ratio in mortality reduction. J Am Coll Surg 2009;209:198-205.
78. Gonzalez E, Pieracci FM, Moore EE, Kashuk JL. Coagulation abnormalities in the trauma patient: The role of point-of-care thromboelastography. Semin Thromb Hemost 2010;36: 723-37.
79. Kashuk J, Moore EE, Sawyer M, et al. Postinjury coagulopathy management: Goal-directed resuscitation via POC thromboelastography. Ann Surg 2010;251:604-14.
80. Jeger V, Zimmerman H, Exadactylos AK. Can RapidTEG accelerate the search for coagulopathies in the patient with multiple injuries? J Trauma 2009;66:1253-7.
81. Kashuk JL, Moore EE, Le T, et al. Noncitrated whole blood is optimal for evaluation of postinjury coagulopathy with point-of-care rapid thromboelastography. J Surg Res 2009;159: 133-8.
82. CRASH-2 Trial Collaborators. Effects of tranexamic acid on death, vascular occlusive events, and blood transfusion in trauma patients with significant haemorrhage (CRASH-2): A randomised, placebo-controlled trial. Lancet 2010;376:23-32.
83. Popovsky MA. Transfusion-related acute lung injury: Incidence, pathogenesis and the role of multicomponent apheresis in its prevention. Transfus Med Hemother 2008;35:76-9.
84. Popovsky MA. Multicomponent apheresis blood collection in the United States: Current status and future directions. Transfus Apher Sci 2005;32:299-304.
85. Zou S, Musavi F, Notari E, et al. Prevalence, incidence, and residual risk of major blood-borne infections among apheresis collections to the American Red Cross Blood Services, 2004-2008. Transfusion 2010;50:1487-94.
86. van Stein D, Beckers EA, Sintnicolaas K, et al. Transfusion-related acute lung injury in the Netherlands: An observational study. Transfusion 2010;50:213-20.
87. Wiersum-Osselton JC, Middelburg RA, Beckers EA, et al. Male-only fresh frozen plasma for transfusion-related acute lung injury prevention: Before-and-after comparative cohort study. Transfusion 2011;51:1278-83.
88. Middelburg RA, le Cessie S, Briet E, et al. A solution to the problem of studying blood-donor-related risk factors when patients have received multiple transfusions. Transfusion 2010;50:1959-66.
89. Win N, Chapman CE, Bowles KM, et al. How much residual plasma may cause TRALI? Transfus Med 2008;18:276-80.
90. Vamvakas EC. The ethics of wasting the donor's gift of buffy coat. Vox Sang 2011;100:256-7.
91. Vamvakas EC. Relative safety of pooled whole-blood-derived versus single-donor (apheresis) platelets in the United States: A systematic review of disparate risks. Transfusion 2009;49: 2743-58.

92. Vamvakas EC. The relative safety of pooled whole-blood-derived platelets prepared by the buffy-coat method versus single-donor (apheresis) platelets. Clin Lab 2010;56:263-79.
93. Winters JL. Complications of donor apheresis. J Clin Apher 2006;21:132-41.
94. Kamel H, Tomasulo P, Bravo M, et al. Delayed adverse reactions to blood donation. Transfusion 2010;50:556-65.
95. Stohlawetz P, Stiegler G, Jilma B, et al. Measurement of the levels of reticulated platelets after plateletpheresis to monitor activity of thrombopoiesis. Transfusion 1998;38:454-8.
96. Lazarus EF, Browning J, Norman J, et al. Sustained decreases in platelet count associated with multiple, regular plateletpheresis donations. Transfusion 2001;41:756-61.
97. Amrein K, Katsching C, Sipurzynski S, et al. Apheresis affects bone and mineral metabolism. Bone 2010;46:789-95.
98. Jacobs MR, Smith D, Heaton WA, Good CE. Detection of bacterial contamination in prestorage culture-negative apheresis platelets on day of issue with the Pan Genera Detection Test. Transfusion 2011;51:2573-82.
99. Vamvakas EC. A patient-centric approach to preventing allergic reactions to platelet transfusions. Transfusion 2011;51:1651-3.
100. Wang SE, Lara PN Jr, Lee-Owa A, et al. Acetaminophen and diphenhydramine as premedication for platelet transfusions: A prospective randomized double blind placebo-controlled trial. Am J Hematol 2002;70:191-4.
101. Kennedy LD, Case LD, Hurd DD, et al. A prospective, randomized, double-blind controlled trial of acetaminophen and diphenhydramine premedication versus placebo for the prevention of transfusion reactions. Transfusion 2008; 48:2285-91.
102. Tobian A, Savage W, Tisch D, et al. Prevention of allergic transfusion reactions to platelets and red blood cells through plasma reduction. Transfusion 2011;51:1676-83.
103. Savage W, Tobian A, Fuller A, et al. Allergic transfusion reactions to platelets are associated more with recipient and donor factors than with product attributes. Transfusion 2011;51:1716-22.
104. Josephson CD, Mullis NC, van Demark C, Hillyer CD. Significant numbers of apheresis derived group O platelet units have "high-titer" anti-A/A, B: Implications for transfusion policy. Transfusion 2004;44:805-8.
105. Azuma H, Hiravayama J, Akino M, et al. Reduction in adverse reactions to platelets by the removal of plasma supernatant and resuspension in a new additive solution (M-sol). Transfusion 2009;49:214-18.
106. Kerkhoffs JLH, van Putten WLJ, Novotny VMJ, et al. Clinical effectiveness of leukoreduced, pooled donor platelet concentrates, stored in plasma or additive solution with and without pathogen reduction. Br J Haematol 2010; 150:209-17.
107. Vamvakas EC. Meta-analysis of the randomized controlled trials of the hemostatic efficacy and capacity of pathogen-reduced platelets. Transfusion 2011;51:1058-71.
108. Vamvakas EC. Meta-analysis of studies of the bleeding complications of platelets pathogen-reduced with the Intercept system. Vox Sang 2012 (in press).
109. Mirasol Clinical Evaluation Study Group. A randomized controlled clinical trial evaluating the performance and safety of platelets treated with MIRASOL pathogen reduction technology. Transfusion 2010;50:2363-75.
110. Lozano M, Knutson F, Tardivel R, et al. A multicenter study of the therapeutic efficacy and safety of platelet components treated with amotosalen and ultraviolet-A pathogen inactivation stored for 6 or 7 days prior to transfusion. Br J Haematol 2011;153:393-401.
111. Snyder E, McCullough J, Slichter SJ, et al. Clinical safety of platelets photochemically treated with amotosalen HCl and ultraviolet A light for pathogen inactivation: The SPRINT trial. Transfusion 2005;45:1864-75.
112. Corash L. The hemostatic efficacy of platelet components prepared with pathogen inactivation. Transfusion 2011;51:1355-6.
113. McCullough J, Vesole DH, Benjamin RJ, et al. Therapeutic efficacy and safety of platelets treated with a photochemical process for pathogen inactivation: The SPRINT trial. Blood 2004;104:1534-41.
114. Friedman RC, Farh KK, Burge CB, Bartel DP. Most mammalian mRNAs are conserved targets of microRNAs. Genome Res 2009;19:92-105.
115. Fabian MR, Sonenberg N, Filipowicz W. Regulation of mRNA translation and stability by microRNAs. Annu Rev Biochem 2010;79:351-79.
116. Bruchova H, Yoon D, Agarwal AM, et al. Regulated expression of microRNAs in normal and polycythemia vera erythropoiesis. Exp Hematol 2007;35:1657-67.

117. Landry P, Plante I, Ouellet DL, et al. Existence of a microRNA pathway in anucleate platelets. Nat Struct Mol Biol 2009:16:961-6.
118. Kondkar AA, Bray MS, Leal SM, et al. VAMP8/endobrevin is overexpressed in hyperreactive human platelets: Suggested role for platelet microRNA. J Thromb Haemost 2010;8:369-78.
119. Booyse FM, Rafelson ME Jr. Studies on human platelets. I. Synthesis of platelet protein in a cell-free system. Biochim Biophys Acta 1968;166:689-97.
120. Kieffer N, Guichard J, Farcet JP, et al. Biosynthesis of major platelet proteins in human blood platelets. Eur J Biochem 1987;164:189-95.
121. Weyrich AS, Lindermann S, Tolley ND, et al. Change in protein phenotype without a nucleus: Translational control in platelets. Semin Thromb Hemost 2004;30:491-8.
122. Hong W, Konkar AA, Nagalla S, et al. Transfection of human platelets with short interfering RNA. Clin Transl Sci 2011;4:180-2.
123. Nagalla S, Shaw C, Kong X, et al. Platelet microRNA-mRNA co-expression profiles correlate with platelet reactivity. Blood 2011;117:5189-97.
124. Edelstein LC, Bray PF. MicroRNAs in platelet production and activation. Blood 2011;117:5289-96.
125. Osman A, Falker K. Characterization of human platelet microRNA by quantitative PCR coupled with an annotation network for predicted target genes. Platelets 2011;22:433-41.
126. Hitzler W, Vamvakas EC. Platelet microRNA profiles and the effect of pathogen reduction on platelet function. Clin Lab 2011;57:451-4.
127. Bruchmuller I, Janetzko K, Bugert P, et al. Polymerase chain reaction inhibition assay documenting the amotosalen-based photochemical pathogen inactivation process of platelet concentrates. Transfusion 2005;45:1464-72.
128. Lozano M, Galan A, Mazzara R, et al. Leukocyte-reduced buffy-coat derived platelet concentrates photochemically treated with amotosalen-HCl and ultraviolet A light stored up to 7 days: Assessment of hemostatic function under flow conditions. Transfusion 2007;47:666-71.
129. Osselaer JC, Cazenave JP, Lambermont M, et al. An active haemovigilance programme characterizing the safety profile of 7437 platelet transfusions prepared with amotosalen photochemical treatment. Vox Sang 2008;94:315-23.
130. Osselaer JC, Messe N, Hervig T, et al. A prospective observational cohort safety study of 5106 platelet transfusions with components prepared with photochemical pathogen inactivation treatment. Transfusion 2008;48:1061-71.
131. Freedman B. Equipoise and the ethics of clinical research. N Engl J Med 1987;317:141-5.
132. Miller FG, Joffee S. Equipoise and the dilemma of randomized clinical trials. N Engl J Med 2011;364:476-80.
133. Food and Drug Administration. Study Designs (Phases 3 and 4) for Product Development of Human Platelets Using the Cerus INTERCEPT Blood System for Pathogen Inactivation. Transcript of the meeting of the Blood Products Advisory Committee, November 16, 2009. Rockville, MD: CBER Office of Community Outreach and Development, 2009:158-345. [Available at http://www.fda.gov/AdvisoryCommittees/CommitteesMeetingMaterials/BloodVaccinesOtherBiologics/BloodProductAdvisoryCommittee/ucm121612.htm.]
134. Kuhn TS. The structure of scientific revolutions. Chicago, IL: University of Chicago Press, 1962.
135. Kuhn TS. The function of measurement in modern physical science. Isis 1961;52:161-93.
136. Etchason J, Petz L, Keeler F, et al. The cost-effectiveness of preoperative autologous blood donations. N Engl J Med 1995;332:719-24.
137. AuBuchon JP, Birkmeyer JD, Busch MP. Cost-effectiveness of expanded human immunodeficiency virus-testing protocols for donated blood. Transfusion 1997;37:45-51.
138. Tengs TO, Adama ME, Pliskin JS, et al. Five hundred life-saving interventions and their cost-effectiveness. Risk Analysis 1995;15:369-90.
139. Kassirer JP, Angell M. The journal's policy on cost-effectiveness analyses. N Engl J Med 1994;331:669-70.
140. Harris J. QALYfying the value of life. J Med Ethics 1987;13:117-23.
141. Busch MP, Korelitz JJ, Kleinman SH, et al. Declining yield of alanine aminotransferase for screening of blood donors for prevention of posttransfusion hepatitis B and C infection. Transfusion 1995;35:903-10.
142. Busch MP, Dodd RY, Lackritz EM, et al. Value and cost-effectiveness of screening blood donors for antibody to hepatitis B core antigen as a way of detecting window-period human immunodeficiency virus type 1 infections. Transfusion 1997;37:1003-11.
143. Tynell E, Anderson S, Lithander E, et al. Screening for human T-cell leukemia/lymphoma virus among blood donors in Sweden: Cost-effectiveness analysis. Br Med J 1998;316:1417-22.

144. AuBuchon JP, Birkmeyer JD. Safety and cost-effectiveness of solvent/detergent-treated plasma: In search of a zero-risk blood supply. JAMA 1994;272:1210-14.

145. Jackson BR, AuBuchon JP, Birkmeyer JD. Update of cost-effectiveness analysis for solvent/detergent-treated plasma. JAMA 1999; 282:329.

146. Pereira A. Cost-effectiveness of transfusing virus-inactivated plasma instead of standard plasma. Transfusion 1999;39:479-87.

147. Advisory Committee on Blood Safety and Availability. Blood safety summary—August 2000. Rockville, MD: Food and Drug Administration, 2000:68-9. [Available at http://www.hhs.gov/ophs/bloodsafety/summaries/sumang00.html.]

Index

Pages designated by italics contain figures or tables.

A

AABB
  guidelines for plasma transfusion, 148-150
  recommendations for TRALI prevention, 37
  standard for bacteria detection in platelets, 36-37, 126
ABLE (Age of Blood Evaluation) trial, 256, 257-258
ABT (allogeneic blood transfusion). *See* Transfusion, allogeneic
Acute lung injury, 46, 252. *See also* Transfusion-related acute lung injury
Acute normovolemic hemodilution, *274*
Acute respiratory distress syndrome
  and pathogen reduction of platelets, 295-296
  and TRALI, 36, 46, 51, 53, 55, 56
Adverse events, transfusion-associated
  decision-making regarding, 24-25
  observational studies and RCTs of, 10-11
  preferential reporting of, 36-39
  underestimation of, 34-35
  and WBC reduction, 2-*4*, 12-24
  See also specific adverse events
Age of Blood Evaluation (ABLE) trial, 256, 257-258
Age of Red Blood Cell in Premature Infants (ARIPI) trial, 256-257, 259
AIDS, 214. *See also* Human immunodeficiency virus
ALARA (as-low-as-reasonably-achievable) risk, 203-204
Allergic reactions, to platelet transfusions, 292-293
Alloantibodies
  red cell, 57, 60-61, 129-130
  white cell, 45-*49*, 50-56, 130, 283, *285*
Allogeneic blood transfusion. *See* Transfusion, allogeneic
Amotosalen-HCl/ultraviolet-A pathogen reduction. *See* Intercept pathogen reduction system
Antigen matching, 60-61, 129-130
Apheresis
  donor reactions to, 132-133, *134*, 287-288
  multicomponent
    cost-effectiveness of, 297, 298-299
    in patient-centric transfusion paradigm, 267, *268*, *269*, 280-288, *291*-292, 297
    protocols for, 280
    to reduce risk of TRALI, 131-*133*, 283, 285, 287
    and TTI, 280-283, *284*, *285*, 296
Apheresis platelets
  bacterial contamination of, 39-45
  detection of bacteria in, 36-*37*, 41-42, *44*-45, 124, 126
  dosages of, *133-134*, *135*, 143-*145*
  and risk of TAS, 41, 42-*44*, 69-*74*, 289
  and risk of TRALI, 50, 126-*128*, 130-131, 218, *221*
  and risk of TTI, 68-69, *72*-74, 125-126, 203-204, 207, *213*, 218, 289, *291*
  See also Pathogen reduction
ARDS. *See* Acute respiratory distress syndrome
ARIPI (Age of Red Blood Cell in Premature Infants) RCT, 256-257, 259
Australia, donor deferrals for MSM in, 201-202, 207, 208
Autologous blood recovery, 141, 275
Autonomy, *273-274*
Average effect, 161

B

Babesiosis, *32*, 34, 39, 88, 89
BacT/Alert system, 41
Bacterial contamination
  organisms involved in, 40
  of platelets, 39-45
    apheresis vs whole-blood derived, 40, 41, 42, *43*
    and component storage time, 40, 266
    detection of, 36-*37*, 41-42, *44*-45, 124, 126
  of red cells, 39, 40, 235, 236
  and WBC reduction, 236

Bacterial infections, 3-4, 12, *14*-15, 16-18, *20*. *See also* Transfusion-associated sepsis
BACTHEM study, 236
Before-and-after studies, 18, *20*, *21-22*
Beneficence, 273-274
Between-studies variation, 179, 180
Bias
  defined, 8
  information, 193
  in meta-analytic research, 192-193
  observation, 8, 178-179
  publication, 193
  selection, 8, 10, 150, 192, 193
  survivor, 279
  "Tower of Babel," 193
Bleeding complications
  of pathogen-reduced platelets
    with Intercept technology, 120, 121, *122*, 185-*186*, 189, 192
    meta-analysis of, 120-121, *122*, *165-175*, 180-185, 189-192, 294
    with Mirasol technology, 121, *183*, 189, 294
  and platelet dosages, *133-134*, 143-*144*, *145*
  and platelet transfusion thresholds, 146-147
Bleeding disorders, and vCJD, 97
Blood component therapy, 265-267, 268-269, 296
Blood inventory, 265, 266, 269, 287
Blood loss, acute, 277-280
Blood management. *See* Patient blood management
Blood recovery, 141, 275
Blood shortages, 265, 266, 287
Bone mineral density, in apheresis donors, 288
Bovine spongiform encephalopathy, 90-91, 92, 97-98

C

Cardiac surgery
  use of "fresh" vs "old" RBC transfusions in
    current RCTs studying, 256
    and mortality, 246, *248*, *249*, *250*
    and organ failure, 252
    and postoperative pneumonia, 253, *254*, *255*
  use of WBC-reduced RBCs in
    and mortality, 124-125, *249*, *251*, 259
    and TRIM effect, *13*, *14*, *15*, 16, 18, *19*, 23, 64, *65*, *66*
CARS (compensatory anti-inflammatory response syndrome), 64
Cause-and-effect relationships, *8*, 9-11
Chagas disease, 89
Chikungunya virus, 67, 88, 89
Circulatory overload. *See* Transfusion-associated circulatory overload
Citrate toxicity, in apheresis donors, 288
Clotting factor concentrates, 97
CMV. *See* Cytomegalovirus
Colorectal cancer, 23
Compensatory anti-inflammatory response syndrome, 64
Component-centric paradigm
  characteristics of, 265-267, *268-269*
  economics of, 266-267
  of platelet transfusions, 288, 289, 290
  premise of, 289
Confounding factors, 6, 10-11, 243, 244, 245, 276
Corrected count increments
  calculation of, *164*
  effect of pathogen-reduced platelets on, *164*, *165*, *167*, *188*-189, 191, 294
  meta-analysis method for, 180
  and platelet storage times, 172, 266
Costs
  of patient-centric transfusion paradigm, 269, 297-299
  per year of life saved from interventions, 296-297
  of using recovered plasma, 266-267
  of using whole-blood-derived platelets, 266-267
Creutzfeldt-Jakob disease, classic, 89
Creutzfeldt-Jakob disease, variant
  assays for detection of, 99-*100*
  codon-129 polymorphism in, 92-93, 94
  incubation period for, 92, 93
  mortality due to, 39
  natural resistance to, 91-93
  number of cases of, 90, 91, 93-95, *105*, *106*
  preventing transmission of
    by minimizing plasma volume in platelets, *106*
    with prion-reduction filters, 100-103
    with washed RBCs, 104-*105*
    with white-cell reduction, 2, 23, 101, 103-104
  and solvent/detergent-treated plasma, 119
  subclinical, prevalence of, 90-95, 99, *105*, 106
  transfusion-transmitted cases of, 95-*100*
Cytomegalovirus, 2, 23, 24

D

Decision-making
  equipoise for, 238-241
  evidence-based medicine in, 4, 5-11, 12, 24-25
  precautionary principle in, 11-12, 24-25
  risk management approach to, 12
Dedicated donors, 256-257
Dengue fever virus, 39, 67, 88, 89
Deviation, systematic, 8
Donor deferrals
  for high-risk heterosexuals, 214-216, 223

for men who have had sex with men
1 year, 201, 202, 203, 204-*205*, 207-212, 223
5 years, 201, 202-203, *205*, 212-216, 223
in Australia, 201-202, 226-227
compared to ALARA risk, 203-204
compared to risk of pooled platelet transfusions, 207, 212, *213*, 218, *220-221*
donors views on, *225*-226
evidence before July 2010, 223-225
evidence since July 2010, 225-227
and HHV-8 transmission, *206*-207, 216-218, 219, *220*, *221*-222
no deferral, 204, 214, *215*
noncompliance with, 202, 208, 209, 214, *215*, 223, 226
relative risk for, 207, 212, 218-221
and risk of TTI, 201-203, 204-*205*, 209, *213*, 218, 222-223
in United Kingdom, 226-227
United States position on, 224-225
Donor exposures, limiting
with multicomponent apheresis, 131-*133*, 280-287, *291*, 296
with patient-centric transfusion paradigm, 266, 267, 268
with platelet transfusions
apheresis, *133*-134
lower dosages, 143-*145*
prophylactic vs therapeutic, *145*-147
in preventing TRALI, 130-*134*
in preventing transfusion-related mortality, 114, *134*-150
in preventing TTI, 222
with prophylactic plasma transfusions, 147-150
with use of evidence-based guidelines, *135*-137
using restrictive vs liberal transfusion strategies, 137-*142*, 274-275
Donors
dedicated, 256-257
prevalence of TTIs in
apheresis vs whole blood, 280-281, 282, 283, 284, 285, 286
first-time vs repeat, 280, *281*, 286
male vs female, 280, *281*
reactions in, 132-*133*, *134*, 287-288

E

eBDS culture system, 41
Emerging transfusion-transmitted infections, 87-90. *See also* specific infections
categories of, 88-89, 218
fatal, impact of, 64-68
and MSM deferrals, 202, *205*, 218, 222-223
precautionary principle regarding, *205*
preventing with pathogen reduction, 116, 118
risk of, due to pooled platelets, 68-69, 71-*74*, *75*, 204, 218, 289, 290-*291*
Epstein-Barr virus, 89, 90
Equipoise
for clinical decision-making, 238-239
defined, 235, 238
for policy decision-making, 239-241
as prerequisite for undertaking RCTs, 237-241
Error, laboratory, *205*, 209-210, 211, 223-224
Erythroid-stimulating agents, 275
Erythropoietin, 141
Ethics
of MSM deferrals, 224
of paradigm shifts, 297
of patient blood management, 272-274
of randomized controlled trials, 25, *240*
of using "fresh" vs "old" blood, 237, 238, 239, 241, 258
euroSPRITE trial, *166*, 178, *183*, *188*-189
Evidence, hierarchy of, 5-*6*, *7*, *8*
Evidence-based medicine
expert opinion in, 238
hierarchy of evidence in, 5-*6*, *7*, *8*
meta-analyses in, *8*-9
overview of, 5
and patient blood management, 270-*271*, 275
for plasma transfusion, 148-150
in policy decision-making, 4, 5, 12, 24-25
randomized controlled trials in, *6*, *8*, 9-11
systematic reviews in, *8*-9
transfusion guidelines, 114, *135*-137
Expert opinion, 238

F

Factor VIII concentrates, 97
Fatalities. *See* Mortality
FDA (US Food and Drug Administration), 31-*32*, *33*-34, 36
Febrile nonhemolytic transfusion reactions, 2, 23
Fixed-effects method, 179, 180
FOCUS RCT, 139, 140
Fresh Frozen Plasma. *See* Plasma transfusions
Functional Outcomes in Cardiovascular Patients Undergoing Surgical Hip Fracture Repair (FOCUS), 139, 140

G

Gastrointestinal surgery, *13*, *14*, *15*, 16
Genotyping, 61
Graft-vs-host disease, transfusion-associated, 31, *32*

H

- Hemoglobin, as transfusion threshold
  - and Jehovah's Witnesses, 274
  - in liberal vs restrictive transfusion strategies, 61, 136, 137-*142*, 270-*271*
- Hemoglobinopathies, 60-61
- Hemolytic transfusion reactions, 57-61
  - delayed, 57
  - mortality due to, 31-*32*, 36, 57, *58*, *59*, 60, *75-76*
  - prevention of, 57-61, 129-130
- Hemophilia, 96-97
- Hemostatic capacity and efficiency of PR platelets
  - defined, 164
  - meta-analysis of
    - fixed-effects vs random-effects method, 180-181
    - medical heterogeneity of, 185-189
    - sources of variation in, *169*-174
    - totality of evidence on, 189-192
    - as unit of observation, *165-169*
- Hemovigilance studies
  - preferential reporting of adverse events by, 36-39
  - underestimation of adverse events by, 34-36
- Hepatitis A virus, 90
- Hepatitis B virus
  - infectious window-period, 204, *205*
  - and MSM deferrals, 207, 209, 212, *213*
  - prevalence in donors
    - apheresis vs whole blood, 69, 280-*281*, *282*, 283, *284*, *285*, *286*
    - fist-time vs repeat, 280, *281*, *286*
    - male vs female, 280, *281*
  - risk of, from pooled platelets, 71, *73*, *75*, 204, 207, *213*
- Hepatitis C virus
  - infectious window-period, 204, *205*
  - mortality due to, 31
  - and MSM deferrals, 207, 212
  - prevalence in donors
    - apheresis vs whole blood, 69, 280-*281*, *282*, 283, *284*, *285*, *286*
    - fist-time vs repeat, 280, *281*, *286*
    - male vs female, 280, *281*
  - risk of, from pooled platelets, 71, *73*, *75*, 204, 207, *213*
- Heterogeneity of effects, 181-182, 185
- HHV-8. *See* Human herpesvirus-8
- Hierarchy of evidence, 5-*6*, *7*, *8*
- HIV. *See* Human immunodeficiency virus
- HLA antibodies, 48-*49*
- Homogeneity of effects, 181-182
- HTLV (human T-cell lymphotropic virus), 236, 241
- Human herpesvirus-8
  - and MSM, 202, *206*-207, 222
  - seroconversion by nontransfusion sources, *217*-218, *219*, *220*
  - transmission by transfusion, *216*-218, *219*, *220*, 221-222
- Human immunodeficiency virus
  - "HIV-like" infections, 67-68
    - and MSM deferrals, *205*
    - predicted prevalence of, 67, 87
    - preventing with pathogen reduction, 116, 118
    - risk of, from pooled platelets, 71, *72*-73, *75*, 204, 289, *291*
  - infectious window-period, 204, *205*
  - mortality due to, 31
  - prevalence in donors
    - apheresis vs whole blood, 69, *281*, *282*, 283, *284*, *285*, *286*
    - first-time vs repeat, 280, *281*, *286*
    - before HIV testing, 67, 87
    - male vs female, 280, *281*
    - MSM, 201, 207-209, 210
  - risk of, from transfusion
    - and MSM deferrals, 201-203, 207, 209-214, 223
    - of "old" RBCs, 236, 241
    - of pooled platelets, 71, *73*, *75*, 204, 207, *213*
  - risk of release of HIV positive units
    - due to false-negative testing results, *205*, 209-210
    - erroneous release, *205*, 209, 210, 211, 223-224
    - and MSM donors, *205*, 209-211, 212, *213*-214, *215*, 223-224
- Human parvovirus 19, 89-90
- Human T-cell lymphotropic virus, 236, 241

I

- I^2 test, 181
- Identification of recipients, 57-60, 129
- Infections
  - bacterial, 3-4, 12, *14-15*, 16-18, *20*
  - nosocomial, 253, 254, 255
  - sexually transmitted, 222
  - *See also* Transfusion-transmitted infections
- Infectious dose, *100*-101, *102*
- Information bias, 193
- Informed consent, 267
- Intensive care unit patients
  - liberal vs restrictive transfusion strategies in, 61-62, 64, 137-140

TRALI in, 35, 51, 52
use of "fresh" vs "old" blood transfusions in, 246, *248*, 252-253, 256, 257-258
Intercept pathogen reduction system
bleeding complications from, 120, 121, *122*, *164*, *166*, *186*, 189, 192, 295
cellular and functional protein losses with, 117
effect on corrected count increments, *164*, *167*
effect on interval between platelet transfusions, *168*
effect on number of platelet transfusions, *169*
and mortality, 117
technology for, 119
Iron overload, 62, *63*

J

Janetzko trial, *166*, *183*, *188*-189
Jehovah's Witnesses, 274
Justice, *273-274*

K

Kaposi's sarcoma, *206*, 222
Kerkhoffs trial
findings of, 189, 190
odd ratios of bleeding complications in, *166*, *188*
patients in study, 187-*188*
quality of, 178-179
reporting bleeding complications in, *183*
Kuru, 92-93

L

Leishmaniasis, 88, 89
Leukocyte reduction. *See* White cell reduction
Liver transplantation, 119

M

Malaria, 89
Massive transfusion
developing protocols for, 279-280
plasma to RBC ratios in, 148-*149*, 277-279
Men who have had sex with men (MSM)
prevalence of undiagnosed HIV infection in, 207-209, *210*
reducing donor deferrals for
to 1 year, 201, 202, 203, 204-*205*, 207-212, 223
to 5 years, 201, 202-203, *205*, 212-216, 223
in Australia, 201-202, 226-227
compared to ALARA risk, 203-204
compared to risk of pooled platelet transfusions, 207, 212, *213*, 218, *220-221*
donors views on, 225-226
evidence before July 2010, 223-225
evidence since July 2010, 225-227
and HHV-8 transmission, 206-207, *216*-218, *219*, *220*, *221*-222
to no deferral, 204, 214, *215*
noncompliance with, 202, 208, 209, 214, *215*, 223
relative risk for, 207, 212, 218-*221*
and risk of emerging agents, 218, 222-223
and risk of transfusion-transmitted diseases, 201-203, 204-*205*, 209, *213*, 218
in the United Kingdom, 226-227
United States position on, 224-225
Meta-analysis, *8*-9
applications of, 161-162
within and between-studies variation in, 179, 180
bias in, 192-193
combinability of reports for, 181-185
defined, 161
eligibility of reports for, 174-176
in evidence hierarchy, *6*, *7*
by fixed-effects method, 179, 180
of individual patient data, *6*, 9
of literature, 9
medical interpretation of, 185-192
qualitative and quantitative components of, 162-*163*
quality of reports in, 162-*163*, 176-179
by random-effects method, 179, 180
rationale for, 179-181
sequence of steps in, *163*
as supplement to RCTs, 162
of TRIM effects, 16-18
unit of observation in, *165-169*
variations in findings of RCTs, *169*-174
vs literature reviews, 161
MicroRNAs, 123, 124, 190-191, 192, 294-295
Military casualties, 277-278, 279
Mirasol pathogen reduction
bleeding complications from, 121, 166, *183*, *186*, 189, 192, 294
effect on corrected count increments, *164*, *167*, 191
effect on interval between platelet transfusions, *168*
effect on number of platelet transfusions, *169*
technology for, 119
Mortality, transfusion-related
due to hemolytic transfusion reactions, 31-*32*, 36, 57, *58*, *59*, 60, *75-76*, 129
due to TACO, *32*, *33*, 56, 113

due to TAS, 31-*32*, *33*, 36-*37*, 39-45, *74*, *76*
due to TRALI, 31-*32*, *33*, 36, *37-38*, 46, 52-57, *74*-75, *76*
due to TTIs, 31, 39, 64-*74*
and "fresh" vs "old" blood transfusions, 241, 246-252, 275-276
in liberal vs restrictive transfusion strategies, 61-62, 64, 137, *138*
passive surveillance studies of, 34-39
and plasma to RBC ratios in trauma, 278-279
preferential reporting of, 36-39
reported to FDA, 31-32, *33*-34
reported to SHOT, 32-34
strategies for reducing, *115*
augmentation of patient identification procedures, 129
extended antigen matching, 129-130
pathogen reduction, 116-124
replacing pooled platelets with apheresis platelets, 125-129
using evidence-based transfusions, *134*-150
using multicomponent apheresis, 131-*133*
using WBC reduction, 124-125
underestimation of, 34-35
and WBC reduction, 4, 12-16, 62, 64
before and after studies of, 18, *21*, *22*
in cardiac surgery, *13*, *14*-15, 19, *22*, *65*, *66*, 124-125
in gastrointestinal surgery, *13*, *14-15*, 16
MSM. *See* Men who have had sex with men
Multicomponent apheresis
cost-effectiveness of, 297, 298-299
donor reactions to, 132-*133*, 134, 287
in patient-centric transfusion paradigm, 267, *268*, *269*, 280-288, *291*-292, 297
protocols for, 280
to reduce risk of TRALI, 131-*133*, 283, *285*, 287
and transfusion-transmitted infections, 280-283, *284*, *285*, *296*
Multiple organ failure, 62, 64, 252-253

N

"N of 1" randomized controlled trials, 6
Neonates, low-birthweight premature, 141-*142*, 256-257
Nonmaleficence, 273-274
Nosocomial infections, 253, *254*, *255*

O

Observation bias, 8, 178-179
Observational studies
before-and-after studies, 18, 20, 21-22
bias in, 8, 192, 193
confounding factors in, 276
in establishing cause-and-effect, 9-10
of "fresh" vs "old" blood transfusions, 237, 243-253, *254*, *255*, 275, 277
in hierarchy of evidence, 6
inclusion in meta-analysis, *163*, 176
of pathogen reduction, 189, 191-192
of plasma transfusions, 148-150
of prophylactic platelet transfusions, 147-148
of TRALI, 35, 50, 51-52, 127, 131
of transfusion-associated sepsis and pooled platelets, 69
of transfusion-related mortality, 34, 276
vs hemovigilance systems, 35
vs randomized controlled studies, 6, 10-11
of WBC reduction, 23
Odds ratio, *8*-9
Organ failure, 62, 64, 252-253

P

Paradigm shifts, 267, 296-299
component-centric vs patient-centric, 265-270, 296, 297-299
multicomponent apheresis, 267, *268*, *269*, 280-288, *291*-292, 297
pathogen reduction of platelets, 293-296
patient blood management, 267, *268-269*, 269, 270-280, 288-293
for platelet transfusions, 288-293
Passive surveillance artifact, 36
Passive surveillance studies, 34-39
Pathogen reduction, 116-124
advantages and disadvantages of, 116-117
of plasma, 116-119
of platelets, 293-296
alternatives to, 124
apheresis vs whole blood-derived, 172
bleeding complications of, 120-123, *164*, *165*-174, 180-181, 182-192, 291, 294-295
cost-effectiveness of, 297, 298-299
effect on corrected count increments, *164*, *165*, *167-169*, 180, 188-189, 191, 294
effect on interval between transfusions, *165*, *167-169*, 180, 294
effect on number of platelet transfusions, *165*, *167-169*, 180, 294
and microRNAs, 123, 124, 190-191, 192, 294-295
platelet additive solutions for, 293-294

and platelet function, 123, 124, 190-191, 192, 294-295
and risk of ARDS, 295-296
in preventing TAS, 124, *164*, 269, 291
in preventing TTIs, 114, *115*, 116-124, 296-297
of red cells, 116
technologies for, 117, 119, *164*
in transfusion paradigms, *269*, 288, 289, 293-296
Patient blood management, 270-280
arguments for, 274-276
cost-effectiveness of, 297, 298-299
defined, 270
elements of, *271*-272
ethics of, 272-*274*
"fresh" vs "old" RBCs in, 275-277
fresh whole blood transfusions in, 277-280
in patient-centric transfusion paradigm, 267, *268-269*, 269-270, 272, *274*-276
of platelet transfusion, 288-293
"three pillars" of, 270
Patient-centric paradigm
characteristics of, *268-269*
informed consent in, 267, *268*, 289
multicomponent apheresis in, 267, *268*, *269*, 280-288, *291*-292, 297
patient blood management in, 267, *268-269*, 270-280, 288-293
of platelet transfusions, 289, 290
Perioperative autologous blood recovery, 141, 275
PINT (Premature Infants in Need of Transfusion) trial, 141-142
PLADO (Prophylactic Platelet Dose on Transfusion Outcomes) trial, 133, *135*, 143, 145
Plasma, recovered, 266-267
Plasma, solvent/detergent-treated, 118-119
Plasma transfusions
guidelines for, 147, 148-150
pathogen-reduced, 116-119
prophylactic, 147-148, 150
ratio to RBCs, in massive transfusion, 148-150, 277-279
and TRALI
due to donor WBC antibodies, 45-49, 51-56
preventing with "male-only" plasma, 36, 37-38, 46, 47, 51-53, 54, 56, *74-75*, 118, 289
preventing with pathogen reduction, 117-118
preventing with screened female donors, *37*, 46, 53, 289
and transfusion of "old" red cells, 253
transmission of vCJD through, 96-97
Plasmapheresis, 133, *134*, 287
Plasmodium sp., 88-89
Platelet additive solutions, 172, 293-294
Platelet transfusions
allergic reactions to, 292-293
informed consent for, 267
pathogen-reduced, 293-296
alternatives to, 124
apheresis vs whole blood-derived, 172
bleeding complications of, 120-123, 164, 165-174, 180-181, 182-192, 291, 294-295
cost-effectiveness of, 297, 298-299
effect on corrected count increments, *164*, *165*, *167-169*, 180, *188*-189, 191, 294
effect on interval between transfusions, *165*, *167-169*, 180, 294
effect on number of platelet transfusions, *165*, *167-169*, 180, 294
and microRNAs, 123, 124, 190-191, 192, 294-295
and mortality, 117
and platelet function, 123, 124, 190-191, 192, 294-295
and risk of ARDS, 295-296
toxic effects of, 117
patient blood management in, 288-293
prophylactic vs therapeutic, 143-148, 173
reducing doses of, *133-134*, 135, 143-*145*
refractoriness to, 2, 23
risk of TAS due to
fatalities due to, 36-37, 39-40
and platelet storage periods, 266
in pooled vs apheresis platelets, 35, 289
projected number of transmissions of, 69-71, *72-73*, *74*
risk-reduction strategies for, 40-42, 291
risk of TRALI due to, 45-46, 49-50, 126-*128*, 130-131, *220-221*
risk of TTIs due to pooled platelets
emerging agents, 68, 71, *74*, 218, 222, 289
exceeds ALARA risk, 203-204
projected number of transmissions, 71-*74*, *75*
reducing risk with apheresis platelets, 68-69, 125-126, *128*-129, 289
relative to risk of reducing MSM deferrals, 207, 212, *213*, 218, *220*, 222, 223
risk reduction strategies for, 291
and storage solutions, 172, 266
transfusion threshold levels, 146-147
use of pooled platelets in US, 126
vCJD infectivity in, *105-106*
washing, 292, 293
Plateletpheresis
citrate toxicity in donors, 288
donor reactions to, *133*, *134*
prevalence of transfusion-transmitted infections in, 69, *281*, 283, *284*, *285*, *286*

- reduction in platelet counts after, 288
- technology for, 280

Platelets
- additive solutions for, 172, 293-294
- bacterial contamination of, 39-45
  - apheresis vs whole-blood-derived, 36-*37*, 40, 41, 42, *43*
  - and component storage time, 40, 266
  - detection of, 36-37, 40, 41-45
- concentrating, 293
- corrected count increments
  - calculation of, 164
  - effect of pathogen-reduced platelets on, *164*, *165*, *167*, *188*-189, 191, 294
  - meta-analysis method for, 180
  - and platelet storage times, 172, 266
- prevalence of TTIs in donors of, 69, *281*, 283, *284*, *285*, *286*

PLX4032, 238-239
Pneumonia, postoperative, 253, 254, 255
Pneumonitis, 295-296
Policy decisions
- evidence-based medicine in, 4, 5, 12, 24-25
- precautionary principle in, 11-12, 24-25
- risk management approach to, 12

Pooled blood components
- risk of TRALI due to, 50, 118, 126-*128*, 130-131, 218, 220-221
- risk of TTIs from
  - emerging agents, 68, 71, *74*, 218, 222, 289
  - exceeds ALARA risk, 203-204
  - projected number of transmissions, 71-*74*, *75*
  - reducing risk with apheresis platelets, 68-69, 125-126, *128*-129, 289
  - relative to risk of reducing MSM deferrals, 207, 212, *213*, 218, 220, 222, 223
  - risk reduction strategies for, *291*
- use in US, 126

Precautionary principle, 11-12, 24-25, *205*
Premature Infants in Need of Transfusion (PINT) trial, 141-*142*
Prion-reduction filters, 100-103, 104, *106*
Prions. *See* Creutzfeldt-Jakob disease, variant
Prophylactic Platelet Dose on Transfusion Outcomes (PLADO) trial, 133, 135, 143, *145*
Protozoal infections, 88-89
Publication bias, 193

Q

Q test statistic, 181, 182
Quality scores for randomized controlled trials, 176-178

R

Random-effects method, 179, 180
Randomized controlled trials, 6, *8*
- drugs that receive approval without, 238-239
- equipoise and prerequisite for, 237-241
- in establishing cause-and-effect, 8, 9-11
- in evidence hierarchy, 6, *7*
- meta-analysis of, *8*-9
  - applications of, 161-162
  - within and between-studies variation in, 179, 180
  - bias in, 192-193
  - combinability of reports for, 181-185
  - defined, 161
  - eligibility of reports for, 174-176
  - by fixed-effects method, 179, 180
  - of individual patient data, *6*, 9
  - of literature, 9
  - medical heterogeneity in, 185-189
  - medical interpretation of, 185-192
  - qualitative and quantitative components of, 162-*163*
  - quality of reports in, 162-*163*, 176-179
  - by random-effects method, 179, 180
  - rationale for, 179-181
  - selection of estimates of effect in, 182-184
  - sequence of steps in, *163*
  - statistical heterogeneity of, 185
  - statistical homogeneity of, 181-182
  - as supplement to RCTs, 162
  - unit of observation in, *165*-169
  - variations in findings of RCTs, 169-174
  - vs literature reviews, 161
- "N of 1," 6
- systematic reviews of, *8*-9
- vs observational studies, 10-11
- *See also* specific trials

RBCs. *See* Red Blood Cells
RCT. See Randomized controlled trials
Recipient identification, 57-60, 129
Recovered plasma, 266-267
Red cell transfusions
- alternatives to, 137, 141
- avoiding, 134-*142*
- evidence-based guidelines for, 114, *135*-137, 270-*271*, 275
- of "fresh" vs "old" blood
  - biologic mechanisms for adverse effects of, 236
  - ethics of, 237, 238, 241, 258
  - and FFP transfusions, 253
  - and mortality, 241, 246-252, 258, *274*-275, 277

observational studies of, 243-253, 254, 255
and organ failure, 252-253
in patient blood management, 276-277
policy decision-making for, 239-241
quality of, 265
randomized controlled trials for, 237-238, 240-243, 253, 256-258
and risk of HIV or HTLV, 236, 241
and risk of TRALI, 236, 266
and risk of transfusion-associated sepsis, 235-236, 265-266
systematic reviews of, 258-259
and illness severity, 10
immunomodulatory effects of, 2-*4*, 12-24
liberal vs restrictive strategies for, 61-62, 64, 137-142, 259, 270-271, 274-275
massive, 148-150, 277-279
for neonates, 141-*142*, 256-257
pathogen-reduced, 116
reporting adverse events related to, 34-35, 36, 39
risks of
competing, 24-25
TA-GVHD, 31, *32*
TACO, 32, 33, 56, 113
See also Transfusion-associated sepsis; Transfusion-related acute lung injury; Transfusion reactions; Transfusion-transmitted infections
for stable adult patients, 140-141
therapeutic vs prophylactic, 134-135, 136
in transfusion medicine paradigms, 265-266, *268-269*
of washed RBCs, 104-105
See also Mortality, transfusion-related
Red Blood Cells (RBCs)
bacterial contamination of, 39, 40, 235, 236
"buffy-coat," 132
storage period for, 235-236, 237, 240
vCJD infectivity in, *105-106*
Red cell alloantibodies, 60-61
Red cell apheresis, double
donor reactions to, *133*, *134*, 287
prevalence of TTIs in, 280-*281*, *282*, 283, *285*, *286*
technology for, 280
Red Cell Storage Duration and Outcomes in Cardiac Surgery Study, 256
Refractoriness to platelet transfusions, 2, 23
Relative risk
of HIV, HBV, or HCV infection, 207, 212
of MSM deferrals and pooled platelet transfusions, 207, 212, *213*, 218, *220-221*
of MSM deferrals and tolerated ABT risk, 203, 204-205
of TRALI from apheresis vs pooled platelets, 131
Renal failure, 252
Riboflavin/UV light pathogen reduction. *See* Mirasol pathogen reduction
Risk management, 12
Risks of transfusion
ALARA (as-low-as-reasonably-achievable), 203-204
competing, 24-25
currently tolerated, 203-*205*
relative risk
of HIV, HBV, or HCV infection, 207, 212
of MSM deferrals and pooled platelet transfusions, 207, 212, *213*, 218, *220-221*
of MSM deferrals and tolerated ABT risk, 203, 204-205
of TRALI from apheresis vs pooled platelets, 131
TA-GVHD, 31, *32*
TACO, *32*, *33*, 56, 113
See also Transfusion-associated sepsis; Transfusion-related acute lung injury; Transfusion reactions; Transfusion-transmitted infections
Rocky Mountain spotted fever, 89

S

Scrapie, 97-98, 104
Selection bias, *8*, 10, 150, 192, 193
Sepsis. *See* Transfusion-associated sepsis
Serious Hazards of Transfusion, *32*-34, 236
Sexually transmitted infections, 222
SLEV (St. Louis encephalitis virus), 88, 89
SPRINT trial
adverse effects reported in, 295
categorization of bleeding in, 182, 183, 184-185
corrected count increments in, *167*
findings of, 120-121, 189, 294
intervals between platelet transfusions in, *168*
odds ratios of bleeding complications in, 166
quality of, 178
total platelet transfusions in, *169*
St. Louis encephalitis virus, 88, 89
Statistical overview. *See* Meta-analysis
Strategies for the Transfusion of Platelets (SToP) RCT, 143-*144*, *145*
Summary effects, *8*-9, 179-180, 181-182, 185
Summary odds ratio, *8*-9
Surgery, 13-16, 18, 19, 274. *See also* Cardiac surgery; Gastrointestinal surgery

Surveillance studies, 34-39
Survivor bias, 279
Syphilis, 204, 222
Systematic reviews of RCTs, *8*-9
Systemic inflammatory response syndrome, 62, *63*, 64

T

TA-GVHD. *See* Transfusion-associated graft-vs-host disease
TACO. *See* Transfusion-associated circulatory overload
TAS. *See* Transfusion-associated sepsis
Thrombocytopenia, hypoproliferative, 143-147, 173, 176
TOPP (Trial of Platelet Prophylaxis), *145*-146
TRACS (Transfusion Requirements After Cardiac Surgery) trial, 139, 140, 270
TRALI. *See* Transfusion-related acute lung injury
Transfusion, allogeneic
  alternatives to, 137, 141
  avoiding, 114, 134-150
    plasma, 147-150
    platelets, 143-148
    red cells, *134-142*
  evidence-based guidelines for, 114, *135*-137, 270-*271*, 275
  of "fresh" vs "old" blood
    biologic mechanisms for adverse effects of, 236
    ethics of, 237, 238, 241, 258
    and FFP transfusions, 253
    and mortality, 241, 246-252, 258, *274*-275, 277
    observational studies of, 243-253, 254, 255
    and organ failure, 252-253
    in patient blood management, 276-277
    policy decision-making for, 239-241
    quality of, 265
    randomized controlled trials for, 237-238, *240*-243, 253, 256-258
    and risk of HIV or HTLV, 236, 241
    and risk of TAS, 235-236, 265-266
    and risk of TRALI, 236, 266
    systematic reviews of, 258-259
  and illness severity, 10
  immunomodulatory effects of, 2-4, 12-24
  massive, 148-149, 277-280
  mortality related to (*See* Mortality, transfusion-related)
  for neonates, 141-142, 256-257
  reporting adverse events related to, 34-39
  restrictive vs liberal strategy for, 61-62, 64, 137-*142*, 259, 270-*271*, *274*-275
  risks of
    competing, 24-25
    currently tolerated vs ALARA, 203-204
    TA-GVHD, 31, *32*
    TACO, *32*, *33*, 56, 113
    See also Transfusion-associated sepsis; Transfusion-related acute lung injury; Transfusion reactions; Transfusion-transmitted infections
  therapeutic vs prophylactic, 134-135, 136
  in transfusion medicine paradigms, 265-267, 268-269, 296
  See also White cell reduction; Mortality, transfusion-related
Transfusion-associated circulatory overload, *32*, *33*, 56, 113
Transfusion-associated graft-vs-host disease, 31, *32*
Transfusion-associated sepsis, 39-45
  and age of red cells, 235-236, 265-266
  contamination rates, 40
  due to platelet transfusion, 39-45, 69-71, 72-*74*, *75*, 204, 208, 266
  due to red cell transfusion, 39, 40, 235, 236
  incidence rates of, 35, 39-40
  increased awareness of, 36
  mortality due to, 31-*32*, *33*, 36-37, 39, 40, 41-42, *74*, *76*
  organisms causing, 40
  recent studies of, 42-45
  reducing risk of
    with bacteria detection, 35, 36-*37*, 39, 41-45, 124, 126
    with pathogen reduction, 124, 164, 269, *291*
  risk of, 89, 207
Transfusion medicine paradigms, 267, 296-299
  component-centric vs patient-centric, 265-270, 296, 297-299
  multicomponent apheresis, 267, *268*, *269*, 280-288, *291*-292, 297
  pathogen reduction of platelets, 293-296
  patient blood management, 267, *268-269*, 269, 270-280, 288-293
  for platelet transfusions, 288-293
Transfusion reactions
  allergic, to platelets, 292-293
  febrile nonhemolytic, 2, 23
  hemolytic, 57-61
    delayed, 57
    mortality due to, 31-*32*, 36, 57, *58*, *59*, 60, *75-76*
    prevention of, 57-61, 129-130
Transfusion-related acute lung injury, 45-57
  and age of RBCs for transfusion, 236, 266
  clinical presentation of, 46

components implicated in, 45, 46, 47
criteria for diagnosing, 35, 46, *55*, 56
definition of, 46
incidence of, *47*
increase in awareness of, 36
mortality due to
after using "male-only" plasma, *37-38*, 56, *74-75*, *77*, 118
and donor WBC antibodies, 51, 52-56, 283
heterogeneity of reports on, *37-38*, 56-57
reported in US and UK, 31-*32*, *33*, 36, *37-38*, 46, *74-75*, *76*
number of cases reported, 34-36
prevention of
AABB recommendation for, *37*
with pathogen reduction, 117-118
by reducing immunologic exposures to donors, 130-134
using "male-only" plasma, 36, *37-38*, 46, *47*, 51-53, *54*, 56, *74-75*, 289
by using multicomponent apheresis, 131-*133*, 283, 285, 287
using screened female donors, 37, 46, 53, 114, 131, 289
risk of
from plasma transfusion, 36, *37-38*, 51
from platelet transfusion, *32*, 49-50, 126-*128*, 130-131, 218, *220-221*
from red cell transfusion, 53, 236
from transfusion of WBC antibodies, 45-*49*
theories of pathogenesis, 50-52
vs transfusion-associated circulatory overload, 56
work-ups for, 46-47
Transfusion-related immunomodulatory effect
in cardiac surgery, *13*, *14*, *15*, 16, 18, 19, 23
in gastrointestinal surgery, *13*, *14*, *15*, 16
mediators and interventions for, 12, *13*
and universal WBC reduction, 2-4, 12-24
Transfusion Requirements After Cardiac Surgery (TRACS) trial, 139, 140, 270
Transfusion Requirements in Critical Care (TRICC) study, 61-62, 64, 136, 137-139, 140, 259, 270
Transfusion thresholds
in liberal vs restrictive transfusion strategies, 61, 136, 137-142, 270-271
for plasma transfusions, 147
for platelet transfusions, 143, 145-148
vs patient blood management, 270
Transfusion-transmitted infections
due to pooled platelets
and ALARA risk, 203-204
emerging agents, 68, 71, *74*, 218, 222, 289
projected number of transmissions, 71-*74*, *75*
relative to risk of reducing MSM deferrals, 207, 212, *213*, 218, *220*, 222, 223
emerging agents, 87-90
categories of, 88-89, 218
fatal, impact of, 64-68
and pooled platelets, 68, 71, 74, 218, 222, 289
morbidity and mortality related to, 31, 39
and MSM deferrals, 202, *205*, 222-223
precautionary principle regarding, *205*
prevalence in donors, 69, 280-*281*, *282*, 283, *284*, *285*
reducing risk of
with multicomponent apheresis, 280-283, *284*, *285*, 296
through pathogen reduction, 114, *115*, 116-124, 291, 296-297
using apheresis platelets vs pooled, 68-69, 125-126, 128-129, 203-204, 289
See also specific infections
Trauma
fresh whole blood use in, 277-280
use of "fresh" vs "old" blood transfusions in, 246, 248, 252, 253
Trial of Platelet Prophylaxis (TOPP) trial, 145-146
TRICC trial, 61-62, 64, 136, 137-139, 140, 259, 270
TRIM effect. *See* Transfusion-related immunomodulatory effect
Trypanosoma cruzi, 88-89
TTI. *See* Transfusion-transmitted infections

U-V

US Food and Drug Administration, 31-*32*, *33*-34, 36
Variation
between-studies, 179, 180
in findings of RCTs, *169*-174
within-studies, 179, 180
vCJD. *See* Creutzfeldt-Jakob disease, variant
Viral encephalitis, tick-borne, 89

W-Y

Washed RBCs, 104-105
Washing platelets, 292, 293
"West-Nile-like" infections
preventing with pathogen reduction, 116, 118
projected transmissions of, 67-68, 88
risk of, from pooled platelets, 71, 73, *74*, *75*, 204, 291
West Nile virus, 39, 67
White cell antibodies, 45-49, 50-56, 130, 283, *285*

White cell reduction
and bacterial contamination of components, 236
and bacterial infections, 3-*4*, 12, *14-15*, 16-18, 20
and colorectal cancer, 23
and Creutzfeldt-Jakob disease, variant, 2, 23, 101, 103-104
definition of, 1-2
indications for, 2, 23
and mortality, 4, 12-16, 62, 64
before and after studies of, 18, 21, *22*
in cardiac surgery, *13*, *14-15*, 19, *22*, *65*, *66*, 124-125
in gastrointestinal surgery, *13*, *14-15*, 16
and multiple organ failure, 62, 64
prestorage vs poststorage, 12-13, 16-18
and transfusion-related immunomodulatory effect, 2-4, 12-24
universal, 2-4, 12-24
and virus activation, 23-24
White cell soluble mediators, 12-14, 16-18, 64
Whole blood donors
prevalence of transfusion-transmitted infections in, 280-*281*, *282*, 283, *284*, *285*, *286*
reactions in, 133, *134*, 287
Whole blood transfusions, *268*, 277-280
Within-studies variation, 179, 180
WNV. *See* West Nile virus
Yersinia enterocolitica, 40, 235, 236